Surgery of coronary artery disease

Surgery of coronary artery disease

Second edition

Edited by

David J Wheatley
MD ChM FRCS (Edin, Glasg, Engl) FRCP (Edin) FMedSci FECTS
British Heart Foundation Professor of Cardiac Surgery
University of Glasgow
UK

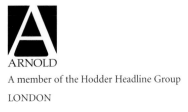

ARNOLD
A member of the Hodder Headline Group
LONDON

First published in Great Britain in 1986 by Chapman & Hall
This second edition published in 2003 by
Arnold, a member of the Hodder Headline Group,
338 Euston Road, London NW1 3BH

http://www.arnoldpublishers.com

Distributed in the United States of America by
Oxford University Press Inc.,
198 Madison Avenue, New York, NY10016
Oxford is a registered trademark of Oxford University Press

Whilst the advice and information in this book are believed to be true
and accurate at the date of going to press, neither the authors nor the
publisher can accept any legal responsibility or liability for any errors or
omissions that may be made. In particular (but without limiting the
generality of the preceding disclaimer) every effort has been made to
check drug dosages; however, it is still possible that errors have been
missed. Furthermore, dosage schedules are constantly being revised and
new side-effects recognized. For these reasons the reader is strongly
urged to consult the drug companies' printed instructions before
administering any of the drugs recommended in this book.

British Library Cataloguing in Publication Data
A catalogue record for this book is available from the British Library

Library of Congress Cataloging-in-Publication Data
A catalog record for this book is available from the Library of Congress

ISBN 0 340 80787 3

1 2 3 4 5 6 7 8 9 10

Commissioning Editor: Joanna Koster
Development Editor: Sarah Burrows
Project Coordinator: Margaret Tolland
Project Editor: Wendy Rooke
Production Controller: Deborah Smith
Cover Design: Lee May Lim

Typeset in 10/12 Minion by Charon Tec Pvt. Ltd, Chennai, India
Printed and bound in Italy

What do you think about this book? Or any other Arnold title?
Please send your comments to **feedback.arnold@hodder.co.uk**

To my father

Contents

List of contributors

Hendrick Barner MD
Professor of Surgery, Division of Cardiothoracic Surgery,
Washington University School of Medicine, St Louis, MO,
USA

Friedhelm Beyersdorf MD PhD FETCS
Professor of Surgery, Chairman of Department of
Cardiovascular Surgery,
Albert-Ludwigs-University, Freiburg, Germany

Eugene H Blackstone MD
Section Head, Clinical Research,
Department of Thoracic and Cardiovascular Surgery
The Cleveland Clinic Foundation, Cleveland, Ohio, USA

Thomas C Bower MD
Professor of Surgery, Mayo Graduate School of Medicine,
Division of Vascular Surgery,
Mayo Clinic, Rochester, MN, USA

Gerald D Buckberg MD
Professor of Surgery, Division of Cardiothoracic Surgery
UCLA Medical Center, Los Angeles, CA, USA

MH Al-Bustami MD
Interventional Cardiologist, RBH & Harefield Trust
Harefield Hospital, Harefield, Middlesex, UK

Brian F Buxton MD
Professor and Director
Department of Cardiac Surgery, Austin Hospital
Melbourne, Victoria, Australia

R Jane Chambers FRCP(C) FRCP(Edin)
Consultant Radiologist, RBH & Harefield Trust
Harefield Hospital, Middlesex, UK

Stanley Chia MB ChB (Hons) MRCP
Registrar, Department of Cardiology,
National Heart Centre, Singapore

W Randolph Chitwood Jr MD FACS FRCS(Engl)
Professor and Chairman, Department of Surgery,
Chief of Cardiothoracic Surgery,
Brody School of Medicine, East Carolina University,
Greenville, North Carolina, USA

Victor F Chu MD FRCS(C)
Assistant Professor, Department of Surgery
Faculty of Health Sciences, McMaster University
Hamilton, Ontario, Canada

Ali Denktas MD
Interventional Cardiology Fellow
Mayo Clinic, Rochester, MN, USA

Eric J Devaney MD
Assistant Professor of Surgery,
Section of Cardiac Surgery
University of Michigan Medical Center, Ann Arbor,
MI, USA

Vincent M Dor MD
Professor, Cardiothoracic Center of Monaco, Monaco

Kim A Eagle MD
Albion Walter Professor of Internal Medicine,
Chief of Clinical Cardiology,
University of Michigan Health System,
Ann Arbor, Michigan, USA

Keith AA Fox BSc (Hons) MB ChB FRCP
Duke of Edinburgh Professor of Cardiology,
Head of Division, Medical and Radiological Sciences
Royal Infirmary of Edinburgh, Edinburgh, UK

OH Frazier MD
Director, Cullen Cardiovascular Surgical Research
Laboratories, Chief of Cardiopulmonary Transplantation,
Texas Heart Institute at St Luke's Episcopal Hospital,
Houston, TX, USA

Gerd Heusch MD FESC FACC FISHR
Direktor, Institut für Pathophysiologie,
Zentrum für Innere Medizin
Universitätsklinikum Essen, Essen, Germany

Stephen Hickey MB ChB FRCA
Consultant and Honorary Clinical Senior Lecturer in
Anaesthesia, Glasgow Royal Infirmary, Glasgow,
Scotland, UK

Michael J Higgins MB ChB PhD FFARCS(I)
British Heart Foundation Senior Lecturer/Honorary
Consultant Anaesthetist, University Department of Cardiac
Surgery, Glasgow Royal Infirmary, Glasgow, UK

David R Holmes Jr MD
Professor of Medicine,
Director, Cardiac Catheterization Laboratory,
Division of Cardiovascular Diseases & Internal Medicine,
Mayo Clinic, Rochester, MN, USA

Stuart W Jamieson MB FRCS
Professor and Head of Cardiothoracic Surgery
Division of Cardiovascular and Thoracic Surgery
UCSD Medical Center, San Diego, CA, USA

Kamuran Kadipasaoglu PhD
Assistant Director, Cullen Cardiovascular Surgical
Research Laboratories, Texas Heart Institute at St Luke's
Episcopal Hospital, Houston, TX, USA

Nicholas T Kouchoukos MD
Attending Surgeon, Division of Cardiovascular and
Thoracic Surgery
Missouri Baptist Medical Center, St Louis, MO, USA

James J Livesay MD FACS FACC
Cardiac Surgeon, Texas Heart Institute, and
Clinical Associate Professor of Surgery, University of
Texas Medical School at Houston, TX, USA

Michael J Mack MD
Director of Cardiovascular Disease, Director of
Transplantation, Medical City Dallas Hospital, and
Chairman, Cardiopulmonary Science Research
Technology Institute, Dallas, TX, USA

Michael M Madani MD
Assistant Professor in Surgery, Division of Cardiothoracic
Surgery, UCSD, University of California San Diego
Medical Center, San Diego, CA, USA

Paolo Masetti MD
Fellow in Cardiovascular Surgery
Missouri Baptist Medical Center, St Louis MO, USA

John McMurray MD FRCP FESC FACC
Professor of Medical Cardiology, Division of
Cardiovascular and Medical Sciences, University of
Glasgow, and Honorary Consultant Cardiologist, Western
Infirmary, Glasgow, UK

Raad H Mohiaddin PhD MRCP FRCR FESC
Consultant and Honorary Clinical Senior Lecturer,
Magnetic Resonance Unit, Royal Brompton Hospital &
National Heart & Lung Institute, London, UK

L Wiley Nifong MD
Assistant Professor of Surgery, Director of Surgical
Research, Department of Surgery, The Brody School of
Medicine, East Carolina University, Greenville, NC, USA

Thomas A Orszulak MD
Professor of Surgery, Division of Cardiovascular Surgery,
Mayo Clinic and Mayo Foundation, Rochester MN, USA

Chris J Packard DSc FRCPath
Top Grade Biochemist, Institute of Biochemistry, Director
of Research and Development, Glasgow Royal Infirmary
University NHS Trust, and
Honorary Professor, Department of Pathological
Biochemistry, University of Glasgow, UK

Stephen K Plume MD
Professor of Surgery, Professor of Community and Family
Medicine, Dartmouth Medical School, Hanover, New
Hampshire, USA

Richard L Prager MD
Clinical Professor of Surgery, Section of Cardiac Surgery,
University of Michigan Medical Center, Ann Arbor, MI,
USA

Shelley L Rahman MRCP BA(Hons)
Research Fellow in Cardiac Imaging, Department of
Nuclear Medicine, Royal Brompton Hospital, London,
UK

Ross M Reul MD
Cardiac Surgeon, Texas Heart Institute, Houston, TX,
USA

Frederick J Schoen MD PhD
Professor of Pathology, Harvard Medical School,
Executive Vice Chairman, Department of Pathology,
Brigham and Women's Hospital, Boston MA, USA

Rainer Schulz MD
Institut für Pathophysiologie,
Zentrum für Innere Medizin
Universitätsklinikum Essen, Essen, Germany

Mandeep Singh MD
Assistant Professor of Medicine
Division of Cardiovascular Diseases & Internal Medicine,
Mayo Clinic, Rochester, MN, USA

Thoralf M Sundt MD
Senior Associate Consultant, Mayo Clinic, Associate
Professor of Surgery, Mayo Medical School, Division of
Cardiovascular Surgery, Department of Surgery, Mayo
Clinic, Rochester MN, USA

James Tatoulis MB BS MS FRACS
Associate Professor and Director, Cardiothoracic Surgery
and Cardiac Services, The Royal Melbourne Hospital,
University of Melbourne, Melbourne, Victoria, Australia

Egemen Tuzun MD
Fellow, Cullen Cardiovascular Surgical Research
Laboratories, Texas Heart Institute at St Luke's Hospital,
Houston, TX, USA

SR Underwood MD FRCP FRCR FESC
Professor of Cardiac Imaging, Royal Brompton Hospital
and Imperial College, London, UK

**David J Wheatley MD ChM FRCS FRCP(Edin)
FMedSci FECTS**
British Heart Foundation Professor of Cardiac Surgery,
University of Glasgow, and Honorary Consultant Cardiac
Surgeon, Glasgow Royal Infirmary, UK

Foreword to second edition

Treatment of atherosclerosis has previously been aimed at what was believed to be an inert collection of cholesterol, fibrosis and calcium that grew unpredictably until it compromised or stopped coronary arterial blood flow. Compared with what we know today, atherosclerosis was *terra incognita* for most of the twentieth century. The latest studies show that atherosclerosis is not degenerative or inevitable. Instead, it is multifactorial, dynamic, episodic and vulnerable to new therapies.

Coronary artery disease remains the leading cause of death in the developed world. But those who have it are dying at an increasingly greater age. By modifying risk factors, and with the selective application of technical innovations, many people have significantly postponed their death from heart disease. It is a notable fact that while epidemiologists report an actual increase in coronary heart disease among all age groups over the past 25 years, there has been no change in the rate of myocardial infarction.

None the less, coronary artery disease remains a major cause of premature death and disability in men and women, and is a killer dependent on genetic predisposition and bad habits. As a last resort, surgeons have had to adapt the operation to treat complicated atherosclerosis to serve an increasingly elderly population. At the same time, less invasive treatments have become more effective, and their success is complemented by vast improvements in patient education and secondary preventive measures.

Coronary artery surgery has been scrutinized and derided more than any procedure. The early randomized trials comparing medicine and surgery suffered from inadequate arteriography and lack of surgical experience. It is now evident that coronary artery surgery has produced benefits far beyond the now seemingly simple construction of a vein conduit between the aorta and the distal arterial system. Surgery has the potential to re-establish normal coronary perfusion and confer long-standing complete revascularization for patients with diffuse disease. Today, surgery may be performed with great safety even in high-risk patients. Long-term symptom relief and freedom from cardiac events are extremely good and consistent, especially with arterial grafting, complete revascularization, and serum lipid control.

The medical profession has never been able to control a disease by only treating the sick. For patients, the greatest danger is that the modification of risk factors comes too late. Atherosclerosis is not inevitable and it may even be reversible. The best time to manage the atherosclerotic profile is early in life, not at the end, which is where the surgeon usually sees the patient.

No one can teach experience; however, the second edition of Dr David Wheatley's *Surgery of Coronary Artery Disease* will help us understand atherosclerosis and the options for diagnosis and treatment more clearly than any text assembled in the past. Perhaps we can then better satisfy the advice offered by Alvin Feinstein in his book, *Clinical Judgment*: 'When I'm sick, I want a doctor that will treat me and not an average. I want a doctor who will recognize the various ways in which I differ … in my particular demographic, clinical and other pertinent attributes. I want the doctor to recognize that the average is obtained as a mixture of different results in different kinds of people. The doctor should then sort out those treatments and apply … the treatment … most suitable to me.'

Dr Wheatley's splendid book will leave the dedicated reader better equipped to mange the complicated patient with all forms of atherosclerosis. The book is an odyssey through epidemiology, natural history, diagnosis and treatment with emphasis on safe and long-lasting coronary artery surgery.

The enterprise of cardiac surgery resembles a grand mansion with many large and sunlit rooms. At any given time, some parts of the mansion are being remodeled based on changing and shifting scientific discoveries. Science has greatly enlarged the pool of light wherein we practice, and the discoveries that are embodied in this text have greatly benefited the patient and surgeon.

A master surgeon and intrepid investigator, Dr Wheatley, has compiled what must now stand as the most comprehensive textbook on coronary atherosclerosis. Physicians and surgeons who absorb the material here, organized by some of the most experienced scientists and clinicians around the world, will come away with a grasp of this complex condition which will prepare them for a lifetime of thoughtful practice.

Floyd D Loop MD
Chief Executive Officer
Chairman, Board of Governors
Cleveland Clinic Foundation
Cleveland, OH, USA

Foreword to first edition

Just a century ago one of the boldest and most intrepid surgeons in the world, Theodor Billroth of Vienna, stated, 'Any man who would undertake an operation on the heart should lose the respect of his colleagues.' His admonition could have been reinforced by Sir Stephen Paget, another recognized leader who in 1896 stated, 'The heart, of all viscera, has reached the limits set by nature toward surgery. No new method and no new technique will overcome the natural obstacles surrounding a wound of the heart.' Progress in cardiac surgery has been so phenomenal, particularly in the past two decades since open-heart techniques were widely employed, that Billroth and Paget's predictions now seem preposterous. Such is the fate of doubters.

Introduction of temporary cardiopulmonary bypass in the 1950s provided the means whereby surgeons could perform elective operations upon the human heart without the pressures of time restrictions and extensive loss of blood. The open-heart era began mostly with operations to repair anatomic defects of the heart, either congenital or acquired.

Before 1960, many crude and indirect methods for treating patients with myocardial ischaemia were employed. Although some were supported by the relief of angina pectoris, none provided objective proof that the technique had done more than interrupt nervous pathways or had produced a 'placebo' effect upon the patient. Introduction of selective coronary arteriography by Mason Sones finally placed the assessment and management of patients with coronary insufficiency on sound bases. At last the precise location and extent of the coronary obstruction could be delineated, and the need for, and anticipated success of, revascularization could be predicted.

Surgeons, led by Rene Favaloro and Dudley Johnson, began to apply the bypass principle to coronary arterial disease. Similar vascular techniques had already been developed for peripheral arterial occlusions in the femoral and popliteal vessels and employed the long saphenous vein as a conduit to extend pulsatile flow to the distal pedal arteries. The aortocoronary bypass using the saphenous vein, or, more recently, the internal mammary artery, has since become the standard means for myocardial revascularization.

While the risk for coronary bypass steadily decreased, skeptics anxiously awaited the results of symptomatic relief and the long-term results. Results from numerous studies now clearly demonstrate that surgically-treated patients have better symptomatic relief and survival rates than patients who are managed with medical treatment alone. In a recent 15-year follow-up study of coronary bypass patients at the Texas Heart Institute, Robert Hall found a decline in early mortality, symptomatic improvement in 94% of patients, and satisfactory survival rates (90% at 5 years and 73% at 10 years). Thus, it is time for misgivings regarding coronary artery bypass to be laid aside. We may take some reassurance from a modern day leader in cardiology, Willis Hurst, who recently wrote, 'When bypass surgery is performed in an excellent fashion, a great deal of "controversy" about this problem vanishes.'

A skilled and talented surgeon, David Wheatley, has organized one of the most outstanding cardiovascular programs in the United Kingdom. This elegant book is a careful, studious approach to the surgical treatment of coronary artery disease and is organized with the same expertise that has made his surgical program known and respected throughout the world. *Surgery of Coronary Artery Disease* is a comprehensive contribution – from evolution to diagnosis, from indications to preoperative management, from surgical treatment to postoperative complications – and will be a reference of inestimable value both to cardiologists and cardiovascular surgeons as they meet the needs of patients with coronary artery disease.

Denton A. Cooley, MD
Surgeon-in-Chief
Texas Heart Institute, Houston, Texas

Preface

The first edition of this book was published in 1986, the year that also saw publication of the landmark paper by Loop and colleagues reporting clear evidence of the clinical benefits of using the thoracic artery as a conduit in coronary surgery. In the intervening years, surgical techniques have evolved: extended use of arterial grafting, beating heart surgery, strategies to minimize the hazard of atheroembolism and other sources of perioperative injury are important examples. A wealth of clinical experience has been accumulated in databases, aiding critical assessment of outcomes.

In 1986 balloon angioplasty was still in its infancy. Since then, advances in percutaneous catheter intervention have been dramatic; non-surgical revascularization now offers an effective, competing strategy for management of many patients formerly considered surgical candidates. Improved understanding of the pathophysiology of coronary atherosclerosis and its clinical manifestations has been paralleled by effective therapies for retardation of disease progression.

Thus it is essential for those involved with the management of coronary atherosclerosis, and the coronary surgeon in particular, to stay abreast of developments and to look critically at current practice and results. Only in this way will it be possible to ensure that surgery is undertaken appropriately in the course of the natural history of coronary disease in the individual patient, to give the best possible outcome in terms of immediate safety and long-term clinical benefit.

A review of coronary surgical practice, in the context of this evolution of knowledge and technology applicable to the management of coronary atherosclerosis, is timely. My own practice spans the era of coronary surgery; I have been privileged to have known, and been influenced by, many of the leaders in this field. The accrued wisdom and experience of such leaders in my own, and related specialties, are presented in this second addition.

David J Wheatley
Glasgow, 2003

Acknowledgments

My colleague, Margaret Tolland, as editorial assistant, has greatly facilitated the task of producing this book. Her role in planning, researching the literature, recruitment of contributors, editing and proof-reading has been inestimable. I am immensely grateful for her contributions.

Ms Tolland was the photographer for the surgical photographs in my own chapter on surgical technique, and she designed and edited the resulting images.

Thanks are also due to AorTech International plc, whose financial sponsorship helped to fund the color sections of the book.

Coronary surgery in the twenty-first century: a perspective

DAVID J WHEATLEY

BACKGROUND

During the first 60 or more years of the twentieth century there were many ingenious attempts to treat angina pectoris with surgery. Many ideas, lacking a secure theoretical basis, soon foundered; others were superseded by evolving drug therapy. The history of these early, pioneering efforts has been well reviewed[1–3] and gives an insight into the justified skepticism that greeted the introduction of coronary bypass grafting.[4] Although a sound physiological basis was claimed for many of the procedures attempted prior to the current era of bypass grafting, there was no convincing evidence that significant increase in myocardial perfusion was produced by any of them.[5] Perhaps of most importance, coronary angiography was not available to confirm the diagnosis, still less to allow rational application of surgery and confirmation of its effectiveness.

Among the milestones in the development of current techniques was the demonstration of the anatomy and pathology of the coronary arteries during life. Selective coronary arteriography was developed and refined in the early 1960s and remains the single most important investigation for revascularization in coronary artery disease. Mason Sones, working at the Cleveland Clinic, was the pioneer of coronary angiography.[6] The Sones technique (using a brachial artery cut down) and the Judkins technique (using a percutaneous femoral artery puncture)[7] rapidly became well established and safe techniques.

THE BEGINNING OF THE MODERN ERA

Although a number of direct coronary surgical procedures had been undertaken before 1967, including endarterectomy,[8,9] use of saphenous vein bypass[10,11] and internal thoracic artery bypass,[12] none of these procedures was widely applied and their potential appears not to have been fully appreciated or exploited. Credit for the introduction, refinement and widespread application of coronary artery bypass grafting (CABG) goes to Rene Favaloro and his colleagues at the Cleveland Clinic. In 1967 he began using saphenous vein, initially as an interposition graft, and shortly afterwards as an aortocoronary bypass graft.[13,14] This form of surgery was rapidly adopted in many centers in North America and around the world.[2] Notable early pioneers were Dudley Johnson and associates from Milwaukee, Cooley and his group in Houston, Urschel and Mitchell in Dallas, Shumway and colleagues in Stanford, and Spencer and Green in New York.[15–17] Green[18] firmly established the use of the internal thoracic artery as a bypass conduit.

The last three decades of the twentieth century saw CABG evolve to become one of the commonest, best documented and most effective of all major surgical procedures.

Percutaneous coronary intervention

Revascularization strategies have not been confined to surgical approaches. Since Andreas Gruentzig initiated balloon dilatation of coronary artery stenoses in the late 1970s, considerable strides have been made in percutaneous coronary intervention (PCI) techniques.[19] The problem of early restenosis of the dilated segment[20] was the subject of intensive research and a number of different stenting devices soon followed.[21] Many inventive percutaneous catheter-based techniques have been developed, including atherectomy devices, systems for laser disobliteration,[22] and intracoronary ultrasound for characterization of lesions and guidance of stenting. The use of intracoronary stents has found widespread application and most balloon dilatation procedures are now combined with stent deployment.[23,24] Antiplatelet therapy in combination with stents has largely eliminated the problem of thrombosis.[25] Methods for retarding or abolishing neointimal proliferation have included localized irradiation and drug-eluting stents. A drug-eluting stent releasing rapamycin has been reported to show considerable promise for prevention of neointimal proliferation and restenosis, with only a 5.8% rate of major cardiac events during the first year.[26]

Evolution of surgical techniques

Spurred on to some extent by competing percutaneous catheter interventional techniques, parallel advances have occurred in the techniques of CABG. Two major drawbacks to coronary surgery are widely recognized. First, discomfort, physiological upset and damage caused by the techniques required for conduit insertion ('injury of access') are disincentives to patients being offered surgery as a treatment option. Second, the critical dependence on bypass grafts for the long-term success of the procedure ('conduit integrity') imposes a limitation on surgical achievements, particularly if saphenous vein is the major conduit in use.

INJURY OF ACCESS

Notable developments of the past few years have included better recognition of the importance and mechanisms of visceral and musculo-skeletal injury accompanying coronary surgery, and the development of strategies to minimize this injury. Minimal or limited access surgery is still evolving, but some of its lessons are applicable to the standard sternotomy approach (limitation of sternal spreading, avoidance of extensive tissue handling and devitalization). Appreciation of the microembolic risk and inflammatory response associated with cardiopulmonary bypass has led to improvements in extracorporeal circuit technology and perioperative management. Recognition of the danger of atheroembolism from the ascending aorta and the coronary arteries has encouraged strategies for minimizing the risks, both for first-time and repeat surgery, with consequent benefit to patients. Attempts to avoid cardiopulmonary bypass-associated risks altogether

have spawned 'beating-heart' or 'off-pump' techniques, which are gaining in popularity as technological aspects improve. Their success in avoiding the problems of the extracorporeal circuit is not yet fully established,[27] but reported outcomes are promising.[28]

CONDUIT INTEGRITY

The vein graft, long the mainstay of coronary surgery, remains a weak link in the procedure.[29] Vein graft failure is well recognized, affects about half of all vein conduits within a decade, and is the major cause of return of symptoms and re-operation. Much is known about the causes of this failure, and at least some preventative measures promise improved future outcome.[30]

There is widespread recognition of the value of the internal thoracic artery conduit. It can be speculated that its value may well be more than simply that of a reliable conduit. Endothelial function is known to be abnormal in atheromatous arteries.[31] Bypass of diseased arteries with an atheroma-free internal thoracic artery may confer benefit for the recipient circulation. Production of biologically vasoactive substances, such as prostacyclin and nitric oxide, which inhibit platelet aggregation and intravascular thrombosis, induce vasodilatation and may have a role in resistance to atherosclerosis,[29] should continue from healthy arterial conduits. These substances may reasonably be expected to act downstream[32] and may therefore influence pathophysiological events in the recipient coronary bed following the use of an artery as a bypass conduit. The clinical value of such a natural 'drug-eluting conduit' has been proven for use of one[33] and recently for both internal thoracic arteries,[34,35] providing a major incentive to the more extensive use of internal thoracic artery conduits.

CABG or PCI for revascularization?

By the beginning of the present century, estimates indicate some 314 000 patients having coronary surgery in 2000 in the USA,[36] a rate of 1116/million population, while in the UK (year end March 2001), 25 127 patients had isolated CABG, a rate of 427/million population (a rate 38% that of the USA). In Europe, the rate of coronary surgery varies considerably amongst countries, but is higher in Western than in Eastern Europe. Rates between 300 (Romania) and 1400 (Germany) per million population are reported for 2000.[37]

While the volume of CABG undertaken in the USA and UK remains impressive, the pattern of annual activity over the last two decades suggests that the growth spurt seen in the mid 1980s–1990s has plateaued (Figure 1.1). Data from Europe are less easy to extract, but the Euro Heart Survey suggests that levels of coronary surgery in Europe have 'stabilized'.[37]

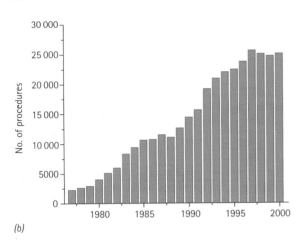

(a)

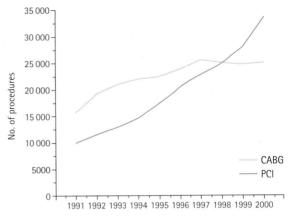

Figure 1.2 *Number of isolated coronary artery bypass graft (CABG) procedures and number of percutaneous coronary intervention (PCI) procedures in the UK, 1991–2000. Graph produced from figures published by the Society of Cardiothoracic Surgeons of Great Britain and Ireland and the British Cardiovascular Intervention Society.*

(b)

Figure 1.1 *(a) Volume of coronary artery bypass surgery in the USA, 1979–2000. Data obtained from annual* National Hospital Discharge Surveys, Advance Data from Vital and Health Statistics. *Hyattsville, MD: National Center for Health Statistics. (b) Number of isolated coronary artery bypass graft procedures in the UK, 1977–2000. Data from* UK Cardiac Surgical Registry, *published by the Society of Cardiothoracic Surgeons of Great Britain and Ireland.*

In parallel with this leveling of coronary surgery activity is the growth in volume of PCI, including stenting. Figure 1.2 illustrates the pattern that had emerged by the end of the twentieth century in the UK, where PCI had overtaken CABG as the commonest interventional revascularization strategy. By the year 2000, stent use had increased to 85% of all percutaneous catheter revascularization procedures (from 2.7% in 1992). Similar trends are evident in the USA. In Europe, PCI utilization ranged from around 100/million population (Romania) to more than 2000/million population (Germany) in 2000.[37] Data from the German Registry of Percutaneous Coronary Interventions over the period 1993–2000 show increasing use of PCI in women, older patients and those with multivessel disease, as well as a substantial increase in stent utilization, from fewer than 5% (1993) to more than 70% (2000).[37]

The increased effectiveness and scope of PCI have affected not only the volume of coronary surgery, but also the patient population to whom it is applied. Localized stenoses in large coronary arteries are more likely to be treated with PCI than surgery. Surgeons are therefore confronted with patients who are older and sicker, with more extensive disease, than in earlier years. This has made the practice of coronary surgery progressively more challenging.

Outcomes

The effectiveness of surgical treatment for coronary artery disease was shown first for symptomatic benefit and later for survival benefit. Immediate relief of angina can be achieved by surgical revascularization in most angina patients, with about 50–60% of patients remaining angina free at 10 years.[38,39] For those with more extensive coronary disease, there is survival benefit when compared with other forms of management, with absolute benefit being greatest for those at highest risk with medical therapy.[38] For those of middle age or beyond, surgery can restore survival expectancy to a level not dissimilar to that of an age-matched and sex-matched general population.[40]

Refinements in physiological monitoring, surgical equipment, extracorporeal perfusion, operative techniques and perioperative management have helped the coronary surgeon to maintain acceptable surgical mortality and morbidity in spite of the changes in patient characteristics that are occurring. Critical assessment of all aspects of operative management to identify particular hazards and to look for ways of enhancing safety and effectiveness is essential. Instead of claiming experimental justification alone, surgeons are nowadays using extensive databases to examine the outcome of particular surgical strategies in a manner far more critical than that pertaining before the current era of coronary surgery.

Systematic documentation of practice has allowed outcome to be predicted with considerable precision. National databases, such as the STS database (which documented nearly 1 400 000 isolated coronary procedures in the 10-year period 1992 to 2001) and the Northern New England Cardiovascular Disease Study Group database in the USA, as well as the National Adult Cardiac Surgical database in the UK and the Euroscore database, record procedure details, together with risk factors and operative outcome. Public and political interest in outcome has resulted in some states in the USA publishing surgeon-specific outcome for coronary surgery, a development imminent in the UK[41] and certain to spread to other countries.

TRENDS IN CORONARY DISEASE PREVALENCE

Mortality from coronary heart disease has fallen since the early 1970s in the USA and since the mid-1970s in Western Europe.[42] On the other hand, the prevalence of coronary heart disease has been predicted to rise by more than 50% in the USA from 2000 to 2030.[43,44] The emergence of obesity and type 2 diabetes in epidemic proportions will ensure that coronary disease stays at the forefront of causes of morbidity and mortality.[43] In some countries of Eastern Europe, mortality from coronary heart disease is rising.[42] Unfortunately the export of certain aspects of the Western lifestyle, including eating habits and cigarette smoking, to the developing world seems likely to assure the continuation of a toll from coronary disease. Thus, there is little prospect of coronary disease disappearing in the forseeable future, though for coronary surgeons in the Western world, the clinical features (especially age and co-morbidity) of patients are changing in a way not conducive to straightforward coronary surgical practice.

THE FUTURE ROLE OF SURGERY

There is better understanding that revascularization, whether by surgery or PCI, is a part of the ongoing treatment of coronary disease. The decision about when to intervene, the choice of the most appropriate intervention, maintenance of patency of stents or bypass conduits, retardation of atheroma, and reduction of the impact of coronary disease on the myocardium all have important roles. The last decade of the twentieth century saw important advances in each of these aspects of the management of coronary disease.

The changing patterns of disease, coupled with the advances in pharmacological and other interventions, must raise questions about the future role of surgery. Even with the most advanced interventional technology, there will be many patients whose coronary pathology precludes safe or effective percutaneous approaches. Those with total occlusion of coronary arteries, or in whom the extent of atheroma is such that effective dilatation is impractical, will probably be candidates for surgery for the forseeable future. One certain way to ensure a bleak future for coronary surgery would be for surgeons to take on 'all comers' who have finally run out of percutaneous interventional options and are at advanced age, when limited life expectancy, diffuse coronary disease and co-morbidity make a worthwhile outcome unlikely.

A re-think of the traditional policy of reserving surgery for the last act in the therapeutic repertoire may be appropriate. In many younger patients (in whom the injury of access is better tolerated), the creation of additional sources of perfusion to the coronary tree in the form of normal, atheroma-free arteries, has undeniable logic. Effective methods for slowing disease progression in surgical patients are available (as they are for PCI recipients). The option of percutaneous intervention for progressive disease later in life would still be available – and perhaps more appropriate, given the lower risk of PCI relative to surgery – for the higher-risk category which these patients would then occupy.

The efficacy of surgery depends on ensuring the effective, consistent use of arterial conduits as well as the application of techniques to avoid visceral injury during the operative procedure. Whether this will involve greater use of beating-heart techniques is still unclear, though answers will certainly emerge in the near future. At present, more than 20% of all coronary surgery is undertaken with off-pump techniques, in the USA at least. There is no doubt that this form of surgery must be in the repertoire of future surgeons. The future role of minimal access and robotic surgery is as yet unclear.

For the future, angiogenesis, myocyte implantation, tissue engineering and cardiac replacement are among the potential therapies that offer a route for surgery to continue its contribution to the management of the manifestations of coronary artery disease. Whether or not alternative, non-surgical interventions or effective preventive strategies will obviate the need for surgery altogether, and whether the pace of technological advance can be matched by the social, political and economic progress necessary for its widespread application, must remain in the realm of speculation for the present.

KEY REFERENCES

Davies MJ. Stability and instability: two faces of coronary atherosclerosis. The Paul Dudley White Lecture 1995. *Circulation* 1996; **94**:2013–20.

This special review, well illustrated and referenced, carries the authority of one of the leaders in the modern understanding of coronary atherosclerosis. It explains the basis of the manifestations of coronary disease, giving insight into the limitations of all current revascularization strategies in its management.

Favaloro RG. Critical analysis of coronary artery bypass graft surgery: a 30 year journey. *J Am Coll Cardiol* 1998; **31**(4 Suppl. B):1B–63B.

A scholarly account of the beginnings of coronary bypass graft surgery and its evolution over 30 years, extensively referenced, from the acknowledged pioneer of this surgery. The impact of percutaneous catheter interventions on coronary surgery is discussed, and the present role of surgery in the management of various manifestations of coronary disease is well described and remains up to date.

King SB III. The development of interventional cardiology. *J Am Coll Cardiol* 1998; **32**(4 Suppl. B):64B–88B.

A comprehensive, well-referenced review of the development of the alternative strategies for revascularization. The contrast between the early, idiosyncratic pioneering efforts of visionary individuals and the current era of acronym-riddled multicenter clinical trials is well shown. No coronary surgeon can risk being ill-informed about advances in interventional cardiology.

Mueller RL, Rosengart TK, Isom OW. The history of surgery for ischemic heart disease. *Ann Thorac Surg* 1997; **63**:869–78.

An interesting review of the history of attempts to treat manifestations of coronary disease by surgery. Some of the earlier techniques that have long been abandoned have their counterparts in current pharmaceutical therapy (e.g. sympathetic blockade), while others are even being proposed afresh for percutaneous application where conventional surgery is impractical.

REFERENCES

1. Vansant JH, Muller WJ Jr. Surgical procedures to revascularize the heart. A review of the literature. *Am J Surg* 1960; **100**:572–83.
2. Mueller RL, Rosengart TK, Isom OW. The history of surgery for ischemic heart disease. *Ann Thorac Surg* 1997; **63**:869–78.
3. Westaby S. *Landmarks in Cardiac Surgery*. Oxford: Isis Medical Media Ltd, 1997.
4. McIntosh HD, Garcia JA. The first decade of aortocoronary bypass grafting, 1967–1977. A review. *Circulation* 1978; **57**:405–31.
5. Miller DW. *The Practice of Coronary Artery Bypass Surgery.* New York and London: Plenum Medical Book Co., 1977.
6. Sones FM Jr, Shirey EK. Cine coronary arteriography. *Mod Conc Cardiovas Dis* 1962; **31**:735–8.
7. Judkins MP. Percutaneous transfemoral selective coronary arteriography. *Radiol Clin N Am* 1968; **6**:467–92.
8. Bailey CP, May A, Lemmon WM. Survival after coronary endarterectomy in man. *J Am Med Assoc* 1957; **164**:641–6.
9. Longmire WP Jr, Cannon JA, Kattus AA. Direct-vision coronary endarterectomy for angina pectoris. *N Engl J Med* 1958; **259**:993–9.
10. Garrett HE, Diethrich EB, DeBakey ME. Myocardial revascularization. *Surg Clin N Am* 1966; **46**:863–71.
11. Sabiston DC Jr. Surgical treatment of coronary artery disease – introduction. *World J Surg* 1978; **2**:673–4.
12. Goetz RH, Rohman M, Haller JD, Dee R, Rosenak SS. Internal mammary-coronary artery anastomosis – a nonsuture method employing tantalum rings. *J Thorac Cardiovasc Surg* 1961; **41**:378–86.
13. Effler DB, Favaloro RG, Groves LK. Coronary artery surgery utilizing saphenous vein graft techniques. Clinical experience with 224 operations. *J Thorac Cardiovasc Surg* 1970; **59**:147–54.
14. Favaloro RG. The present era of myocardial revascularization – some historical landmarks. *Int J Cardiol* 1983; **4**:331–44.
15. Cannom DS, Miller DC, Shumway NE, Fogarty TJ, Daily PO, Hu M, *et al.* The long-term follow-up of patients undergoing saphenous vein bypass surgery. *Circulation* 1974; **49**:77–85.
16. Cooley DA, Dawson JT, Hallman GL, Sandiford FM, Wukasch DC, Garcia E, *et al.* Aortocoronary saphenous vein bypass. Results in 1,492 patients, with particular reference to patients with complicating features. *Ann Thorac Surg* 1973; **16**:380–90.
17. Johnson WD, Flemma RJ, Lepley D Jr, Ellison EH. Extended treatment of severe coronary artery disease: a total surgical approach. *Ann Surg* 1969; **170**:460–70.
18. Green GE, Stertzer SH, Reppert EH. Coronary arterial bypass grafts. *Ann Thorac Surg* 1968; **5**:443–50.
19. King SB III. The development of interventional cardiology. *J Am Coll Cardiol* 1998; **31**:64B–88B.
20. Holmes DR Jr, Vlietstra RE, Smith HC, Vetrovec GW, Kent KM, Cowley MJ, *et al.* Restenosis after percutaneous transluminal coronary angioplasty (PTCA): a report from the PTCA Registry of the National Heart, Lung, and Blood Institute. *Am J Cardiol* 1984; **53**:77C–81C.
21. Sigwart U, Puel J, Mirkovitch V, Joffre F, Kappenberger L. Intravascular stents to prevent occlusion and restenosis after transluminal angioplasty. *N Engl J Med* 1987; **316**:701–6.
22. Mehran R, Dangas G, Mintz GS, Waksman R, Abizaid A, Satler LF, *et al.* Treatment of in-stent restenosis with excimer laser coronary angioplasty versus rotational atherectomy: comparative mechanisms and results. *Circulation* 2000; **101**:2484–9.
23. Kelly RF. New developments in percutaneous coronary intervention. *Crit Care Clin* 2001; **17**:303–20.
24. Popma JJ, Wang JC. Advances in percutaneous coronary intervention. *Adv Intern Med* 2001; **46**:307–58.
25. Cutlip DE, Baim DS, Ho KK, Popma JJ, Lansky AJ, Cohen DJ, *et al.* Stent thrombosis in the modern era: a pooled analysis of multicenter coronary stent clinical trials. *Circulation* 2001; **103**:1967–71.
26. Morice MC, Serruys PW, Sousa JE, Fajadet J, Ban HE, Perin M, *et al.* A randomized comparison of a sirolimus-eluting stent with a standard stent for coronary revascularization. *N Engl J Med* 2002; **346**:1773–80.
27. Bonchek LI. Off-pump coronary bypass: is it for everyone? *J Thorac Cardiovasc Surg* 2002; **124**:431–4.
28. Mack M, Bachand D, Acuff T, Edgerton J, Prince S, Dewey T, *et al.* Improved outcomes in coronary artery bypass grafting with beating-heart techniques. *J Thorac Cardiovasc Surg* 2002; **124**:598–607.

29. Shuhaiber JH, Evans AN, Massad MG, Geha AS. Mechanisms and future directions for prevention of vein graft failure in coronary bypass surgery. Review. *Eur J Cardiothorac Surg* 2002; **22**:387–96.

30. Motwani JG, Topol EJ. Aortocoronary saphenous vein graft disease: pathogenesis, predisposition, and prevention. [Review –133 refs.] *Circulation* 1998; **97**:916–31.

31. Davies MJ. Stability and instability: two faces of coronary atherosclerosis. The Paul Dudley White Lecture 1995. *Circulation* 1996; **94**:2013–20.

32. Nwasokwa ON. Coronary artery bypass graft disease. [Review –148 refs.] *Ann Intern Med* 1995; **123**:528–45.

33. Loop FD, Lytle BW, Cosgrove DM, Stewart RW, Goormastic M, Williams GW, *et al.* Influence of the internal-mammary-artery graft on 10-year survival and other cardiac events. *N Engl J Med* 1986; **314**:1–6.

34. Lytle BW, Blackstone EH, Loop FD, Houghtaling PL, Arnold JH, Akhrass R, *et al.* Two internal thoracic artery grafts are better than one. *J Thorac Cardiovasc Surg* 1999; **117**:855–72.

35. Endo M, Nishida H, Tomizawa Y, Kasanuki H. Benefit of bilateral over single internal mammary artery grafts for multiple coronary artery bypass grafting. *Circulation* 2001; **104**:2164–70.

36. Hall MJ, Owings MF. *2000 National Hospital Discharge Survey. Advance data from vital and health statistics 2002*; **No. 329**. Hyattsville, MD: National Center for Health Statistics, 2002.

37. Boersma E, Manini M, Wood DA, Bassand J-P, Simoons ML (eds). *Cardiovascular Diseases in Europe. Euro Heart Survey and National Registries of Cardiovascular Diseases and Patient Management – 2002.* Sophia Antipolis: European Society of Cardiology, 2002.

38. Eagle KA, Guyton RA, Davidoff R, Ewy GA, Fonger J, Gardner TJ, *et al.* ACC/AHA guidelines for coronary artery bypass graft surgery: a report of the American College of Cardiology/ American Heart Association Task Force on Practice Guidelines (Committee to Revise the 1991 Guidelines for Coronary Artery Bypass Graft Surgery). American College of Cardiology/American Heart Association. [Review – 753 refs.] *J Am Coll Cardiol* 1999; **34**:1262–347.

39. Sergeant P, Blackstone E, Meyns B. Is return of angina after coronary artery bypass grafting immutable, can it be delayed, and is it important? *J Thorac Cardiovasc Surg* 1998; **116**:440–53.

40. Sergeant P, Blackstone E, Meyns B. Validation and interdependence with patient-variables of the influence of procedural variables on early and late survival after CABG. K.U. Leuven Coronary Surgery Program. *Eur J Cardiothorac Surg* 1997; **12**:1–19.

41. Keogh BE, Kinsman R. National adult cardiac surgical database report 2000–2001. Society of Cardiothoracic Surgeons of Great Britain and Ireland. Henley-on-Thames: Dendrite Clinical Systems Ltd, 2002.

42. Levi F, Lucchini F, Negri E, La Vecchia C. Trends in mortality from cardiovascular and cerebrovascular diseases in Europe and other areas of the world. *Heart* 2002; **88**:119–24.

43. Beller GA. Coronary heart disease in the first 30 years of the 21st century: challenges and opportunities: The 33rd Annual James B. Herrick Lecture of the Council on Clinical Cardiology of the American Heart Association. *Circulation* 2001; **103**: 2428–35.

44. Foot DK, Lewis RP, Pearson TA, Beller GA. Demographics and cardiology, 1950–2050. *J Am Coll Cardiol* 2000; **35**:1067–81.

2

The physiology and pathophysiology of myocardial perfusion

RAINER SCHULZ AND GERD HEUSCH

This review will attempt:

- to characterize the mechanical, metabolic and neurohumoral factors that control coronary blood flow and its distribution under normal circumstances and during myocardial ischemia/reperfusion, and
- to define the quantitative relationship of blood flow and contractile function in various scenarios of myocardial ischemia/reperfusion.

CORONARY AND MYOCARDIAL BLOOD FLOW

Anatomy

Most individuals possess two coronary arteries originating from the left and the right aortic sinuses, respectively. The main left coronary artery varies in length before the two branches, the left anterior descending (LAD) and the left circumflex (LCx) coronary arteries, originate. In most cases, the LAD coronary artery supplies approximately 50% of the left ventricular mass ($\sim$150 g), including two-thirds of the interventricular septum and the anterior free wall of the left ventricle. The right coronary artery supplies up to 30% of the left ventricular mass ($\sim$90 g), including the posterior third of the interventricular septum and half of the posterior wall. The remaining 20% of the left ventricular mass ($\sim$60 g) is supplied by the LCx coronary artery.[1]

Mechanical determinants of coronary blood flow: coronary perfusion pressure

As in any other perfusion circuit, in the coronary circulation myocardial blood flow is related to the available driving pressure. Under physiological conditions, diastolic aortic pressure is the input pressure of the coronary circulation.[2] Systolic aortic pressure, on the other hand, together with cardiac dimensions, determines left ventricular afterload and thus myocardial work and oxygen consumption. Therefore, any increase in aortic pressure will increase not only the available perfusion pressure for coronary blood flow but also the metabolic needs for coronary blood flow.

In elderly patients with a decreased compliance of the arterial windkessel leading to an increase in systolic and a decrease in diastolic aortic pressure, in particular when associated with arterial hypertension, the situation is even less favorable for matching coronary blood flow to myocardial oxygen demand. Likewise, aortic stenosis (i.e. increased systolic left ventricular pressure and relatively decreased diastolic aortic pressure) and aortic regurgitation (i.e. decreased diastolic aortic pressure) are conditions which favor a mismatch between coronary blood flow and myocardial oxygen demand.[3,4]

In the presence of a coronary stenosis, post-stenotic coronary pressure is the input pressure for myocardial perfusion. Post-stenotic pressure still depends to some extent on aortic pressure, but also on the severity of the coronary stenosis. Stenosis severity, in turn, is dependent upon stenosis morphology as well as on the distending pressure since most stenoses are compliant and their luminal cross-section depends on the pre-stenotic and post-stenotic pressures.[5]

The site and nature of the output pressure of the coronary circulation are not clear. When coronary perfusion pressure is systematically lowered, coronary inflow ceases at pressures substantially above right atrial pressure, i.e. at about 20–40 mmHg.[6,7] Two main factors appear to contribute to the relatively high zero-flow pressure in the coronary circulation. First, the coronary circulation has some properties of a Starling resistor which have been termed the 'vascular waterfall mechanism'.[8] When intramyocardial pressure exceeds the pressure at the venous outflow site, this intramyocardial pressure becomes the limiting outflow pressure, potentially by a partial vascular collapse. For example, in heart failure patients, increased left ventricular end-diastolic pressure is associated with an increased zero-flow pressure.[9] Second, the coronary circulation has a small but significant capacitance.[10] Thus, when coronary perfusion pressure is related to coronary arterial inflow measured in an epicardial conduit coronary artery, coronary arterial inflow may cease at surprisingly high perfusion pressures, whereas the capacitance may discharge the 'stored' blood volume into the microcirculation, thus maintaining myocardial perfusion.

Extravascular coronary compression

The squeezing effect of cardiac contraction that enhances venous outflow is active during beat-to-beat variations in coronary blood flow and particularly important for its phasic pattern.[11] However, during steady state conditions over several cardiac cycles, myocardial contraction impedes myocardial perfusion, and this is the clinically more relevant aspect of extravascular coronary compression during myocardial ischemia. After elimination of coronary vasomotor tone with maximal pharmacological dilatation, increases in heart rate increase coronary resistance.[12,13] A rise in left ventricular end-diastolic pressure also augments the extravascular component of coronary resistance.[7,12,14]

Extravascular compression is not uniformly distributed across the left ventricular wall, decreasing from sub-endocardium to sub-epicardium. Thus, extravascular compression is of particular importance for the transmural distribution of myocardial blood flow.[15] In the presence of intact coronary vasomotor tone, this endocardial–epicardial gradient of extravascular compression is fully compensated by a reverse epicardial–endocardial gradient in coronary autoregulatory reserve[16] and vascularization,[17] thus maintaining a uniform transmural myocardial blood flow distribution.

However, in the presence of a coronary stenosis, the effects of extravascular coronary compression on transmural myocardial blood flow distribution become fully apparent.[18] Any increase in heart rate[16] or left ventricular end-diastolic pressure[19] will then predominantly compromise the perfusion of sub-endocardial layers. Thus, extravascular compression is of major importance for the transmurally non-uniform, preferentially subendocardial manifestation of myocardial ischemia.[2,20]

Myocardial and coronary blood flow

Myocardial blood flow at rest averages 0.8–0.9 mL $min^{-1} g^{-1}$, which sums up to a total coronary blood flow of approximately 250 mL min^{-1} or 5% of cardiac output. Left ventricular intramyocardial blood flow occurs during diastole, flow in systole being prevented by the compressive effect of ventricular contraction (see above); the epicardial coronary arteries are not subject to this compression and fill in diastole. Therefore, LAD and LCx coronary blood flow mainly occurs in diastole and to a lesser extent during systole (Figure 2.1). In the right coronary artery, where aortic pressure represents the input pressure but extravascular compression is less pronounced, diastolic and systolic coronary blood flows are not substantially different and their cyclic variation is less than in the left ventricle.

Myocardial blood flow displays a spatial heterogeneity,[21–23] which is not simply related to temporal fluctuations as the heterogeneous flow pattern is stable over at least a few minutes.[23] The spatial heterogeneity of resting myocardial blood flow is not correlated to the heterogeneity of maximal myocardial blood flow,[23] and small patchy areas with and without persistent coronary dilator reserve (see below) coexist in ischemic myocardium.[24] The spatial heterogeneity of myocardial blood flow is

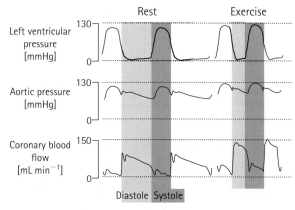

Figure 2.1 *Schematic diagram of left ventricular pressure, aortic pressure and coronary blood flow. Most of the coronary blood flow occurs during diastole.*

associated with similar heterogeneity in oxidative metabolism,[25] but not in morphology.[26]

Autoregulation of coronary blood flow

Autoregulation refers to the intrinsic mechanisms keeping blood flow constant when perfusion pressure is varied.[27] The coronary circulation exhibits a substantial autoregulatory capacity. In anesthetized dogs, coronary blood flow is maintained relatively constant when perfusion pressure is varied between 70 and 130 mmHg (Figure 2.2).[28] However, in the awake dog, the lower limit of autoregulation may even be as low as 40 mmHg.[29] Thus, anesthesia influences the lower limit of the autoregulatory range. When coronary perfusion pressure falls below this lower limit, myocardial blood flow becomes nearly linearly related to perfusion pressure, so that further decreases result in myocardial ischemia and contractile dysfunction.[29–31]

Autoregulation varies in different parts of the heart even when perfused by the same coronary artery. Both autoregulatory gain and the range of autoregulation are greater in the right than in the left ventricular perfusion territories of the right coronary artery, which perfuses parts of both ventricles.[32] Within the left ventricle, there is a transmural variation in autoregulatory capacity such that flow becomes pressure-dependent at higher perfusion pressures in the sub-endocardium than in the sub-epicardium,[29,33,34] thus again favoring a sub-endocardial manifestation of myocardial ischemia.

Whereas the existence and importance of coronary autoregulation are beyond doubt, the underlying mechanisms are less clear. First, increases in perfusion pressure may transiently increase coronary blood flow and a metabolic feedback signal may then increase vascular resistance to limit the increase in coronary blood flow, an explanation strengthened by the close coupling of coronary autoregulatory capacity to coronary venous PO_2.[35] Second, increases in perfusion pressure may induce a *myogenic response*, i.e. an increase in vasomotor tone opposing a transient vascular stretch secondary to an increase in perfusion pressure. Stretch, in particular dynamic stretch of a vessel, increases its electrical and in consequence its mechanical activity.[36] Finally, increases in perfusion pressure may increase capillary filtration, increase tissue pressure and thereby limit increases in coronary blood flow, but identical changes in tissue pressure do not mediate autoregulation after maximal pharmacological dilatation.[37]

Coronary reserve, i.e. the potential for increasing coronary blood flow above the instantaneous resting flow, is a measure of autoregulatory capacity.[38,39] The human coronary circulation has a coronary reserve of up to seven-fold, i.e. at unchanged coronary perfusion pressure coronary blood flow can be increased by up to seven-fold.[40,41] Whereas autoregulatory mechanisms maintain resting coronary blood flow constant over a range of perfusion pressures, blood flow during maximal coronary dilatation is pressure-dependent (Figure 2.2), as are, therefore, all ratios of maximal to resting blood flow.[38,39]

In the presence of a coronary stenosis, autoregulatory mechanisms try to maintain resting myocardial blood flow within the normal range. With a stenosis of less than 50% diameter reduction, neither resting myocardial blood flow nor flow reserve is impaired (Figure 2.3). With a stenosis of 50–80% diameter reduction, resting myocardial blood flow is maintained but flow reserve is significantly impaired: in patients this will result in signs of exercise-induced or stress-induced myocardial ischemia. As soon as the stenosis becomes more severe, both resting myocardial blood flow and flow reserve are decreased.

The assessment of coronary reserve in patients may provide useful clinical information (either on the risk of developing myocardial ischemia during stress situations[42,43] or on microvascular patency[44,45]). However, there are potential limitations, in that (a) different techniques to measure coronary blood flow (coronary sinus thermodilution, contrast angiography, Doppler flow, argon technique) have limited reliability, (b) there is spatial heterogeneity of resting blood flow and coronary reserve,[23] and (c) it is uncertain whether or not different techniques of inducing maximum coronary dilatation (reactive hyperemia, adenosine, papaverine, dipyridamole,

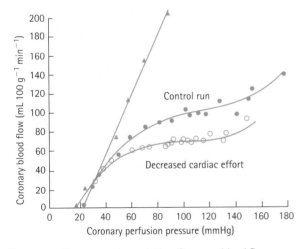

Figure 2.2 *Coronary autoregulation. Coronary blood flow varies in a linear fashion with instantaneous changes in coronary perfusion pressure ( ). Autoregulation develops over time, and during steady state conditions coronary blood flow is fairly constant in a range of perfusion pressures from about 70 to 130 mmHg ( ). The whole autoregulatory curve is displaced downwards at decreased cardiac performance ( ), emphasizing the coupling of coronary autoregulation to the myocardial metabolic state. Reproduced with permission.[28]*

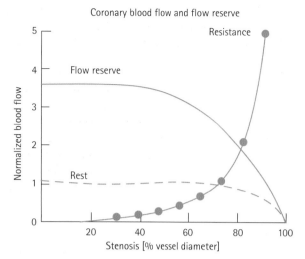

Coronary blood flow and flow reserve

Figure 2.3 *With a vessel diameter stenosis of less than 50%, neither resting myocardial blood flow nor flow reserve is impaired. Between 50% and 80% vessel diameter stenosis, resting myocardial blood flow is maintained but flow reserve is significantly impaired: in patients this will result in signs of exercise-induced or stress-induced myocardial ischemia. As soon as vessel diameter stenosis becomes more severe, both resting myocardial blood flow and flow reserve are decreased. Reprinted from Gould KL, Lipscomb K. Effects of coronary stenosis on coronary flow reserve and resistance. Am J Cardiol 1974; 34:48–55, with permission from Excerpta Medica Inc.*

contrast medium) do indeed achieve maximum coronary blood flow at a given perfusion pressure.

SUMMARY

In the normal left ventricle, blood flow to the inner myocardial layers occurs during diastole due to systolic extravascular compression. The driving pressure for perfusion is thus the diastolic aortic pressure. Profound hypotension (by reducing the driving pressure), profound tachycardia (by shortening diastolic duration and increasing extravascular compression and oxygen demand) and hypertension (by increasing extravascular compression and oxygen demand) therefore impair myocardial blood flow. This situation is aggravated in the presence of a coronary stenosis.

Local metabolic regulation of coronary blood flow

Only when coronary venous PO_2 is substantially reduced does arterial hypoxia cause coronary dilatation.[46] Although the involvement of increased PCO_2 in local metabolic regulation of myocardial blood flow has been suggested,[47] the effects are not very pronounced and are difficult to separate from simultaneous changes in pH. Even a synergistic action of PO_2 and PCO_2 would account for no more than 40% of changes in coronary blood flow in response

to changes in myocardial oxygen consumption.[48] A workload-induced release of K^+ is transient and may only be involved in the initial but not the sustained dilatation during increased cardiac work.[49] A metabolic feedback signal through protons also appears not to be important in metabolic coronary regulation, as intracoronary infusion of sodium bicarbonate restores a normal intracellular and coronary venous pH, but does not interfere with post-stenotic coronary vasodilatation.[50]

There may be a contribution of adenosine (which on a molar basis is one of the most powerful coronary dilators)[51] to initial transient coronary flow adaptations during rapid changes in cardiac performance[52,53] as well as to hypoxic and ischemic coronary vasodilatation. However, under physiological conditions,[51,54] adenosine is probably of minor importance for local metabolic coronary regulation, as the effective degradation of endogenous adenosine does not alter resting coronary blood flow[55] and coronary autoregulation.[56] Opening of ATP-sensitive K^+ channels and subsequent smooth muscle hyperpolarization are also involved in coronary dilatation.[57,58] In fact, the immediate and close coupling of changes in myocardial oxygen consumption to changes in coronary blood flow suggests a multistage controlled system.[59]

Persistence of coronary dilator reserve in ischemic myocardium

In ischemic myocardium, some coronary vasomotor tone persists, which can be removed by pharmacological dilatation. At a coronary perfusion pressure as low as 35 mmHg[60–62] or even 30 mmHg,[24,63] when a significant reduction in regional myocardial blood flow,[24,60–63] ischemic contractile dysfunction[24,60,62] and net lactate production[24,62] are present, intracoronary infusion of adenosine still significantly increases regional myocardial blood flow. Sub-epicardial vasodilator reserve persists even down to a perfusion pressure as low as 25 mmHg.[61] The resulting effects of a pharmacological recruitment of coronary dilator reserve on the contractile function of ischemic myocardium remain controversial.[24,60,62,64] In a true resting situation, no dilator reserve can be pharmacologically recruited in ischemic myocardium, suggesting that the persistent dilator reserve is related to increased vasoconstrictor tone, in particular α-adrenergic vasoconstrictor tone which becomes apparent during sympathetic activation.[64]

Collaterals and steal phenomena

In contrast to the canine heart, which has an extensive, mainly epicardial innate collateral circulation, the human (like the porcine) heart has only a sparse, primarily sub-endocardial innate collateral circulation.[65]

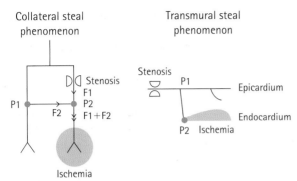

Figure 2.4 *Mechanisms of collateral and transmural steal. For detailed description, see text. P_1 = pressure at the origin of collaterals; P_2 = pressure at the orifice of collaterals into the ischemic terminal vascular bed; F_1 = flow through stenosis; F_2 = collateral blood flow. Reprinted from Baumgart D et al. A proischemic action of nisoldipine: relationship to a decrease in perfusion pressure and comparison to dipyridamole. Cardiovasc Res 1993;27:1254–9, with permission from Elsevier.*

Collateral growth and the development of a collateral circulation sufficient to provide a significant amount of myocardial blood flow occur in response to myocardial ischemia and/or to a pressure gradient across the collaterals,[65,66] and a number of growth factors are potentially involved in collateral angiogenesis.[67–71]

Coronary vasomotion even in mature collaterals differs somewhat from that in native vessels. Mature collateral vessels do not respond with constriction to α-adrenoceptor activation,[72] but dilate during β-adrenoceptor activation,[73] thus favoring collateral vasodilatation during sympathetic activation. Well-developed collateral vessels dilate in response to atrial natriuretic peptide[74] and constrict in response to serotonin and thromboxane A_2.[75] Vasopressin not only constricts collaterals,[76] but the vasoconstrictor response to vasopressin is particularly pronounced in the collateral-dependent microcirculation.[77] A well-developed collateral circulation provides significant protection during myocardial infarction. The amount of collateral circulation determines the time frame for effective thrombolysis in patients with acute myocardial infarction, and the outcome for patients with angiographically visible collaterals undergoing reperfusion after myocardial infarction is improved.[66,78] Whereas collaterals certainly have a cardioprotective function, they can also be the underlying morphological substrate for an aggravation of myocardial ischemia when steal phenomena occur (Figure 2.4).

In the presence of a flow-limiting coronary stenosis, flow into the ischemic terminal vascular bed is the sum of coronary arterial inflow through the stenosis and of collateral inflow from adjacent non-ischemic or less ischemic regions. Collateral inflow is dependent on the pressure gradient between the origin of collaterals in the intact donor vessels and their orifice into the ischemic recipient vessels. When the dilator reserve of the ischemic recipient vessels is fully exhausted and flow is therefore pressure-dependent, any dilatation of the non-ischemic donor terminal vascular bed during enhanced metabolic demand[13] or in response to dilator agents[79–83] will decrease the driving pressure gradient across the collaterals and, in consequence, decrease collateral flow. This phenomenon was termed collateral steal.[84] A similar situation is found with respect to the transmural distribution of myocardial blood flow when sub-endocardial autoregulatory reserve is exhausted but some sub-epicardial autoregulatory reserve persists.[33] The dilatation of sub-epicardial vessels during enhanced metabolic demand will then compromise sub-endocardial perfusion,[85] a phenomenon termed transmural steal. A transmural steal phenomenon can be considered as the major cause of the preferential sub-endocardial manifestation of myocardial ischemia and infarction. Finally, a steal situation also develops when a stenotic coronary artery perfuses parts of both the left and right ventricles. During increased myocardial metabolic demand, a redistribution from the left to the right ventricular perfusion territory, i.e. a right ventricular steal phenomenon, may occur.[32] The presence of a well-developed collateral circulation often maintains sufficient blood flow to the post-stenotic myocardium at rest, but steal phenomena contribute to the precipitation of myocardial ischemia during exercise.[64,86,87] For diagnostic purposes, such unfavorable blood flow redistribution is induced by dipyridamole and detected as reversible perfusion defects using thallium scintigraphy.[88,89]

Thus, in the presence of a flow-limiting stenosis, vasodilatation and/or inotropic stimulation can induce a collateral, transmural and/or interventricular steal phenomenon, thereby aggravating myocardial ischemia and contractile dysfunction. Pharmacological induction of steal phenomena may help to identify the existence, and quantify the severity, of coronary stenoses in patients.

Endothelial control of coronary blood flow

Several endothelial signaling agents promote coronary vasodilatation: nitric oxide (NO), prostanoids and endothelium-dependent hyperpolarizing factor (EDHF). These endothelium-dependent vasodilators can interact with other vasodilating substances (adenosine) and mechanisms (activation of ATP-sensitive potassium channels) as well as with constrictor signals (endothelin, angiotensin, catecholamines, see below). There is a continuous, basal NO production from the amino acid L-arginine by the constitutively expressed NO synthase located in coronary endothelial cells.[90,91] This basal release is maintained by a number of circulating substances such as norepinephrine, acetylcholine, ATP, bradykinin, histamine and thrombin. The most important stimulus for NO release is probably the laminar shear stress, or viscous drag, of the circulating blood[92] and the pulsatile stretching of the endothelial lining,[93] whereas increases in the perfusion pressure alone have no effect. Shear stress-dependent Ca^{2+} and K^+ channels have been characterized,[94,95] and a rise in the intracellular Ca^{2+} concentration is a prerequisite for NO formation.[96]

Endothelial NO release impacts on the tone of coronary conduit and resistance vessels at rest and during exercise.[97] There is evidence that endogenous NO preferentially controls the tone of epicardial vessels, with a declining gradient of action along the coronary vascular bed towards the periphery, whereas exogenously administered NO induces uniform dilatation throughout the coronary vascular bed. Furthermore, NO also has a tonic influence on the diameter of collateral vessels. Constitutive expression of the endothelial NO synthase is evident mainly in the conduit vessels and large resistance arteries and decreases towards the capillaries. In addition, stimulation of endothelial NO synthase preferentially increases flow in the sub-endocardial regions.[98]

Endothelium-independent myogenic mechanisms[99] and endothelium-dependent, flow-mediated dilatation interact in the microvascular control of coronary vasomotor tone[100] and in the autoregulatory adjustment of coronary blood flow.

There are numerous potential disturbances of endothelial L-arginine–NO metabolism, resulting in reduced NO synthesis:

- lack of the substrate of NO synthase, L-arginine,
- lack of co-factors such as tetrahydrobiopterin (BH4),
- reduced expression of the enzyme,
- increase in endogenous inhibitors of the enzyme such as asymmetrically dimethylated arginine derivatives.[98]

Furthermore, reduced bioavailability of NO can be caused by increased inactivation of NO as a result of increased production of oxygen-dependent radicals such as superoxide anions and hydroxyl radicals. Thus, reduced antioxidant capacity can induce NO-dependent endothelial dysfunction.

The principal risk factors for disturbances of endothelial NO metabolism in the coronary circulation are: arterial hypertension, hypercholesterolemia, diabetes mellitus, environmental factors such as sedentary lifestyle and cigarette smoking, and genetic determinants. The specific pathomechanism that finally culminates in reduced bioavailability of NO appears to vary with the individual risk factors.[101–105]

Responses to endothelium-dependent dilators such as acetylcholine,[106] substance P[107] or bradykinin[108] can be taken as an index of the functional integrity of coronary endothelium. In the absence of coronary artery disease, intracoronary injection of acetylcholine results in an endothelium-dependent dilator response of the large coronary arteries and of the resistance vessels.[109] This dilatation of resistance vessels results in an increased myocardial perfusion, which in turn adds to the large artery dilator response through a shear-stress-mediated augmentation of NO release. In the presence of coronary artery disease, NO release in response to acetylcholine is impaired, resulting in an attenuation of dilatation or even constriction due to the prevailing effects of activation of muscarinic smooth muscle receptors.[106] The flow-mediated dilator response is also substantially reduced, with impairment of endothelial function in patients with coronary artery disease.[110] The impairment of coronary dilator responses to acetylcholine is associated with an increased sensitivity to coronary constrictor responses to catecholamines[111,112] and exercise-induced ischemia[113] in patients with endothelial dysfunction. The degree of abnormality of epicardial vasomotor responses to intracoronary acetylcholine is related to the number of risk factors.[114] Abnormal vasomotor responses of atherosclerotic vessels can be restored by exogenous administration of L-arginine in the experimental[115] and clinical settings[116,117] as well as by application of co-factors of NO synthase.[118] An abnormal function of the bradykinin receptor might contribute to the abnormal flow-mediated coronary vasomotion observed in humans,[119] and abnormalities of coronary vasomotion secondary to endothelial dysfunction can be attenuated by angiotensin-converting enzyme (ACE) inhibition and angiotensin-1-receptor antagonism.[120,121]

Humoral control of coronary blood flow

In response to vasopressin, endothelium-dependent dilatation may prevail in epicardial coronary arteries,[122] but overall coronary resistance is increased.[123] Such vasopressin-induced constrictor response persists during coronary hypoperfusion[124] and is also apparent in collaterals.[76] Atrial natriuretic peptide (ANP) can cause endothelium-independent coronary dilatation.[125] However, the plasma ANP concentration required to induce coronary dilatation is probably not even reached under pathological conditions.

Angiotensin II (AGT II) in supraphysiological doses increases coronary tone both in large coronary conduit vessels and in resistance vessels.[126] The formation of AGT II depends on renin activity, the enzyme that splits off the decapeptide AGT I from the α-globulin angiotensinogen. AGT I, in turn, is converted into its active form, AGT II (an octapeptide), either by an endothelial ACE or the enzyme chymase, especially in human hearts.[127,128]

Simultaneously, ACE inactivates another octapeptide, bradykinin, which is an endothelium-dependent dilator (see above). ACE inhibitors can reduce coronary tone and increase myocardial perfusion, although under normal conditions the dilator effect of ACE inhibitors is minimal.[120] Experimentally, the coronary vasodilatation induced by ACE inhibition is mediated primarily by bradykinin and it is completely blocked by blockade of the bradykinin-B_2-receptor with HOE 140.[129]

With a low-sodium diet[130] or possibly during experimental myocardial ischemia[131] when renin secretion is stimulated, AGT II-mediated constrictor tone becomes more pronounced and the dilator effects of ACE inhibitors are more apparent.[132] Also, in patients with coronary artery disease or hypertension, ACE inhibitors exert an anti-ischemic effect.[133,134]

The exogenous infusion of endothelin-1 induces coronary constriction,[135] which in principle is strong enough to precipitate myocardial ischemia.[136] Distal portions of human coronary arteries are more sensitive to the constrictor effects of endothelin-1 than proximal regions and there is pharmacological evidence that this constriction is mediated by different endothelin receptors.[137] Both endothelin$_A$ (ETA) and endothelin$_B$ (ETB) receptors exist in human coronary arteries, with ETA receptors dominating on proximal epicardial coronary arteries and ETB receptors in medial and distal parts of the coronary circulation. Human coronary endothelial cells express only ETB receptors. Activation of both ETA and ETB receptors on vascular smooth muscle cells induces constriction, while activation of endothelial ETB receptors mediates dilatation through NO.[138]

Blockade of ETA receptors with BQ-123 reduces the coronary vasomotor tone of normal arteries by approximately 7%.[139] In patients with coronary artery disease, the reduction in the coronary vasomotor tone is more pronounced (16%), especially at the site of the coronary stenosis (22%).[139] Such increased endothelin-1-induced coronary vasoconstriction might relate to loss of endothelium-dependent vasodilatation and/or increased plasma endothelin-1 levels, which have been reported in patients with myocardial infarction.[140,141]

Prostacyclin (PGI$_2$), which is mainly synthesized in endothelial cells, acts via a receptor-mediated activation of adenylyl cyclase; the resulting increase in cAMP causes vasodilatation. PGI$_2$-synthesis is stimulated by a number of endogenous and exogenous substances.[142] Thromboxane (Tx A$_2$) is mainly synthesized in platelets and only to a small extent in the vasculature. Thromboxane increases the cytosolic concentration of calcium via the formation of inositol-1, 4,5-trisphosphate (IP$_3$) and a protein kinase C-mediated mechanism.[143]

Although PGI$_2$ can induce coronary dilatation and Tx A$_2$ coronary constriction, their contribution to the regulation of myocardial perfusion under physiological conditions is only minor. Coronary vasomotor tone of functionally intact vessels is not substantially changed by blockade of eicosanoid formation.[144,145] However, mature collateral vessels are under a tonic dilator influence

of prostaglandins, which is removed by cyclo-oxygenase inhibition with indomethacin.[146] In patients with endothelial dysfunction secondary to atherosclerosis, however, blockade of cyclo-oxygenase and subsequent prostaglandin production with aspirin decreased coronary blood flow.[91]

Constrictor effects of Tx A$_2$ and other platelet release products such as serotonin may be involved in cyclical critical coronary flow reductions superimposed on severe coronary stenoses.[147] Although it is tempting to link an uncontrolled release or action of Tx A$_2$ or other platelet products such as serotonin in the presence of endothelial damage[148,149] to the initiation of ischemic episodes, it remains to be established whether the increased Tx B$_3$ (a key metabolite of Tx A$_2$) levels are cause or consequence of myocardial ischemia.[150]

Neuronal control of coronary blood flow

Neurogenic mechanisms underlying changes in coronary vasomotor tone have attracted particular interest, as they might provide a causal link for the acute initiation of myocardial ischemia in situations of exercise and excitement[151] as well as for the apparently paradoxical initiation of myocardial ischemia in resting situations characterized by low myocardial oxygen demand.[152] Both sympathetic and vagal vasomotion occur at the level of epicardial coronary arteries, in the resistive microcirculation, and in the collateral circulation.

Cholinergic control of coronary blood flow

In dogs in which heart rate and left ventricular pressure were carefully controlled, coronary arteries dilated in response to exogenous acetylcholine[153] or electrical and reflex vagal activation.[153–155] Intracoronary acetylcholine increases blood flow more in the sub-endocardium than in the sub-epicardium, whereas electrical vagal stimulation induces uniform dilatation across the left ventricular wall.[156] However, there are obvious species differences of acetylcholine-induced coronary constrictor responses in calves, baboons and pigs.[157–159]

Whereas cholinergic coronary constriction is observed in isolated human vascular preparations,[160] the predominant response of angiographically normal coronary arteries to intracoronary acetylcholine appears to be dilatation.[106,114] In atherosclerotic segments, however, the predominant response is constriction.[104,106,110,161] It has to be kept in mind, though, that these studies did not demonstrate cholinergic regulation of coronary vasomotor tone but responses to exogenous acetylcholine reaching the coronary vascular smooth muscle from the luminal rather than the adventitial site. Thus, there is neither evidence for a physiological role of vagal regulation of coronary blood flow nor for a pathophysiological role in the initiation of myocardial ischemia in man.

Adrenergic control of coronary blood flow

Reflex sympathetic activation during exercise and excitement is beyond doubt.[151] The activation of cardiac β-adrenoceptors mediates an increase in heart rate and myocardial inotropic state. The resulting increase in myocardial oxygen demand is adequately matched by an augmented oxygen supply after metabolic dilatation of the coronary vasculature under normal conditions.[53,162] However, the direct effect of the sympathetic neurotransmitter norepinephrine on the coronary vascular smooth muscle is vasoconstriction that is mediated by activation of α-adrenoceptors.[151,163] Even under normal conditions in the presence of a substantial coronary dilator reserve, α-adrenergic constriction acts to limit metabolic coronary dilatation by about 30%, such that myocardial oxygen extraction increases together with coronary blood flow during sympathetic activation to match oxygen supply to the increased myocardial oxygen demand.[164–166]

A direct β-adrenergic coronary dilatation independent of metabolic factors has been demonstrated both in large epicardial and small resistive coronary arteries *in situ*.[167–169] The direct coronary dilatation of epicardial coronary arteries is mediated by both β$_1$-adrenoceptors and β$_2$-adrenoceptors.[168,169] However, the physiological significance of β-adrenoceptor-mediated coronary dilatation during sympathetic activation appears to be minimal.[167,170] In epicardial coronary arteries, β-adrenoceptor activation may also exert indirect dilator effects through an ascending mechanism[171,172] secondary to increases in coronary blood flow after metabolically mediated small vessel dilatation.[109] The lack of this indirect dilator effect may be responsible for the large vessel constriction observed after pharmacological β-blockade, rather than unopposed α-adrenergic constrictor tone.[173] Mature canine coronary collateral vessels express a mixed population of β$_1$-adrenoceptors and β$_2$-adrenoceptors mediating relaxation.[73]

In animal experiments, there is little α-adrenergic coronary vasomotor tone at rest, and the increase in coronary blood flow during sympathetic activation is only somewhat blunted. During supramaximal cardiac sympathetic nerve stimulation in the presence of β-blockade, epicardial coronary resistance contributes only about 5% to total coronary resistance, which amounts to 20–30%.[174,175] The microvascular coronary constrictor response to α-adrenoceptor activation is non-uniform, with a significant constriction of arterial and larger arteriolar segments and a dilatation of arterioles with a resting diameter of less than 100 μm.[176,177] These findings indicate a different coronary vascular site for metabolic dilatation and α-adrenergic constriction and a redistribution of coronary vascular resistance towards larger coronary vessels during α-adrenoceptor activation. The simultaneous constriction and dilatation of various coronary vascular segments may explain the weak net constrictor effect of α-adrenoceptor activation in the coronary circulation. There is a gradient of α$_1$-adrenergic coronary constriction, being more pronounced in larger vascular segments, and a reverse gradient of α$_2$-adrenergic coronary constriction, being more pronounced in the distal circulation.[175,177] Coronary collaterals are not responsive to α-adrenoceptor activation.[72,178–180]

In normal volunteers without signs, symptoms or risk factors of coronary artery disease, resting perfusion before and after 10 days of oral treatment with the selective α$_1$-antagonist doxazosin did not differ.[181] Intracoronary infusion of the non-selective α-antagonist phentolamine following β-blockade of angiographically normal coronary arteries induced minimal changes in diameter and resistance, both in normally innervated and denervated hearts. Similarly, neither epicardial diameter nor coronary blood flow velocity was altered by intracoronary phentolamine in another study in cardiac transplant recipients.[182]

The response of angiographically normal coronary arteries to sympathetic activation by the cold pressor test, mental stress or exercise is vasodilatation of both epicardial coronary arteries and microvessels.[183] In contrast to animal studies,[184] there is no evidence that vasodilatation is limited by α-adrenergic coronary vasoconstriction and consequently enhanced by α-blockade in healthy humans.[182,185]

While there appears to be no α-adrenergic coronary constrictor tone at rest in humans, coronary arteries respond to α$_2$-adrenergic stimulation; intracoronary infusion of the selective α$_2$-agonist BHT 933 does not affect epicardial coronary artery diameter, but induces a dose-dependent microvascular constriction.[186]

α–Adrenergic vasoconstriction in disease

Intact endothelium opposes α-adrenergic vasoconstriction,[112] and both shear stress and activation of endothelial α$_2$-adrenoceptors contribute to the inhibition of α-adrenergic vasoconstriction in the experimental setting.[187] Early stages of endothelial dysfunction already impair coronary dilator responses and predispose to constrictor responses.[188] When the coronary circulation is further impaired by hypercholesterolemia,[189] exhaustion of autoregulation[177] or severe coronary stenosis,[190,191] α-adrenergic vasoconstriction becomes unrestrained and powerful enough to reduce coronary blood flow and initiate myocardial ischemia.[151] Indeed, a progressive reversal from vasodilatation to vasoconstriction was demonstrated during the cold pressor test[192,193] and intracoronary acetylcholine[193] in both epicardial and resistive vessels with increasing severity of atherosclerosis. Exercise-induced dilatation of angiographically normal epicardial vessels was largely attenuated in the presence of hypercholesterolemia[194] or hypertension.[195] Patients with endothelial dysfunction in one protocol tended to experience exercise-induced ischemia during another protocol, as judged by thallium scintigraphy and anginal symptoms.[196]

In patients with established coronary artery disease, coronary resistance increases during the cold pressor test[197–199] and exercise[185] and this is prevented by intravenous phentolamine[185,197] or intravenous trimazosin, a selective α_1-antagonist.[199] Also, intracoronary infusion of the selective α_2-antagonist yohimbine with concomitant β-blockade increases coronary sinus norepinephrine levels and reduces both epicardial diameter and coronary blood flow velocity.[200] Similarly, coronary vascular resistance index increases in response to intravenous norepinephrine in patients with coronary artery disease.[201] Finally, intracoronary infusion of the selective α_2-agonist BHT 933 induces constriction of atherosclerotic epicardial segments sufficient to induce net myocardial lactate production and EKG signs of ischemia[186] (Figure 2.5). α-Adrenergic coronary vasoconstriction also occurs during coronary interventions,[183] not only at the site of the culprit segment and a distal segment of the vessel undergoing percutaneous transluminal coronary angioplasty (PTCA) also in the non-manipulated control vessel. This vasoconstriction is abolished by α-blockade with intracoronary phentolamine.[202] Similarly in patients undergoing PTCA, phentolamine prevents constriction distal to the site of PTCA, but not in the control segment.[203] These findings have been interpreted as evidence of a cardio-cardiac sympatho-excitatory reflex initiated by coronary stretch and/or myocardial ischemia and resulting in α-adrenergic coronary vasoconstriction, as previously demonstrated in animal experiments.[204,205] Also, in patients undergoing rotational atherectomy and PTCA, intracoronary infusion of the selective α_1-antagonist urapidil administered after atherectomy/PTCA reverses the observed decrease in epicardial diameter, and pretreatment with urapidil prevents any decrease in diameter.[206] Prevention of the decreases in the diameter of the distal post-stenotic and control vessels, and in coronary blood flow, also reverses the decreases in systolic wall thickening in the previously ischemic and non-ischemic myocardium that would otherwise occur.[207] Finally, in patients with recent acute myocardial infarction and subsequent thrombolysis who then undergo PTCA and stent implantation, intracoronary phentolamine and intravenous urapidil reverse the observed α-adrenergic vasoconstriction and also the reduction in systolic wall thickening, both in the infarct-related and in the non-infarct-related artery territories; the improvements seen

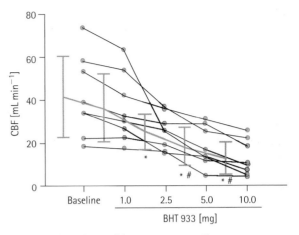

Figure 2.5 *In patients with coronary artery disease, intracoronary infusion of the selective α_2-agonist BHT 933 dose-dependently reduced coronary blood flow (CBF). The reduction at the highest dose was sufficient to induce net myocardial lactate production and EKG signs of ischemia. Reproduced with permission.[186]*

with urapidil are slightly attenuated by concomitant β-blockade.[208]

β-Adrenergic mechanisms in myocardial ischemia

Myocardial ischemia augments the impact of sympathetic activation on the coronary vasculature and the myocardium, and a situation of 'sympathetic over-stimulation' develops. Energy depletion of sympathetic nerve terminals and a resulting increase in intracellular sodium reverse the transport direction of the uptake carrier, which then transports large amounts of norepinephrine into the extracellular space.[209,210] The β-adrenoceptor density at the cellular surface[211,212] and the activity of adenylyl cyclase[213] are increased. This over-stimulation of the myocardial β-adrenoceptor cascade is largely responsible for the initiation of early ischemic arrhythmias, and the unmasking of α-adrenoceptor-mediated constriction in ischemic myocardium tends to further aggravate ischemia.[151] Furthermore, the β-adrenergic mechanisms contribute to myocardial ischemia through an unfavorable redistribution of coronary blood flow away from the ischemic sub-endocardium, i.e. through a collateral as well as a transmural steal mechanism (see above). β-Blockade decreases heart rate at rest and attenuates the exercise-induced increases in heart rate, left ventricular dP/dt and function of the non-ischemic myocardium. In consequence, the increases in blood flow to the non-ischemic myocardium and the post-stenotic sub-epicardium are attenuated. However, sub-endocardial blood flow of the ischemic myocardium is increased, thus resulting in improved regional myocardial function.[214] The beneficial effects of β-blockade in exercise-induced myocardial ischemia are almost exclusively due to the attenuation of the increase in heart rate. When this reduction in heart rate is prevented by atrial pacing, ischemic regional myocardial blood flow and function are even slightly reduced as compared to the untreated situation, possibly due to an unmasking of α-adrenergic constriction in the ischemic coronary microcirculation.[86] The hemodynamic severity of a dynamic coronary stenosis is reduced by β-blockade. The β-blockade-induced autoregulatory decrease in flow to non-ischemic regions results in an increase in post-stenotic coronary perfusion pressure. Increased perfusion pressure, in turn, reduces stenotic resistance, thus finally improving blood flow to ischemic regions.[215] These favorable effects on ischemic regional myocardial blood flow as well as additional anti-arrhythmic properties[216] are probably responsible for the fact that, among all anti-anginal agents, only β-blockers improve the prognosis of patients with coronary artery disease.[217]

RELATIONSHIP BETWEEN FLOW AND FUNCTION

In the normal heart, increases in contractile function are associated with increased metabolism, and the increased metabolic demands are met by increased oxygen extraction (to a smaller extent) and by increased myocardial blood flow (to a larger extent);[59] this is clearly a situation of perfusion–contraction matching. Whether or not perfusion–contraction matching holds true on the microregional level as well, i.e. whether or not the substantial spatial heterogeneity of myocardial blood flow (see above) is associated with a similar spatial heterogeneity of contractile function, is currently unclear due to the insufficient spatial resolution of current techniques to measure contractile function. Therefore, the hypothesis that hibernation at the microregional level is a physiological phenomenon, permitting some myocardium to rest in the otherwise continuously working heart,[218] appears somewhat far-fetched at present.

While an increase in myocardial contractile function will lead to a metabolically mediated increase in myocardial blood flow, several studies suggest that increases in coronary perfusion *per se* (Gregg phenomenon,[219] 'garden hose' phenomenon[220]) within or above the coronary autoregulatory range also increase myocardial contractile function. While on a global ventricular level the existence of a Gregg or garden hose phenomenon remains controversial, there is no evidence for the existence of a Gregg or garden hose phenomenon on a regional myocardial level in anesthetized swine[221] or conscious dogs[29] as long as autoregulation is operative.

Acute (minutes) ischemia: ischemic region

Upon acute coronary artery inflow reduction, contractile function in the ischemic region is rapidly decreased.[222] As soon as a steady state has developed (2–3 minutes), a consistent relation between the reduced regional myocardial blood flow and contractile function is apparent. Although the shape of this flow–function relationship has been a matter of some controversy in the past,[30,31,223,224] at present the consistent, close perfusion–contraction matching appears more important than subtle differences in the shape of such a relationship, which may be attributable to differences in experimental conditions, segment shortening versus wall thickening, data presentation and statistical phenomena.

The relationship between ischemic regional myocardial blood flow and contractile function varies with the hemodynamic situation. There is a higher blood flow for a given level of function during exercise than at rest.[31] However, when myocardial blood flow is normalized for heart rate, i.e. expressed as blood flow per beat rather than per minute, and thus related to the same temporal reference as contractile function, i.e. one arbitrary average cardiac cycle, the relationships at rest and during exercise[31] (Figure 2.6) and those at different heart rates[225,226] are superimposable.

The mechanisms/biochemical signals that underlie the rapid development of perfusion–contraction matching in acutely ischemic myocardium are still unclear. Endogenous NO is not the biochemical signal for perfusion–contraction matching, but sets the level for such matching, i.e. with inhibition of NO synthesis, regional myocardial function for any level of blood flow and oxygen consumption is reduced in anesthetized open-chest[227] (Figure 2.7) and sedated, chronically instrumented pigs[228] subjected to 90 minute acute ischemia.

As originally outlined by Ross,[229] perfusion–contraction matching with maintenance of viability occurs only as long as there is some residual blood flow. In fact, the lower limits for the maintenance of viability are at 50% and 25% of baseline for transmural and sub-endocardial blood flow, respectively, during 90 minute ischemia in anesthetized open-chest pigs.[230] A similar flow threshold for infarct development has also been obtained in patients using positron emission tomography (PET).[231]

Acute (minutes) ischemia: non-ischemic region

Regional myocardial ischemia also impacts on the non-ischemic myocardium. During acute coronary artery occlusion in anesthetized swine[232] and in both anesthetized[233] and conscious dogs,[234,235] the ischemic region is surrounded by a narrow zone of normally perfused

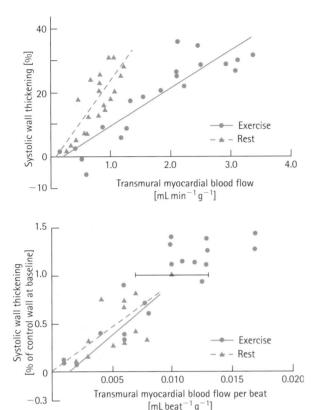

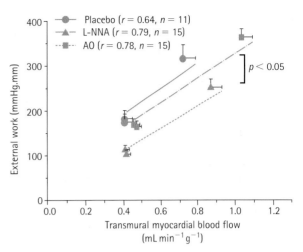

Figure 2.7 *Symbols represent mean values (± SEM) before and at 10 minutes and 85 minutes ischemia. The relationship between the external work index and transmural blood flow in placebo is shifted rightwards with L-NNA (▲), but not with aortic constriction (AO, ■). P-value indicates significant difference of relationship with L-NNA from both placebo and AO. Reproduced with permission.[277]*

Figure 2.6 *Relationship between mean transmural blood flow and transmural systolic wall thickening. When myocardial work increases during exercise, the relationship between flow and function is shifted to the right as compared to the relationship at rest, but it converges to a point similar to that of the resting relationship when flow restriction is severe and wall motion akinetic. However, when myocardial blood flow is normalized for heart rate, i.e. expressed as blood flow per beat rather than per minute, and thus related to the same temporal reference as contractile function, i.e. one arbitrary average cardiac cycle, the relationships at rest and during exercise are superimposable. Reproduced with permission.[31]*

myocardium with depressed systolic wall thickening or segment shortening. This depressed contractile function in the immediate border zone surrounding the ischemic region is attributed to more or less well defined mechanical 'tethering' between non-ischemic and ischemic myocardial fibers.[236] The mechanism of such 'tethering' probably relates to the existence of high regional wall stresses present at the border between ischemic and dysfunctional versus normal myocardium.[237] Such dysfunctional border zone leads to the over-estimation of the ischemic region from a diagnostic point of view. The extent and severity of dysfunction in the non-ischemic border zone are unaltered by changes in afterload.[238] Whether the size of the dysfunctional border zone is decreased by inotropic stimulation[239] or not[240] remains

controversial at present. The size of the dysfunctional border zone resulting from acute occlusion of the LAD or of the LCx coronary artery is considerably different, with a larger dysfunctional zone[236] and a greater reduction in contractile function[241] in the anterior region during LAD occlusion than in the posterior region during LCx occlusion. Such a larger dysfunctional non-ischemic border zone surrounding an anterior ischemic region may in part explain the more pronounced impairment of global left ventricular function during anterior versus inferior ischemia.[242]

A dysfunctional non-ischemic border zone may not only extend laterally from an ischemic region during complete coronary occlusion, but may also overlie the ischemic inner myocardial layers during non-transmural ischemia. The sub-epicardium became dysfunctional when ischemia was restricted to the sub-endocardium and sub-epicardial perfusion was normal,[243,244] and outer wall dysfunction was out of proportion to the outer wall flow reduction during treadmill exercise in dogs with coronary stenosis.[245] Transmural tethering – like lateral tethering – is non-uniform throughout the left ventricle, with more pronounced non-ischemic epicardial dysfunction during sub-endocardial ischemia of the anterior as compared to the posterior myocardium.[246] Whereas lateral and transmural tethering create a non-ischemic dysfunctional border zone in the immediate vicinity of the ischemic region, more remote non-ischemic regions are characterized by enhanced contractile function.[247–250] Whether an increase in remote non-ischemic zone function can be considered as compensatory, in that it acts to preserve global left ventricular function,[247,250,251] is not completely clear, as a major part of non-ischemic zone hyperfunction occurs during isovolumic systole and does not contribute to ejection.[248] The increase in function in the remote non-ischemic zone is associated with a moderate, presumably metabolically mediated increase in blood flow to this region.[247,252] However, the relationship of regional myocardial blood flow and function in remote, hyper-functioning, non-ischemic myocardium has not yet been systematically analyzed.

Subacute (hours) ischemia

When moderate ischemia, defined by a reduction of systolic wall thickening to 60% of baseline, is extended to 5 hours in chronically instrumented, conscious dogs, perfusion–contraction is still maintained,[253] and this situation is associated with complete recovery of contractile function following reperfusion and the lack of infarction in the previously dysfunctional myocardium. Likewise, 2 hours of moderate coronary stenosis in chronically instrumented, conscious dogs induces matched 50% reductions in regional blood flow and contractile function.[254,255] However, when ischemia, defined by a reduction in transmural blood flow to 60% of baseline, is extended to 24 hours duration in anesthetized, open-chest pigs with constant flow perfusion, perfusion–contraction matching is lost after more than 90 minutes and contractile function is progressively reduced without any further reduction in blood flow[256] (Figure 2.8). This situation of progressive contractile dysfunction with sub-acute moderate ischemia is still associated with maintained viability; however, some animals develop patchy necrosis.

Likewise, in sedated, chronically instrumented pigs subjected to 24 hours moderate ischemia by manipulation of a hydraulic occluder at a reduction of myocardial blood flow to 60% of baseline, there is loss of perfusion–contraction matching. However, in this study, multifocal patchy necrosis developed, and those microregions (on average 150 mg) with necrosis had decreased blood flow, whereas the viable ones had maintained normal blood flow, reflecting a substantial spatial heterogeneity of blood flow during sustained moderate ischemia.[257] The partial discrepancy between the latter two studies with respect to the development of patchy necrosis may be related to the use of an anesthetized, open-chest preparation with controlled coronary inflow versus a sedated, chronically instrumented preparation with a manipulated hydraulic stenosis that has a better, more physiological inotropic state, but possibly also episodes of superimposed stress-induced ischemia. Despite this discrepancy, both studies agree on the loss of perfusion–contraction matching with time. In contrast, in two other

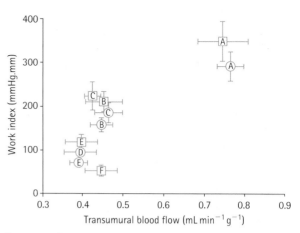

Figure 2.8 *Relation between flow and function during 12 hours ( ) or 24 hours hypoperfusion ( ) in pigs with viable myocardium. A close matching between reduced transmural myocardial blood flow and the reduced work index existed in both groups during the first 90 minutes hypoperfusion. However, when hypoperfusion was prolonged for 6 hours or more, the work index decreased further, although transmural myocardial blood flow did not change significantly – i.e. perfusion–contraction mismatch developed. A: baseline; B: 5-min hypoperfusion; C: 90-min hypoperfusion; D: 6-h hypoperfusion; E: 12-h hypoperfusion; F: 24-h hypoperfusion. Reproduced with permission.[256]*

studies in anesthetized, closed-chest pigs subjected to moderate ischemia at 60% of inflow by a hydraulic occluder for 24 hours, the relation of reduced blood flow to reduced wall thickening appeared to be maintained; however, in these studies coronary inflow varied substantially during the protocol, some animals developed patchy necrosis, and regional myocardial blood flow data were not reported, such that the existence of perfusion–contraction matching on a regional level cannot be evaluated.[258,259]

Acute reperfusion

Brief periods of ischemia, not causing irreversible damage, nevertheless result in prolonged impairment of contractile function upon reperfusion, i.e. stunning.[260–264] Almost by definition, the close relationship of reduced myocardial blood flow and function observed during the preceding ischemia is lost, as blood flow is restored by reperfusion – often there is even reactive hyperemia – whereas function remains depressed. Although sub-endocardial blood flow in stunned myocardium may be somewhat reduced (after reactive hyperemia has subsided),[265–268] this finding is not consistent.[269–271] As is the case with normally perfused myocardium, increases in myocardial perfusion induce no increase in contractile function, excluding a causal role of the possibly somewhat reduced sub-endocardial blood flow in the observed contractile dysfunction.[272]

Thus, stunned myocardium is apparently characterized by perfusion–contraction mismatch. However, as mentioned before, hypokinetic and dyskinetic myocardium may develop substantial wall stress, such that the true contractile function and its energetic equivalent may be underestimated and the mismatch between perfusion and contraction be over-estimated in stunned myocardium.

Whereas there is no apparent relationship between regional myocardial blood flow and contractile function in stunned myocardium during reperfusion, there is a relationship between regional myocardial contractile function during reperfusion and the severity of regional myocardial blood flow reduction during the preceding ischemia. The rate of recovery of function in stunned myocardium during 24 hours of reperfusion depends on the severity of blood flow reduction during the 15 minutes of the preceding ischemia.[265] Function in the inner myocardial layers where ischemia is more severe recovers more slowly than that in outer, less ischemic myocardial layers.[273] Dependence of post-ischemic dysfunction on the severity of the preceding reduction in blood flow per beat was also demonstrated during recovery from a bout of exercise-induced ischemia.[274]

Coronary microembolization

Embolization of atherosclerotic and thrombotic material is a frequent and important consequence of spontaneous and interventional plaque rupture.[275–277] Experimental coronary microembolization in anesthetized dogs induces regional contractile dysfunction.[278,279] However, at a spatial resolution of 300 mg myocardial tissue using microspheres, there is no measurable reduction in regional myocardial blood flow in the dysfunctional myocardium, i.e. clearly a perfusion–contraction mismatch[280] (Figure 2.9). The slight amount of patchy microinfarction is unlikely to account for the observed dysfunction; however, there is a marked inflammatory response that is possibly responsible for the observed dysfunction, through mediators such as TNFα [281–283] and free radicals.[279] Undoubtedly coronary microembolization is a factor in perfusion–contraction mismatch distinct from stunning.

Experimental chronic stenosis

In pigs with an implanted hydraulic stenosis that reduced coronary blood flow velocity by 50% during the initial surgery, but did not reduce regional myocardial blood flow (microspheres) either during the initial surgery or at a second surgery 4 days later, segment shortening was reduced by 50%. This scenario of perfusion–contraction

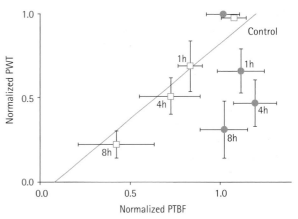

Figure 2.9 *Relationships between normalized posterior transmural blood flow (PTBF) and normalized posterior systolic wall thickening (PWT) with an epicardial coronary stenosis (□) and with coronary microembolization (●) at control, 1, 4 and 8 hours (h) of ischemia. Values are mean ± SD. With stenosis but not with coronary microembolization, there was a good linear relationship between PWT and PTBF (y = 0.90, x = −0.07, r = 0.82). Reproduced with permission.[280]*

mismatch led the authors to speculate on intermittent episodes of ischemia and reperfusion which also induced metabolic alterations such as decreased fatty acid oxidation and increased glucose utilization.[284] Chen *et al.* also used a hydraulic occluder in pigs that reduced resting coronary inflow by 30–40%[285,286] and restudied these pigs 7 days[285] and 4 weeks[286] later. They observed proportionate reductions in coronary inflow and systolic wall thickening (echocardiography) at 7 days[285] and at 4 weeks,[286] which were associated with patchy necrosis in some[285,286] and patchy apoptosis in all pigs,[286] indicating the inability of downregulation of contractile function fully to prevent loss of viable cardiomyocytes. Similarly, reduction of coronary inflow by 90% using a hydraulic occluder reduced both post-stenotic blood flow (PET) and function (echocardiogram, wall motion score) and induced patchy necrosis over 30 days in chronically instrumented pigs.[287]

Canty and Klocke[288] implanted an ameroid constrictor on the LCx coronary artery in dogs after ligation of visible epicardial collaterals and followed regional myocardial blood flow and contractile function over 2–4 weeks. They observed a temporal pattern of flow–function relationship, with function being reduced in excess of blood flow prior to and at ameroid closure, then matching of reduced blood flow and function later after ameroid closure, and finally return of both blood flow and function to control. They proposed a complex adjustment to progressive coronary stenosis, initially involving stunning as a consequence of episodic, transient ischemia and subsequently hibernation.[288] Similarly, using an ameroid constrictor in pigs,

Shen and Vatner[289] found decreased systolic wall thickening after 3 weeks, but no decrease in regional blood flow; subsequently, function returned to normal after 5 weeks, again with no change in blood flow. They observed occasional episodes of transient excitement followed by stunning and patchy necrosis post mortem in some pigs[289,290] and concluded that the phenotype of hibernating myocardium is the result of cumulative stunning rather than of a downregulation of contractile function in response to a persistent reduction in resting flow. After implantation of multiple ameroid constrictors in dogs, Firoozan et al.[291] also found decreased systolic wall thickening before decreased regional myocardial blood flow after 2 weeks, but at the final study after 6 weeks there were both regions with proportionate decreases in blood flow and contractile function (perfusion–contraction match) and others with decreased function but without decreased blood flow (perfusion–contraction mismatch). Although no episodes of stunning were documented, these authors also proposed a temporal progression from stunning to hibernation.[291]

Using a model of a chronic fixed stenosis that is implanted in juvenile pigs which are studied several weeks after having grown,[292] McFalls et al.[293] found proportionate decreases in regional myocardial blood flow and systolic wall thickening after 5 weeks, consistent with the concept of hibernation. Using this same model, Fallavollita again characterized a typical time course of adaptation to this chronic coronary stenosis.[294,295] One to 2 months after stenosis placement, regional myocardial blood flow at rest was still normal, whereas an echocardiographic wall motion score was reduced, associated with increased sub-endocardial fluoro-deoxyglucose (FDG) uptake, consistent with chronic stunning.[295] However, 3–4 months after stenosis placement, there was both decreased resting blood flow and contractile function, again associated with increased FDG uptake, consistent with hibernation.[294] Fallavollita et al. emphasize the hypothesis of a temporal progression from stunning to hibernation in which reduced resting flow is the result rather than the cause of chronic contractile dysfunction.[295]

Finally, Shivalkar et al.[296] combined the implantation of multiple ameroid constrictors with the creation of a chronic fixed stenosis in dogs and over 8 weeks observed decreases in systolic wall thickening, initially episodic but subsequently becoming more persistent, with no decreases in resting blood flow. Importantly, they also observed recovery of contractile function with revascularization and only minor morphological changes in some dogs. These authors also interpret their findings as a progression from stunning to hibernation where flow is decreased in response to decreased demand.[296]

Taken together, the experimental studies with chronic coronary stenosis that suggest a temporal progression from stunning (perfusion–contraction mismatch) to hibernation (perfusion–contraction match) where blood flow is reduced in response to reduced function are indeed intriguing. However, in none of these studies were regional myocardial blood flow and contractile function continuously monitored, were episodes of stunning systematically recorded, or was stunning systematically induced finally to produce the phenotype of hibernation.

Clinical chronic coronary stenosis

Using inert gas techniques, Arani et al.[297] measured decreased blood flow draining into the great cardiac vein in collateral-dependent myocardium of patients with coronary artery disease and suggested that this flow reduction might be an adaptation to reduced local metabolic demand, consistent with Rahimtoola's concept of myocardial hibernation. Currently, a number of studies in patients with chronic coronary artery disease exist that quantify regional myocardial blood flow with PET and regional contractile function with various techniques. Unfortunately, no consistent picture emerges from the available data. Several studies find no decreases in resting regional blood flow in dysfunctional, viable myocardium, whereas the majority of studies – and patients studied – show decreased blood flow at rest in dysfunctional myocardium. Canty and Fallavollita estimated in their review[298] that some of those studies without a significant reduction in resting blood flow were statistically underpowered. In the other studies, the degree of contractile dysfunction appears to be in excess of the reduction in blood flow; however, this may reflect to some extent the limited spatial resolution of PET and its inability to measure sub-endocardial blood flow. However, all available studies, with[299,300] and without[301,302] reduced baseline blood flow agree on a reduced coronary dilator reserve.

The available clinical data therefore provide no solution to the ongoing controversy about whether chronic hibernation is an adaptation to a reduced baseline blood flow with perfusion–contraction match, as originally proposed by Rahimtoola, or whether it is a manifestation of cumulative stunning, or whether finally there is a temporal progression from cumulative stunning to a state of hibernation where reduced blood flow is the consequence rather than the cause of contractile dysfunction. This situation is based on the obvious impossibility of continuously or even frequently monitoring both blood flow and function in the natural course of coronary artery disease. Clearly, there are many scenarios with different relationships of flow and function in coronary artery disease.[303]

Although this situation is disappointing from a mechanistic point of view, it may not impact too badly on clinical decisions: patients with contractile dysfunction and normal baseline flow but reduced coronary reserve will certainly benefit from revascularization. Likewise, patients with contractile dysfunction and moderately reduced baseline flow, particularly when associated with increased FDG uptake and maintained inotropic responsiveness, are likely to benefit from revascularization.[304] The extent of fibrosis, as a consequence of loss of cardiomyocytes and myofilaments[305,306] and/or increased apoptosis,[286,307] appears to be the major determinant of postoperative functional recovery after revascularization.[307,308]

In conclusion, coronary blood flow and its regional distribution are controlled by a complex interactive system of mechanical, metabolic, endothelial and neurohumoral factors, the contribution of which varies with the actual situation, i.e. at rest versus exercise or in health versus atherosclerosis. Various scenarios of myocardial ischemia and reperfusion are characterized by different quantitative relationships of regional blood flow and contractile function. The exact mechanisms determining perfusion–contraction match or mismatch and their interrelationship remain to be defined.

KEY REFERENCES

Erbel R, Heusch G. Brief review: coronary microembolization. *J Am Coll Cardiol* 2000; **36**:22–4.

Atheromatous thromboembolism is now recognized as an important feature not only of acute coronary events, but also of stable atheroma and interventional procedures. Small infarcts, contractile dysfunction and arrhythmias are probably due to this phenomenon. This is of relevance to the etiology/prevention of low output syndrome following coronary surgery.

Guth BD, Schulz R, Heusch G. Time course and mechanisms of contractile dysfunction during acute myocardial ischemia. *Circulation* 1993; **87**(Suppl. IV):35–42.

Evidence for a potentially harmful effect of inotropic stimulation of ischemic myocardium in which contractile function is downregulated – of particular relevance to coronary surgery in the presence of impaired left ventricular function.

Heusch G. α-Adrenergic mechanisms in myocardial ischemia. *Circulation* 1990; **81**:1–13.

Review of evidence for multiple α-adrenergic mechanisms contributing to myocardial ischemia.

Heusch G, Baumgart D, Camici P, Chilian W, Gregorini L, Hess O, *et al.* α-Adrenergic coronary vasoconstriction and myocardial ischaemia in humans. *Circulation* 2000; **101**:689–94.

α-Adrenergic coronary constriction may occur during coronary interventions and may cause myocardial ischemia. This review links experimental findings with clinical studies, using recently available techniques.

Ross J Jr. Myocardial perfusion–contraction matching. Implications for coronary heart disease and hibernation. *Circulation* 1991; **83**:1076–83.

Account of the role of perfusion–contraction matching in acute and chronic ischemic states, with potential implications for clinical therapy.

REFERENCES

1. Weaver ME, Pantely GA, Bristow JD, Ladley HD. A quantitative study of the anatomy and distribution of coronary arteries in swine in comparison with other animals and man. *Cardiovasc Res* 1986; **20**:907–17.
2. Buckberg GD, Fixler DE, Archie JP Jr, Hoffman JIE. Experimental subendocardial ischemia in dogs with normal coronary arteries. *Circ Res* 1972; **30**:67–81.
3. Buckberg G, Eber L, Herman M, Gorlin R. Ischemia in aortic stenosis: hemodynamic prediction. *Am J Cardiol* 1975; **35**:778–84.
4. Trenouth RS, Phelps NC, Neill WA. Determinants of left ventricular hypertrophy and oxygen supply in chronic aortic valve disease. *Circulation* 1976; **53**:644–50.
5. Schwartz JS, Carlyle PF, Cohn JN. Effect of coronary arterial pressure on coronary stenosis resistance. *Circulation* 1980; **61**:70–6.
6. Klocke FJ, Weinstein IR, Klocke JF, Ellis AK, Kraus DR, Mates RE, *et al.* Zero-flow pressures and pressure–flow relationships during single long diastoles in the canine coronary bed before and during maximum vasodilation. *J Clin Invest* 1981; **68**:970–80.
7. Aldea GS, Mori H, Husseini WK, Austin RE, Hoffman JI. Effects of increased pressure inside or outside ventricles on total and regional myocardial blood flow. *Am J Physiol Heart Circ Physiol* 2000; **279**:H2927–38.
8. Downey JM, Kirk ES. Inhibition of coronary blood flow by a vascular waterfall mechanism. *Circ Res* 1975; **36**:753–60.
9. Traverse JH, Chen Y-J, Crampton M, Voss S, Bache RJ. Increased extravascular forces limit endothelium-dependent and -independent coronary vasodilation in congestive heart failure. *Cardiovasc Res* 2001; **52**:454–61.
10. Chilian WM, Eastham CL, Layne SM, Marcus ML. Small vessel phenomena in the coronary microcirculation: phasic intramyocardial perfusion and coronary microvascular dynamics. *Progr Cardiovasc Dis* 1988; **31**:17–38.
11. Spaan JAE, Breuls NPW, Laird JD. Diastolic–systolic coronary flow differences are caused by intramyocardial pump action in anesthetized dog. *Circ Res* 1981; **49**:584–93.
12. Raff WK, Kosche F, Lochner W. Extravascular coronary resistance and its relation to microcirculation. *Am J Cardiol* 1972; **29**:598–603.
13. Heusch G, Yoshimoto N. Effects of heart rate and perfusion pressure on segmental coronary resistances and collateral perfusion. *Pflügers Arch* 1983; **397**:284–9.
14. Heusch G, Yoshimoto N. Effects of cardiac contraction on segmental coronary resistances and collateral perfusion. *Int J Microcirc* 1983; **2**:131–41.
15. Hoffman JIE. Transmural myocardial perfusion. *Progr Cardiovasc Dis* 1987; **29**:429–64.
16. Bache RJ, Cobb FR. Effect of maximal coronary vasodilation on transmural myocardial perfusion during tachycardia in the awake dog. *Circ Res* 1977; **41**:648–53.
17. Downey HF, Bashour FA, Boatwright RB, Parker PE. Uniformity of transmural perfusion in anesthetized dogs with maximally dilated coronary circulations. *Circ Res* 1975; **37**:111–17.

18. Raff WK, Kosche F, Goebel H, Lochner W. Coronary extravascular resistance at increasing left ventricular pressure. *Pflügers Arch* 1972; 333:352–61.

19. Kjekshus JK. Mechanisms for flow distribution in normal and ischemic myocardium during increased ventricular preload in the dog. *Circ Res* 1973; 33:489–99.

20. Bache RJ, Cobb FR, Greenfield JC Jr. Myocardial blood flow distribution during ischemia-induced coronary vasodilation in the unanesthetized dog. *J Clin Invest* 1974; 54:1462–72.

21. Franzen D, Conway RS, Zhang H, Sonnenblick EH, Eng C. Spatial heterogeneity of local blood flow and metabolic content in dog hearts. *Am J Physiol Heart Circ Physiol* 1988; 254:H344–53.

22. Bassingthwaighte JB, King RB, Roger SA. Fractal nature of regional myocardial blood flow heterogeneity. *Circ Res* 1989; 65:578–90.

23. Austin RE Jr, Aldea GS, Coggins DL, Flynn AE, Hoffman JI. Profound spatial heterogeneity of coronary reserve. Discordance between patterns of resting and maximal myocardial blood flow. *Circ Res* 1990; 67:319–31.

24. Coggins DL, Flynn AE, Austin RE Jr, Aldea GS, Muehrcke D, Goto M, *et al.* Nonuniform loss of regional flow reserve during myocardial ischemia in dogs. *Circ Res* 1990; 67:253–64.

25. Schwanke U, Deussen A, Heusch G, Schipke JD. Heterogeneity of local myocardial flow and oxidative metabolism. *Am J Physiol Heart Circ Physiol* 2000; 279:H1029–35.

26. Sonntag M, Deussen A, Schultz J, Loncar R, Hort W, Schrader J. Spatial heterogeneity of blood flow in the dog heart. I. Glucose uptake, free adenosine and oxidative/glycolytic enzyme activity. *Pflügers Arch* 1996; 432:439–50.

27. Dole WP. Autoregulation of the coronary circulation. *Progr Cardiovasc Dis* 1987; 29:293–323.

28. Mosher P, Ross J Jr, McFate PA, Shaw RF. Control of coronary blood flow by an autoregulatory mechanism. *Circ Res* 1964; 14:250–9.

29. Canty JM. Coronary pressure–function and steady-state pressure–flow relations during autoregulation in the unanesthetized dog. *Circ Res* 1988; 63:821–36.

30. Vatner SF. Correlation between acute reductions in myocardial blood flow and function in conscious dogs. *Circ Res* 1980; 47:201–7.

31. Gallagher KP, Matsuzaki M, Osakada G, Kemper WS, Ross J Jr. Effect of exercise on the relationship between myocardial blood flow and systolic wall thickening in dogs with acute coronary stenosis. *Circ Res* 1983; 52:716–29.

32. Guth BD, Schulz R, Heusch G. Pressure–flow characteristics in the right and left ventricular perfusion territories of the right coronary artery in swine. *Pflügers Arch* 1991; 419:622–8.

33. Guyton RA, McClenathan JH, Newman GE, Michaelis LL. Significance of subendocardial S-T segment elevation caused by coronary stenosis in the dog. Epicardial S-T segment depression, local ischemia and subsequent necrosis. *Am J Cardiol* 1977; 40:373–80.

34. Rouleau J, Boerboom LE, Surjadhana A, Hoffman JIE. The role of autoregulation and tissue diastolic pressures in the transmural distribution of left ventricular blood flow in anesthetized dogs. *Circ Res* 1979; 45:804–15.

35. Dole WP, Nuno DW. Myocardial oxygen tension determines the degree and pressure range of coronary autoregulation. *Circ Res* 1986; 59:202–15.

36. Johansson B, Mellander S. Static and dynamic components in the vascular myogenic response to passive changes in length as revealed by electrical and mechanical recordings from the rat portal vein. *Circ Res* 1975; 36:76–83.

37. Driscol TE, Moir TW, Eckstein RW. Vascular effect of changes in perfusion pressure in the nonischemic and ischemic heart. *Circ Res* 1964; 14/15 (Suppl. I):I94–I102.

38. Hoffman JIE. Maximal coronary flow and the concept of coronary vascular reserve. *Circulation* 1984; 70:153–9.

39. Klocke FJ. Measurements of coronary flow reserve: defining pathophysiology versus making decisions about patient care. *Circulation* 1987; 76:1183–9.

40. Marcus M, Wright C, Doty D, Eastham C, Laughlin D, Krumm P, *et al.* Measurements of coronary velocity and reactive hyperemia in the coronary circulation of humans. *Circ Res* 1981; 49:877–91.

41. Uren NG, Melin JA, de Bruyne B, Wijns W, Baudhuin T, Camici PG. Relation between myocardial blood flow and the severity of coronary artery stenosis. *N Engl J Med* 1994; 330:1782–8.

42. Strauer B-E. Myocardial oxygen consumption in chronic heart disease: role of wall stress, hypertrophy and coronary reserve. *Am J Cardiol* 1979; 44:730–40.

43. Opherk D, Mall G, Zebe H, Schwarz F, Weihe E, Manthey J, *et al.* Reduction of coronary reserve: a mechanism for angina pectoris in patients with arterial hypertension and normal coronary arteries. *Circulation* 1984; 69:1–7.

44. Nanto S, Kodama K, Hori M, Mishima M, Hirayama A, Inoue M, *et al.* Temporal increase in resting coronary blood flow causes an impairment of coronary flow reserve after coronary angioplasty. *Am Heart J* 1992; 123:28–36.

45. Herrmann J, Haude M, Lerman A, Schulz R, Volbrach L, Ge J, *et al.* Abnormal coronary flow velocity reserve following coronary intervention is associated with cardiac marker elevation. *Circulation* 2001; 103:2339–45.

46. Berne RM, Blackmon JR, Gardner TH. Hypoxemia and coronary blood flow. *J Clin Invest* 1957; 36:1101–6.

47. Case RB, Greenberg H. The response of canine coronary vascular resistance to local alterations in coronary arterial PCO_2. *Circ Res* 1976; 39:558–66.

48. Broten TP, Romson JL, Fullerton DA, Van Winkle DM, Feigl EO. Synergistic action of myocardial oxygen and carbon dioxide in controlling coronary blood flow. *Circ Res* 1991; 68:531–42.

49. Murray PA, Belloni FL, Sparks HV. The role of potassium in the metabolic control of coronary vascular resistance of the dog. *Circ Res* 1979; 44:767–80.

50. Gewirtz H, Weeks G, Nathanson M, Sharaf B, Fedele F, Most AS. Tissue acidosis. Role in sustained arteriolar dilatation distal to a coronary stenosis. *Circulation* 1989; 79:890–8.

51. Berne RM. Cardiac nucleotides in hypoxia: possible role in regulation of coronary blood flow. *Am J Physiol* 1963; 204:317–22.

52. DeWitt DF, Wangler RD, Thompson CI, Sparks HV Jr. Phasic release of adenosine during steady state metabolic stimulation in the isolated guinea pig heart. *Circ Res* 1983; 53:636–43.

53. Miller WL, Belardinelli L, Bacchus A, Foley DH, Rubio R, Berne RM. Canine myocardial adenosine and lactate production, oxygen consumption, and coronary blood flow during stellate ganglia stimulation. *Circ Res* 1979; 45:708–18.

54. Gerlach E, Deuticke B, Dreisbach RH. Der Nucleotid-Abbau im Herzmuskel bei Sauerstoffmangel und seine mögliche Bedeutung für die Coronardurchblutung. *Naturwissenschaften* 1963; 6:228–9.

55. Kroll K, Feigl EO. Adenosine is unimportant in controlling coronary blood flow in unstressed dog hearts. *Am J Physiol Heart Circ Physiol* 1985; 249:H1176–87.

56. Dole WP, Yamada N, Bishop VS, Olsson RA. Role of adenosine in coronary blood flow regulation after reductions in perfusion pressure. *Circ Res* 1985; 56:517–24.

57. Daut J, Maier-Rudolph W, von Beckerath N, Mehrke G, Gunther K, Goedel-Meinen L. Hypoxic dilation of coronary arteries is mediated by ATP-sensitive potassium channels. *Science* 1990; 247:1341–4.

58. Aversano T, Ouyang P, Silverman H. Blockade of the ATP-sensitive potassium channel modulates reactive hyperemia in the canine coronary circulation. *Circ Res* 1991; 69:618–22.

59. Bassenge E, Heusch G. Endothelial and neuro-humoral control of coronary blood flow in health and disease. *Rev Physiol Biochem Pharmacol* 1990; **116**:77–165.

60. Aversano T, Becker LC. Persistence of coronary vasodilator reserve despite functionally significant flow reduction. *Am J Physiol Heart Circ Physiol* 1985; **248**:H403–11.

61. Canty JM, Klocke FJ. Reduced regional myocardial perfusion in the presence of pharmacologic vasodilator reserve. *Circulation* 1985; **71**:370–7.

62. Pantely GA, Bristow JD, Swenson LJ, Ladley HD, Johnson WB, Anselone CG. Incomplete coronary vasodilation during myocardial ischemia in swine. *Am J Physiol Heart Circ Physiol* 1985; **249**:H638–47.

63. Grattan MT, Hanley FL, Stevens MB, Hoffman JIE. Transmural coronary flow reserve patterns in dogs. *Am J Physiol Heart Circ Physiol* 1986; **250**:H276–83.

64. Heusch G, Guth BD, Seitelberger R, Ross J Jr. Attenuation of exercise-induced myocardial ischemia in dogs with recruitment of coronary vasodilator reserve by nifedipine. *Circulation* 1987; **75**:482–90.

65. Schaper W, Görge G, Winkler B, Schaper J. The collateral circulation of the heart. *Prog Cardiovasc Dis* 1988; **31**:57–77.

66. Sasayama S, Fujita M. Recent insights into coronary collateral circulation. *Circulation* 1992; **85**:1197–204.

67. Kass RW, Kotler MN, Yazdanfar S. Stimulation of coronary collateral growth: current developments in angiogenesis and future clinical applications. *Am Heart J* 1992; **123**:486–96.

68. Weihrauch D, Tessmer J, Warltier DC, Chilian WM. Repetitive coronary artery occlusions induce release of growth factors into the myocardial interstitium. *Am J Physiol Heart Circ Physiol* 1998; **44**:H969–76.

69. Kersten JR, Pagel PS, Chilian WM, Warltier DC. Multifactorial basis for coronary collateralization: a complex adaptive response to ischemia. *Cardiovasc Res* 1999; **43**:44–57.

70. Buschmann I, Schaper W. Arteriogenesis versus angiogenesis: two mechanisms of vessel growth. *News Physiol Sci* 1999; **14**:121–5.

71. Buschmann I, Schaper W. The pathophysiology of the collateral circulation (arteriogenesis). *J Pathol* 2000; **190**:338–42.

72. Harrison DG, Chilian WM, Marcus ML. Absence of functioning α-adrenergic receptors in mature canine coronary collaterals. *Circ Res* 1986; **59**:133–42.

73. Feldman RD, Christy JP, Paul ST, Harrison DG. β-adrenergic receptors on canine coronary collateral vessels: characterization and function. *Am J Physiol Heart Circ Physiol* 1989; **257**:H1634–9.

74. Foreman B, Dai X-Z, Homans DC, Laxson DD, Bache RJ. Effect of atrial natriuretic peptide on coronary collateral blood flow. *Circ Res* 1989; **65**:1671–8.

75. Wright L, Homans DC, Laxson DD, Dai XZ, Bache RJ. Effect of serotonin and thromboxane A2 on blood flow through moderately well developed coronary collateral vesels. *J Am Coll Cardiol* 1992; **19**:687–93.

76. Peters KG, Marcus ML, Harrison DG. Vasopressin and the mature coronary collateral circulation. *Circulation* 1989; **79**:1324–31.

77. Sellke FW, Quillen JE, Brooks LA, Harrison DG. Endothelial modulation of the coronary vasculature in vessels perfused via mature collaterals. *Circulation* 1990; **81**:1938–47.

78. Topol EJ, Ellis SG. Coronary collaterals revisited. Accessory pathway to myocardial preservation during infarction. *Circulation* 1991; **83**:1084–6.

79. Ertl G, Simm F, Wichmann J, Fuchs M, Lochner W. The dependence of coronary collateral blood flow on regional vascular resistances. *Naunyn Schmiedebergs Arch Pharmacol* 1979; **308**:265–72.

80. Seiler C, Fleisch M, Meier B. Direct intracoronary evidence of collateral steal in humans. *Circulation* 1997; **96**:4261–7.

81. Billinger M, Fleisch M, Eberli FR, Meier B, Seiler C. Collateral and collateral-adjacent hyperemic vascular resistance changes and the

psilateral coronary flow reserve: documentation of a mechanism causing coronary steal in patients with coronary artery disease. *Cardiovasc Res* 2001; **49**:600–8.

82. Holmvang G, Fry S, Skopicki HA, Abraham SA, Alpert NM, Fischman AJ, *et al.* Relation between coronary 'steal' and contractile function at rest in collateral-dependent myocardium of humans with ischemic heart disease. *Circulation* 1999; **99**:2510–16.

83. Kyriakides ZS, Kremastinos DT, Kolettis TM, Tasouli A, Antoniadis A, Webb DJ. Acute endothelin-A receptor antagonism prevents normal reduction of myocardial ischemia on repeated balloon inflations during angioplasty. *Circulation* 2000; **102**:1937–43.

84. Rowe GG. Inequalities of myocardial perfusion in coronary artery disease ('coronary steal'). *Circulation* 1970; **42**:193–4.

85. Gallagher KP, Folts JD, Shebuski RJ, Rankin JH, Rowe GG. Subepicardial vasodilator reserve in the presence of critical coronary stenosis in dogs. *Am J Cardiol* 1980; **46**:67–73.

86. Guth BD, Heusch G, Seitelberger R, Ross J Jr. Mechanism of beneficial effect of β-adrenergic blockade on exercise-induced myocardial ischemia in conscious dogs. *Circ Res* 1987; **60**:738–46.

87. Guth BD, Heusch G, Seitelberger R, Ross J Jr. Elimination of exercise-induced regional myocardial dysfunction by a bradycardic agent in dogs with chronic coronary stenosis. *Circulation* 1987; **75**:661–9.

88. Gould KL. Noninvasive assessment of coronary stenoses by myocardial perfusion imaging during pharmacologic coronary vasodilation. I. Physiologic basis and experimental validation. *Am J Cardiol* 1978; **41**:267–78.

89. Albro PC, Gould KL, Westcott RJ, Hamilton GW, Ritchie JL, Williams DL. Noninvasive assessment of coronary stenoses by myocardial imaging during pharmacologic coronary vasodilation. III. Clinical trial. *Am J Cardiol* 1978; **42**:751–60.

90. Kelm M, Schrader J. Nitric oxide release from the isolated guinea pig heart. *Eur J Pharmacol* 1988; **155**:317–21.

91. Duffy SJ, Castle SF, Harper RW, Meredith IT. Contribution of vasodilator prostanoids and nitric oxide to resting flow, metabolic vasodilation, and flow-mediated dilation in human coronary circulation. *Circulation* 1999; **100**:1951–7.

92. Pohl U, Holtz J, Busse R, Bassenge E. Crucial role of endothelium in the vasodilator response to increased flow *in vivo*. *Hypertension* 1986; **8**:37–44.

93. Pohl U, Busse R, Kuon E, Bassenge E. Pulsatile perfusion stimulates the release of endothelial autacoids. *J Appl Cardiol* 1986; **1**:215–35.

94. Lansman JB, Hallam TJ, Rink TJ. Single stretch-activated ion channels in vascular endothelial cells as mechanotransducers? *Nature* 1987; **325**:811–13.

95. Olesen S-P, Clapham DE, Davies PF. Haemodynamic shear stress activates a K^+ current in vascular endothelial cells. *Nature* 1988; **331**:168–70.

96. Lückhoff A, Busse R. Calcium influx into endothelial cells and formation of endothelium-derived relaxing factor is controlled by the membrane potential. *Pflügers Arch* 1990; **416**:305–11.

97. Kelm M, Schrader J. Control of coronary vascular tone by nitric oxide. *Circ Res* 1990; **66**:1561–75.

98. Kelm M, Rath J. Endothelial dysfunction in human coronary circulation: relevance of the L-arginine–NO pathway. *Basic Res Cardiol* 2001; **96**:107–27.

99. Kuo L, Chilian WM, Davies MJ. Coronary arteriolar myogenic response is independent of endothelium. *Circ Res* 1990; **66**:860–6.

100. Kuo L, Davis MJ, Chilian WM. Endothelium-dependent, flow-induced dilation of isolated coronary arterioles. *Am J Physiol Heart Circ Physiol* 1990; **259**:H1063–70.

101. Harrison DG, Marcus ML, Dellsperger KC, Lamping KG, Tomanek RJ. Pathophysiology of myocardial perfusion in hypertension. *Circulation* 1991; **83** (Suppl. III):III14–18.

102. Brush JE Jr, Faxon DP, Salmon S, Jacobs AK, Ryan TJ. Abnormal endothelium-dependent coronary vasomotion in hypertensive patients. *J Am Coll Cardiol* 1992; 19:809–15.

103. Flavahan NA. Atherosclerosis or lipoprotein-induced endothelial dysfunction? Potential mechanisms underlying reduction in EDRF/nitric oxide activity. *Circulation* 1992; 85:1927–38.

104. Zeiher AM, Drexler H, Saurbier B, Just H. Endothelium-mediated coronary blood flow modulation in humans. Effects of age, atherosclerosis, hypercholesterolemia, and hypertension. *J Clin Invest* 1993; 92:652–62.

105. Quyyumi AA, Dakak N, Andrews NP, Husain S, Arora S, Gilligan DM, et al. Nitric oxide activity in the human coronary circulation. Impact of risk factors for coronary atherosclerosis. *J Clin Invest* 1995; 95:1747–55.

106. Ludmer PL, Selwyn AP, Shook TL, Wayne RR, Mudge GH, Aldexander RW, et al. Paradoxical vasoconstriction induced by acetylcholine in atherosclerotic coronary arteries. *N Engl J Med* 1986; 315:1046–51.

107. Crossman DC, Larkin SW, Fuller RW, Davies GJ, Maseri A. Substance P dilates epicardial coronary arteries and increases coronary blood flow in humans. *Circulation* 1989; 80:475–84.

108. Kuga T, Mohri M, Egashira K, Hirakawa Y, Tagawa T, Shimokawa H, et al. Bradykinin-induced vasodilation of human coronary arteries in vivo: role of nitric oxide and angiotensin-converting enzyme. *J Am Coll Cardiol* 1997; 30:108–12.

109. Quyyumi AA, Dakak N, Andrews NP, Gilligan DM, Panza JA, Cannon RO 3rd. Contribution of nitric oxide to metabolic coronary vasodilation in human heart. *Circulation* 1995; 92:320–6.

110. Drexler H, Zeiher AM, Wollschläger H, Meinertz T, Just H, Bonzel T. Flow-dependent coronary artery dilatation in humans. *Circulation* 1989; 80:466–74.

111. Zeiher AM, Drexler H, Wollschläger H, Saurbier B, Just H. Coronary vasomotion in response to sympathetic stimulation in humans: importance of the functional integrity of the endothelium. *J Am Coll Cardiol* 1989; 14:1181–90.

112. Vita JA, Treasure CB, Yeung AC, Vekshtein VI, Fantasia GM, Fish RD, et al. Patients with evidence of coronary endothelial dysfunction as assessed by acetylcholine infusion demonstrate marked increase in sensitivity to constrictor effects of catecholamines. *Circulation* 1992; 85:1390–7.

113. Tsao PS, McEvoy LM, Drexler H, Butcher EC, Cooke JP. Enhanced endothelial adhesiveness in hypercholesterolemia is attenuated by L-arginine. *Circulation* 1994; 89:2176–82.

114. Vita JA, Treasure CB, Nabel EG, McLenachan JM, Fish RD, Yeung AC, et al. Coronary vasomotor response to acetylcholine relates to risk factors for coronary artery disease. *Circulation* 1990; 81:491–7.

115. Kuo L, Davis MJ, Cannon MS, Chilian WM. Pathophysiological consequences of atherosclerosis extend into the coronary microcirculation. *Circ Res* 1992; 70:465–76.

116. Drexler H, Zeiher AM, Meinzer K, Just H. Correction of endothelial dysfunction in coronary microcirculation of hypercholesterolaemic patients by L-arginine. *Lancet* 1991; 338:1546–50.

117. Panza JA, Casino PR, Badar DM, Quyyumi AA. Effect of increased availability of endothelium-derived nitric oxide precursor on endothelium-dependent vascular relaxation in normal subjects and in patients with essential hypertension. *Circulation* 1993; 87:1475–81.

118. Tiefenbacher CP. Tetrahydrobiopterin: a critical cofactor for eNOS and a strategy in the treatment of endothelial dysfunction? *Am J Physiol Heart Circ Physiol* 2001; 280:H2484–8.

119. Prasad A, Husain S, Schenke W, Mincemoyer R, Epstein N, Quyyumi AA. Contribution of bradykinin receptor dysfunction to abnormal coronary vasomotion in humans. *J Am Coll Cardiol* 2000; 36:1467–73.

120. Prasad A, Husain S, Quyyumi AA. Abnormal flow-mediated epicardial vasomotion in human coronary arteries is improved by angiotensin-converting enzyme inhibition. A potential role of bradykinin. *J Am Coll Cardiol* 1999; 33:796–804.

121. Prasad A, Tupas-Habib T, Schenke WH, Mincemoyer R, Panza JA, Waclawin MA, et al. Acute and chronic angiotensin-1 receptor antagonism reverses endothelial dysfunction in atherosclerosis. *Circulation* 2000; 101:2349–54.

122. Myers PR, Banitt PF, Guerra R, Harrison DG. Characteristics of canine coronary resistance arteries: importance of endothelium. *Am J Physiol* 1989; 257:H603–10.

123. Heyndrickx GR, Boettcher DH, Vatner SF. Effects of angiotensin, vasopressin, and methoxamine on cardiac function and blood flow distribution in conscious dogs. *Am J Physiol* 1976; 231:1579–87.

124. Pantely GA, Ladley HD, Anselone CG, Bristow JD. Vasopressin-induced coronary constriction at low perfusion pressures. *Cardiovasc Res* 1985; 19:433–41.

125. Chu A, Morris K, Kuehl WD, Cusma J, Navetta F, Cobb FR. Effects of atrial natriuretic peptide on the coronary arterial vasculature in humans. *Circulation* 1989; 80:1627–35.

126. Cohen MV, Kirk ES. Differential response of large and small coronary arteries to nitroglycerin and angiotensin. *Circ Res* 1973; 33:445–53.

127. Balcells E, Meng QC, Johnson WH Jr, Oparil S, Dell'Italia LJ. Angiotensin II formation from ACE and chymase in human and animal hearts: methods and species considerations. *Am J Physiol Heart Circ Physiol* 1997;42:H1769–74.

128. Jalowy A, Schulz R, Heusch G. AT1 receptor blockade in experimental myocardial ischemia/reperfusion. *J Am Soc Nephrol* 1999; 10:S129–39.

129. Weidenbach R, Schulz R, Gres P, Behrends M, Post H, Heusch G. Enhanced reduction of myocardial infarct size by combined ACE inhibition and AT_1-receptor antagonism. *Br J Pharmacol* 2000; 131:138–44.

130. Holtz J, Busse R, Sommer O, Bassenge E. Dilation of epicardial arteries in conscious dogs induced by angiotensin-converting enzyme inhibition with enalaprilat. *J Cardiovasc Pharmacol* 1987; 9:348–55.

131. Ertl G. Coronary vasoconstriction in experimental myocardial ischemia. *J Cardiovasc Pharmacol* 1987; 9(Suppl. 2):S9–17.

132. Yanagishita T, Tomita M, Itoh S, Mukae S, Arata H, Ishioka H, et al. Protective effect of captopril on ischemic myocardium. *Jpn Circ J* 1997; 61:161–9.

133. Remme WJ, Bartels GL. Anti-ischaemic effects of converting enzyme inhibitors: underlying mechanisms and future prospects. *Eur Heart J* 1995; 16(Suppl. I):87–95.

134. Prasad A, Mincemoyer R, Quyyumi AA. Anti-ischemic effects of angiotensin-converting enzyme inhibition in hypertension. *J Am Coll Cardiol* 2001; 38:1116–22.

135. Pernow J, Ahlborg G, Lundberg JM, Kaijser L. Long-lasting coronary vasoconstrictor effects and myocardial uptake of endothelin-1 in humans. *Acta Physiol Scand* 1997; 159:147–53.

136. Clozel J-P, Clozel M. Effects of endothelin on the coronary vascular bed in open-chest dogs. *Circ Res* 1989; 65:1193–200.

137. Godfraind T. Evidence for heterogeneity of endothelin receptor distribution in human coronary artery. *Br J Pharmacol* 1993; 110:1201–5.

138. Dashwood MR, Timm M, Muddle JR, Ong AC, Tippins JR, Parker R, et al. Regional variations in endothelin-1 and its receptor subtypes in human coronary vasculature: pathophysiological implications in coronary disease. *Endothelium* 1998; 6:61–70.

139. Kinlay S, Behrendt D, Wainstein M, Beltrame J, Fang JC, Creager MA, et al. Role of endothelin-1 in the active constriction

of human atherosclerotic coronary arteries. *Circulation* 2001; **104**:1114–18.

140. Miyauchi T, Yanagisawa M, Tomizawa T, Sugishita Y, Suzuki N, Fujino M, *et al.* Increased plasma concentrations of endothelin-1 and big endothelin-1 in acute myocardial infarction. *Lancet* 1989; **2**:53–4.

141. Yanagisawa M, Masaki T. Endothelin, a novel endothelium-derived peptide. Pharmacological activities, regulation and possible roles in cardiovascular control. *Biochem Pharmacol* 1989; **38**:1877–83.

142. Simmet T, Peskar BA. Eicosanoids and the coronary circulation. *Rev Physiol Biochem Pharmacol* 1986; **104**:1–64.

143. Schrör K. The effect of prostaglandins and thromboxane A2 on coronary vessel tone – mechanisms of action and therapeutic implications. *Eur Heart J* 1993; **14** (Suppl.):34–41.

144. Holtz J, Förstermann U, Pohl U, Giesler M, Bassenge E. Flow-dependent, endothelium-mediated dilation of epicardial coronary arteries in conscious dogs: effects of cyclooxygenase inhibition. *J Cardiovasc Pharmacol* 1984; **6**:1161–9.

145. Dai X-Z, Bache RJ. Effect of indomethacin on coronary blood flow during graded treadmill exercise in the dog. *Am J Physiol Heart Circ Physiol* 1984; **247**:H452–8.

146. Altman J, Dulas D, Bache RJ. Effect of cyclooxygenase blockade on blood flow through well-developed coronary collateral vessels. *Circ Res* 1992; **70**:1091–8.

147. Gallagher KP, Osakada G, Kemper WS, Ross J Jr. Cyclical coronary flow reductions in conscious dogs equipped with ameroid constrictors to produce severe coronary narrowing. *Basic Res Cardiol* 1985; **80**:100–6.

148. Cohen RA, Shepherd JT, Vanhoutte PM. Inhibitory role of the endothelium in the response of isolated coronary arteries to platelets. *Science* 1983; **221**:273–4.

149. Houston DS, Shepherd JT, Vanhoutte PM. Aggregating human platelets cause direct contraction and endothelium-dependent relaxation of isolated canine coronary arteries. Role of serotonin, thromboxane A2, and adenine nucleotides. *J Clin Invest* 1986; **78**:539–44.

150. Hirsh PD, Hillis LD, Campbell WB, Firth BG, Willerson JT. Release of prostaglandins and thromboxane into the coronary circulation in patients with ischemic heart disease. *N Engl J Med* 1981; **304**:685–91.

151. Heusch G. α-Adrenergic mechanisms in myocardial ischemia. *Circulation* 1990; **81**:1–13.

152. Heusch G, Guth BD. Neurogenic regulation of coronary vasomotor tone. *Eur Heart J* 1989; **10**(Suppl. F):6–14.

153. Feigl EO. Parasympathetic control of coronary blood flow in dogs. *Circ Res* 1969; **25**:509–19.

154. Hackett JG, Abboud FM, Mark AL, Schmid PG, Heistad DD. Coronary vascular responses to stimulation of chemoreceptors and baroreceptors. *Circ Res* 1972; **31**:8–17.

155. Zucker IH, Cornish KG, Hackley J, Bliss K. Effects of left ventricular receptor stimulation on coronary blood flow in conscious dogs. *Circ Res* 1987; **61**(Suppl. II):II54–60.

156. Reid JVO, Ito BR, Huang AH, Buffington CW, Feigl EO. Parasympathetic control of transmural coronary blood flow in dogs. *Am J Physiol Heart Circ Physiol* 1985; **249**:H337–43.

157. Young MA, Knight DR, Vatner SF. Autonomic control of large coronary arteries and resistance vessels. *Prog Cardiovasc Dis* 1987; **30**:211–34.

158. van Winkle DM, Feigl EO. Acetylcholine causes coronary vasodilation in dogs and baboons. *Circ Res* 1989; **65**:1580–93.

159. Knight DR, Shen Y-T, Young MA, Vatner SF. Acetylcholine-induced coronary vasoconstriction and vasodilation in tranquilized baboons. *Circ Res* 1991; **69**:706–13.

160. Kalsner S. Cholinergic mechanisms in human coronary artery preparations: implications of species differences. *J Physiol* 1985; **358**:509–26.

161. Zeiher AM, Drexler H, Wollschläger H, Just H. Modulation of coronary vasomotor tone in humans. Progressive endothelial dysfunction with different early stages of coronary atherosclerosis. *Circulation* 1991; **83**:391–401.

162. Berne RM, DeGeest H, Levy MN. Influence of the cardiac nerves on coronary resistance. *Am J Physiol* 1965; **208**:763–9.

163. Berne RM. Effect of epinephrine and norepinephrine on coronary circulation. *Circ Res* 1958; **6**:644–55.

164. Feigl EO. Control of myocardial oxygen tension by sympathetic coronary vasoconstriction in the dog. *Circ Res* 1975; **37**:88–95.

165. Mohrman DE, Feigl EO. Competition between sympathetic vasoconstriction and metabolic vasodilation in the canine coronary circulation. *Circ Res* 1978; **42**:79–86.

166. Murray PA, Vatner SF. α-Adrenoceptor attenuation of coronary vascular response to severe exercise in the conscious dog. *Circ Res* 1979; **45**:654–60.

167. Hamilton FN, Feigl EO. Coronary vascular sympathetic β-receptor innervation. *Am J Physiol* 1976; **230**:1569–76.

168. Vatner SF, Hintze TH, Macho P. Regulation of large coronary arteries by β-adrenergic mechanisms in the conscious dog. *Circ Res* 1982; **51**:56–66.

169. Vatner DE, Knight DR, Homcy CJ, Vatner SF, Young MA. Subtypes of β-adrenergic receptors in bovine coronary arteries. *Circ Res* 1986; **59**:463–73.

170. McRaven DR, Mark AL, Abboud FM, Mayer HE. Responses of coronary vessels to adrenergic stimuli. *J Clin Invest* 1971; **50**:773–8.

171. Holtz J, Giesler M, Bassenge E. Two dilatory mechanisms of anti-anginal drugs on epicardial coronary arteries *in vivo*: indirect, flow-dependent, endothelium-mediated dilation and direct smooth muscle relaxation. *Z Kardiol* 1983; **72**(Suppl. 3): 98–106.

172. Hintze TH, Vatner SF. Reactive dilation of large coronary arteries in conscious dogs. *Circ Res* 1984; **54**:50–7.

173. Vatner SF, Hintze TH. Mechanism of constriction of large coronary arteries by β-adrenergic receptor blockade. *Circ Res* 1983; **53**:389–400.

174. Kelley KO, Feigl EO. Segmental α-receptor-mediated vasoconstriction in the canine coronary circulation. *Circ Res* 1978; **43**:908–17.

175. Heusch G, Deussen A, Schipke J, Thämer V. α₁- and α₂-adrenoceptor-mediated vasoconstriction of large and small canine coronary arteries *in vivo*. *J Cardiovasc Pharmacol* 1984; **6**:961–8.

176. Chilian WM, Layne SM, Eastham CL, Marcus ML. Heterogeneous microvascular coronary α-adrenergic vasoconstriction. *Circ Res* 1989; **64**:376–88.

177. Chilian WM. Functional distribution of α₁- and α₂-adrenergic receptors in the coronary microcirculation. *Circulation* 1991; **84**:2108–22.

178. Hautamaa PV, Dai XZ, Homans DC, Robb JF, Bache RJ. Vasomotor properties of immature canine coronary collateral circulation. *Am J Physiol Heart Circ Physiol* 1987; **252**:H1105–11.

179. Hautamaa PV, Dai X-Z, Homans DC, Bache RJ. Vasomotor activity of moderately well-developed canine coronary collateral circulation. *Am J Physiol Heart Circ Physiol* 1989; **256**:H890–7.

180. Bache RJ, Foreman B, Hautamaa PV. Response of canine coronary collateral vessels to ergonovine and α-adrenergic stimulation. *Am J Physiol Heart Circ Physiol* 1991; **261**:H1019–25.

181. Lorenzoni R, Rosen SD, Camici PG. Effect of α₁-adrenoceptor blockade on resting and hyperemic myocardial blood flow in normal humans. *Am J Physiol Heart Circ Physiol* 1996; **40**:H1302–6.

182. Aptecar E, Dupouy P, Benvenuti C, Mazzucotelli JP, Teiger E, Geschwind H, *et al.* Sympathetic stimulation overrides

flow-mediated endothelium-dependent epicardial coronary vasodilation in transplant patients. *Circulation* 1996; 94:2542–50.

183. Heusch G, Baumgart D, Camici P, Chilian W, Gregorini L, Hess O, et al. α-Adrenergic coronary vasoconstriction and myocardial ischemia in humans. *Circulation* 2000; 101:689–94.

184. Chilian WM, Harrison DG, Haws CW, Synder WD, Marcus ML. Adrenergic coronary tone during submaximal exercise in the dog is produced by circulating catecholamines. Evidence for adrenergic denervation supersensitivity in the myocardium but not in coronary vessels. *Circ Res* 1986; 58:68–82.

185. Julius BK, Vassalli G, Mandinov L, Hess OM. α-Adrenoceptor blockade prevents exercise-induced vasoconstriction of stenotic coronary arteries. *J Am Coll Cardiol* 1999; 33:1499–505.

186. Baumgart D, Haude M, Gorge G, Liu F, Ge J, Grosse-Eggebrecht C, et al. Augmented α-adrenergic constriction of atherosclerotic human coronary arteries. *Circulation* 1999; 99:2090–7.

187. Tesfamariam B, Cohen RA. Inhibition of adrenergic vasoconstriction by endothelial cell shear stress. *Circ Res* 1988; 63:720–5.

188. Jones CJH, DeFily DV, Patterson JL, Chilian WM. Endothelium-dependent relaxation competes with α1- and α2-adrenergic constriction in the canine epicardial coronary microcirculation. *Circulation* 1993; 87:1264–76.

189. Rosendorff C, Hoffman JIE, Verrier ED, Rouleau J, Boerboom LE. Cholesterol potentiates the coronary artery response to norepinephrine in anesthetized and conscious dogs. *Circ Res* 1981; 48:320–9.

190. Heusch G, Deussen A. The effects of cardiac sympathetic nerve stimulation on the perfusion of stenotic coronary arteries in the dog. *Circ Res* 1983; 53:8–15.

191. Seitelberger R, Guth BD, Heusch G, Lee JD, Katayama K, Ross J Jr. Intracoronary α2-adrenergic receptor blockade attenuates ischemia in conscious dogs during exercise. *Circ Res* 1988; 62:436–42.

192. Nabel EG, Ganz P, Gordon JB, Alexander RW, Selwyn AP. Dilation of normal and constriction of atherosclerotic coronary arteries caused by the cold pressor test. *Circulation* 1988; 77:43–52.

193. Zeiher AM, Drexler H, Wollschläger H, Just H. Endothelial dysfunction of the coronary microvasculature is associated with impaired coronary blood flow regulation in patients with early atherosclerosis. *Circulation* 1991; 84:1–10.

194. Seiler C, Hess OM, Buechi M, Suter TM, Krayenbuehl HP. Influence of serum cholesterol and other coronary risk factors on vasomotion of angiographically normal coronary arteries. *Circulation* 1993; 88:2139–48.

195. Frielingsdorf J, Seiler C, Kaufmann P, Vassalli G, Suter T, Hess OM. Normalization of abnormal coronary vasomotion by calcium antagonists in patients with hypertension. *Circulation* 1996; 93:1380–7.

196. Zeiher AM, Krause T, Schächinger V, Minners J, Moser E. Impaired endothelium-dependent vasodilation of coronary resistance vessels is associated with exercise-induced myocardial ischemia. *Circulation* 1995; 91:2345–52.

197. Mudge GH, Grossman W, Mills RM Jr, Lesch M, Braunwald E. Reflex increase in coronary vascular resistance in patients with ischemic heart disease. *N Engl J Med* 1976; 295:1333–7.

198. Mudge GH Jr, Goldberg S, Gunther S, Mann T, Grossman W. Comparison of metabolic and vasoconstrictor stimuli on coronary vascular resistance in man. *Circulation* 1979; 59:544–50.

199. Kern MJ, Horowitz JD, Ganz P, Gaspar J, Colucci WS, Lorell BH, et al. Attenuation of coronary vascular resistance by selective α1-adrenergic blockade in patients with coronary artery disease. *J Am Coll Cardiol* 1985; 5:840–6.

200. Indolfi C, Piscione F, Villari B, Russolillo E, Rendina V, Golino P, et al. Role of α2-adrenoceptors in normal and atherosclerotic human coronary circulation. *Circulation* 1992; 86:1116–24.

201. White CW, Chierchia S, Wilson RF, Porter A, Maseri A. Coronary vasoconstrictor effects of norepinephrine in patients with coronary atherosclerosis: evidence from selective measurement of coronary flow velocity. *J Am Coll Cardiol* 1985; 5:432.

202. Gregorini L, Fajadet J, Robert G, Cassagneau B, Bernis M, Marco J. Coronary vasoconstriction after percutaneous transluminal coronary angioplasty is attenuated by antiadrenergic agents. *Circulation* 1994; 90:895–907.

203. Indolfi C, Piscione F, Rapacciuolo A, Esposito G, Esposito N, Ceravolo R, et al. Coronary artery vasoconstriction after successful single angioplasty of the left anterior descending artery. *Am Heart J* 1994; 128:858–64.

204. Heusch G, Deussen A, Thämer V. Cardiac sympathetic nerve activity and progressive vasoconstriction distal to coronary stenoses: feed-back aggravation of myocardial ischemia. *J Auton Nerv Syst* 1985; 13:311–26.

205. Malliani A, Schwartz PJ, Zanchetti A. A sympathetic reflex elicited by experimental coronary occlusion. *Am J Physiol* 1969; 217:703–9.

206. Gregorini L, Marco J, Bernies M, Cassagneau B, Pomidossi G, Anguissola GB, et al. The α1-adrenergic blocking agent urapidil counteracts postrotational atherectomy 'elastic recoil' where nitrates have failed. *Am J Cardiol* 1997; 79:1100–3.

207. Gregorini L, Marco J, Palombo C, Kozakova M, Anguissola GB, Cassagneau B, et al. Postischemic left ventricular dysfunction is abolished by α-adrenergic blocking agents. *J Am Coll Cardiol* 1998; 31:992–1001.

208. Gregorini L, Marco J, Kozàkovà M, Palombo C, Anguissola GB, Marco I, et al. α-Adrenergic blockade improves recovery of myocardial perfusion and function after coronary stenting in patients with acute myocardial infarction. *Circulation* 1999; 99:482–90.

209. Schömig A, Fischer S, Kurz T, Richardt G, Schömig E. Nonexocytotic release of endogenous noradrenaline in the ischemic and anoxic rat heart: mechanism and metabolic requirements. *Circ Res* 1987; 60:194–205.

210. Schömig A, Kurz T, Richardt G, Schömig E. Neuronal sodium homoeostasis and axoplasmic amine concentration determine calcium-independent noradrenaline release in normoxic and ischemic rat heart. *Circ Res* 1988; 63:214–26.

211. Maisel AS, Motulsky HJ, Insel PA. Externalization of β-adrenergic receptors promoted by myocardial ischemia. *Science* 1985; 230:183–6.

212. Vatner DE, Knight DR, Shen Y-T, Thomas JX Jr, Homcy CJ, Vatner SF. One hour of myocardial ischemia in conscious dogs increases β-adrenergic receptors, but decreases adenylate cyclase activity. *J Mol Cell Cardiol* 1988; 20:75–82.

213. Strasser RH, Krimmer J, Braun-Dullaeus R, Marquetant R, Kübler W. Dual sensitization of the adrenergic system in early myocardial ischemia: independent regulation of the β-adrenergic receptors and the adenylyl cyclase. *J Mol Cell Cardiol* 1990; 22:1405–23.

214. Matsuzaki M, Patritti J, Tajimi T, Miller M, Kemper WS, Ross J Jr. Effects of β-blockade on regional myocardial flow and function during exercise. *Am J Physiol Heart Circ Physiol* 1984; 247:H52–60.

215. Buck JD, Hardman HF, Warltier DC, Gross GJ. Changes in ischemic blood flow distribution and dynamic severity of a coronary stenosis induced by β-blockade in the canine heart. *Circulation* 1981; 64:708–15.

216. Menken U, Wiegand V, Bucher P, Meesmann W. Prophylaxis of ventricular fibrillation after acute experimental coronary occlusion by chronic β-adrenoceptor blockade with atenolol. *Cardiovasc Res* 1979; 13:588–94.

217. Rauch B, Kübler W. Antianginal medication. *Curr Opin Cardiol* 1991; 6:511–23.

218. Schipke JD, Birkenkamp-Demtröder K, Schwanke U. Myokardiale Hibernation: eine andere Sicht. *Z Kardiol* 2000; 89:259–63.

219. Gregg DE. Effect of coronary perfusion pressure or coronary flow on oxygen usage of the myocardium. *Circ Res* 1963; 13:497–500.

220. Arnold G, Kosche F, Miessner E, Neitzert A, Lochner W. The importance of the perfusion pressure in the coronary arteries for the contractility and the oxygen consumption of the heart. *Pflügers Arch* 1968; 299:339–56.

221. Schulz R, Guth BD, Heusch G. No effect of coronary perfusion on regional myocardial function within the autoregulatory range in pigs: evidence against the Gregg phenomenon. *Circulation* 1991; 83:1390–403.

222. Guth BD, Schulz R, Heusch G. Time course and mechanisms of contractile dysfunction during acute myocardial ischemia. *Circulation* 1993; 87(Suppl. IV):IV35–42.

223. Gallagher KP, Matsuzaki M, Koziol JA, Kemper WS, Ross J Jr. Regional myocardial perfusion and wall thickening during ischemia in conscious dogs. *Am J Physiol Heart Circ Physiol* 1984; 247:H727–38.

224. Weintraub WS, Hattori S, Agarwal JB, Bodenheimer MM, Banka VS, Helfant RH. The relationship between myocardial blood flow and contraction by myocardial layer in the canine left ventricle during ischemia. *Circ Res* 1981; 48:430–8.

225. Indolfi C, Guth BD, Miura T, Miyazaki S, Schulz R, Ross J Jr. Mechanisms of improved ischemic regional dysfunction by bradycardia. Studies on UL-FS 49 in swine. *Circulation* 1989; 80:983–93.

226. Indolfi C, Ross J Jr. The role of heart rate in myocardial ischemia and infarction: implications of myocardial perfusion–contraction matching. *Prog Cardiovasc Dis* 1993; 36:61–74.

227. Heusch G, Post H, Michel MC, Kelm M, Schulz R. Endogenous nitric oxide and myocardial adaptation to ischemia. *Circ Res* 2000; 87:146–52.

228. Kudej RK, Kim SJ, Shen YT, Jackson JB, Kudej AB, Yang GP, *et al.* Nitric oxide, an important regulator of perfusion–contraction matching in conscious pigs. *Am J Physiol Heart Circ Physiol* 2000; 279:H451–6.

229. Ross J Jr. Myocardial perfusion–contraction matching. Implications for coronary heart disease and hibernation. *Circulation* 1991; 83:1076–83.

230. Schulz R, Rose J, Martin C, Brodde OE, Heusch G. Development of short-term myocardial hibernation: its limitation by the severity of ischemia and inotropic stimulation. *Circulation* 1993; 88:684–95.

231. Gewirtz H, Fischman AJ, Abraham S, Gilson M, Strauss HW, Alpert NW. Positron emission tomographic measurements of absolute regional myocardial blood flow permits identification of nonviable myocardium in patients with chronic myocardial infarction. *J Am Coll Cardiol* 1994; 23:851–9.

232. Guth BD, White FC, Gallagher KP, Bloor CM. Decreased systolic wall thickening in myocardium adjacent to ischemic zones in conscious swine during brief coronary artery occlusion. *Am Heart J* 1984; 107:458–64.

233. Gallagher KP, Gerren RA, Stirling MC, Choy M, Dysko RC, McManimon SP, *et al.* The distribution of functional impairment across the lateral border of acutely ischemic myocardium. *Circ Res* 1986; 58:570–83.

234. Gallagher KP, Gerren RA, Ning XH, McManimon SP, Stirling MC, Shlafer M, *et al.* The functional border zone in conscious dogs. *Circulation* 1987; 76:929–42.

235. Buda AJ, Shlafer M, Gallagher KP. Spatial and temporal characteristics of circumferential flow–function relations during acute myocardial ischemia in the conscious dog. *Am Heart J* 1988; 116:1514–23.

236. Gallagher KP. Regional myocardial flow–function relationship in ischemia. In: *Pathophysiology and Rational Pharmacotherapy of Myocardial Ischemia*, Heusch G (ed.). Darmstadt, New York: Steinkopff, Springer; 1990.

237. Bogen DK, Rabinowitz SA, Needleman A, McMahon TA, Abelmann WH. An analysis of the mechanical disadvantage of myocardial infarction in the canine left ventricle. *Circ Res* 1980; 47:728–41.

238. Gallagher KP, Ning XH, Gerren RA, Drake DH, Dunham WR. Effect of aortic constriction on the functional border zone. *Am J Physiol Heart Circ Physiol* 1987; 252:H826–35.

239. Buda AJ, Zotz RJ, Gallagher KP. The effect of inotropic stimulation on normal and ischemic myocardium after coronary occlusion. *Circulation* 1987; 76:163–72.

240. Drake DH, McClanahan TB, Ning XH, Gerren RA, Dunham WR, Gallagher KP. Changes in contractility fail to alter the size of the functional border zone in anesthetized dogs. *Circ Res* 1987; 61:166–80.

241. Marino PN, Kass DA, Becker LC, Lima JA, Weiss JL. Influence of site of regional ischemia on nonischemic thickening in anesthetized dogs. *Am J Physiol* 1989; 256:H1417–25.

242. Schneider RM, Morris KG, Chu A, Roberts KB, Coleman RE, Cobb FR. Relation between myocardial perfusion and left ventricular function following acute coronary occlusion: disproportionate effects of anterior vs. inferior ischemia. *Circ Res* 1987; 60:60–71.

243. Gallagher KP, Osakada G, Hess OM, Koziol JA, Kemper WS, Ross J Jr. Subepicardial segmental function during coronary stenosis and the role of myocardial fiber orientation. *Circ Res* 1982; 50:352–9.

244. Stirling MC, Choy M, McClanahan TB, Schott RJ, Gallagher KP. Effects of ischemia on epicardial segment shortening. *J Surg Res* 1991; 50:30–9.

245. Homans DC, Sublett E, Lindstrom P, Nesbitt T, Bache RJ. Subendocardial and subepicardial wall thickening during ischemia in exercising dogs. *Circulation* 1988; 78:1267–76.

246. Gallagher KP, Stirling MC, Choy M, Szpunar CA, Gerren RA, Botham MJ, *et al.* Dissociation between epicardial and transmural function during acute myocardial ischemia. *Circulation* 1985; 71:1279–91.

247. Deussen A, Heusch G. Einfluss einer akuten Myokardischaemie auf die haemodynamischen Parameter des Restmyokards. *Herzmedizin* 1984; 7:32–5.

248. Lew WYW, Chen Z, Guth BD, Covell JW. Mechanisms of augmented segment shortening in nonischemic areas during acute ischemia of the canine left ventricle. *Circ Res* 1985; 56:351–8.

249. Heusch G, Guth BD, Widmann T, Peterson KL, Ross J Jr. Ischemic myocardial dysfunction assessed by temporal Fourier transform of regional myocardial wall thickening. *Am Heart J* 1987; 113:116–24.

250. Buda AJ, Lefkowitz CA, Gallagher KP. Augmentation of regional function in nonischemic myocardium during coronary occlusion measured with two-dimensional echocardiography. *J Am Coll Cardiol* 1990; 16:175–80.

251. Grines CL, Topol EJ, Califf RM, Stack RS, George BS, Kereiakes D, *et al.* Prognostic implications and predictors of enhanced regional wall motion of the noninfarct zone after thrombolysis and angioplasty therapy after acute myocardial infarction. *Circulation* 1989; 80:245–53.

252. Gascho JA, Beller GA. Adverse effects of circumflex coronary artery occlusion on blood flow to remote myocardium supplied by stenosed left anterior descending coronary artery in anesthetized open-chest dogs. *Am Heart J* 1987; 113:679–83.

253. Matsuzaki M, Gallagher KP, Kemper WS, White F, Ross J Jr. Sustained regional dysfunction produced by prolonged coronary stenosis: gradual recovery after reperfusion. *Circulation* 1983; **68**:170–82.

254. Sherman AJ, Harris KR, Hedjbeli S, Yaroshenko Y, Schafer D, Shroff S, *et al.* Proportional reversible decreases in systolic function and myocardial oxygen consumption after modest reduction in coronary flow: hibernation versus stunning. *J Am Coll Cardiol* 1997; **29**:1623–31.

255. Sherman AJ, Klocke FJ, Decker RS, Decker ML, Kozlowski KA, Harris KR, *et al.* Myofibrillar disruption in hypocontractile myocardium showing perfusion–contraction matches and mismatches. *Am J Physiol Heart Circ Physiol* 2000; **278**:H1320–34.

256. Schulz R, Post H, Neumann T, Gres P, Lüss H, Heusch G. Progressive loss of perfusion–contraction matching during sustained moderate ischemia in pigs. *Am J Physiol Heart Circ Physiol* 2001; **280**:H1945–53.

257. Kudej RK, Ghaleh B, Sato N, Shen YT, Bishop SP, Vatner SF. Ineffective perfusion–contraction matching in conscious, chronically intstrumented pigs with an extended period of coronary stenosis. *Circ Res* 1998; **82**:1199–205.

258. Chen C, Li L, Chen LL, Prada JV, Chen MH, Fallon JT, *et al.* Incremental doses of dobutamine induce a biphasic response in dysfunctional left ventricular regions subtending coronary stenoses. *Circulation* 1995; **92**:756–66.

259. Chen C, Chen L, Fallon JT, Ma L, Li L, Bow L, *et al.* Functional and structural alterations with 24-hour myocardial hibernation and recovery after reperfusion. A pig model of myocardial hibernation. *Circulation* 1996; **94**:507–16.

260. Bolli R. Mechanism of myocardial 'stunning'. *Circulation* 1990; **82**:723–38.

261. Bolli R, Marban E. Molecular and cellular mechanisms of myocardial stunning. *Physiol Rev* 1999; **70**:609–34.

262. Braunwald E, Kloner RA. The stunned myocardium: prolonged, postischemic ventricular dysfunction. *Circulation* 1982; **66**:1146–9.

263. Heyndrickx GR, Millard RW, McRitchie RJ, Maroko PR, Vatner SF. Regional myocardial functional and electrophysiological alterations after brief coronary artery occlusion in conscious dogs. *J Clin Invest* 1975; **56**:978–85.

264. Marban E. Myocardial stunning and hibernation. The physiology behind the colloquialisms. *Circulation* 1991; **83**:681–8.

265. Bolli R, Zhu W-X, Thornby JI, O'Neill PG, Roberts R. Time course and determinants of recovery of function after reversible ischemia in conscious dogs. *Am J Physiol Heart Circ Physiol* 1988; **254**:H102–14.

266. Bolli R, Triana JF, Jeroudi MO. Prolonged impairment of coronary vasodilation after reversible ischemia. *Circ Res* 1990; **67**:332–43.

267. Guth BD, Martin JF, Heusch G, Ross J Jr. Regional myocardial blood flow, function and metabolism using phosphorus-31 nuclear magnetic resonance spectroscopy during ischemia and reperfusion. *J Am Coll Cardiol* 1987; **10**:673–81.

268. Heyndrickx GR, Baig H, Nellens P, Leusen I, Fishbein MC, Vatner SF. Depression of regional blood flow and wall thickening after brief coronary occlusions. *Am J Physiol Heart Circ Physiol* 1978; **234**:H653–9.

269. Laxson DD, Homans DC, Dai X-Z, Sublett E, Bache RJ. Oxygen consumption and coronary reactivity in postischemic myocardium. *Circ Res* 1989; **64**:9–20.

270. Stahl LD, Weiss HR, Becker LC. Myocardial oxygen consumption, oxygen supply/demand heterogeneity, and microvascular patency in regionally stunned myocardium. *Circulation* 1988; **77**:865–72.

271. Thaulow E, Guth BD, Heusch G, Gilpin E, Schulz R, Kroeger K, *et al.* Characteristics of regional myocardial stunning after exercise in dogs with chronic coronary stenosis. *Am J Physiol Heart Circ Physiol* 1989; **257**:H113–19.

272. Schulz R, Janssen F, Guth BD, Heusch G. Effect of coronary hyperperfusion on regional myocardial function and oxygen consumption of stunned myocardium in pigs. *Basic Res Cardiol* 1991; **86**:534–43.

273. Bolli R, Patel BS, Hartley CJ, Thornby JI, Jeroudi MO, Roberts R. Nonuniform transmural recovery of contractile function in stunned myocardium. *Am J Physiol Heart Circ Physiol* 1989; **257**:H375–85.

274. Heusch G, Guth BD, Gilpin E, Oudiz R, Matsuzaki M, Ross J Jr, *et al.* Determinants of recovery of regional contractile function after exercise-induced ischemia in conscious dogs. *Fed Proc* 1987; **46**:834 (Abstract).

275. Erbel R, Heusch G. Brief review: coronary microembolization. *J Am Coll Cardiol* 2000; **36**:22–4.

276. Topol EJ, Yadav JS. Recognition of the importance of embolization in atherosclerotic vascular disease. *Circulation* 2000; **101**:570–80.

277. Heusch G, Schulz R, Baumgart D, Haude M, Erbel R. Coronary microembolization. *Prog Cardiovasc Dis* 2001; **44**:217–30.

278. Hori M, Inoue M, Kitakaze M, Koretsune Y, Iwai K, Tamai J, *et al.* Role of adenosine in hyperemic response of coronary blood flow in microcirculation. *Am J Physiol Heart Circ Physiol* 1986; **250**:H509–18.

279. Hori M, Gotoh K, Kitakaze M, Iwai K, Iwakura K, Sato H, *et al.* Role of oxygen-derived free radicals in myocardial edema and ischemia in coronary microvascular embolization. *Circulation* 1991; **84**:828–40.

280. Dörge H, Neumann T, Behrends M, Skyschally A, Schulz R, Kasper C, *et al.* Perfusion–contraction mismatch with coronary microvascular obstruction: role of inflammation. *Am J Physiol Heart Circ Physiol* 2000; **279**:H2587–92.

281. Yokoyama T, Vaca L, Rossen RD, Durante W, Hazarika P, Mann DL. Cellular basis for the negative inotropic effects of tumor necrosis factor-α in the adult mammalian heart. *J Clin Invest* 1993; **92**:2303–12.

282. Frangogiannis NG, Lindsey ML, Michael LH, Youker KA, Bressler RB, Mendoza LH, *et al.* Resident cardiac mast cells degranulate and release preformed TNF-α, initiating the cytokine cascade in experimental canine myocardial ischemia/reperfusion. *Circulation* 1998; **98**:699–710.

283. Dörge H, Schulz R, Belosjorow S, Post H, van de Sand A, Konietzka I, *et al.* Coronary microembolization: the role of TNF-α in contractile dysfunction. *J Mol Cell Cardiol* 2002; **34**:51–62.

284. Liedtke AJ, Renstrom B, Nellis SH, Hall JL, Stanley WC. Mechanical and metabolic functions in pig hearts after 4 days of chronic coronary stenosis. *J Am Coll Cardiol* 1995; **26**:815–28.

285. Chen C, Ma L, Dyckman W, Santos F, Lai T, Gillam LD, *et al.* Left ventricular remodeling in myocardial hibernation. *Circulation* 1997; **96**(Suppl. II):II46–50.

286. Chen C, Ma L, Linfert DR, Lai T, Fallon JT, Gillam LD, *et al.* Myocardial cell death and apoptosis in hibernating myocardium. *J Am Coll Cardiol* 1997; **30**:1407–12.

287. St. Louis JD, Hughes GC, Kypson AP, DeGrado TR, Donovan CL, Coleman RE, *et al.* An experimental model of chronic myocardial hibernation. *Ann Thorac Surg* 2000; **69**:1351–7.

288. Canty JM, Klocke FJ. Reductions in regional myocardial function at rest in conscious dogs with chronically reduced regional coronary artery pressure. *Circ Res* 1987; **61**(Suppl. II):107–16.

289. Shen Y-T, Vatner SF. Mechanism of impaired myocardial function during progressive coronary stenosis in conscious pigs. Hibernation versus stunning. *Circ Res* 1995; **76**:479–88.

290. Shen Y-T, Kudej RK, Bishop SP, Vatner SF. Inotropic reserve and histological appearance of hibernating myocardium in conscious pigs with ameroid-induced coronary stenosis. *Basic Res Cardiol* 1996; **91**:479–85.

291. Firoozan S, Wei K, Linka A, Skyba D, Goodman NC, Kaul S. A canine model of chronic ischemic cardiomyopathy: characterization of regional flow–function relations. *Am J Physiol Heart Circ Physiol* 1999; **276**:H446–55.

292. Mills I, Fallon JT, Wrenn D, Sasken H, Gray W, Bier J, et al. Adaptive responses of coronary circulation and myocardium to chronic reduction in perfusion pressure and flow. *Am J Physiol Heart Circ Physiol* 1994; **266**:H447–57.

293. McFalls EO, Baldwin D, Palmer B, Marx D, Jaimes D, Ward HB. Regional glucose uptake within hypoperfused swine myocardium as measured by positron emission tomography. *Am J Physiol Heart Circ Physiol* 1997; **41**:H343–9.

294. Fallavollita JA, Perry BJ, Canty JM. 18F-2-deoxyglucose deposition and regional flow in pigs with chronically dysfunctional myocardium. Evidence for transmural variations in chronic hibernating myocardium. *Circulation* 1997; **95**:1900–9.

295. Fallavollita JA, Canty JM. Differential 18F-2-deoxyglucose uptake in viable dysfunctional myocardium with normal resting perfusion. *Circulation* 1999; **99**:2798–805.

296. Shivalkar B, Flameng W, Szilard M, Pislaru S, Borgers M, Vanhaecke J. Repeated stunning precedes myocardial hibernation in progressive multiple coronary artery obstruction. *J Am Coll Cardiol* 1999; **34**:2126–36.

297. Arani DT, Greene DG, Bunnell IL, Smith GL, Klocke FJ. Reductions in coronary flow under resting conditions in collateral-dependent myocardium of patients with complete occlusion of the left anterior descending coronary artery. *J Am Coll Cardiol* 1984; **3**:668–74.

298. Canty JM, Fallavollita JA. Resting myocardial flow in hibernating myocardium: validating animal models of human pathophysiology. *Am J Physiol Heart Circ Physiol* 1999; **277**:H417–22.

299. Sambuceti G, Parodi O, Marzullo P, Giorgetti A, Fusani L, Puccini G, et al. Regional myocardial blood flow in stable angina pectoris associated with isolated significant narrowing of either the left anterior descending or left circumflex coronary artery. *Am J Cardiol* 1993; **72**:990–4.

300. Vanoverschelde JL, Wijns W, Depré C, Essamri B, Heyndrickx GR, Borgers M, et al. Mechanisms of chronic regional postischemic dysfunction in humans. New insights from the study of noninfarcted collateral-dependent myocardium. *Circulation* 1993; **87**:1513–23.

301. Pagano D, Townend JN, Parums DV, Bonser RS, Camici PG. Hibernating myocardium: morphological correlates of inotropic stimulation and glucose uptake. *Heart* 2000; **83**:456–61.

302. Fath-Ordoubadi F, Beatt KJ, Spyrou N, Camici PG. Efficacy of coronary angioplasty for the treatment of hibernating myocardium. *Heart* 1999; **82**:210–16.

303. Bolli R. Myocardial 'stunning' in man. *Circulation* 1992; **86**:1671–91.

304. Heusch G. Hibernating myocardium. *Physiol Rev* 1998; **78**:1055–85.

305. Borgers M, Ausma J. Structural aspects of the chronic hibernating myocardium in man. *Basic Res Cardiol* 1995; **90**:44–6.

306. Elsässer A, Schaper J. Hibernating myocardium: adaptation or degeneration? *Basic Res Cardiol* 1995; **90**:47–8.

307. Elsässer A, Schlepper M, Klövekorn W-P, Cai WJ, Zimmermann R, Muller KD, et al. Hibernating myocardium. An incomplete adaptation to ischemia. *Circulation* 1997; **96**:2920–31.

308. Shivalkar B, Maes A, Borgers M, Ausma J, Scheys I, Nuyts J, et al. Only hibernating myocardium invariably shows early recovery after coronary revascularization. *Circulation* 1996; **94**:308–15.

309. Gould KL, Lipscomb K. Effects of coronary stenoses on coronary flow reserve and resistance. *Am J Cardiol* 1974; **34**:48–55.

310. Baumgart D, Ehring T, Krajcar M, Heusch G. A proischemic action of nisoldipine: relationship to a decrease in perfusion pressure and comparison to dipyridamole. *Cardiovasc Res* 1993; **27**:1254–9.

3

Pathology of coronary artery and ischemic heart disease

FREDERICK J SCHOEN

Ischemic myocardial damage generally results from obstructive coronary artery disease owing to atherosclerosis and the subsequent events that occur in plaque.[1–3] This chapter reviews the causes and myocardial consequences of coronary arterial obstruction, focusing on the morphology and dynamic evolution of atherosclerotic plaque, the events that occur in reversible and irreversible myocardial injury, myocardial infarction and its consequences, and pathological considerations pertinent to therapeutic revascularization.

CORONARY ARTERY DISEASE

Over 90% of patients with ischemic heart disease have advanced stenosing coronary atherosclerosis (*fixed obstructions*) and nearly all cases of acute myocardial infarction occur in patients with pre-existing coronary atherosclerosis. Atherosclerosis in the heart typically involves the epicardial coronary arteries but not the intramural branches. Coronary atherosclerosis tends to be most severely obstructive in the proximal half of the left anterior descending and circumflex arteries (and their proximal branches) and variable along the right coronary artery. Severe distal stenosis generally occurs only following severe proximal disease, and distal lesions are typically shorter and more discrete than those observed proximally. However, severe obstruction of the left main coronary artery generally follows severe disease in the other major epicardial vessels. Some arteries are consistently spared (such as the internal thoracic [mammary] artery), yet venous bypass grafts interposed within branches of the arterial system (such as autologous saphenous veins used as bypass grafts) can also develop intimal thickening and ultimately atherosclerotic obstructions.

Non-atherosclerotic causes of coronary artery obstruction can occur; the most common causes are infectious disease (e.g. tuberculosis), autoimmune diseases (e.g. systemic lupus erythematosus and rheumatoid arthritis), vasculitis (e.g. Buerger's and Kawasaki disease), fibromuscular dysplasia and embolism. Isolated ostial stenosis may occur, owing to calcification of the aortic sinotubular junction, aortitis, congenital malformations, or following coronary arterial perfusion. Obstruction of the intramural coronary arteries is seen in several disease states, including diabetes, deposition diseases (e.g. Fabry disease and amyloidosis), progressive systemic sclerosis (scleroderma), and as a proliferative intimal lesion in the coronary arteries of cardiac allografts that can cause distal ischemic injury. Graft coronary arteriosclerosis, a predominantly but not exclusively intramural (small arterial) lesion, is the major limitation to long-term graft success and recipient survival following heart transplantation.[4,5]

Atherogenesis and plaque growth

The characteristic lesion of atherosclerosis, atheroma or plaque, forms primarily through two key processes: *intimal thickening* (mediated predominantly by smooth

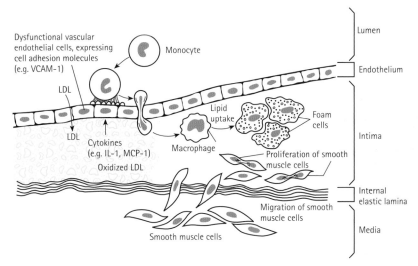

Figure 3.1 *Hypothetical sequence of cell-level events and cellular interactions in atherosclerosis. Hyperlipidemia and other risk factors are thought to cause endothelial injury, resulting in adhesion of platelets and monocytes and release of growth factors, including platelet-derived growth factor (PDGF), which leads to smooth muscle cell migration and proliferation. Smooth muscle cells produce large amounts of extracellular matrix, including collagen and proteoglycans. Foam cells of atheromatous plaques are derived from both macrophages and smooth muscle cells – from macrophages via the very-low-density lipoprotein (VLDL) receptor and low-density lipoprotein (LDL) modifications recognized by scavenger receptors (e.g. oxidized LDL), and from smooth muscle cells by less certain mechanisms. Extracellular lipid accumulates by insudation from the vessel lumen, particularly in the presence of hypercholesterolemia, and also from degenerating foam cells. Cholesterol accumulation in the plaque reflects an imbalance between influx and efflux; high-density lipoprotein (HDL) probably helps clear cholesterol from plaque. VCAM-1, vascular cell adhesion molecule 1; MCP-1, monocyte chemotactic protein 1. Reprinted from Schoen FJ. Pathologic considerations (in the surgery of adult heart disease). In: Cardiac Surgery in the Adult, Edmunds LH (ed.). New York: McGraw-Hill, 1997, 85–144, with permission of The McGraw-Hill Companies.*

muscle cell proliferation) and *lipid accumulation* (mediated primarily by monocyte phagocytosis).

The contemporary understanding of the pathogenesis of atherosclerosis is embodied in the *response-to-injury hypothesis*, which envisions an interaction of the cells of the blood vessel wall (especially smooth muscle cells and endothelial cells), circulating blood cells (platelets and monocytes) and plasma lipoproteins (Figure 3.1). The initiating event is a subtle, non-denuding injury to endothelial cells caused by the cumulative effects of chronic hypercholesterolemia, homocystinemia, chemicals in cigarette smoke, localized hemodynamic forces, systemic hypertension, hyperglycemia or the local effects of cytokines.[6,7] This type of endothelial cell injury (termed *endothelial dysfunction*) is characterized by:

1 abnormalities in vasoreactivity favoring vasoconstriction, caused in part by depressed production of vasorelaxants such as nitric oxide (NO),
2 alteration or loss of the selective permeability barrier with entry of plasma lipoproteins into the vessel wall,
3 induction of a thrombogenic surface on endothelial cells (through membrane expression of tissue factor), and/or
4 adherence of inflammatory cells or platelets, mediated by injury-induced surface expression of molecules that increase endothelial cell–monocyte adhesion.[8]

Nevertheless, early atherosclerotic lesions remain covered by endothelial cells.

Lesion progression involves the following events.

1 Blood monocytes adhere to endothelial cells and emigrate into the sub-endothelial space and transform into tissue macrophages.
2 Smooth muscle cells migrate from the media into the intima, where they proliferate and secrete collagen and other extracellular matrix components.
3 Lipid accumulates, intracellularly in macrophages and smooth muscle cells (*foam cells*) and extracellularly.
4 Lipoproteins undergo oxidative modification, generating potent biological stimuli (including chemoattractants) within the vessel wall.
5 Cells die, releasing intracellular lipids (mostly cholesterol esters).
6 Chronic inflammation continues, particularly at the junction of the lesion with uninvolved wall.
7 Calcification may ensue.

Inflammation associated with advanced plaque may also be prominent in the adventitia. The location of lesions is largely determined by mechanical factors, as evidenced by the initiation of lesions at branch points, although the specific mechanisms are only beginning to be understood.[9]

Inflammatory mechanisms clearly play a role in lesion infiltration and progression.[10] There has been recent interest in the possible role of infections in causing atherosclerosis or potentiating the action of traditional risk factors.[11,12] The agents most frequently implicated are *Chlamydia pneumoniae* and *Cytomegalovirus*. However, despite some evidence in support of this concept and hope for therapeutic potential, proof of a causal role for infection in atherosclerosis or its complications remains elusive.

In mild and moderate disease, the plaque bulges outward at the expense of the media, and the arterial lumen remains circular in cross-section (Figure 3.2). Early plaque progression does not substantially alter luminal architecture; with plaque formation causing up to 40–50% obstruction, the arterial lumen is not reduced in caliber. Thus, the vessel increases in diameter, in a process often called *vascular remodeling*.[13,14] Moreover, approximately two-thirds of plaques are eccentric in location, leaving a proportion of the circumference plaque free. Although atherosclerosis begins as an intimal disease, the media may subsequently become thinned due to necrosis or atrophy; the resultant weakening can lead to aneurysm formation.

Mature atheromatous plaque is composed of lipid and cholesterol crystals, macrophages, foam cells, necrotic cell debris, plasma proteins and degenerating blood elements (collectively comprising the *core*), separated from the lumen by a layer of fibrous tissue (*fibrous cap*). The composition of atheromas can vary considerably, among individuals, among arteries in the same individual, or among regions of one artery, particularly in the relative proportion of lipid to connective tissue. An individual plaque region can be characterized structurally by intravascular ultrasound.[15] The natural history of atheromatous plaque and the efficacy and safety of interventional therapies probably depend on relative plaque composition, the spatial distribution of the constituents and especially, as discussed later, the integrity of the fibrous cap.[16–18] A natural plane of weakness exists between the atherosclerotic intima and the internal elastic lamina; this potential site of cleavage is used in surgical endarterectomy.

The predominant clinical effects of advanced atherosclerotic plaques in most medium-sized arteries, including the coronary arteries, are due either to their progressive and chronic encroachment of the lumen or to acute plaque disruption with thrombosis (Figure 3.3). Acute obstruction can also result from spasm or embolization (which itself can be a consequence of complicated atherosclerotic lesions).

Under normal conditions, coronary arterial flow provides adequate myocardial perfusion at rest and compensatory vasodilatation provides flow reserve that is generally more than sufficient to accommodate transient and occasional increased myocardial metabolic demands, such as during vigorous exertion. When the fixed luminal cross-sectional area is decreased by approximately 75% or more, coronary blood flow generally becomes limited

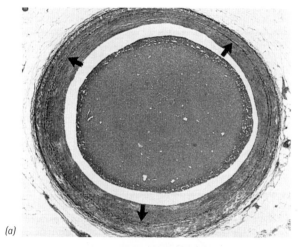

(a)

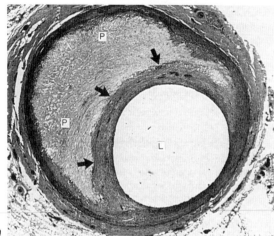

(b)

Figure 3.2 *Distended normal artery (a) and artery with moderate atherosclerotic plaque (b) correspond with maximal vasodilatation in life in cross-section. In both cases the lumen is circular and distended by a gelatin/barium suspension injected at physiological pressures. The injection material retracts away from the intima in tissue processing. The elastic lamina (arrows) marking the junction of intima and media is straight in such preparations. (b) Shows lipid-rich plaque in cross-section. The artery has been distended at physiological pressure and the lumen (L) is round. The plaque (P) is a crescentic clear area within the intima. The plaque lipid is dissolved out in processing for histology. The contents of the plaque are separated from the lumen by the fibrous cap (arrows). Reprinted from Davies MJ. Pathology of ischemic heart disease. In:* Surgery of Coronary Artery Disease, *Wheatley DJ (ed.). London: Chapman & Hall, 1986, 52.*

with exertion. Indeed, such coronary stenoses are the hallmark pathology of stable angina. With approximately 90% or greater reduction in cross-sectional area, coronary flow may be inadequate at rest. However, high-grade but slowly developing occlusions can stimulate collateral vessels over time that may protect against distal myocardial ischemia and infarction.

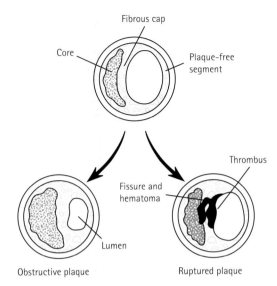

Figure 3.3 *Progression of fibrous atheromatous plaque with core of extracellular lipid and necrotic debris covered by intact fibrous cap (top) either to severe chronic stenosis (lower left) or to acute plaque fissuring, resulting in a complex lesion with a surface defect, hematoma or mural thrombus (lower right). Reprinted from Schoen FJ. Pathologic considerations (in the surgery of adult heart disease). In:* Cardiac Surgery in the Adult, *Edmunds LH (ed.). New York: McGraw-Hill, 1997, 85–144, with permission of The McGraw-Hill Companies.*

Acute coronary syndromes

The arteriographically determined extent and severity of fixed coronary artery disease do not precisely predict the onset and prognosis of ischemic heart disease and other complications of atherosclerosis.[19–21] Considerable evidence exists that dynamic vascular changes, most frequently a precipitous fracture in the protective fibrous cap of the plaque, cause coronary thrombosis, the condition that is usually responsible for the conversion of chronic stable angina or an asymptomatic state to acute ischemic heart disease (*unstable angina, myocardial infarction* or *sudden coronary death*; Figure 3.4). Plaque disruption causes both interference with flow and exposure of the luminal blood to a thrombogenic surface (collagen, lipid and necrotic debris), thereby setting the stage for mural or total thrombosis. In transmural infarction, the thrombi tend to be occlusive; in unstable angina, sub-endocardial infarction and sudden coronary death, they are generally non-occlusive. Moreover, microembolization may play a role in the induction of symptoms, ventricular arrhythmias and the formation of microinfarcts (see later).

In a minority of cases, thrombosis in coronary arteries results from a superficial erosion of the intima without a frank rupture through the plaque fibrous cap.[22] Endothelial cells, like smooth muscle cells, may undergo apoptosis in response to inflammatory mediators, and loss of endothelial cells can uncover the thrombogenic sub-endothelial matrix. Even in the absence of actual sloughing of endothelial cells, an altered balance between prothrombotic and fibrinolytic properties of the endothelium may underlie thrombosis *in situ*.

Fissures and ruptures most frequently occur at the junction of the fibrous cap with the adjacent plaque-free segment of the arterial wall and less frequently at the center of the lesion. Vasospasm, tachycardia, hypercholesterolemia or intraplaque hemorrhage are likely contributors, as are stresses induced by blood flow and/or coronary intramural pressure or tone in plaque.

Pathological and clinical studies have shown that coronary occlusion and myocardial infarction evolve from plaques with highly variable pre-existing obstructions. Most frequently, however, lesions causing mild to moderate stenosis (and therefore likely to be asymptomatic) undergo abrupt disruption and superimposed thrombosis leading to acute ischemic heart disease (Figure 3.5). Overall, approximately two-thirds of plaques that rupture (and in which a totally occlusive thrombus subsequently develops) cause occlusion of only 50% or less before plaque rupture, and in 85% of patients, stenosis is initially less than 70%.[23,24] The reasons for this disturbing reality are uncertain. Nevertheless, it has been suggested that less advanced plaques have a higher lipid fraction and are thereby more vulnerable, are more numerous and are less likely to be associated with collateral circulation. Moreover, plaque fissures have been found at autopsy in nearly 10% of patients without acute coronary syndromes.[25] Thus, it is presently impossible reliably to predict plaque disruption or subsequent thrombosis in an individual patient.

Imaging of coronary artery disease is an area of substantial current interest and importance. Invasive x-ray coronary angiography remains the gold standard. However, the trend is toward both non-invasive testing and modalities that elucidate wall structure and especially indicate plaque vulnerable to rupture and other markers of prognosis. Calcification of the coronary arteries can be detected non-invasively by electron beam computed tomography.[26,27] Radiographically visible calcium in the epicardial coronary arteries predicts the extent of atherosclerotic disease, and as plaque burden correlates with cardiovascular risk, coronary calcium tends to be a good prognostic indicator of future myocardial ischemic events. However, the correlation fails in patients younger than 50 years, in whom calcification is relatively uncommon, and at present imaging of coronary calcium does not permit identification of unstable coronary plaques. In contrast, three-dimensional coronary magnetic resonance angiography may permit reliable detection of coronary artery disease, whether or not calcification is present.[28] Moreover, this technique has the potential to visualize both the coronary lumen and the atherosclerotic plaques in the arterial wall. Intravascular ultrasound and optical

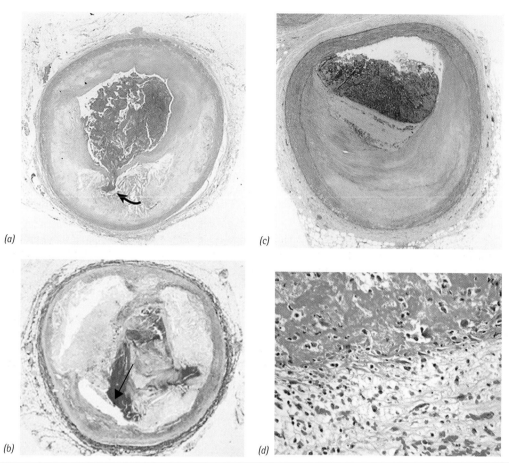

(a)

(c)

(b)

(d)

Figure 3.4 *Acute changes in atherosclerotic plaque precipitating coronary events: rupture and erosion. (a) Acute coronary thrombosis superimposed on an atherosclerotic plaque with focal disruption of the fibrous cap, triggering fatal myocardial infarction. (b) Massive plaque rupture with superimposed thrombus, also triggering a fatal myocardial infarction (special stain highlighting fibrin in red). In both (a) and (b), an arrow points to the site of plaque rupture. (c) Sudden death owing to erosion at the surface of an eccentric plaque, with non-occlusive luminal thrombus (Movat pentachrome). (d) A higher magnification of (c) demonstrates the surface erosion, without disruption of the fibrous cap. There is smooth muscle cell proliferation in a proteoglycan-rich matrix (hematoxylin & eosin). (a) and (b)* Reprinted from Schoen FJ. The heart. In: Robbins Pathologic Basis of Disease, 6th edn, Cotran RS, Kumar V, Collins T (eds). Philadelphia: WB Saunders, 1999, 543–99, with permission from Elsevier Science. *(c) and (d)* Reprinted from Virmani R, Burke AP, Farb A. Sudden cardiac death. Cardiovasc Pathol 2001;*10:211–18*, with permission from Elsevier Science.

coherence tomography are catheter-based techniques that visualize local arterial wall structure in substantial detail.[29,30]

The events that trigger abrupt changes in plaque configuration and superimposed thrombosis are complex and poorly understood.[31] Influences both intrinsic (i.e. plaque structure and composition) and extrinsic to the plaque (i.e. blood pressure, platelet reactivity) are probably important. Surface erosions, fissures and ruptures are more likely to involve soft and eccentric plaques than hard and concentric lesions, those that contain large areas of foam cells and extracellular lipid, and those in which the fibrous caps are thin or contain clusters of inflammatory cells. Conversely, there is evidence that lipid lowering by diet or drugs such as statins can reduce the onset of coronary thrombotic complications in experimental models, with potential clinical benefits. The

mechanisms include stabilizing plaque through reducing the accumulation of macrophages expressing matrix-degrading enzymes and tissue factor, reducing the activation of smooth muscle cells and endothelial cells, and suppressing macrophage growth.[32–34] The pronounced circadian periodicity for the time of onset of acute myocardial infarction and other acute coronary syndromes, with a peak incidence between 9:00 and 11:00 a.m., suggests that the usual morning surge in blood pressure and heightened platelet reactivity may contribute to plaque disruption.

Considerable evidence supports the concept that the fibrous cap is a highly dynamic tissue that can undergo continuous remodeling, and that the balance of collagen synthetic and degradative activity determines stability and prognosis (Figure 3.6). Lesions with fatal thrombosis overlying plaque rupture typically have few smooth

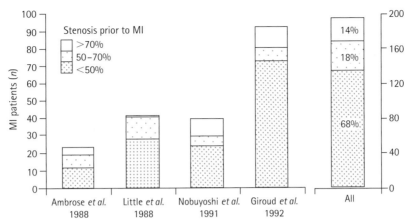

Figure 3.5 *Myocardial infarction usually evolves from plaques that are only mildly to moderately obstructive months to years before infarction. The bar graphs are constructed from published data: Nobuyoshi M, Tanaka M, Nosaka H, Kimura T, Yokoi H, Hamasaki N, et al. Progression of coronary atherosclerosis: is coronary spasm related to progression? J Am Coll Cardiol 1991; 18:904–10. Giroud D, Li JM, Urban P, Meier B, Rutishauser W. Relation of the site of acute myocardial infarction to the most severe coronary arterial stenosis at prior angiography. Am J Cardiol 1992; 69:729–32. Ambrose JA, Tannenbaum MA, Alexopoulos D, Hjemdahl-Monsen CE, Leavy J, Weiss M, et al. Angiographic progression of coronary artery disease and the development of myocardial infarction. J Am Coll Cardiol 1988; 12:56–62. Little WC, Constantinescu M, Applegate RJ, Kutcher MA, Burrows MT, Kahl FR, et al. Can coronary angiography predict the site of a subsequent myocardial infarction in patients with mild-to-moderate coronary artery disease? Circulation 1988; 78:1157–66. Reproduced by permission from Falk E, Shah PK, Fuster V. Coronary plaque disruption. Circulation 1995; 92:657–71.*

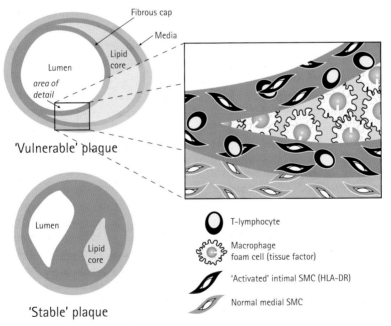

Figure 3.6 *Comparison of the characteristics of 'vulnerable' and 'stable' plaques. Vulnerable plaques often have a well-preserved lumen, because plaques grow outward initially. The vulnerable plaque typically has a substantial lipid core and a thin fibrous cap separating the thrombogenic macrophages bearing tissue factor from the blood. At sites of lesion disruption, smooth muscle cells (SMCs) are often activated, as detected by their expression of the transplantation antigen HLA-DR (see text). In contrast, the stable plaque has a relatively thick fibrous cap protecting the lipid core from contact with the blood. Clinical data suggest that stable plaques more often show luminal narrowing detectable by angiography than do vulnerable plaques. Reproduced by permission from Libby P. Molecular bases of the acute coronary syndromes. Circulation 1995; 91:2844–50.*

muscle cells – the cells that repair and maintain the all-important collagenous matrix of the fibrous cap and are a rich source of extracellular matrix macromolecules in the artery wall.[35] Smooth muscle cells and macrophages undergo apoptosis within the plaque.[36] Indeed, plaques that rupture generally have thin and friable fibrous caps because of the paucity of collagen. Matrix metalloproteinases, including interstitial collagenases and gelatinases, which degrade collagen and other extracellular matrix components and are largely synthesized and released by macrophages, can degrade the collagen fibrils that lend strength to the plaque's fibrous cap.[37]

Inflammation is a central mechanism in both atherogenesis and the initiation of the acute coronary syndromes. The role of inflammation in plaque formation has been discussed above. The balance between the synthesis and degradation of collagen is largely controlled by inflammatory mediators; for example, pro-inflammatory cytokines and *fas* ligand – factors over-expressed in atherosclerotic plaques – can trigger the complex mechanisms of smooth muscle cell loss by apoptosis. Cytokines can induce the expression of metalloproteinases. Inflammation may also contribute to coronary thrombosis by altering the balance between prothrombotic and fibrinolytic properties of the endothelium. For example, endothelial cells exposed to pro-inflammatory cytokines express tissue factor procoagulant, and plaque rupture may expose necrotic and apoptotic cells and cell debris to the circulating blood.[38] It is thus not surprising that several serum markers of inflammation have been linked to atherosclerosis and the acute coronary syndromes.[39] For example, C-reactive protein has multiple direct atherothrombotic effects and increases the risk of acute coronary events.[40] Moreover, it has recently been shown that pregnancy-associated plasma protein A (PAPP-A), a metalloproteinase and prothrombotic inflammatory marker, is expressed in ruptured and eroded but not stable plaque.[41] This raises the possibility of the early detection of plaques at risk for rupture or erosion.

The consequences of plaque rupture and secondary thrombosis are variable. Potential outcomes for unstable lesions include acute thrombotic occlusion, healing with organization of non-occlusive thrombus at the site of plaque disruption, distal atheroembolization or thromboembolization, and organization of the thrombotic mass, with varying degrees of recanalization. Coronary arterial occlusion also induces ischemia of the distal myocardium.

ISCHEMIC MYOCARDIAL INJURY

In ischemia, the supply of blood is insufficient to meet the demand of tissue.[42] Ischemia induces cellular hypoxia, decreased availability of nutrient substrates and accumulation of cellular wastes. Cardiac ischemia is most commonly caused by decreased perfusion owing to obstruction (caused by atherosclerosis, thrombosis, embolism or spasm). However, decreased perfusion resulting from global hypotension (owing to shock or cardiopulmonary bypass) or increased cardiac demand (owing to exercise, tachycardia, hyperthyroidism or ventricular hypertrophy and/or dilatation) also shifts the balance in favor of ischemia. Moreover, patients with coronary artery disease show not only signs of coronary plaque rupture and thrombus formation, but also microemboli and embolic microinfarcts.[43] Microembolization also occurs during percutaneous transluminal coronary angioplasty (PTCA), as evidenced by elevations of troponin T and I and elevations of the ST segment in the electrocardiogram. Indeed, myocardial 'infarctlets', as microinfarcts are often termed, also occur after apparently successful coronary interventions and contribute to an adverse long-term prognosis, and particularly to an increase in late mortality.[44]

The consequences of ischemia depend on severity and duration, and on the pre-existing adaptive and nutritional/metabolic state of the affected cells and tissues. Ischemic injury is potentiated by anemia, hypoxemia or cardiac failure. Moreover, cardiac or ventricular hypertrophy increases vulnerability to myocardial ischemic injury through the combined effects of increased numbers of cells requiring perfusion coupled with relatively decreased vascularity and increased myocardial wall stress. Prolonged severe ischemia can induce *infarction*, a term that implies a loss of cardiac myocytes by necrosis.[45] In contrast, chronic ischemia insufficient to induce infarction may permit development of collateral circulation. Moreover, there is strong evidence that brief episodes of ischemia (lasting 5–15 minutes or so and insufficient to induce necrosis) with intervening reperfusion in patients with coronary artery disease may cause important changes in myocardial metabolism and function (see later). One such change is *stunned myocardium*, which represents 'prolonged post-ischemic contractile dysfunction of myocardium salvaged by reperfusion'.[46] Brief periods of ischemia may also protect against subsequent, more severe, myocardial ischemic injury (a phenomenon termed *preconditioning*)[47] (Figure 3.7). The progressive effects of ischemia are summarized in Figure 3.8 and discussed below.

Progression of damage

The cellular changes following the onset of myocardial ischemia are multifaceted and sequential.[48,49] Severe ischemia of cardiac myocytes (as induced by reduction of blood flow to <10% of normal) induces a transition from aerobic metabolism to anaerobic glycolysis within a few seconds, leading to both inadequate production of high-energy phosphates (e.g. creatine phosphate and adenosine

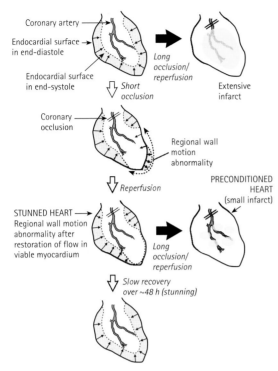

Figure 3.7 *Diagram to illustrate stunning and preconditioning. Short coronary artery occlusions result in stunning, in which there is prolonged regional wall motion abnormality, despite the presence of reperfusion and viable myocardial cells. Brief episodes of ischemia/reperfusion also precondition heart. When heart is then exposed to a longer duration of ischemia and reperfusion, myocardial infarct size is reduced. Reproduced by permission from Kloner RA, Jennings RB. Consequences of brief ischemia: stunning, preconditioning, and their clinical implications: Part 1.* Circulation 2001; *104:2981–9.*

triphosphate [ATP]) and the accumulation of potentially noxious breakdown products (such as lactic acid), thereby causing intracellular acidosis. Owing to the sensitivity of myocardial function to these biochemical consequences of severe ischemia, a striking contractility defect is evident within seconds and virtual cessation of contraction occurs in less than 2 minutes.

Nevertheless, cell death does not occur immediately. Indeed, and owing to the progressive nature of the injury, ischemic changes in an individual cell are potentially *reversible* if the duration of ischemia is short and perfusion is restored prior to the onset of irreversible lesions (approximately 15–20 minutes). *Irreversible* (lethal) injury of cardiac myocytes (associated with irreparable structural defects in the cell membrane) occurs at least focally in the most severely ischemic region only after 20–40 minutes of severe ischemia. Following ischemic injury of sufficient severity and duration, groups of involved cells die and myocardial infarction results.

Largely as a result of collateral flow at the lateral and sub-epicardial margins of the zone or region suffering loss

of perfusion and thereby vulnerable to injury (the so-called *area at risk*), a gradient of ischemia exists across the myocardium. Thus, not all cells are equally affected, cardiac ischemia being most severe in the sub-endocardium at the center of the ischemic zone and in the papillary muscles. In addition, myocytes are more vulnerable than endothelial and connective tissue cells. With prolonged ischemia, a progressive *wavefront* of cell death moves outward from the mid sub-endocardial region toward, and eventually encompassing, the lateral borders and less ischemic sub-epicardial and peripheral regions.[50] The mechanism of cell death in myocardial infarction is historically considered to be *coagulation necrosis*, but evidence suggests that apoptotic cell death may also play an important role.[51] However, some protection at the endocardial surface may accrue owing to perfusion from the blood in the left ventricular chamber, leading to an approximately 1-mm rim of viable myocardium. In dog and sheep experimental models and in humans, approximately half of the necrosis occurs in 3–4 hours; most of the clinically relevant transmural extent of an infarct is typically established within 6–12 hours. The outcome is altered by the restoration of flow to (*reperfusion of*) severely ischemic myocardium at risk of becoming necrotic. The specific result depends greatly on the time interval between the onset of ischemia and the intervention (Figure 3.9; see below).

During cardiopulmonary bypass or organ procurement for transplantation, susceptibility to ischemic injury is global. Although, as stated above, hypertrophy and coronary obstructions tend to enhance injury, decreased tissue temperature and cardioplegic arrest slow intramyocardial chemical reactions and thereby protect against progressive ischemic damage.

Pathological demonstration of very early myocardial infarction is challenging. The histological changes of myocardial necrosis that occurred less than approximately 6 hours prior to death are generally not visible by gross examination or light microscopy. However, in many cases pathologists can observe the presence of a necrotic region at autopsy as a region that does not stain with triphenyl tetrazolium chloride, a dye which turns myocardium a brick-red color on reaction with intact myocardial dehydrogenases (indicating viability) as early as 2–3 hours following the onset of infarction (Figure 3.10).[52]

The earliest changes of reversible ischemic injury can be demonstrated by transmission electron microscopy, including glycogen depletion, cellular and mitochondrial swelling, myofibrillar relaxation and margination of nuclear chromatin. Prolonged ischemia induces irreversible changes: amorphous mitochondrial densities and sarcolemmal disruption. Capillary injury may also occur, with endothelial swelling and eventually necrosis. Although transmission electron microscopy can be used

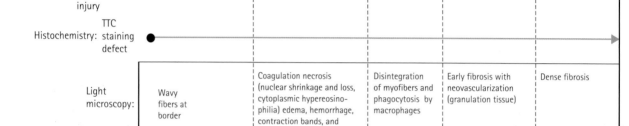

Figure 3.8 *Temporal sequence of biochemical, ultrastructural, histochemical and histological findings after onset of severe myocardial ischemia. Substantial depletion of ATP and accumulation of lactate occur within a few minutes, long prior to cardiac myocyte death by apoptosis and/or necrosis. These biochemical changes are accompanied by profound functional impairment (see text). For approximately half an hour following the onset of even the most profound ischemia, myocardial injury is potentially reversible; subsequently there is progressive loss of viability that is largely complete by 6–12 hours. The benefits of reperfusion are greatest when it is achieved early, with progressively lesser benefits occurring as reperfusion is delayed. The time-dependent progression of the light microscopic histological and other morphological changes that accompany and occur following myocardial infarction are summarized below the graph. TTC, triphenyl tetrazolium chloride. Reprinted from Schoen FJ. Pathologic considerations (in the surgery of adult heart disease). In:Cardiac Surgery in the Adult, Edmunds LH (ed.). New York: McGraw-Hill, 1997, 85–144, with permission of The McGraw-Hill Companies.*

to study these changes in a research setting, persons who die undergo rapid autolysis of all tissues (including morphological changes similar to those of ischemia), and electron microscopy cannot be used to demonstrate early myocardial changes in the clinical setting.

Following infarction, the progression of histological changes generally follows a predictable sequence (Figure 3.11). The earliest features observable by light microscopy are clusters of irreversibly ischemic (necrotic) myocardial cells, which initially exhibit intense sarcoplasmic eosin staining, nuclear pyknosis and loss and, occasionally, stretched and wavy myocytes. Approximately 6–12 hours following the onset of injury, early inflammatory exudation initiates the stereotyped sequence of tissue

changes. The inflammatory reaction is characterized initially by an infiltrate of polymorphonuclear leukocytes (most prominent at 1–3 days), removal of necrotic tissue by macrophages (beginning at approximately 3–5 days), followed by a fibroblastic reparative response with neovascularization (*granulation tissue*) beginning at the margins of preserved tissue (after 1–2 weeks). The infarcted tissue is ultimately replaced by scar; maturation of the scar is usually complete in approximately 6 weeks. Although conventional wisdom considers cardiac muscle cells incapable of meaningful spontaneous regeneration, this concept has recently been challenged by the demonstration of active mitosis of cardiac myocytes at the borders of human myocardial infarcts.[53]

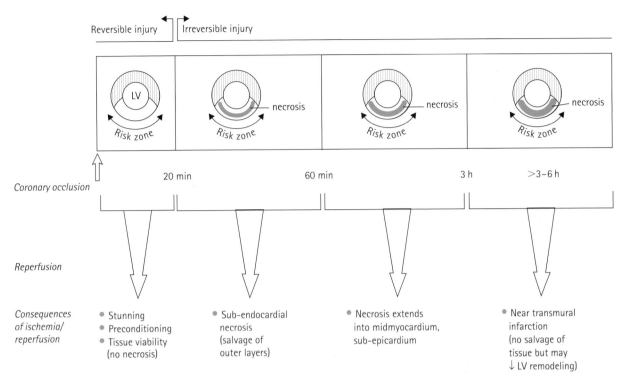

Figure 3.9 *Effects of ischemia and reperfusion on heart based on studies in a dog model of proximal coronary artery occlusion. Brief periods of ischemia of <20 minutes followed by reperfusion are not associated with the development of necrosis (reversible injury). If the duration of coronary occlusion is extended beyond 20 minutes, a wavefront of necrosis marches from sub-endocardium to sub-epicardium over time. Reperfusion before 3 hours of ischemia salvages ischemic but viable tissue. (This salvaged tissue may demonstrate stunning.) Reperfusion beyond 3–6 hours in this model does not reduce myocardial infarct size. Late reperfusion may still have a beneficial effect on reducing or preventing myocardial infarct expansion and left ventricular (LV) remodeling. Brief ischemia/reperfusion results only in phenomena of stunning and preconditioning. Reproduced by permission from Kloner RA, Jennings RB. Consequences of brief ischemia: stunning, preconditioning, and their clinical implications: Part 1. Circulation 2001; 104:2981–9.*

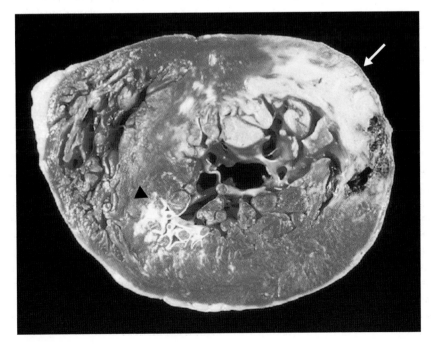

Figure 3.10 *Acute myocardial infarct, predominantly of the postero-lateral wall ventricle (arrow), demonstrated histochemically by a lack of staining by the triphenyltetrazolium chloride stain in areas of necrosis. The staining defect is due to the enzyme leakage that follows cell death. The infarct is of approximately 4 days' duration, and transmural. There is an area of old infarct (scar) in the antero-septal region (arrowhead). (Specimen oriented with posterior wall up.) Reprinted from Schoen FJ. The heart. In: Robbins Pathologic Basis of Disease, 6th edn, Cotran RS, Kumar V, Collins T (eds). Philadelphia: WB Saunders, 1999, 543–99, with permission from Elsevier Science.*

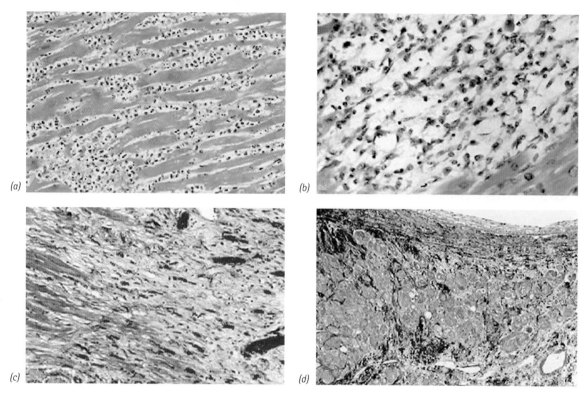

Figure 3.11 *Microscopic features of myocardial infarction. (a) Coagulation necrosis in a large infarct of 3–4 days' duration. Widened spaces between the dead fibers contain edema fluid and dense polymorphonuclear leukocytic infiltrate. (b) Nearly complete removal of necrotic myocytes by phagocytosis (approximately 7–10 days). (c) Granulation tissue with neovascularization and early collagen deposition. (d) Well-healed myocardial infarct with replacement of the necrotic fibers by dense collagenous scar. A few residual cardiac muscle cells are present. (a) and (b) Hematoxylin & Eosin. (c) and (d) Masson's trichrome stain (collagen blue). Reprinted from Schoen FJ. The heart. In: Robbins Pathologic Basis of Disease, 6th edn, Cotran RS, Kumar V, Collins T (eds). Philadelphia: WB Saunders, 1999, 543–99, with permission from Elsevier Science.*

Effects of reperfusion

The progression of myocardial ischemic injury can be modified by the restoration of blood flow to jeopardized myocardium (*reperfusion*). Reperfusion salvages reversibly injured myocytes; thus, reperfusion occurring early before the onset of irreversibility (generally less than 20 minutes in the most severely ischemic regions) may substantially limit infarct size or prevent cell death altogether. In contrast, later reperfusion (20 minutes to 6 hours or more) does not prevent infarction entirely, but myocytes (beyond the leading edge of the 'wavefront') that are only reversibly injured at the time of reflow may be salvaged. Late reperfusion beyond the interval of potential myocyte salvage (i.e. following completion of necrosis) may also be beneficial, by mechanisms that are poorly understood.[54,55]

Owing to the injury to the vasculature that follows myocyte injury in regions of prolonged severe ischemia, reperfusion may lead to hemorrhage in some areas and the inability to perfuse others (*no-reflow*). The reperfused areas in which hemorrhage occurs have a characteristic gross and microscopic appearance (Figure 3.12). Gross myocardial hemorrhage may be prominent owing to ischemia-induced vascular weakness and incompetence; the microscopic pattern is necrosis with contraction bands, which are broad transverse eosinophilic lines across cardiac myocytes visible microscopically. Contraction bands reflect the cellular response to irreversible injury – irreversible ischemic damage to the cell membranes, followed by flooding with high calcium-containing blood concentrations that cause tetanic contraction of sarcomeres. Contraction bands are clusters of contracted sarcomeres. In severe cases of reperfused global ischemia, the entire left ventricular myocardium undergoes a massive contraction to a small, hard mass (*stone heart syndrome*).[56]

In no-reflow, alleviation of an acute coronary occlusion or global ischemia by reperfusion does not alleviate ischemia in at least a portion of the vulnerable region of myocardium, because the microvasculature is obstructed. Several factors are thought to contribute to no-reflow, including interstitial and endothelial edema, ischemic contracture of myocytes with compression of adjacent capillary channels, and plugging of the local microcirculation with neutrophils and platelets.

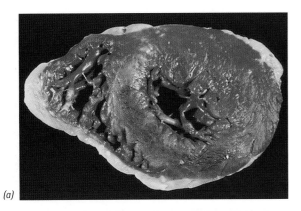

(a)

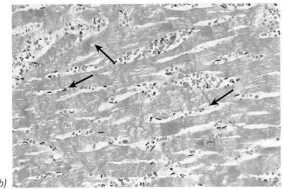

(b)

Figure 3.12 *Gross and microscopic appearance of myocardium modified by reperfusion. (a) Large, densely hemorrhagic, anterior wall acute myocardial infarction from a patient with left anterior descending artery thrombus treated with streptokinase intracoronary thrombolysis (triphenyltetrazolium chloride [TTC]-stained heart slice). (b) Myocardial necrosis with hemorrhage and contraction bands (arrows), visible as dark bands staining the myofibers. This is the characteristic appearance of markedly ischemic myocardium that has been reperfused. (Gross specimen oriented with posterior wall up.) Reprinted from Schoen FJ. The heart. In: Robbins Pathologic Basis of Disease, 6th edn, Cotran RS, Kumar V, Collins T (eds). Philadelphia: WB Saunders, 1999, 543–99, with permission from Elsevier Science.*

There is evidence that the process of reperfusion may damage some of the myocytes that were not already dead at the time at which reflow occurred (a phenomenon called *reperfusion injury*).[57] In most cases, the myocardium affected by reperfusion injury is less than that salvaged by reperfusion. Reperfusion injury is mediated primarily by toxic oxygen species (such as free radicals) that are over-produced by myocytes or polymorphonuclear leukocytes upon restoration of oxygen supply to the tissues; complement activation may also contribute. Consequently, injury may be ameliorated by free radical scavengers such as superoxide dismutase and catalase, inhibitors of polymorphonuclear leukocyte endothelial cell adhesion, or drugs that regulate complement.[58,59] Thus, no-reflow and reperfusion injury may mitigate some of the beneficial effects

achieved by reperfusion in limiting ischemic myocardial damage. In addition, arrhythmias often occur after reperfusion therapy; myocyte injury caused by oxygen free radicals, excessive intracellular calcium or post-procedural microembolization may contribute.

Although successfully reperfused myocardium retains viability, its metabolic and functional recovery may not be instantaneous. Indeed, post-ischemic myocardial dysfunction (*myocardial stunning*) may continue for hours to several days following brief periods of ischemia (see Figure 3.8). The mechanism of stunning involves the generation of oxygen radicals as well as alteration in calcium homeostasis and possibly alteration in contractile protein structure. Stunning has been observed in several clinical scenarios, including unstable angina, stress-induced ischemia, and after PTCA, thrombolysis and cardiopulmonary bypass. The persistent but ultimately recoverable functional abnormalities of reversibly injured myocardium may have important clinical implications, thereby providing the pathophysiological rationale for the use of cardiac assist in some such instances.[60–62] The effects of reperfusion on infarct healing are still unclear.[63]

Although brief periods of ischemia can contribute to prolonged left ventricular dysfunction and even heart failure, they paradoxically play a cardioprotective role. Episodes of ischemia as short as 5 minutes, followed by reperfusion, protect the heart from a subsequent longer coronary artery occlusion (see Figure 3.8) by *ischemic preconditioning*. The mechanism of ischemic preconditioning involves adenosine, adenosine receptors, protein kinase C and ATP-dependent potassium channels. The development of pharmacological agents that stimulate pathways thought to be involved in preconditioning, but without causing ischemia, could result in novel approaches to treating ischemia.

Viable regions of myocardium with impaired function in the setting of chronically reduced coronary blood flow are said to be *hibernating*.[64–66] A major rationale for myocardial revascularization is the potential improvement of the contractile function of hibernating myocardium, with return toward normal blood flow or reduction of oxygen demand. Myocardial hibernation is characterized by:

1 persistent wall motion abnormality,
2 low myocardial blood flow,
3 evidence of viability of at least some of the affected areas, and
4 functional improvement following the restoration of normal coronary blood flow.

Indeed, recovery of flow to regions of hibernation is a likely mechanism for the reversal of longstanding defects in ventricular wall motion following coronary bypass graft surgery or angioplasty. A major challenge is the non-invasive demonstration of viable but severely ischemic myocardium.[67,68]

MYOCARDIAL INFARCTION AND ITS COMPLICATIONS

In a *transmural infarct*, ischemic necrosis involves at least one-half and usually the full or nearly full thickness of the ventricular wall, usually in the distribution of a single coronary artery; coronary atherosclerosis with acute plaque change and superimposed thrombosis is most frequently responsible. In contrast, a *sub-endocardial (non-transmural) infarct* constitutes one or more areas of ischemic necrosis limited to the inner half of the ventricular wall, which may extend beyond the perfusion territory of a single coronary artery. A sub-endocardial infarct may result from a non-occlusive coronary thrombus or one that lyses before myocardial necrosis becomes transmural. Circumferential sub-endocardial infarcts are commonly associated with diffuse stenosing coronary atherosclerosis without acute plaque rupture or superimposed thrombosis, in the setting of episodic hypotension, global ischemia or hypoxemia.

Transmural infarcts are usually associated clinically with ST segment elevation and the development of abnormal Q waves (*Q-wave infarct*). In contrast, sub-endocardial infarcts are usually characterized by ST and T wave changes without abnormal Q waves. Clinical enzymatic estimations of infarct size, which correlate well with pathological determinations, indicate that Q-wave infarcts are generally larger than non-Q-wave lesions. The short-term prognosis is better for non-Q-wave than for Q-wave infarctions. Regardless of the type of infarction, however, a thin rim (1–2 mm) of sub-endocardium may survive, as a result of diffusion of nutrients from the ventricular blood, unless hindered by overlying mural thrombus. Focal small infarcts not limited to the sub-endocardium can be caused by coronary embolization, most commonly due to valvular vegetations or fragments of atherosclerosis or thrombus from the proximal coronary vessels, which may be dislodged during intervention.

Concurrent with the marked decrease in the overall mortality of ischemic heart disease since the 1960s, the in-hospital death rate has declined from approximately 30% to 10–13% today overall, and to only approximately 7% in those receiving aggressive reperfusion therapy.[69] Nevertheless, half of the deaths associated with acute myocardial infarction occur within 1 hour of onset, and these individuals never reach a hospital. Factors associated with a poor prognosis include advanced age, female gender, diabetes mellitus and a history of previous myocardial infarction. The long-term prognosis after myocardial infarction depends on many factors, the most important of which are the quality of left ventricular function and the extent of vascular obstructions in vessels that perfuse viable myocardium. The total mortality within the first year is about 30%; thereafter there is a 3–4% mortality among survivors with each passing year.

Important and frequent complications of myocardial infarction include ventricular dysfunction, cardiogenic shock, arrhythmias, myocardial rupture, extension and expansion, papillary muscle dysfunction, right ventricular involvement, ventricular aneurysm, pericarditis and systemic arterial embolism. Some of these complications are illustrated in Figure 3.13. Among patients with a diagnosis of acute myocardial infarction, approximately one-half will experience one or more complications.[70] The type of complication is primarily related to the size, location and transmurality of the infarction. For example, heart failure is more likely to complicate transmural infarcts, whereas angina and recurrent infarction occur more often with sub-endocardial lesions. Mechanical complications are more common with antero-septal infarctions, but conduction disturbances are more frequent with inferior ones. Overall prognosis worsens with increasing infarct size, and large, transmural anterior infarcts have the worst prognosis.

Myocardial dysfunction

Myocardial infarcts cause functional abnormalities approximately proportional to their size. However, scar caused by previous infarcts and areas of viable but poorly functioning (e.g. stunned or hibernating) myocardium may also contribute to ventricular dysfunction. Large infarcts yield a higher probability of cardiogenic shock, arrhythmias and late congestive heart failure. Patients with anterior infarcts are at greatest risk for regional dilatation, mural thrombus and a poor clinical course. In contrast, posterior infarcts are more likely to cause serious conduction blocks and right ventricular involvement. Although the relative prognosis of patients with sub-endocardial versus transmural infarcts is controversial, mechanical complications are clearly more frequent and significant in patients with transmural lesions. Occurring in 10–15% of patients following myocardial infarction, *cardiogenic shock* is generally indicative of a large infarct (often greater than 40% of the left ventricle).[71] The mortality of myocardial dysfunction and cardiogenic shock has benefited from the use of intra-aortic balloon pumps and ventricular assist devices to manage patients through phases of prolonged but reversible ventricular functional abnormalities associated with infarction.

Arrhythmias

Some abnormality of cardiac rhythm occurs in the majority of hospitalized patients with acute myocardial infarction. Cardiac arrhythmias during acute myocardial

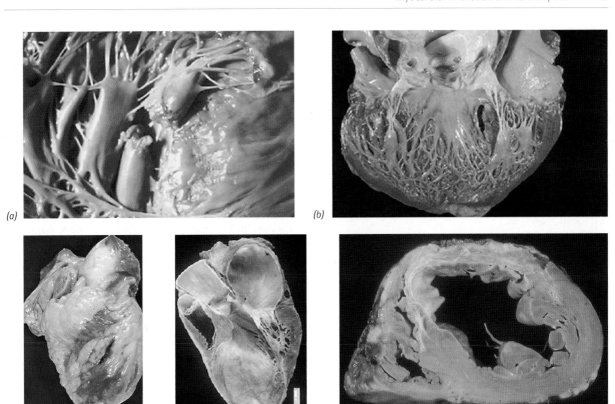

Figure 3.13 *Complications of myocardial infarction. (a), (b) and (c) Cardiac rupture syndromes. (a) Complete rupture of a necrotic papillary muscle. (b) Rupture of the ventricular septum. (c) Anterior myocardial rupture in an acute infarct. (d) Large apical left ventricular aneurysm with laminated mural thrombus in remote infarct. The left ventricle is on the right in this apical, four-chamber view of the heart. (e) End-stage heart failure with large healed remote antero-septal infarct necessitating heart transplantation. (Specimen oriented with anterior wall up.) (e) courtesy of Gayle L. Winters, Brigham and Women's Hospital.*

infarction are of three types: electrical instability, pump failure with excessive sympathetic stimulation and brady-arrhythmias, and conduction disturbances. Arrhythmias occurring in patients with acute myocardial infarction require aggressive treatment when they:

1 impair hemodynamics,
2 compromise myocardial viability by augmenting myocardial oxygen requirements, or
3 predispose to malignant ventricular arrhythmias (i.e. ventricular tachycardia, ventricular fibrillation or asystole).

All forms of bradycardia and tachycardia may depress the cardiac output in patients with acute myocardial infarction. Arrhythmias associated with acute myocardial infarction appear to be related to electrically unstable ischemic ventricular myocardium at the border of the infarction, to arrhythmogenic metabolites released by the infarcted tissues, or to microembolization from a thrombosed coronary artery. Heart block following myocardial infarction is usually transient, but conduction block in the proximal atrioventricular conduction

system may necessitate pacemaker implantation. A leading hypothesis for a major mechanism of arrhythmias in the acute phase of coronary occlusion is micro-reentry due to inhomogeneity of the electrical characteristics of ischemic myocardium. The cellular electrophysiological mechanisms for reperfusion arrhythmias appear to include washout of various ions such as potassium and lactate, and toxic metabolic substances that have accumulated in the ischemic zone. Arrhythmias that develop late after infarction may originate in ischemic myocardium at the border of or within the infarct scar.

Cardiac rupture

Cardiac rupture syndromes comprise three entities:

1 rupture of the ventricular free wall (most common), usually with hemopericardium and cardiac tamponade,
2 rupture of the ventricular septum (less common), leading to an acquired ventricular septal defect with a left-to-right shunt,
3 papillary muscle rupture (least common), resulting in the acute onset of severe mitral regurgitation.

In 8–10% of patients with fatal acute transmural myocardial infarcts, cardiac rupture is the cause of death noted at autopsy.

Free-wall ruptures tend to occur when coagulative necrosis, neutrophilic infiltration and lysis of the myocardial connective tissue have appreciably weakened the infarcted myocardium (mean approximately 4–5 days; range 1–10 days). However, as many as one-quarter of cardiac ruptures occur within 24 hours.[72] The lateral wall at the mid-ventricular level is the most common site for post-infarction free-wall rupture. Risk factors for free-wall rupture include age greater than 60 years, female gender, pre-existing hypertension, absence of left ventricular hypertrophy and no prior myocardial infarction. Acute free-wall ruptures are usually rapidly fatal; repair is rarely possible.[73]

A strategically located pericardial adhesion that aborts a rupture may result in the formation of a *false aneurysm* (i.e. a contained rupture with a hematoma communicating with the ventricular cavity). The wall of a false aneurysm contains no myocardial elements and consists only of blood clot, epicardium and adherent parietal pericardium. Many false aneurysms are filled with mural thrombus and half ultimately rupture.

Post-infarction rupture of septal myocardium causing an (*acute*) *ventricular septal defect* complicates 1–2% of infarcts. Infarct-related septal defects are of two types:

1 single or multiple, sharply localized, jagged, linear passageways that connect the ventricular chambers, most frequently at the antero-apical aspect of the septum (*simple* type), and
2 defects that tunnel serpiginously through the septum to a somewhat distant opening on the right side (*complex* type).[74]

In simple lesions, neither gross hemorrhage nor peripheral laceration is usually present. In contrast, the track of complex lesions, including the entry site of blood into the right side of the heart, may extend into regions remote from the site of the infarct, including the right ventricular free wall. Complex ruptures most frequently involve the infero-septal wall, especially basally. Without surgery, the prognosis following infarct-related septal rupture is poor: 50% of patients die within the first week (half of these within 24 hours), and only 15–20% survive beyond 2 months.

Post-infarction ruptures of the mitral papillary muscles are less frequent than free-wall and septal ruptures and may occur with either sub-endocardial or transmural infarcts. The resulting mitral regurgitation is sudden in onset and its severity is variable, depending on the extent of papillary muscle involvement. Rupture near the tip, with only partial involvement of a papillary muscle group, causes less severe regurgitation than disruption of an entire muscle. Since chordae tendineae arising from the heads of both papillary muscles provide continuity with each of the valve leaflets, interference with the structure or function of one papillary muscle can result in dysfunction of both mitral valve leaflets.

In about 85% of the cases, the postero-medial muscle is the site of rupture, probably owing to its blood supply from only one source, the dominant coronary artery. In contrast, the antero-lateral muscle is nourished by arterial branches from both the left anterior descending artery and the left circumflex coronary artery. Perfused with blood that has traversed the entire transmural extent of the myocardium, papillary muscles are particularly vulnerable to ischemic injury. Papillary muscle rupture can also occur later than other rupture syndromes (i.e. as late as 1 month), since healing in this area can be particularly retarded because of the limited vasculature and resultant inaccessibility to inflammatory cells. Rarely, right ventricular infarction may be associated with rupture of a tricuspid papillary muscle.

Other mechanisms can produce mitral regurgitation in the setting of ischemic heart disease. They include a non-contractile ischemic papillary muscle that fails to tighten the chordae during systole and a previously infarcted papillary muscle that undergoes fibrosis and shortening that fixes the chordae deeply within the ventricle. Moreover, in left ventricular failure, ventricular dilatation can cause distortion and malalignment of the papillary muscle axes, yielding *functional mitral regurgitation*.

Right ventricular infarction

Isolated *right ventricular infarction* is rare. However, clinically important involvement of the right ventricular myocardium occurs in approximately 10% of transmural infero-septal infarcts. The functional consequences can include right ventricular failure with or without tricuspid regurgitation and arrhythmias.[75] Whether or not right ventricular infarction is present, right ventricular dysfunction appears to be an independent risk factor for prognosis following myocardial infarction.[76]

Extension and expansion

Infarct extension is characterized by new/recurrent necrosis in the same distribution as a completed recent infarct.[77,78] Extension is associated with an incremental increase in the amount of necrotic myocardium and may involve either ventricle. Risk factors for infarct extension include sub-endocardial infarction, female gender, previous infarctions and a large infarction associated with cardiogenic shock. Extension most often occurs between 2 and 10 days after the initial infarction and tends to form along its lateral and sub-epicardial borders. Microscopically, necrotic myocardium in an area of extension appears younger than the original infarction and occurs outside its peripheral border of neutrophilic macrophages or granulation tissue.

In contrast, *infarct expansion* is disproportionate thinning and dilatation of the infarcted region[79] owing to its inherent structural weakness and leading to significant increase in ventricular diameter and thereby increase in wall stress and workload of non-infarcted myocardium. A combination of an abnormality in local myocardial contractility (causing stasis), endocardial damage (causing thrombogenicity) and systemic hypercoagulability can potentiate intracardiac mural thrombosis with its attendant risk of embolism. Moreover, infarct expansion is the early precursor to late aneurysm formation (see below).

Geometrical changes following infarction: ventricular remodeling and aneurysm formation

Dynamic structural changes occur in both the necrotic zone and the non-infarcted segments of the ventricle after acute myocardial infarction. The composite process, called *ventricular remodeling*, occurs by a combination of changes, including left ventricular dilatation, early wall thinning, healing and potentially late aneurysm formation in the infarct zone, and compensatory hypertrophy of non-infarcted myocardium.[80–82] Compensatory hypertrophy is hemodynamically beneficial, but the adaptive effect of remodeling may be overwhelmed by depression of contractile function owing to degenerative changes. Ventricular remodeling probably begins at the time of acute infarction and probably continues for months to years, until either a stable hemodynamic state is achieved or progressively severe cardiac decompensation occurs. When the overall function of non-scarred, viable myocardium can no longer maintain an adequate cardiac output, ischemic congestive heart failure (*ischemic cardiomyopathy*) may ensue.[83] Moreover, hyperfunctioning but failing residual myocardium is particularly vulnerable to ischemic injury.

A *ventricular aneurysm* is a large area of thin scar tissue that paradoxically bulges during ventricular systole; it usually develops in the area of infarction and usually follows expansion of a large transmural infarct that heals into scar tissue. The majority of ventricular aneurysms (80%) involve the antero-septal region.[84] Although they are often very thin (only 1 mm in some cases), left ventricular aneurysms are not prone to rupture since they have tough fibrous or fibrocalcific walls. This contrasts with the instability and vulnerability of false aneurysms to rupture. Approximately half of patients with chronic fibrous aneurysms have mural thrombus contained within the ventricle, and systemic embolization may occur. Pharmacological approaches previously considered to limit infarct size, such as steroids and non-steroidal anti-inflammatory agents, were implicated

in exacerbating infarct expansion and aneurysm formation.[85,86]

THERAPEUTIC CORONARY AND MYOCARDIAL INTERVENTIONS

Since myocardial ischemia and infarction are the consequences of critically obstructive coronary artery disease, the primary goal is to perfuse the myocardium. In the acute phase of myocardial infarction, reperfusion therapy is done to limit infarct size, improve myocardial function, prevent future infarctions and improve survival by bypassing or dissolving, disrupting or dislodging the thrombotic material. In the longer term, the aim is to prevent infarction of, and elicit maximal function from, viable yet ischemic and thereby jeopardized myocardium. The pathology of therapeutic coronary and myocardial interventions has recently been reviewed in detail.[87]

Thrombolysis

Revascularization by thrombolysis in early acute myocardial infarction limits infarct size and enhances function and survival.[88,89] Thrombolytic therapy is motivated by several clinicopathological principles:

1 untreated thrombotic occlusion of a coronary artery usually causes transmural infarction,
2 the extent of necrosis during an evolving myocardial infarction progresses as a wavefront and becomes complete only 6 hours or more following coronary occlusion (see Figure 3.8),
3 both early and long-term mortality following acute myocardial infarction correlate strongly with the amount of residual functioning myocardium, and
4 early reperfusion prevents necrosis of at least some jeopardized myocardium.

The benefits of thrombolytic therapy – assessed by the amount of myocardium salvaged, recovery of left ventricular function and resultant reduction in mortality – are largely determined by the time interval between onset of symptoms and successful intervention, adequacy of early coronary reflow, and the degree of residual stenosis of the infarct vessel. Recanalization rates vary from 60% to 90%; the best efficacy relates to the earliest time of infusion of thrombolytic agents (most commonly streptokinase, urokinase or tissue-derived plasminogen activator). The critical time within which lysis must occur in order to achieve substantial myocardial salvage is approximately 4 hours for intracoronary and 3 hours for intravenous administration. Nevertheless, studies also suggest that at least some benefit can occur following later reperfusion, usually within 12 hours of symptoms. Although spontaneous thrombolysis can be beneficial to left ventricular function, and has been well documented within 24 hours of infarct onset, it occurs in less than 10% of patients within the critical 3–4 hours after symptom onset.

Successful thrombolytic therapy re-establishes antegrade flow in the infarct-related coronary artery but does not reverse factors responsible for initiating the original thrombosis, such as advanced atherosclerotic plaque, intimal rupture, enhanced platelet adhesiveness or coronary spasm. Indeed, the nidus that caused thrombosis (such as plaque rupture) still remains, and constitutes an unstable lesion until re-endothelialization takes place. Thus, balloon angioplasty, usually with stenting, or surgical revascularization during infarct evolution constitutes more effective management of the underlying disease process than thrombolysis alone.

The most common complications of thrombolytic reperfusion are failure to achieve clot lysis, so-called reperfusion arrhythmias, coronary rethrombosis and myocardial and systemic hemorrhage. Failure of therapy to effect thrombolysis occurs in 20–30% of patients and is related to the presence of critical plaques, recently disrupted and with complex geometry, plaque rupture with luminal obstruction by thromboatheromatous debris, and old organizing thrombus. Acute reocclusion occurs in 15–35% of patients and appears to be related to incomplete thrombolysis and the unstable nature of the underlying atherosclerotic plaque. Other complications include coronary embolism and hemopericardium. The most frequent and potentially the most serious complication of thrombolytic therapy is bleeding, with hemorrhage at sites of vascular punctures the most common (>70%) and intracranial hemorrhage (~1%) the most dreaded.

Angioplasty, atherectomy and stents

Percutaneous transluminal coronary angioplasty is widely used in patients with stable angina, unstable angina or acute myocardial infarction.[90] PTCA is successful in 85–95% of cases and is associated with a mortality rate of 1%. The characteristic pathological features are summarized in Figure 3.14.

In PTCA, the progressive and substantial expansile force induced by an intravascular balloon causes the essentially non-distensible atherosclerotic plaque to split at its weakest point, but this is not necessarily the site most severely involved by stenosis. The split extends at least to the intimal–medial border and often into the media, with consequent circumferential and longitudinal dissection of the media.[91] Balloon angioplasty is associated with rates of initial failure of 2–20%, early closure up to 15%, and restenosis 30–50% (luminal diameter reduction of <50% compared with proximal reference

segment) at 6 months. Abrupt closure after PTCA occurs in 5–10% of patients. Exposure of sub-endothelial vascular wall components, coupled with the stasis engendered by medial flaps, induces platelet deposition and potentially obstructive thrombus. Acute dissection may contribute. For example, a dissection that involves a considerable portion of the circumference can generate a 'flap', which may impinge on the lumen. Alternatively, a dissection that involves a substantial proximal-to-distal segment of the vessel, which traverses a large plaque-free wall segment, can induce compression of the vessel at a point of minimal disease. Thus, with local flow abnormalities and generation of new, thrombogenic blood-contacting surfaces, an atherosclerotic plaque following angioplasty has many features of a spontaneously disrupted plaque, namely those associated with the acute coronary syndromes. Dissimilar plaques respond differently to balloon dilatation, and the composition and configuration of the original atherosclerotic lesion play a key role in the outcome of angioplasty.[92] Immediate success is enhanced in arteries having eccentric plaques with large lipid-rich necrotic cores and/or calcification, in contrast to concentric fibrotic lesions. The immediate post-angioplasty healing process in either arteries or bypass grafts is not well understood, but dissolution of soft atheromatous material, retraction of the split plaque, thrombus formation and intimal healing with re-endothelialization probably occur.

The long-term success of angioplasty is limited by the development of progressive, proliferative restenosis over a period of months to years.[93] Clinically significant restenosis occurs in approximately 30–40% of patients within the first 4–6 months following coronary balloon angioplasty. Restenosis probably represents a fundamental and complex[94–96] vascular healing response that only achieves clinical significance in some patients. The major process leading to restenosis is excessive smooth muscle proliferation as a response to angioplasty-induced injury and its repair. Vessel wall recoil and organization of thrombus may contribute. There is considerable interest in locally delivered pharmacological and molecular therapies to mitigate restenosis; regrettably, success has so far been limited.[97–101]

Angioplasty has also been applied to obstructions in saphenous vein grafts, internal mammary artery grafts and coronary arteries in transplanted hearts. The success rate is about 90% for vein grafts and 95% for internal mammary arteries. For vein grafts less than 1 year old, intimal tears and wall stretching represent the primary alterations, and for older grafts, plaque rupture is the most common lesion observed. Angioplasty of old saphenous vein grafts that are involved by atherosclerosis and by aneurysmal dilatation poses a particular risk for significant atheromatous embolization and myocardial infarction. Restenosis occurs in about 40% and involves the same mechanisms described for native coronary arteries.

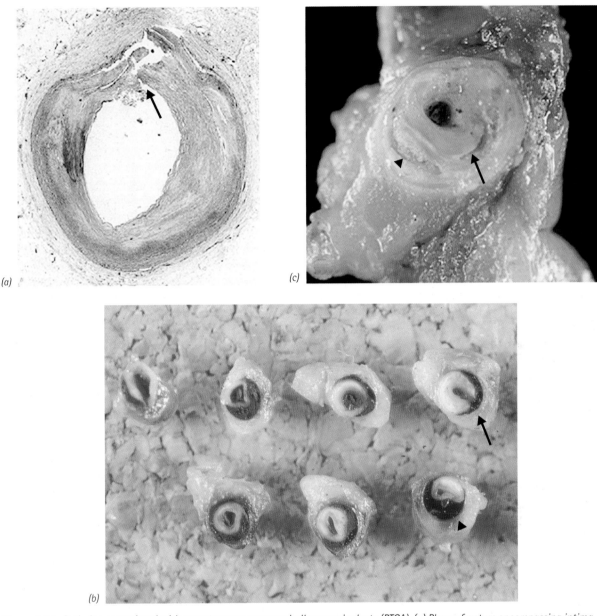

Figure 3.14 *Pathology associated with percutaneous coronary balloon angioplasty (PTCA). (a) Plaque fracture encompassing intima and media (arrow) and partial circumferential wall dissection induced by PTCA. These features account for both mechanisms of efficacy and potential complications. (b) Acute thrombotic occlusion of localized atherosclerotic coronary stenosis with extensive dissection extending both proximal and distal to plaque fracture of lesion ballooned (arrow), including and probably compressing a minimally stenotic distal vessel segment (arrowhead). (c) Restenosis following balloon angioplasty. Gross photograph demonstrates residual atherosclerotic plaque (arrowhead) and a new, glistening proliferative lesion (arrow). (a) and (c) Reprinted from Schoen FJ. Blood vessels. In: Robbins Pathologic Basis of Disease, 6th edn, Cotran RS, Kumar V, Collins T (eds). Philadelphia: WB Saunders, 1999, 538, with permission from Elsevier Science. (b) Reprinted from Schoen FJ.* Interventional and Surgical Cardiovascular Pathology: Clinical Correlations and Basic Principles. *Philadelphia: WB Saunders, 1989, 77, with permission from Elsevier Science.*

Coronary atherectomy of primary or restenosis lesions is achieved percutaneously with a catheter that mechanically removes obstructive tissue by excision. Deep arterial resection, including medial and even adventitial elements, occurs frequently but has not been associated with acute symptomatic complications. The morphology of arterial vessel healing after directional or rotational atherectomy is similar to that following angioplasty.[102,103]

Metallic balloon-expandable and self-expanding coronary stents are expandable tubes of metallic mesh that are inserted percutaneously to preserve luminal patency, particularly at sites of balloon angioplasty. They may reverse the untoward effects of PTCA by providing a larger and more regular lumen, initially acting as a scaffold to support the intimal flaps and dissections that occur in PTCA, limit elastic recoil, mechanically prevent vascular spasm, and increase blood flow. Stenting has been applied to both coronary arteries and saphenous vein grafts. Such devices could provide a larger and more regular lumen by acting as a scaffold to support the intimal dissections that occur in PTCA, mechanically prevent vascular spasm and increase blood flow, all of which could minimize thrombus formation and reduce the impact of post-angioplasty restenosis.[104–107]

Stent implantation is accompanied by damage to the endothelial lining and stretching of the vessel wall, stimulating early adherence and accumulation of platelets and leukocytes. Covered initially by a variable platelet-fibrin coating, stent wires may eventually become completely covered by an endothelium-lined neointima, with the wires embedded in a layer of intimal thickening consisting of α-actin-positive smooth muscle cells in a collagenous matrix (Figure 3.15).[108–110] Nevertheless, the neointima may thicken, and proliferative restenosis is currently not necessarily prevented by stenting.[111] Important questions remain with regard to the determinants of healing and the potential for late complications of endovascular stents, such as migration, perforation or infection.

The complications and limitations of stenting include initial failure, early thrombosis and late restenosis. Subacute stent thrombosis occurs in 1–3% of patients, usually within 7–10 days of the procedure. Antiplatelet treatment minimizes the risk of subacute stent thrombosis. Attempts to reduce within-stent restenosis include evaluation of intracoronary radiotherapy, the delivery of recombinant vascular endothelial growth factor with a balloon catheter to speed endothelialization of a stent, gene therapy and local drug delivery.[112–115] In particular, recent clinical studies using sirolimus- and paclitaxel-eluting stents show favourable results.

Coronary artery bypass graft surgery

Coronary artery bypass graft surgery (CABG) improves survival in patients with significant left main coronary artery disease, three-vessel disease or reduced ventricular function. CABG prolongs and improves the quality of life in patients with 'left main equivalent' disease (proximal left anterior descending and proximal left circumflex), but does not protect them from the risk of subsequent myocardial infarction.[116] Major relief of angina pectoris occurs in more than 90% of appropriately selected patients after CABG. Three major randomized trials into which patients were enrolled during the 1970s shaped current clinical practice – the Veterans Administration (VA) Study, the European Coronary Surgery Study (ECSS) and the

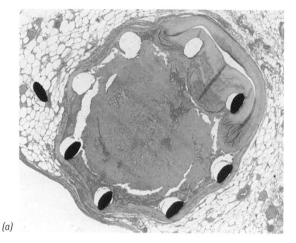

(a)

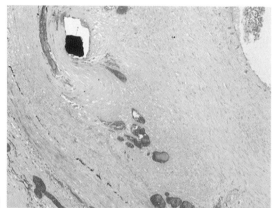

(b)

Figure 3.15 *Pathology associated with metallic coronary stents. (a) Low-power view of stent occluded by thrombosis early following placement. Hematoxylin & eosin. (b) Coronary arterial metallic stent implanted long term, demonstrating thickened proliferative neointima separating the stent wires from the lumen. Masson's trichrome stain (collagen blue). Adapted from Schoen FJ, Edwards WD. Pathology of cardiovascular interventions, including endovascular therapies, revascularization, vascular replacement, cardiac assist/replacement, arrhythmia control and repaired congenital heart disease. In: Cardiovascular Pathology, 3rd edn, Silver MD, Gotlieb AI, Schoen FJ (eds). New York: Churchill Livingstone/WB Saunders, 2001, 678–723, with permission from Elsevier Science.*

National Institutes of Health-supported Coronary Artery Surgery Study (CASS). The most important mechanism of improved survival and left ventricular function after CABG is the reperfusion of viable but non-contractile or poorly contracting hibernating myocardium.

The hospital mortality rate for coronary bypass operations may be less than 1% in low-risk patients; perioperative myocardial infarction occurs in less than 3%; and the 5-year survival rate is about 90%. Overall mortality for elective first bypass procedures in the US from 1980 to 1990 was 2.2% in 58 384 patients in the Society of

Thoracic Surgeons database. More recently, there may have been a slight overall increase in morbidity and mortality, reflecting the tendency to treat an older and sicker population of patients, in which a greater proportion have unstable angina, three-vessel disease, prior coronary revascularization with either coronary bypass surgery or PTCA, left ventricular dysfunction, and/or co-morbid conditions, including hypertension, diabetes and peripheral vascular disease. Many series have demonstrated a markedly higher perioperative morbidity (including myocardial infarction, respiratory failure and stroke) and mortality in coronary surgery in women than in men.

The most consistent predictors of mortality after coronary artery surgery are urgency of operation, age, prior heart surgery, female sex, left ventricular ejection fraction, percentage stenosis of the left main coronary artery, and number of major coronary arteries with significant stenoses – with the first three factors being of greatest importance. The benefit of surgery is greatest in the highest risk patients with the most advanced disease. In contrast, in low-risk and moderate-risk patients, medical therapy or PTCA have results comparable to those of CABG.

Acute cardiac failure is the most common mode of early death after CABG. However, when early cardiac failure with low output or arrhythmias occurs following uncomplicated coronary artery bypass surgery, the underlying cause is often uncertain. Many such patients have no detectable myocardial necrosis, either clinically or at autopsy. In others, the extent of necrosis noted at autopsy seems insufficient to account for the profound ventricular dysfunction encountered clinically. Possible explanations include:

1 evolving myocardial necrosis either undetectable clinically or too recent to detect at autopsy,
2 post-ischemic dysfunction of viable myocardium, for which no morphological markers of the dysfunctional state are known, or
3 a metabolic cause, such as hypokalemia, for which there is no morphologic counterpart.

Thus, although established myocardial necrosis causes cardiac dysfunction in many patients with postoperative failure, it may not be the predominant lesion or the cause or death. However, when such necrosis is detected at autopsy, it may indicate that a potentially larger volume of adjacent myocardium was biochemically and functionally deranged (but not necessarily morphologically abnormal).[117]

The long-term patency of saphenous vein grafts is 60% or less at 10 years, owing to pathological changes, including thrombosis (early), intimal thickening (several months to several years postoperatively) and graft atherosclerosis (years) (Figure 3.16).[118,119] In contrast, the internal mammary (internal thoracic) artery has a greater than 90% patency rate at 10 years (Figure 3.17).[120] The primary complication of bypass grafts is obstruction, which may occur at the aortic anastomosis site, within the body of the graft, or at the distal coronary artery anastomosis site. Graft occlusion occurs with a frequency of approximately

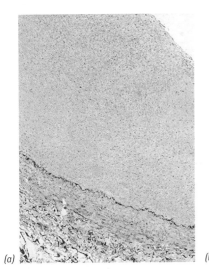
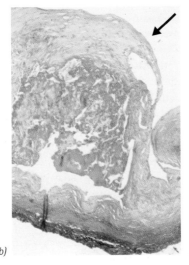
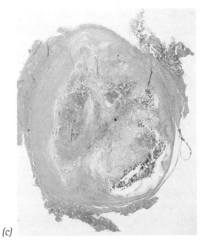

(a) (b) (c)

Figure 3.16 *Pathology associated with coronary artery bypass grafts. (a) Intimal hyperplasia of saphenous vein. Residual lumen is at upper right. Movat stain. (b) Atherosclerosis in saphenous vein coronary artery bypass graft, demonstrating the poorly developed fibrous cap (arrow) and large necrotic core, with calcification. Lumen is at upper right. Elastin stain. (c) Late thrombosis of saphenous vein coronary artery bypass graft initiated by rupture of graft atherosclerotic plaque. Masson's trichrome stain. Reprinted from Schoen FJ, Edwards WD. Pathology of cardiovascular interventions, including endovascular therapies, revascularization, vascular replacement, cardiac assist/replacement, arrhythmia control and repaired congenital heart disease. In: Cardiovascular Pathology, 3rd edn, Silver MD, Gotlieb AI, Schoen FJ (eds). New York: Churchill Livingstone/WB Saunders, 2001, 678–723, with permission from Elsevier Science.*

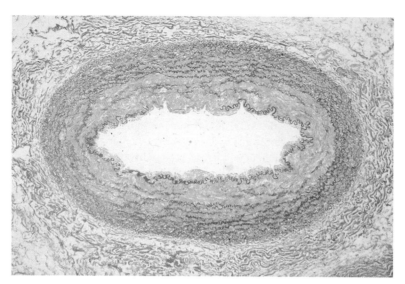

Figure 3.17 *Internal mammary artery as coronary artery bypass graft following long-term implantation (13 years) demonstrating near-normal structure with preservation of the elastic arterial media. Elastin stain. Reprinted from Schoen FJ, Edwards WD. Pathology of cardiovascular interventions, including endovascular therapies, revascularization, vascular replacement, cardiac assist/replacement, arrhythmia control and repaired congenital heart disease. In: Cardiovascular Pathology, 3rd edn, Silver MD, Gotlieb AI, Schoen FJ (eds). New York: Churchill Livingstone/WB Saunders, 2001, 678–723, with permission from Elsevier Science.*

10–15% at 1 month, 20% at 1 year, 30% at 5 years and 40% at 10 years. Antiplatelet therapy has resulted in improved patency rates. Risk factors for graft occlusion include pre-existing phlebosclerosis, operative injury to the vein graft, low blood flow in the graft, small luminal size of the grafted artery, atheromatous plaques or arterial branching at the coronary anastomosis site, mechanical factors (such as graft compression or kinking) and postoperative hyperlipidemia or continued smoking.

Early thrombotic occlusion is predominantly due to inadequate distal run-off into extremely small distal native coronaries, frequently further compromised by partial atherosclerotic occlusions. Other factors in the acute occlusion of aortocoronary bypass grafts (with or without superimposed thrombus) include anastomotic compression by atherosclerosis, suboptimal insertion site, graft or native vessel mural dissection at the anastomotic site, and distortion of a graft that is too short or too long for the intended bypass. In some cases, thrombosis occurring early postoperatively involves only the distal portion of the graft, suggesting that early graft thrombosis is most frequently initiated at the distal anastomosis. Progression of obstructive atherosclerosis in non-bypassed coronary artery segments and graft obstruction are major factors in late symptom recurrence.

The pathology of graft changes is summarized in Figure 3.16.[101,102] Between 1 month and 1 year postoperatively, intimal hyperplasia is the most frequent cause of graft stenosis. Some degree of intimal thickening develops in all vein grafts; however, it is excessive in some, consisting of an exuberant proliferation of smooth muscle cells, with a few fibroblasts, and deposition of variable amounts of extracellular glycosaminoglycans and collagen. The microscopic appearance of intimal thickening in this situation is similar to that observed following angioplasty.

After 1–3 years, atherosclerosis of vein grafts becomes more important than intimal proliferation as a cause of stenosis. As in the coronary arteries, atherosclerosis in aortocoronary bypass grafts can cause myocardial ischemia through progressive luminal stenosis or plaque rupture with secondary thrombotic obstruction. The potential for disruption and embolization of atherosclerotic lesions in vein grafts exceeds that for native coronary atherosclerotic lesions. Plaques in grafts generally involve dilated segments, often have poorly developed fibrous caps, have large necrotic cores, and develop secondary dystrophic calcific deposits that may be closer to the lumen than in typical native arterial atherosclerosis. Finally, atheroembolization may occur; balloon angioplasty or intraoperative manipulation of grafts may stimulate atheroembolism.[121,122]

Multiple factors probably contribute to the remarkably higher long-term patency of internal mammary artery grafts compared to vein grafts. Free saphenous vein grafts sustain not only disruption of their vasa vasora during autotransplantation, but also endothelial damage, medial ischemia and acutely increased internal pressure. In contrast, the internal mammary artery generally has minimal pre-existing atherosclerosis, requires minimal surgical manipulation, maintains its nutrient blood supply, is accustomed to arterial pressures, needs no proximal anastomosis, and has an artery-to-artery distal anastomosis. The sizes of graft and recipient vessel are comparable with the internal mammary artery but disparate (graft substantially larger) with saphenous vein.

Transmyocardial laser revascularization

Transmyocardial revascularization (TMR) may be an attractive alternative therapy for a subset of patients having coronary artery disease with intractable angina who are refractory to medical therapy but not candidates for direct revascularization procedures such as CABG or

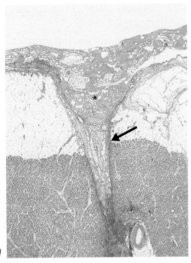
(a)

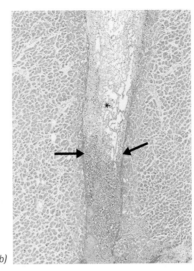
(b)

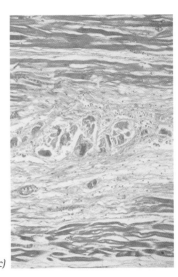
(c)

Figure 3.18 *Transmyocardial laser revascularization channels. (a) and (b) Early thrombotic occlusion of lumen of myocardial channel created by transmyocardial laser revascularization in a patient who died 2 days following the procedure. The edge of the channel is denoted by arrows. The thrombus is designated by an asterisk (*). Myocardium adjacent to the channel shows a thin zone of necrosis. (c) Organizing thrombus in channel 18 days following transmyocardial laser revascularization. (a) and (b) Hematoxylin & eosin. (c) Masson's trichrome stain. Reprinted from Schoen FJ, Edwards WD. Pathology of cardiovascular interventions, including endovascular therapies, revascularization, vascular replacement, cardiac assist/replacement, arrhythmia control and repaired congenital heart disease. In: Cardiovascular Pathology, 3rd edn, Silver MD, Gotlieb AI, Schoen FJ (eds). New York: Churchill Livingstone/WB Saunders, 2001, 678–723, with permission from Elsevier Science.*

PTCA. Candidates for TMR often have diffuse or small-vessel atherosclerotic or other obstructions and lack of distal targets for bypass and are not suitable for cardiac transplant. TMR is a surgical procedure that uses a laser to create transmural channels through the myocardial wall to the left ventricular chamber intended to enhance intramyocardial perfusion. TMR is based on the hypothesis that myocardial sinusoids comprise a vascular network that could communicate between the ventricular chambers and the coronary arteries. In reptiles, it has been postulated that the myocardium receives a substantial supply of blood directly via a meshwork of branching vessels that communicate with and are filled from the ventricular cavity and not from epicardial vessels.

Performed on a beating heart through a left thoracotomy, the operation employs a high-energy laser to bore transmural channels (1 mm in diameter) into the left ventricle. Possible risks include ventricular perforation, pericardial effusion and tamponade, and ventricular septal perforation. Although experimental and clinical trials suggest benefit,[123–127] the mechanism of efficacy is still uncertain.[128]

Although blood flows through channels immediately after they are made, as demonstrated by the pulsatile spurts of blood that frequently come from epicardial channel openings, a clot soon forms at the epicardial surface and the new channels typically occlude. Early claims of prolonged channel patency and resultant direct transmyocardial perfusion of blood have largely been refuted. Indeed, examination of hearts from patients who have died at various post-mortem intervals generally fails to reveal patent channels (Figure 3.18).

Regardless of the type of laser used, intramyocardial channels generated by TMR initially have a central region of vaporized myocardium surrounded by a thin rim of necrosis due to thermal damage. Acute changes (within 24 hours) typically consist of circular to elliptic channels with a lumen filled to varying degrees with thrombus composed of blood and fibrin. This is surrounded by a zone of thermocoagulated myocytes with contraction bands, well demarcated from the adjacent normal myocytes. At 2–3 weeks, the channels are usually filled with loosely arranged granulation tissue rich in capillaries and small muscular arterioles embedded within the connective tissue matrix. Intensive clinical and animal studies, including canine, porcine and ovine models in both acute and chronic ischemic injury, have not demonstrated long-term channel patency.[129–131] The leading hypothesis for efficacy suggests that TMR stimulates angiogenesis,[132–134] the normal inflammatory responses that result in the formation of new vessels in granulation tissue that are triggered following myocardial injury. An additional possible mechanism of action of TMR is denervation of the heart. Current and future investigation is directed at a clearer elucidation of the mechanism(s) of action of TMR and the clinical indications for its use.

FUTURE DIRECTIONS

An understanding of pathology, anatomy and mechanisms has contributed greatly to the spectacular 60% decline in the mortality from both coronary heart disease and stroke in the second half of the twentieth century. The formidable challenges that remain in the early twenty-first century necessitate both innovative research and breakthroughs in clinical care for patients with or at risk for coronary heart disease. Potential improvements that are beyond the scope of this chapter include genetic screening for future risk of coronary heart disease, subclinical detection of coronary atherosclerosis and vulnerable plaques, and therapeutic interventions for chronic ischemic heart disease, including gene therapy,[135,136] myocardial transplantation and regeneration,[137] tissue-engineered myocardium,[138,139] mechanical hearts and assist devices,[140,141] and xenotransplantation.[142] Continued insights derived from cardiovascular pathology and applied cardiovascular biology will be critical in moving these exciting innovations forward.

KEY REFERENCES

Anversa P, Nadal-Ginard B. Myocyte renewal and ventricular remodelling. *Nature* 2002; **415**:240–3.

Continuous cell renewal in the adult myocardium, previously thought impossible, may occur following injury. Thus, it becomes a potentially realistic goal to stimulate multipotent cardiac stem cells to renew the myocardium and repair the heart after infarction.

Libby P, Aikawa M. Stabilization of atherosclerotic plaques: new mechanisms and clinical targets. *Nature Med*, 2002; **11**:1257–309.

Lipid-lowering statins substantially reduce acute coronary events resulting from atherosclerosis, but only modestly reduce arterial stenosis. This apparent paradox has shifted the goal of therapy towards the stabilization of plaque against rupture or erosion by intrinsic structural modification rather than enlargement of the lumen.

Menasche P. Cell transplantation for the treatment of heart failure. *Semin Thorac Cardiovasc Surg* 2002; **14**:157–66.

Cell transplantation is a new treatment that could potentially improve the outcome for patients with cardiac failure. Experimental and clinical data suggest that implantation of contractile cells into fibrous scars following infarction can allow them to gain some functionality. Autologous skeletal myoblasts have been the first to be tested in a clinical trial, but other cell types can be considered, among which bone marrow stromal and hematopoietic stem cells are of particular interest because of their presumed pluripotentiality.

Rabkin E, Schoen FJ. Cardiovascular tissue engineering. *Cardiovasc Pathol* 2002; **11**:305–17.

The term *tissue engineering* describes approaches at the interface of the biomedical and engineering sciences intended to produce medical devices that have living cells or attract endogenous cells to aid tissue regeneration. In the most widely explored paradigm, cells are seeded on a scaffold composed of synthetic polymer or natural material (collagen or chemically treated tissue), a tissue is matured *in vitro*, and the resultant construct is implanted in the appropriate anatomic location, where remodeling occurs. This review summarizes the evolving approaches to engineering cardiovascular tissues, including living patches of myocardium, substitute cardiac valves and vascular grafts.

Young JB. Healing the heart with ventricular assist device therapy: mechanisms of cardiac recovery. *Ann Thorac Surg* 2001; **71**:S210–19.

In some patients with cardiogenic shock treated by mechanical circulatory assist, myocardial recovery occurs and device removal is permitted. Benefit appears related to amelioration of circulatory insufficiency, attenuation of perturbed humoral networks and reduction of myocardial wall stress.

REFERENCES

1. Schoen FJ, Cotran RS. Blood vessels. In: *Robbins Pathologic Basis of Disease*, 6th edn, Cotran RS, Kumar V, Collins T (eds). Philadelphia: W.B. Saunders, 1999, 493–541.
2. Gotlieb AI. Atherosclerosis. In: *Cardiovascular Pathology*, 3rd edn, Silver MD, Gotlieb AI, Schoen FJ (eds). New York: Churchill Livingstone, 2001, 68–106.
3. Libby P. The vascular biology of atherosclerosis. In: *Heart Disease*, 6th edn, Braunwald E, Zipes DP, Libby P (eds). Philadelphia: W.B. Saunders, 2001, 995–1009.
4. Weis M, von Scheidt W. Cardiac allograft vasculopathy. *Circulation* 1997; **96**:2069–77.
5. Julius BK, Attenhofer Jost CH, Sutsch G, Brunner HP, Kuenzli A, *et al.* Incidence, progression and functional significance of cardiac allograft vasculopathy after heart transplantation. *Transplantation* 2000; **69**:847–53.
6. Ross R. The pathogenesis of atherosclerosis. A perspective for the 1990s. *Nature* 1993; **362**:801–9.
7. Ross R. Atherosclerosis. An inflammatory disease. *N Engl J Med* 1999; **340**:115–26.
8. Price DT, Loscalzo J. Cellular adhesion molecules and atherogenesis. *Am J Med* 1999; **107**:85–97.
9. Gimbrone MA Jr, Nagel T, Topper JN. Biomechanical activation: an emerging paradigm in endothelial adhesion biology. *J Clin Invest* 1997; **99**:1809–13.
10. Hansson GK. Immune mechanisms in atherosclerosis. *Arterioscler Thromb Vasc Biol* 2001; **21**:1876–90.
11. Mehta JL, Saldeen TGP, Rand K. Interactive role of infection, inflammation and traditional risk factors in atherosclerosis and coronary artery disease. *J Am Coll Cardiol* 1998; **31**:1217–25.
12. Kol A, Libby P. The mechanisms by which infectious agents may contribute to atherosclerosis and its clinical manifestations. *Trends Cardiovasc Med* 1998; **8**:191–9.
13. Gibbons GH, Dzau VJ. The emerging concept of vascular remodeling. *N Engl J Med* 1994; **330**:1431–8.

14. Schoenhagen P, Ziada KM, Vince DG, Nissen SE, Tuzcu EM. Arterial remodeling and coronary artery disease: the concept of 'dilated' vs. 'obstructive' coronary atherosclerosis. *J Am Coll Cardiol* 2001; **38**:297–306.

15. Nissen SE, Yock P. Intravascular ultrasound. Novel pathophysiological insights and current clinical applications. *Circulation* 2001; **103**:604–16.

16. Richardson PD, Davies MJ, Born GVR. Influence of plaque configuration and stress distribution on fissuring of coronary atherosclerotic plaques. *Lancet* 1989; **21**:941–4.

17. Loree HM, Kamm RD, Stringfellow RG, Lee RT. Effects of fibrous cap thickness on peak circumferential stress in model atherosclerotic vessels. *Circ Res* 1992; **71**:850–8.

18. Davies MJ, Richardson PD, Woolf N, Katz DR, Mann J. Risk of thrombosis in human atherosclerotic plaques: role of extracellular lipid, macrophage, and smooth muscle cell content. *Br Heart J* 1993; **69**:377–81.

19. Falk E, Shah PK, Fuster V. Coronary plaque disruption. *Circulation* 1995; **92**:657–71.

20. Libby P. Current concepts of the pathogenesis of the acute coronary syndromes. *Circulation* 2001; **104**:365–72.

21. Rentrop KP. Thrombi in acute coronary syndromes. Revisited and revised. *Circulation* 2000; **101**:1619–26.

22. Burke AP, Farb A, Malcom GT, Liang YH, Smialek J, Virmani R. Coronary risk factors and plaque morphology in men with coronary disease who died suddenly. *N Engl J Med* 1997; **336**:1276–82.

23. Davies MJ. A macro and micro view of coronary vascular insult in ischemic heart disease. *Circulation* 1990; **82**:II38–46.

24. Little WC, Constantinescu M, Applegate RJ, Kutcher MA, Burrows MT, Kahl FR, *et al.* Can coronary angiography predict the site of a subsequent myocardial infarction in patients with mild-to-moderate coronary artery disease? *Circulation* 1988; **78**:1157–66.

25. Davies MJ. Stability and instability: two faces of coronary atherosclerosis. The Paul Dudley White Lecture 1995. *Circulation* 1996; **94**:2013–20.

26. Keelan PC, Bielak LF, Ashai K, Jamjoum LS, Denktas AE, Rumberger JA, *et al.* Long-term prognostic value of coronary calcification detected by electron-beam computed tomography in patients undergoing coronary angiography. *Circulation* 2001; **104**:412–17.

27. Schmermund A, Erbel R. Unstable coronary plaque and its relation to coronary calcium. *Circulation* 2001; **104**:1682–7.

28. Kim WY, Danias PG, Stubber M, Flamm SD, Plein S, Nagel E, *et al.* Coronary magnetic resonance angiography for the detection of coronary stenoses. *N Engl J Med* 2001; **345**:1863–9.

29. Fayad ZA, Fuster V. Clinical imaging of the high-risk or vulnerable atherosclerotic plaque. *Circ Res* 2001; **89**:305–16.

30. Jang IK, Bouma BE, Kang DH, Park SJ, Park SW, Seung KB, *et al.* Visualization of coronary atherosclerotic plaques in patients using optical coherence tomography: comparison with intravascular ultrasound. *J Am Coll Cardiol* 2002; **39**:604–9.

31. Muller JE, Abela GS, Nesto RW, Tofler GH. Triggers, acute risk factors and vulnerable plaques: the lexicon of a new frontier. *J Am Coll Cardiol* 1994; **23**:809–13.

32. Aikawa M, Rabkin E, Sugiyama S, Voglic SJ, Fukumoto Y, Furukawa Y, *et al.* An HMG-CoA reductase inhibitor, cerivastatin, suppresses growth of macrophages expressing matrix metalloproteinases and tissue factor *in-vivo* and *in-vitro*. *Circulation* 2001; **103**:276–83.

33. Rabbani R, Topol EJ. Strategies to achieve coronary arterial plaque stabilization. *Cardiovasc Res* 1999; **41**:402–17.

34. Libby P, Aikawa M. Stabilization of atherosclerotic plaques: New mechanisms and clinical targets. *Nature Med* 2002; **8**:1257–62.

35. Schwartz SM, Virmani R, Rosenfeld ME. The good smooth muscle cells in atherosclerosis. *Curr Atheroscler Rep* 2000; **2**:422–9.

36. Kolodgie FD, Narula J, Burke AP, Haider N, Farb A, Hui-Liang Y, *et al.* Localization of apoptotic macrophages at the site of plaque rupture in sudden coronary death. *Am J Pathol* 2000; **157**:1259–68.

37. Shah PK, Galis ZS. Matrix metalloproteinase hypothesis of plaque rupture. Players keep piling up but questions remain. *Circulation* 2001; **104**:1878–80.

38. Mallat Z, Tedgui A. Current perspective on the role of apoptosis in atherothrombotic disease. *Circ Res* 2001; **88**:998–1003.

39. Blake GJ, Ridker PM. Novel clinical markers of vascular wall inflammation. *Circ Res* 2001; **89**:763–71.

40. Ridker PM, Cushman M, Stamfer MJ, Tracy RP, Hennekens CH. Inflammation, aspirin, and the risk of cardiovascular disease in apparently healthy men. *N Engl J Med* 1997; **336**:973–9.

41. Bayes-Genis A, Conover CA, Overgaard MT, Bailey KR, Christiansen M, Holmes DR Jr, *et al.* Pregnancy-associated plasma protein A as a marker of acute coronary syndromes. *N Engl J Med* 2001; **345**:1022–9.

42. Schoen FJ. The heart. In: *Robbins Pathologic Basis of Disease*, 6th edn, Cotran RS, Kumar V, Collins T (eds). Philadelphia: W.B. Saunders, 1999, 543–99.

43. Erbel R, Heusch G. Coronary microembolization – its role in acute coronary syndromes and interventions. *Herz* 1999; **24**:558–75.

44. Abdelmeguid AE, Topol EJ. The myth of the myocardial 'infarctlet' during percutaneous coronary revascularization procedures. *Circulation* 1996; **94**:3369–75.

45. Anonymous. Myocardial infarction redefined – a consensus document of The Joint European Society of Cardiology/American College of Cardiology Committee for the Redefinition of Myocardial Infarction. *J Am Coll Cardiol* 2000; **36**:959–69.

46. Kloner RA, Jennings RB. Consequences of brief ischemia: stunning, preconditioning, and their clinical implications. *Circulation* 2001; **104**:2981–9, 3158–67.

47. Murry CE, Jennings RB, Reimer KA. Preconditioning with ischemia: a delay of lethal cell injury in ischemic myocardium. *Circulation* 1986; **74**:1124–36.

48. Buja LM. Modulation of the myocardial response to ischemia. *Lab Invest* 1998; **78**:1345–73.

49. Jennings RB, Steenbergen C, Reimer KA. Myocardial ischemia and reperfusion. In: *Cardiovascular Pathology: Clinicopathologic Correlations and Pathogenetic Mechanisms*, Schoen FJ, Gimbrone MA (eds). Philadelphia: Williams & Wilkins, 1995, 47–80.

50. Reimer KA, Jennings RB. The 'wavefront phenomenon' of myocardial ischemic cell death. II. Transmural progression of necrosis within the framework of ischemic bed size (myocardium at risk) and collateral flow. *Lab Invest* 1979; **40**:633–44.

51. James TN. Apoptosis in cardiac disease. *Am J Med* 1999; **107**:606–20.

52. Vargas SO, Sampson BA, Schoen FJ. Pathologic detection of early myocardial infarction: a critical review of the evolution and usefulness of modern techniques. *Mod Pathol* 1999; **12**:635–45.

53. Beltrami AP, Urbanek K, Kajstura J, Yan SM, Finato N, Bussani R, *et al.* Evidence that human cardiac myocytes divide after myocardial infarction. *N Engl J Med* 2001; **344**:1750–7.

54. Brodie BR, Stuckey TD, Hansen C, Muncy D, Weintraub RA, LeBauer EJ, *et al.* Benefit of late coronary reperfusion in patients with acute myocardial infarction and persistent ischemic chest pain. *Am J Cardiol* 1994; **74**:538–43.

55. Richard V, Murry CE, Reimer KA. Healing of myocardial infarcts in dogs. Effects of late reperfusion. *Circulation* 1995; **92**:1891–901.

56. Hutchins GM, Silverman KJ. Pathology of the stone heart syndrome. Massive myocardial contraction band necrosis and widely patent coronary arteries. *Am J Pathol* 1979; **95**:745–52.

57. Granger DN, Korthuis RJ. Physiologic mechanisms of postischemic tissue injury. *Ann Rev Physiol* 1995; **57**:311–32.

58. Talbott GA, Sharar SR, Harlan JM, Winn RK. Leukocyte–endothelial interactions and organ injury: the role of adhesion molecules. *New Horiz* 1994; **2**:545–54.

59. Homeister JW, Lucchesi BR. Complement activation and inhibition in myocardial ischemia and reperfusion injury. *Annu Rev Pharmacol Toxicol* 1994; **34**:17–40.

60. Leavitt JI, Better N, Tow DE, Rocco TP. Demonstration of viable, stunned myocardium with technetium-99m-sestamibi. *J Nucl Med* 1994; **35**:1805–7.

61. Schoen FJ, Palmer DC, Bernhard WF, Pennington DG, Haudenschild CC, Ratliff NB, *et al*. Clinical temporary ventricular assist. *J Thorac Cardiovasc Surg* 1986; **92**:1071–81.

62. Kern KB, Hilwig RW, Rhee KH, Berg RA. Myocardial dysfunction after resuscitation from cardiac arrest: an example of global myocardial stunning. *J Am Coll Cardiol* 1996; **28**:232–40.

63. Cowan MJ, Reichenbach D, Turner P, Hostenson C. Cellular response of the evolving myocardial infarction after therapeutic coronary artery reperfusion. *Hum Pathol* 1991; **22**:154–63.

64. Rahimtoola SH. The hibernating myocardium. *Am Heart J* 1989; **117**:211–21.

65. Heusch G, Schulz R. The biology of myocardial hibernation. *Trends Cardiovasc Med* 2000; **10**:108–14.

66. Vanoverschelde JL, Melin JA. The pathophysiology of myocardial hibernation: current controversies and future directions. *Prog Cardiovasc Dis* 2001; **43**:387–98.

67. Kim RJ, Wu E, Rafael A, Chen EL, Parker MA, Simonetti O, *et al*. The use of contrast-enhanced magnetic resonance imaging to identify reversible myocardial dysfunction. *N Engl J Med* 2000; **343**:1445–53.

68. Perrone-Filardi P, Chiariello M. The identification of myocardial hibernation in patients with ischemic heart failure by echocardiography and radionuclide studies. *Prog Cardiovasc Dis* 2001; **43**:419–32.

69. Beller GA. Coronary heart disease in the first 30 years of the 21st century: challenges and opportunities. *Circulation* 2001; **103**:2428–35.

70. Antman, EM, Braunwald E. Acute myocardial infarction. In: *Heart Disease,* 6th edn, Braunwald E, Zipes DP, Libby P (eds). Philadelphia: W.B. Saunders, 2001, 1114–231.

71. Hasdai D, Topol EJ, Califf RM, Berger PB, Holmes DR Jr. Cardiogenic shock complicating acute coronary syndromes. *Lancet* 2000; **356**:749–56.

72. Batts KP, Ackermann DM, Edwards WD. Postinfarction rupture of the left ventricular free wall: clinicopathologic correlates in 100 consecutive autopsy cases. *Hum Pathol* 1990; **21**:530–5.

73. Sutherland FWH, Guell FJ, Pathi VL, Naik SK. Postinfarction ventricular free wall rupture: strategies for diagnosis and treatment. *Ann Thorac Surg* 1996; **61**:1281–5.

74. Edwards BS, Edwards WD, Edwards JE. Ventricular septal rupture complicating acute myocardial infarction: identification of simple and complex types in 53 autopsied hearts. *Am J Cardiol* 1984; **54**:1201–5.

75. Zehender M, Kasper W, Kauder E, Schönthaler M, Geibel A, Olschewski M, *et al*. Right ventricular infarction as an independent predictor of prognosis after acute inferior myocardial infarction. *N Engl J Med* 1993; **328**:981–8.

76. Zornoff LA, Skali H, Pfeffer MA, St. John Sutton M, Rouleau JL, Lamas GA, *et al*. Right ventricular dysfunction and risk of heart failure and mortality after myocardial infarction. *J Am Coll Cardiol* 2002; **39**:1450–5.

77. Muller JE, Rude RE, Braunwald E, Hartwell TD, Roberts R, Sobel BE, *et al*. Myocardial infarct extension: occurrence, outcome, and risk factors in the multicenter investigation of limitation of infarct size. *Ann Intern Med* 1988; **108**:1–6.

78. Weisman HF, Healy B. Myocardial infarct expansion, infarct extension, and reinfarction: pathophysiologic concepts. *Prog Cardiovasc Dis* 1987; **30**:73–110.

79. Weiss JL, Marino PN, Shapiro EP. Myocardial infarct expansion: recognition, significance and pathology. *Am J Cardiol* 1991; **68**:35D–40D.

80. Sonnenblick EH, Anversa P. Models and remodeling: mechanisms and clinical implications. *Cardiologia* 1999; **44**:609–19.

81. Swynghedauw B. Molecular mechanisms of myocardial remodeling. *Physiol Rev* 1999; **79**:215–62.

82. Pfeffer MA, Braunwald E. Ventricular remodeling after myocardial infarction. Experimental observations and clinical implications. *Circulation* 1990; **81**:1161–72.

83. Anversa P, Sonnenblick EH. Ischemic cardiomyopathy: pathophysiologic mechanisms. *Prog Cardiovasc Dis* 1990; **33**:49–70.

84. Cabin HS, Roberts WC. True left ventricular aneurysm and healed myocardial infarction: clinical and necropsy observations including quantification of degrees of coronary arterial narrowing. *Am J Cardiol* 1980; **46**:754–63.

85. Hammerman H, Kloner RA, Hale S, Schoen FJ, Braunwald E. Dose-dependent effects of short-term methylprednisolone on myocardial infarction extent, scar formation and ventricular function. *Circulation* 1983; **68**:446–52.

86. Brown EJ, Schoen FJ, Hammerman H, Hale S, Braunwald E. Scar thinning due to ibuprofen administration following experimental myocardial infarction. *Am J Cardiol* 1983; **51**:877–83.

87. Schoen FJ, Edwards WD. Pathology of cardiovascular interventions, including endovascular therapies, revascularization, vascular replacement, cardiac assist/replacement, arrhythmia control and repaired congenital heart disease. In: *Cardiovascular Pathology*, 3rd edn, Silver MD, Gotlieb AL, Schoen FJ (eds). Philadelphia: W.B. Saunders, 2001, 678–723.

88. Laffel GL, Braunwald E. Thrombolytic therapy. A new strategy for the treatment of acute myocardial infarction. *N Engl J Med* 1984; **311**:710–17, 770–6.

89. Cairns JA, Fuster V, Gore J, Kennedy JW. Coronary thrombolysis. *Chest* 1995; **108**:401S.

90. Landau C, Lange RA, Hillis LD. Percutaneous transluminal coronary angioplasty. *N Engl J Med* 1994; **330**:981–93.

91. Waller BF. Pathology of new cardiovascular interventional procedures. In: *Cardiovascular Pathology*, Silver MD (ed.). New York: Churchill Livingstone, 1991, 1683–781.

92. Virmani R, Farb A, Burke AP. Coronary angioplasty from the perspective of atherosclerotic plaque: morphologic predictors of immediate success and restenosis. *Am Heart J* 1994; **127**:163–79.

93. Kuntz RE, Baim DS. Defining coronary restenosis. Newer clinical and angiographic paradigms. *Circulation* 1993; **88**:1310–23.

94. Haudenschild CC. Pathobiology of restenosis after angioplasty. *Am J Med* 1993; **94**(Suppl.):40–4S.

95. Epstein SE, Speir E, Unger EF, Guzman RJ, Finkel T. The basis of molecular strategies for treating coronary restenosis after angioplasty. *J Am Coll Cardiol* 1994; **23**:1278–88.

96. Libby P, Sukhova G, Brogi E, Schoen FJ, Tanaka H. Restenosis as an example of vascular hyperplastic disease: reassessment of potential mechanisms. *Adv Vasc Surg* 1995; **3**:279–90.

97. Riessen R, Isner JM. Prospects for site-specific delivery of pharmacologic and molecular therapies. *J Am Coll Cardiol* 1994; **23**:1234–44.

98. Lincoff AM, Topol EJ, Ellis SG. Local drug delivery for the prevention of restenosis. *Circulation* 1994;**90**:2070–84.

99. Casscells W. Growth factor therapies for vascular injury and ischemia. *Circulation* 1995; **91**:2699–702.

100. Bennett MR, Schwartz SM. Antisense therapy for angioplasty restenosis. *Circulation* 1995; **92**:1981–93.

101. Kibbe MR, Billiar TR, Tzeng E. Gene therapy for restenosis. *Circ Res* 2000; **86**:829–33.

102. Diethrich EB. Classical and endovascular surgery: indications and outcomes. *Surg Today* 1994; **24**:949–56.

103. Stertzer SH, Rosenblum J, Shaw RE, Sugeng I, Hidalgo B, Ryan C, et al. Coronary rotational ablation: initial experience in 302 procedures. J Am Coll Cardiol 1993; 21:287–95.

104. Serruys PW, de Jaegere P, Kiemeneij F, Macaya C, Rutsch W, Heyndrickx G, et al. A comparison of balloon-expandable-stent implantation with balloon angioplasty in patients with coronary artery disease. N Engl J Med 1994; 331:489–95.

105. Topol EJ. Caveats about elective coronary stenting (Editorial). N Engl J Med 1994; 331:539–41.

106. Eeckhout E, Kappenberger L, Goy J-J. Stents for intracoronary placement: current status and future directions. J Am Coll Cardiol 1996; 27:757–65.

107. Al Suwaidi J, Berger PB, Holmes DR Jr. Coronary artery stents. J Am Med Assoc 2000; 284:1828–36.

108. Anderson PG, Bajaj RK, Baxley WA, Roubin GS. Vascular pathology of balloon-expandable flexible coil stents in humans. J Am Coll Cardiol 1992; 19:372–81.

109. van Beusekom HMM, van der Giessen WJ, van Suylen RJ, Bos E, Bosman FT, Serruys PW. Histology after stenting of human saphenous vein bypass grafts: observations from surgically excised grafts 3 to 320 days after stent implantation. J Am Coll Cardiol 1993; 21:45–54.

110. Farb A, Sangiorgi G, Carter AJ, Walley VM, Edwards WD, Schwartz RS, et al. Pathology of acute and chronic coronary stenting in humans. Circulation 1999; 99:44–52.

111. Virmani R, Farb A. Pathology of in-stent restenosis. Curr Opin Lipidol 1999; 10:499–506.

112. Salame MY, Verheye S, Cracker IR, Chronos NA, Robinson KA, King SB 3rd. Intracoronary radiation therapy. Eur Heart J 2001; 22:629–47.

113. Williams DO, Sharaf BL. Intracoronary radiation: it keeps on glowing. Circulation 2000; 101:350–4.

114. Morice MC, Serruys PW, Sousa JE, Fajadet J, Ban Hayashi E, Perin M, et al. A randomized comparison of a sirolimus-eluting stent with a standard stent for coronary revascularization. N Engl J Med 2002; 346:1773–80.

115. Park SJ, Shim WH, Ho DS, Raisner AE, Park SW, Hong MK, et al. A paclitaxel-eluting stent for the prevention of coronary restenosis. N Engl J Med 2003; 348:1537–45.

116. Lytle BW, Cosgrove DM. Coronary artery bypass surgery. Curr Probl Surg 1992; 29:733.

117. Schoen FJ. Interventional and Surgical Cardiovascular Pathology: Clinical Correlations and Basic Principles. Philadelphia: W.B. Saunders, 1989.

118. Bourassa MG. Long-term vein graft patency. Curr Opin Cardiol 1994; 9:685–91.

119. Nwasokwa ON. Coronary artery bypass graft disease. Ann Intern Med 1995; 123:528–45.

120. Loop FD, Lytle BW, Cosgrove DM, Stewart RW, Goormastic M, Williams GW, et al. Influence of the internal-mammary-artery graft on 10-year survival and other cardiac events. N Engl J Med 1986; 314:1–6.

121. Saber RS, Edwards WD, Holmes DR Jr, Vlietstra RE, Reeder GS. Balloon angioplasty of aortocoronary saphenous vein bypass grafts: a histopathologic study of six grafts from five patients, with emphasis on restenosis and embolic complications. J Am Coll Cardiol 1988; 12:1501–9.

122. Webb JG, Carere RG, Virmani R, Baim D, Teirstein PS, Whitlow P, et al. Retrieval and analysis of particulate debris after saphenous vein graft intervention. J Am Coll Cardiol 1999; 34:468–75.

123. Cooley DA, Frazier OH, Kadipasaoglu KA, Pehlivanoglu S, Shannon RL, Angelini P. Transmyocardial laser revascularization.

Anatomic evidence of long-term channel patency. Tx Heart Inst J 1994; 21:22–4.

124. Horvath KA, Smith WJ, Laurence RG, Schoen FJ, Appleyard RF, Cohn LH. Recovery and viability of an acute myocardial infarct after transmyocardial laser revascularization. J Am Coll Cardiol 1995; 25:258–63.

125. Cooley DA, Frazier OH, Kadipasaoglu KA, Lindenmeir MH, Pehlivanoglu S, Kolff JW, et al. Transmyocardial laser revascularization: clinical experience with twelve-month follow-up. J Thorac Cardiovasc Surg 1996; 111:791–7.

126. Horvath KA, Mannting F, Cummings N, Sherman SK, Cohn LH. Transmyocardial laser revascularization: operative techniques and clinical results at two years. J Thorac Cardiovasc Surg 1996; 111:1047–53.

127. Horvath KA. Results of clinical trials of transmyocardial laser revascularization versus medical management for end-stage coronary disease. J Clin Laser Med Surg 2000; 18:247–52.

128. Whittaker P, Rakusan K, Kloner RA. Transmural channels can protect ischemic tissue. Circulation 1996; 93:143–52.

129. Fleischer KJ, Goldschmidt-Clermont PJ, Fonger JD, Hutchins GM, Hruban RH, Baumgartner WA. One-month histologic response of transmyocardial laser channel with molecular intervention. Ann Thorac Surg 1996; 62:1051–8.

130. Kohmoto T, Fisher PE, Gu A, Zhu SM, DeRosa CM, Smith CR, et al. Physiology, histology, and 2-week morphology of acute transmyocardial channels made with a CO_2 laser. Ann Thorac Surg 1997; 63:1275–83.

131. Kohmoto T, DeRosa CM, Yamamoto N, Fisher PE, Failey P, Smith CR, et al. Evidence of vascular growth associated with laser treatment of normal canine myocardium. Ann Thorac Surg 1998; 65:1360–7.

132. Whittaker P. Transmyocardial revascularization. The fate of myocardial channels. Ann Thorac Surg 1999; 68:2376–82.

133. Bridges CR. Myocardial laser revascularization. The controversy and the data. Ann Thorac Surg 2000; 69:655–62.

134. Malekan R, Reynolds C, Narula N, Kelley ST, Suzuki Y, Bridges CR. Angiogenesis in transmyocardial laser revascularization. A nonspecific response to injury. Circulation 1998; 98:II62–5.

135. Braunwald E. Shattuck lecture – Cardiovascular medicine at the turn of the millennium: triumphs, concerns, and opportunities. N Engl J Med 1997; 337:1360–9.

136. Flower J, Dreifus LS, Bove AA, Weintraub WS. Technological advances and the next 50 years of cardiology. J Am Coll Cardiol 2000; 35:1082–91.

137. El Oakley RM, Ooi OC, Bongso A, Yacoub MH. Myocyte transplantation for myocardial repair: a few good cells can mend a broken heart. Ann Thorac Surg 2001; 71:1724–33.

138. Mann BK, West JL. Tissue engineering in the cardiovascular system: progress toward a tissue engineered heart. Anat Rec 2001; 263:367–71.

139. Fuchs JR, Nasseri BA, Vacanti JP. Tissue engineering: a 21st century solution to surgical reconstruction. Ann Thorac Surg 2001; 72:577–91.

140. Stevenson LW, Kormos RL. Mechanical cardiac support 2000: current applications and future trial design. J Am Coll Cardiol 2001; 37:340–70.

141. Rose EA, Gelijns AC, Moskowitz AJ, Heitjan DF, Stevenson LW, Dembitsky W, et al. Long-term use of a left ventricular assist device for end-stage heart failure. N Engl J Med 2001; 345:1435–43.

142. Adams DH, Chen RH, Kadner A. Cardiac xenotransplantation: clinical experience and future directions. Ann Thorac Surg 2000; 70:320–6.

4

Clinical manifestations of coronary artery disease

STANLEY CHIA AND KEITH AA FOX

Cardiovascular disease is the principal cause of death in adults in the industrialized world as well as in many developing countries, and coronary artery disease (CAD) accounts for half of these deaths. In the US alone, more than 11 million people are estimated to suffer from CAD. Although there has been encouraging evidence over the last three decades that the incidence, mortality and in-hospital case fatalities are declining in the Western world,[1] there continues to be an escalation in the cardiovascular events in Asia and in central and eastern Europe.[2] It is estimated that cardiovascular disease will be the leading cause of death among emerging nations by the year 2020.[3] The overall prevalence of CAD is rising as a consequence of the ageing populations, signifying a growing burden on health and economic resources in many countries.

In recent years, we have witnessed an unparalleled evolution in the understanding of CAD. Developments in vascular biology have unravelled important fundamentals of disease processes leading to significant advances in the diagnosis and treatment of CAD. The publication of several landmark trials has also revolutionized the management of CAD, and population studies suggest that the decrease in CAD mortality may be due in significant part to the improvement in the treatment of myocardial infarction (MI) and to secondary prevention.[4]

Decisions on the medical or surgical management of patients cannot be made without a thorough understanding of the clinical manifestations of CAD and of the underlying pathophysiology and natural history of the disease process. This is often complicated by the heterogeneity of the clinical presentations of CAD where there is no uniform presenting syndrome. The condition can be classified broadly into acute or chronic CAD. Acute CAD may present as the acute coronary syndromes (ACS – this encompasses unstable angina, non-ST-elevation MI and ST-elevation MI), acute heart failure and arrhythmia. Chronic CAD includes chronic stable angina, congestive heart failure (CHF) and the related complications. Although chest pain is the predominant complaint in most patients with CAD, in sudden cardiac death (SCD) or silent myocardial ischemia, pain may be absent. Furthermore, ischemia may manifest atypically as chest pressure or dyspnea, and the presentation may be occult in certain groups of patients, including the elderly and diabetics. Two other conditions, syndrome X and variant angina, are not strictly due to atheromatous CAD, but are discussed in this chapter.

ACUTE CORONARY SYNDROMES

The acute coronary syndromes define a spectrum of clinical manifestations of CAD that extends from acute transmural MI (ST-elevation MI, STEMI) through minimal myocardial injury (non-ST-elevation MI, NSTEMI) to unstable angina. This spectrum shares common underlying pathophysiological mechanisms involving acute or subacute primary reduction of myocardial supply caused by the fissuring or erosion of an atherosclerotic plaque with superimposed platelet aggregation and thrombosis, usually associated with vasoconstriction, microfragmentation and distal embolization.[5] As a consequence, clinical manifestations are dependent upon the severity and location of the obstruction in the affected coronary artery, the presence or absence of collateral blood supply and the myocardial oxygen demand within the affected territory. Thus the spectrum extends from abrupt vessel occlusion with acute ischemia leading to infarction, through partial coronary obstruction and distal ischemia with minor enzyme release, to non-occlusive thrombosis with normal cardiac enzymes.

Non-ST-elevation myocardial infarction (NSTEMI) and unstable angina

EPIDEMIOLOGY

The pathophysiology, clinical presentation and management of unstable angina are similar to those of NSTEMI and, in the broad context of ischemic heart disease, these two syndromes are usually considered together. The distinction between the two conditions can be made only several hours or even days after the initial presentation, based upon cardiac enzyme levels and markers of myocyte injury (troponins).

The prevalence of recognized unstable angina appears to be increasing and may now be more common than acute MI.[6,7] In the US alone, unstable angina and NSTEMI accounted for 1.43 million hospitalizations in 1996, compared to the estimated 350 000 hospitalizations for STEMI.[8] Based upon the Global Registry of Acute Coronary Events (GRACE) registry,[9] 36% of ACS present as ST-elevation MI, 44% as unstable angina and 20% as chest pain of uncertain etiology. The risk of death or MI from unstable angina and NSTEMI is approximately 10% at 6 months, and almost a quarter of patients sustain these events or acute refractory angina within 6 months of the initial presentation.[10,11]

CLINICAL PRESENTATION

Patients with an ACS usually present with prolonged anginal pain at rest, new-onset severe angina (class III of the Canadian Cardiac Society (CCS) Classification[12]), or recent destabilization of previously stable angina with at least CCS III angina characteristics (crescendo angina).[13] Atypical presentation may include epigastric pain, recent-onset indigestion, stabbing chest pain or increasing dyspnea. Atypical symptoms are usually more common in younger (25–40 years) and older (>75 years) patients, diabetic patients or women. Although most patients with ACS may present directly to emergency departments, some may also present to rapid access chest pain clinics, care of the elderly units or primary care physicians.[14]

CLASSIFICATION OF ACS

Based on recent trial data and prospective registries,[9–11,15] patients with ACS are now identified by the criteria stated in Table 4.1. Patients with typical clinical features of unstable angina but a normal electrocardiogram (ECG) and no prior documented coronary disease have a suspected ACS until cardiac enzymes and further ECGs confirm or refute the diagnosis.

The most frequently cited classification of patients with unstable angina is that proposed by Braunwald in 1989 based on clinical symptoms.[16] This system has been validated in numerous prospective studies and correlates with prognosis and is also linked to angiographic and histological findings. As this pre-dates modern enzymatic measures, a revised classification has recently been proposed to subclassify patients who present with angina at rest within 48 hours into those who are troponin positive or negative.[17] The risk of death and MI at 30 days is up to 20% in patients with troponin elevation, compared to less than 2% in those without troponin release (Table 4.2).[18,19] The GRACE registry of ACS has provided prospective international data on outcome of patients with the full spectrum of ACS. Whereas in-hospital mortality figures for those who survive to reach hospital alive are 7% for STEMI, 6% for NSTEMI and 3% for unstable angina, the mortality rates from admission to 6 months are 12%, 13% and 8%, respectively.[9]

Table 4.1 *Acute coronary syndromes: criteria required to establish a working diagnosis on admission*[9–11]

- Ischemic chest pain (discomfort) at rest or on minimal exertion or emotion (2 × 5-minute episodes or 1 episode >10 minutes) and
- Evidence of underlying coronary artery disease (at least one of the following):
  - ECG: ST-segment depression, T-wave inversion or transient ST elevation
  - enzyme elevation: troponin I or T, creatine kinase (CK) or CK-MB
  - evidence of coronary artery disease on angiography or perfusion scanning

Table 4.2 *Revised Braunwald classification of unstable angina*

Classification	A. Secondary unstable angina	B. Primary unstable angina	C. Post-infarction (<2 weeks) unstable angina
I New onset, severe or accelerated angina	IA	IB	IC
II Subacute rest angina (>48 hours ago)	IIA	IIB	IIC
III Acute rest angina within 48 hours	IIIA	IIIB – troponin negative IIIB – troponin positive	IIIC

Data from Hamm C, Braunwald E. *Circulation* 2000; **102**:118–22.[17]

TRIAGE OF PATIENTS WITH SUSPECTED ACS

In patients presenting with suspected ACS, the following investigations should be undertaken.

- An ECG should ideally be obtained immediately and repeated if the initial changes are not diagnostic or if symptoms change. Continuous ST segment analysis allows optimal assessment of ischemic episodes in higher risk patients with ACS.
- Troponin T or troponin I are the preferred serum markers of myocardial injury and elevated concentrations reflect myocardial cellular necrosis. They are more cardiac specific and reliable than the traditional marker, creatine kinase or its isoenzyme CK-MB.[20] In order to demonstrate or exclude myocardial damage, blood sampling is required, ideally on arrival and 6–12 hours after admission, and 4–6 hours after any further episodes of severe chest pain. Increased plasma concentrations of C-reactive protein[21] and interleukin-6[22] are also markers of increased risk and in particular of long-term risk.
- Coronary angiography and percutaneous intervention (PCI) or surgical revascularization (coronary artery bypass grafting surgery) have been shown to improve outcome in those with ECG evidence of ischemia and especially those with elevated biomarkers or C-reactive protein.[23,24]
- After stabilization and prior to discharge from hospital, echocardiography and exercise stress test are appropriate to detect evidence of ventricular impairment and for future risk assessment. Echocardiography may be useful in establishing a diagnosis in those with suspected ischemia. Normal

left ventricular function indicates that significant ischemia is unlikely, while left ventricular dysfunction may reflect new ischemia or previous MI.

RISK STRATIFICATION AND INITIAL MANAGEMENT

The key to the management of patients with an established diagnosis is to select the appropriate strategy based on the perceived risk of progression to MI or death. This can be divided into acute and long-term risks.

The markers of acute thrombotic risk are recurrence of chest pain, ST-segment depression on ECG, dynamic ST-segment changes, elevated level of cardiac troponins and the presence of thrombus on coronary angiography. These should be differentiated from the markers of underlying disease, which are determinants of long-term risk of disease progression. The latter clinical markers include age, history of prior MI or severe angina and diabetes. Other factors are the levels of plasma C-reactive protein and interleukin-6 and the presence of left ventricular dysfunction or extensive CAD on coronary angiography.

Patients with suspected acute ischemia or ACS should be admitted directly to hospital to differentiate non-cardiac and low-risk patients from intermediate/high-risk patients, as the latter require specific anti-thrombotic therapy and possible surgical or percutaneous revascularization.

ANTI-THROMBIN THERAPY

Antiplatelet therapy with aspirin is indicated in all patients with CAD unless there is clear evidence of aspirin allergy. In patients with unstable angina, aspirin almost halves the risk of cardiac death or non-fatal MI.[25] The platelet adenosine diphosphate inhibitor clopidogrel has further beneficial effects when combined with aspirin in patients with unstable angina or NSTEMI, although there is a modest increase in the risk of bleeding.[26] For those proceeding to coronary artery bypass graft surgery, the risk of major bleeding is increased from 6% to 9% if clopidogrel was administered within the preceding 5 days. There was no increase in those in whom the drug was stopped for more than 5 days.

Glycoprotein IIb/IIIa inhibitors such as abciximab, eptifibatide or tirofiban are indicated in high-risk patients, especially those with marked ischemia and those proceeding to PCI.[27] Anti-thrombin drugs (unfractionated heparin or low-molecular-weight heparin) can reduce thrombus formation and stimulate thrombus resolution and should be initiated early. A significant reduction in death or new MI at 6 days (1.8% vs 4.8%), sustained at 42 days, has been reported when patients were treated with a low-molecular-weight heparin (compared with placebo) in the presence of aspirin therapy.[28]

ANTI-ISCHEMIC THERAPY

Anti-ischemic treatment is aimed at reducing myocardial oxygen demand, inducing coronary vasodilatation and reducing ischemia. Patients should therefore be commenced on a β-adrenoceptor antagonist in the first instance. Meta-analysis has suggested that β-adrenoceptor antagonist treatment was associated with a 13% relative reduction in the risk of progression to acute MI.[29] In the presence of contraindications, calcium channel antagonists with heart-rate-limiting properties (diltiazem, verapamil) may be suitable alternatives. Intravenous nitrates should also be administered and the dose titrated upwards until symptoms are relieved or side effects occur. For patients with recurrent ischemia despite the above treatment or those at high thrombotic risk at presentation, urgent coronary revascularization should be considered.[23,24]

The European Society of Cardiology and the American College of Cardiology/American Heart Association have both issued detailed recommendations on the management of ACS without persistent ST-segment elevation and these should be referred to for a more detailed account of the management of these patients.[30,31]

Acute myocardial infarction (ST-elevation MI, STEMI)

EPIDEMIOLOGY

We have seen major advances in the diagnosis and management of acute MI in the last few decades. The establishment of coronary care units, introduction of invasive hemodynamic monitoring, thrombolytic therapy and primary percutaneous intervention, and preventative cardiology have all contributed to the steady decline in the morbidity and mortality of MI. Nevertheless, MI is still a potentially fatal disease with devastating consequences. Although the in-hospital mortality has been drastically reduced from 25–30% in the 1960s to 6–7% in recent large-scale trials and registries,[2,32] the overall fatality rate of acute MI in the community in the first month may be as high as 30–50%. It should be recognized that at least half of these fatalities occur within the first 2 hours and many occur prior to any contact with the medical services.

CLINICAL PRESENTATION

About half of the patients with acute MI are aware of non-specific prodromal symptoms, and short episodes of chest discomfort may precede the event by up to 4 weeks. Patients presenting with acute MI classically describe severe retrosternal chest pain or pressure lasting more than 30 minutes. The pain may have a crushing or squeezing quality or may be described as an intense weight on the chest which is not relieved by nitroglycerine. Radiation of the pain to the jaw, neck and left arm is common, and occasionally to the back. In patients with pre-existing chronic stable angina, the pain may be similar in quality but much more intense, severe and persistent than their typical angina. Autonomic symptoms such as nausea, vomiting, dizziness and perspiration are frequently present due to activation of the vagal reflex. Especially in the elderly, autonomic symptoms may sometimes be the only presenting features. A sense of impending doom may also be experienced. There is a marked circadian rhythm in the time of onset of acute MI, with a peak incidence in the early hours of the morning, possibly due to an increase in sympathetic tone and platelet aggregation. Differential diagnoses that have to be considered at the time of presentation include aortic dissection, pericarditis, esophageal and gastric pain, musculo-skeletal pain and pulmonary embolism.

About 25% of patients with non-fatal acute MI may be completely asymptomatic, or may only experience modest chest discomfort, weakness and fatigue.[33] Silent MI is more common in the elderly and in patients with diabetes and hypertension, and the diagnosis is often only made on subsequent routine ECG or on post-mortem examinations.

Acute MI with ST elevation is almost always caused by an acute reduction in coronary blood flow due to atherosclerosis with superimposed thrombosis that is occlusive and persistent (Figure 4.1).[5] Prolonged ischemia subsequently leads to the necrosis of cardiac myocytes. About 65–75% of fatal coronary thrombi are precipitated by sudden rupture of a vulnerable lipid-rich atheromatous plaque, and the remainder are mostly due to plaque erosion (see Chapter 3).

ESTABLISHING THE DIAGNOSIS

Acute evolving MI is defined clinically by the presence of appropriate symptoms, new ST-segment elevation greater than 0.2 mV in two adjacent chest leads or two limb leads as recorded on the 12-lead ECG, and confirmed subsequently by elevated biochemical markers of myocardial necrosis (troponin I, troponin T, creatine kinase and its isoenzyme CK-MB). Regional wall motion abnormalities are often detectable on echocardiography and may be apparent within seconds after coronary occlusion. Clinically established MI may also be identified by the presence of Q waves on ECG. NSTEMI has already been discussed in the previous section.

In patients with suspected acute MI, a 12-lead ECG must be recorded immediately. Early diagnosis is necessary to allow emergency treatment to relieve the patient's discomfort and to minimize the extent of myocardial damage. Confirmation of the diagnosis is sometimes only possible following sequential ECGs and biochemical

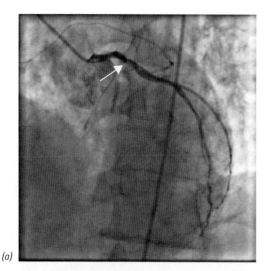

(a)

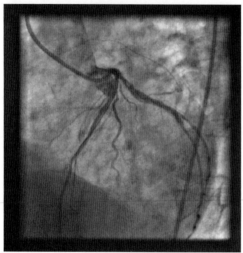

(b)

Figure 4.1 *Coronary angiograms from a patient presenting with acute myocardial infarction. (a) Left coronary angiogram showing complete occlusion of the left anterior descending artery (arrow). (b) Left coronary angiogram from the same patient following angioplasty to the left anterior descending artery.*

markers. The management of acute MI is beyond the scope of this chapter, but the principles of management can be summarized as follows.

- Pre-hospital and immediate care: the main objectives are to relieve pain (usually with opiate analgesia), to administer aspirin and oxygen, and to prevent or treat arrhythmias (including cardiac arrest).
- Early care: the priority is to initiate reperfusion with thrombolytic therapy or primary coronary angioplasty in order to limit infarct size and to prevent infarct extension and expansion. The aim is also to treat immediate complications such as cardiac failure, shock and malignant arrhythmias.

- Subsequent care: management of complications, further investigation, and strategies to minimize progression of CAD and inhibit new infarction, heart failure and death (secondary prevention measures).
- Cardiac rehabilitation: aimed at restoring the patient to as full a life as possible and including reassurance and advice on physical, psychological and socio-economic factors. A significant reduction in mortality is shown in rehabilitation programs that included exercise.[34]

A more detailed account of the management of acute MI can be found in the recently published (2003) practice guidelines by the European Society of Cardiology and the 1999 update on guidelines by the American College of Cardiology/American Heart Association Task Force.[35,36]

SUDDEN CARDIAC DEATH AND FATAL ARRHYTHMIAS

In more than a quarter of patients with CAD, the first clinical manifestation is sudden death. SCD is the commonest cause of sudden death in the community, and half of all SCDs occur in individuals with no previous history of CAD.

Sudden cardiac death is defined as witnessed death within 1 hour of onset of acute symptoms that is attributed to the consequences of acute myocardial ischemia or infarction, post-infarction scarring, left ventricular hypertrophy or cardiac failure. Pre-existing heart disease may or may not have been known to be present, but the time and mode of death are unexpected.

Sudden cardiac death is precipitated by an abrupt disturbance of cardiac function or arrhythmia such that cerebral blood flow is inadequate and cardiac arrest ensues. The trigger for SCD is commonly ventricular fibrillation. This may originate in scarred myocardium following prior MI, or may be precipitated by acute myocardial ischemia or necrosis. The initial arrhythmia is usually ventricular tachycardia, ventricular fibrillation or, more rarely, severe bradyarrhythmias. SCD is more common in men and the prevalence increases with age. Marked impairment in left ventricular systolic function is the most powerful predictor of SCD in patients with chronic ischemic heart disease, and the incidence of SCD increases markedly with successive classes of the New York Heart Association classification of CHF.[37] Although most premature ventricular complexes are prognostically benign, frequent and complex ventricular ectopics in survivors of MI predict an increased risk of SCD.

Acute myocardial ischemia often causes a broad range of arrhythmias and complicates the course of patients with ACS. This may be attributed to a variety of mechanisms that include enhanced sympathetic activity due to activation of atrial and ventricular receptors, systemic and local release of catecholamines, increased sensitivity of the ischemic myocardium to catecholamines and interruption to the electrical innervation of the heart following transmural MI. The common arrhythmias during acute myocardial ischemia are ventricular premature beats, ventricular tachycardia, ventricular fibrillation, accelerated idioventricular rhythm, sinus tachycardia and atrioventricular block. In patients with chronic CAD, cardiac arrhythmias such as paroxysmal ventricular tachycardia and atrioventricular block may be the dominant manifestation of the disease. There is generally good correlation between the frequency and severity of ventricular arrhythmias induced during exercise tests and ambulatory monitoring with the degree of angiographically documented CAD.

Individuals with suspected cardiac arrest should be managed according to the Advanced Cardiovascular Life Support algorithms recommended by the International Liaison Committee on Resuscitation 2000[38] and also modified by the European Resuscitation Council.[39] Basic life support should be initiated promptly and should include checking for responsiveness, airway patency and respiratory movements, followed by giving effective breaths, a quick assessment of circulation and commencing chest compression if circulation is absent. The key to management is to identify the underlying arrhythmia and attempt defibrillation as soon as possible if appropriate. A summary of the algorithm is shown in Table 4.3.

CHRONIC STABLE ANGINA

EPIDEMIOLOGY AND CLINICAL PRESENTATION

Chronic stable angina and acute MI are the most common clinical manifestations of CAD. Primary care diagnoses and nitrate prescriptions suggest a 2% prevalence of stable angina pectoris in the general population.[40] The incidence of angina pectoris in men and women aged 61–70 years as determined by a cardiologist and non-invasive testing is 2.6 and 0.9 per 1000 patients per annum, respectively.[41] Patients have a 4–6% risk of death or non-fatal MI each year and 30% of those with recent-onset angina will have a significant cardiac event (death, non-fatal MI or coronary revascularization) within a year of presentation.[41]

The classical description of angina pectoris as a 'sense of strangling and anxiety' by Heberden in the eighteenth century continues to be pertinent today. Patients typically complain of a retrosternal chest discomfort that may be described as a heavy, constricting or gripping sensation. The discomfort may reside exclusively in the chest or radiate to the jaws, epigastrium, back and left or both arms. It is often initiated by physical or emotional

Table 4.3 *Adult Advanced Cardiovascular Life Support Algorithm*

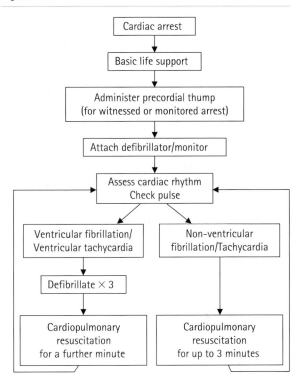

During cardiopulmonary resuscitation, the resuscitation team should check for paddle and electrode position, gain intravenous access and secure airway patency. Epinephrine should be administered either intravenously or via the tracheal tube every 3 minutes. The use of anti-arrhythmics, pacing, atropine and buffers should also be considered. Potentially reversible causes such as hypoxia, hypovolemia, hypothermia, hypo/hyperkalemia, tension pneumothorax, cardiac tamponade, pulmonary thromboembolism and toxins (drugs) should be excluded.
Data from de Latorre F *et al*. European Council Guidelines 2000 for Adult Advanced Life Support. *Resuscitation* 2000; 48:211–21.[39]

stress, persists for 3–5 minutes and is relieved by rest or the administration of nitroglycerin. The anginal pain precipitated by exertion may actually improve in some patients as they persevere at the same level of activity, possibly a manifestation of ischemic preconditioning. Angina 'equivalents' such as breathlessness, fatigue and dizziness may also be manifestations of myocardial ischemia in the absence of chest pain.

CLASSIFICATION OF ANGINA

The symptomatic discomfort that represents angina pectoris is a result of mismatch between myocardial oxygen demand and supply. This usually reflects underlying atheromatous stenoses of the coronary arteries that limit perfusion (Figure 4.2) and the imbalance between maximal blood flow during exercise or emotional stress and the myocardial oxygen demand.[42] Although the vast

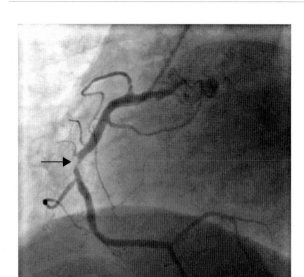

Figure 4.2 *Right coronary angiogram in a patient with stable angina showing severe stenosis of the proximal right coronary artery (arrow).*

Table 4.4 *Causes of anginal chest pain not attributed to a fixed atheromatous stenosis of the coronary artery*

Aortic stenosis
Hypertensive heart disease and left ventricular hypertrophy
Atheroma-associated vasospasm and variant angina
Syndrome X (microvascular angina)
Hypertrophic cardiomyopathy
Mitral valve prolapse
Severe pulmonary hypertension and right ventricular hypertrophy

Table 4.5 *Canadian Cardiovascular Society functional classification of stable angina pectoris*

Grade 1 Ordinary physical activity does not cause angina
Grade 2 Slight limitation of ordinary activity
Grade 3 Marked limitation of ordinary activity
Grade 4 Inability to carry on any physical activity without discomfort

Data from Campeau L. Grading of angina pectoris. *Circulation* 1976; 55:522–3.[12]

majority of angina is caused by atheromatous coronary disease, there are other causes of the symptom (Table 4.4).

The severity of angina is traditionally graded according to the CCS system.[12,43] This widely accepted functional classification is dependent on accurate patient reporting and is influenced by the extent of tolerance of symptoms. Patients are classified into four grades according to the level of physical activity at which angina is experienced (Table 4.5).

The diagnosis of chronic stable angina can usually be made with a degree of confidence based on the clinical history. The probability of angina is supported by the presence of risk factors that predispose to atherosclerosis. Non-modifiable risk factors include advanced age, male gender and a positive family history of CAD (in first-degree relatives aged <60 years). The identification of modifiable risk factors such as hypercholesterolemia, smoking, hypertension, diabetes mellitus and prior documented CAD not only lends weight to the diagnosis, but will also be influential in prognosis and long-term management.

ESTABLISHING THE DIAGNOSIS

Several non-invasive investigations are used to confirm the diagnosis of CAD and to identify patients at increased risk.[44]

- A resting ECG should always be recorded, although this may be entirely normal in half of the patients with chronic stable angina. The most common abnormalities are non-specific ST T wave changes and Q waves suggestive of previous MI. Other abnormalities include left bundle branch block, conduction disturbances and arrhythmias.
- Exercise electrocardiography is the most widely used non-invasive test for the assessment of myocardial ischemia and involves recording the 12-lead ECG before, during and after exercise on a treadmill or bicycle ergometer. The test consists of a standardized incremental increase in external workload while the patient's ECG, symptoms and blood pressure are continuously monitored. Performance is usually symptom limited, and the test is discontinued upon evidence of chest discomfort, severe shortness of breath, dizziness, fatigue, ST-segment depression of greater than 0.2 mV (2 mm), a fall in blood pressure exceeding 10 mmHg, or the development of a ventricular tachyarrhythmia. There are a number of treadmill protocols available, and the Bruce protocol is by far the most common (Table 4.6).[45] The interpretation of the results is based on ECG changes (notably ST-segment shift), the provocation of symptoms during exercise, exercise capacity and hemodynamic changes. The Duke treadmill score (Table 4.7) is a simple quantitative score that can improve the test's prognostic accuracy when it is considered in conjunction with data from the clinical evaluation, the results of coronary angiography and the ejection fraction.[46] It is important to note that the exercise stress test is an inappropriate test for ischemic heart disease when used in isolation. In a population with a low prevalence of ischemic heart disease, the false-positive rate is high, particularly in the absence of symptoms. The false-positive rate is also higher in younger individuals and in women.

Table 4.6 *Bruce protocol*

Stage	Speed (mph)	Gradient (%)	Time (min)	Cumulative time (min)
1	1.7	10	3	3
2	2.5	12	3	6
3	3.4	14	3	9
4	4.2	16	3	12
5	5.0	18	3	15
6	5.5	20	3	18

Table 4.7 *Duke treadmill score*

Duration of exercise in minutes − (5 × the maximal net
ST-segment deviation during or after exercise, in mm) −
(4 × the treadmill angina index)
The angina index is assigned:
  0 if angina is absent during exercise
  1 if typical angina occurs during exercise
  2 if angina is the reason the patient stopped exercise

- Stress echocardiography is useful in the evaluation of patients with CAD by assessing changes in left ventricular dimensions and regional wall motion abnormalities before and immediately after exercise. It has better sensitivity and specificity than exercise ECG but requires highly trained operators. It can also identify the presence of left ventricular hypertrophy, associated valve abnormalities and those patients with left ventricular dysfunction or hibernating myocardium who would potentially benefit from coronary revascularization.
- The sensitivity and specificity of treadmill exercise testing for the detection of CAD can be enhanced by the addition of myocardial perfusion imaging. This is particularly helpful in diagnosing ischemic heart disease in those individuals who have equivocal exercise ECG changes, abnormal resting ECG, suspected false-positive or false-negative exercise ECG, or submaximal exercise tolerance. It also assists in identifying the territory of ischemia in patients with multivessel disease for revascularization (see Chapter 6).
- Ischemia can be provoked with pharmacological agents followed by either myocardial perfusion scanning or echocardiography. Dobutamine is a positive inotropic agent that provokes ischemia by increasing myocardial work, whereas adenosine and dipyridamole are vasodilators that unmask coronary stenosis by causing relative increases in flow in coronary arteries that are not diseased as well as increases in cardiac work.

THERAPEUTIC MANAGEMENT

The principles of medical management of angina are to alleviate the symptoms of angina, establish the risk for future acute coronary events and modify disease progression (including risk factor modification and revascularization).

Pharmacological treatment of chronic stable angina can be divided into anti-ischemic therapy and measures of secondary prevention. There are four classes of anti-ischemic agents: β-adrenoceptor antagonists, nitrates, calcium-channel antagonists and potassium-channel activators. These drugs are equally efficacious and there is no convincing evidence that one class is clinically superior to another.[47] However, β-adrenoceptor antagonists should usually be initiated first, if tolerated, due to the inferred benefits of secondary prevention. If a single drug does not control the anginal symptoms, the introduction of a second agent often provides significant benefits. However, there is scarce evidence to support the addition of multiple anti-anginal therapies in those that remain symptomatic. They should be considered for revascularization. The targets of secondary prevention include lipid lowering with statins,[48] antiplatelet treatment with aspirin[25] and/or clopidogrel,[49] and angiotensin-converting enzyme (ACE) inhibitors.[50] The symptomatic management of patients with chronic stable angina should also include a rehabilitation process that encompasses patient education, exercise and vocational advice. Patients enrolled in exercise and rehabilitation programmes have fewer cardiovascular events as well as better cardiorespiratory fitness and vocational status.[51]

Risk stratification is an essential part of the management of a patient with chronic stable angina and this includes clinical and non-invasive indicators of risks. The principal factors determining risks are the same as those for the longer term risk of ACS (age, hypertension, diabetes, evidence of ischemia, left ventricular dysfunction and the extent of CAD). A number of risk scoring systems have been developed that incorporate both clinical characteristics and non-invasive investigations. Patients who are considered to be at high risk of future cardiac events, or those who have limiting angina despite medical therapy, should be considered for coronary angiography with a view to coronary revascularization. This is discussed further in Chapter 9.

Lifestyle and risk factor modifications are integral parts of, and complementary to, the treatment of patients and this is discussed further in Chapter 25.

IMPAIRED LEFT VENTRICULAR FUNCTION

Patients with CAD frequently present with symptoms of CHF. Dyspnea on activity or chronic fatigue may be the predominant feature of impaired left ventricular function caused by myocardial ischemia, left ventricular aneurysm or mitral regurgitation associated with papillary muscle dysfunction.

Table 4.8 *New York Heart Association functional classification of symptoms*

Class 1	Cardiac disease without symptoms on ordinary effort
Class 2	Minor limitation of activity by symptoms
Class 3	Marked limitation of activity by symptoms
Class 4	Symptoms at rest or on minimal exertion

Congestive heart failure is predominantly characterized by impaired left ventricular systolic function leading to diminished cardiac output and reserve. A minority of patients exhibit isolated diastolic dysfunction. CHF induces neurohumoral reflexes, principally involving the sympathetic nervous system and renin–angiotensin–aldosterone system, with consequent increases in peripheral vascular resistance and water and sodium reabsorption. A well-accepted classification system has been proposed by the New York Heart Association (NYHA) (Table 4.8).[52]

Congestive heart failure is associated with high morbidity and mortality, with a 30–50% 1-year survival for advanced heart failure (NYHA class IV) and a 45–50% 5-year survival in less severe cases (NYHA class II–III).[53,54] Although the incidence of most cardiovascular disorders has declined in Western countries in the past 10–20 years, the prevalence and incidence of CHF are increasing and it currently affects 1–2% of the general population.[56] The initial Framingham Study indicated that hypertension was the most common cause of CHF,[57] but more effective treatment of hypertension in the last three decades has resulted in CAD emerging as the predominant cause of CHF.[58]

In patients with CAD and stable angina, scattered myocardial fibrosis, previous MI or non-contractile ischemic (hibernating) myocardium may lead to left ventricular dysfunction. Although patients may initially present with angina, the symptoms of cardiac failure can become more prominent as fibrous scars replace ischemic myocardium. Left ventricular dilatation (remodeling) is common. CHF may appear immediately after an extensive acute MI, or may present some years later as left ventricular function gradually deteriorates. In approximately 15% of patients who survive MI, the infarcted ventricular wall may progressively expand over several weeks, resulting in a thinned fibrous ventricular aneurysm. As a consequence, the myocardium expands paradoxically in systole, and ventricular contraction becomes ineffective, causing symptoms of heart failure as well as angina and tachyarrhythmias.

Mitral regurgitation may be an acute and dramatic complication of MI secondary to rupture of the papillary muscles, causing massive regurgitation and acute cardiac failure. Chronic mitral regurgitation is more commonly caused by papillary muscle dysfunction due to ischemia or fibrosis in patients with evidence of previous MI.

Treatment is aimed at improving the symptoms, enhancing survival and delaying the progression of CHF. Diuretics are well established in the treatment of CHF and act by relieving the symptoms through the induction of natriuresis and decreasing pulmonary congestion. In the Vasodilator Heart Failure Trial I (V-HeFT-I), the combination of nitrates and hydralazine was shown to be beneficial in improving the survival and exercise tolerance in patients with CHF.[59] ACE inhibitors such as enalapril were subsequently shown to be associated with a greater improvement in survival than nitrates and hydralazine, and are now considered the first-line treatment.[60] However, the underlying mechanism is still not completely understood and may be related to afterload reduction, blocking the effects of angiotensin on resistance vessels or angiotensin II on myocardial hypertrophy and fibrosis. Digoxin, a positive inotrope, does not appear to influence survival, but its use is associated with a decrease in hospitalization rate.[61] Two major advances in the treatment of CHF are the addition of spironolactone and β-adrenoceptor antagonists such as bisoprolol and carvedilol in combination with ACE inhibitors.[62–64] Both have been shown to attenuate disease progression by reducing hospitalization, symptomatology and mortality. β-Adrenoceptor antagonists should be introduced with caution in patients with CHF, and never in the acute decompensated phase. The initial dose should be low and progressively titrated upwards.

In spite of these advances, the outlook for patients with ischemic CHF treated medically remains poor and the prognosis is worse for those with associated ventricular arrhythmias. However, patients whose CHF is due to hibernating myocardium associated with reversible ischemia have better outcomes following revascularization. Therefore these patients should be identified and considered for coronary revascularization where possible.[65] In patients with large left ventricular aneurysms, surgical aneurysmectomy, sometimes combined with coronary artery bypass grafting, may lead to improvement in symptoms of cardiac failure or even angina. Left ventricular function and exercise capacity have also been reported to improve following aneurysmectomy. Patients with papillary rupture also require immediate surgery where possible. Finally, in suitable patients with refractory symptoms, cardiac transplantation may be considered.

SYNDROME X (MICROVASCULAR ANGINA)

The term syndrome X is often used to describe the clinical presentation of typical angina-like chest pains, positive exercise tolerance tests, but normal coronary angiograms. Patients in this category probably represent a heterogeneous group with a variety of cardiac as well as non-cardiac pathology. They should be differentiated from patients with CAD because their long-term survival is not adversely affected, although they may have an impaired quality of life and many develop recurrent chest pain in spite of therapy.[66] Management is often difficult and any intervention is unlikely to improve outcome because the prognosis is good. Therefore the aim is relief of symptoms and improvement in quality of life. It is important to rule out any extracardiac and treatable causes of pain. The currently available therapeutic agents for cardiac syndrome X are β-adrenoceptor antagonists, calcium-channel antagonists and nitrates.[67] However, clinical response is variable and not always sustained. In post-menopausal women, hormone replacement therapy should also be considered for symptomatic relief.

VARIANT ANGINA

Originally described in 1959, Prinzmetal angina or variant angina is an unusual syndrome of myocardial ischemia that occurs almost exclusively at rest, is not precipitated by physical or emotional exertion, and is associated with ST-segment elevation on the ECG.[68] The underlying mechanism has been demonstrated to be focal coronary artery spasm and may result in localized myocardial perfusion and functional abnormalities and ECG changes. The syndrome may occur in normal or diseased coronary arteries, and the site of spasm may be adjacent to atherosclerotic plaques. The key to diagnosis in these patients is documented transient ST elevation on ECG at the time of chest pain. Coronary angiography may demonstrate significant fixed proximal coronary obstruction of at least one major vessel in the majority of patients, and different provocation tests for coronary spasm have been developed. Management is usually with high-dose calcium-channel antagonists and long-acting nitrates. The prognosis for variant angina is good, although this is also dependent on the extent and severity of the underlying CAD.

KEY REFERENCES

Bertrand ME, Simoons ML, Fox KA, Wallentin LC, Hamm CW, McFadden E, *et al.* Management of acute coronary syndromes: acute coronary syndromes without persistent ST segment elevation; recommendations of the Task Force of the European Society of Cardiology. *Eur Heart J* 2000; **21**:1406–32.

This is a detailed guideline on the management of patients with suspected acute coronary syndromes without persistent ST-segment elevation based upon a comprehensive review of evidence from clinical trials.

Fox KA, Goodman SG, Klein W, Brieger D, Steg PG, Dabbous O, *et al.* Management of acute coronary syndromes. Variations in practice and outcome: findings from Global Registry of Acute Coronary Events (GRACE). *Eur Heart J* 2002; **23**:1177–89.

The GRACE project provides important and extensive insights into patient demographic and clinical characteristics, current practice patterns, and outcomes for patients with acute coronary syndromes from a number of countries throughout the world. The results of GRACE provide a multinational perspective on these important outcomes and identify practice variations that will allow new opportunities to improve patient care.

Lee TH, Boucher CA. Noninvasive tests in patients with stable coronary artery disease. *N Engl J Med* 2001; **344**:1840–5.

This is a brief review of the strategies and evidence for non-invasive investigations in patients with stable coronary artery disease that include exercise electrocardiography, radionuclide imaging and stress echocardiography.

The American Heart Association in collaboration with the International Liaison Committee on Resuscitation. Guidelines 2000 for Cardiopulmonary Resuscitation and Emergency Cardiovascular Care. Part 6: Advanced Cardiovascular Life Support: 7C: A guide to the International ACLS Algorithms. *Circulation* 2000; **102** (8 Suppl.):I142–57.

The International Advanced Cardiovascular Life Support (ACLS) Algorithm represents a groundbreaking effort to unify and simplify the essential information of adult ACLS and demonstrates the integration of the steps of basic life support, early defibrillation and ACLS.

Van de Werf F, Ardissino D, Betriu A, Cokkinos DV, Falk E, Fox KA, *et al.* Management of acute myocardial infarction in patients presenting with ST-segment elevation. *Eur Heart J* 2003; **24**:28–66.

The new guidelines from the European Society of Cardiology provide a detailed and updated review of the management of acute myocardial infarction and have attempted to define which treatment strategies are based upon unequivocal evidence and which are open to genuine differences of opinion.

REFERENCES

1. Sytkowski PA, Kannel WB, D'Agostino RB. Changes in risk factors and the decline in mortality from cardiovascular disease. The Framingham Heart Study. *N Engl J Med* 1990; 322:1635–41.
2. Tunstall-Pedoe H, Kuulasmaa K, Mahonen M, Tolonen H, Ruokokoski E, Amouyel P, for the WHO MONICA Project. Contribution of trends in survival and coronary event-rates to

changes in coronary heart disease mortality: 10-year results from 37 WHO MONICA Project populations. *Lancet* 1999; **353**:1547–57.

3. WHO. *The World Health Report 1998. Life in the 21st Century – a Vision for All.* Geneva: WHO, 1998.

4. Tunstall-Pedoe H, Vanuzzo D, Hobbs M, Mahonen M, Cepaitis Z, Kuulasmaa K, *et al.* Estimation of contribution of changes in coronary care to improving survival, event rates, and coronary heart disease mortality across the WHO MONICA Project populations. *Lancet* 2000; **355**:688–700.

5. Davies MJ. The pathophysiology of acute coronary syndromes. *Heart* 2000; **83**:361–6.

6. Theroux P, Lidon RM. Unstable angina: pathogenesis, diagnosis, and treatment. *Curr Probl Cardiol* 1993; **18**:157–231.

7. Fox KA, Cokkinos DV, Deckers J, Keil U, Maggioni A, Steg G. The ENACT study: a pan-European survey of acute coronary syndromes. European Network for Acute Coronary Treatment. *Eur Heart J* 2000; **21**:1440–9.

8. Detailed diagnoses, and procedures, National Hospital Discharge Survey 1996. National Center for Health Statistics. *Vital Health Stat* 1998; **13**:138.

9. Fox KA, Goodman SG, Klein W, Brieger D, Steg PG, Dabbous O, *et al.* Management of acute coronary syndromes. Variations in practice and outcome: findings from Global Registry of Acute Coronary Events (GRACE). *Eur Heart J* 2002; **23**:1177–89.

10. Yusuf S, Flather M, Pogue J, Hunt D, Varigos J, Piegas L, *et al.* Variations between countries in invasive cardiac procedures and outcomes in patients with suspected unstable angina or myocardial infarction without initial ST elevation. OASIS (Organisation to Assess Strategies for Ischemic Syndromes) Registry Investigators. *Lancet* 1998; **352**:507–14.

11. Collinson J, Flather MD, Fox KA, Findlay I, Rodrigues E, Dooley P, *et al.* Clinical outcomes, risk stratification and practice patterns of unstable angina and myocardial infarction without ST elevation: Prospective Registry of Acute Ischemic Syndromes in the UK (PRAIS-UK). *Eur Heart J* 2000; **21**:1450–7.

12. Campeau L. Grading of angina pectoris. *Circulation* 1976; **55**:522–3.

13. Fox KA. Coronary disease. Acute coronary syndromes: presentation – clinical spectrum and management. *Heart* 2000; **84**:93–100.

14. Newby DE, Fox KA, Flint LL, Boon NA. A 'same day' direct-access chest pain clinic: improved management and reduced hospitalization. *QJM* 1998; **91**:333–7.

15. The Global Use of Strategies to Open Occluded Coronary Arteries (GUSTO) IIb investigators. A comparison of recombinant hirudin with heparin for the treatment of acute coronary syndromes. *N Engl J Med* 1996; **335**:775–82.

16. Braunwald E. Unstable angina. A classification. *Circulation* 1989; **80**:410–14.

17. Hamm CW, Braunwald E. A classification of unstable angina revisited. *Circulation* 2000; **102**:118–22.

18. Hamm CW, Goldmann BU, Heeschen C, Kreymann G, Berger J, Meinertz T. Emergency room triage of patients with acute chest pain by means of rapid testing for cardiac troponin T or troponin I. *N Engl J Med* 1997; **337**:1648–53.

19. Antman EM, Tanasijevic MJ, Thompson B, Schactman M, McCabe CH, Cannon CP, *et al.* Cardiac-specific troponin I levels to predict the risk of mortality in patients with acute coronary syndromes. *N Engl J Med* 1996; **335**:1342–9.

20. Lindahl B, Venge P, Wallentin L. The FRISC experience with troponin T. Use as decision tool and comparison with other prognostic markers. *Eur Heart J* 1998; **19**(Suppl. N):N51–8.

21. Toss H, Lindahl B, Siegbahn A, Wallentin L. Prognostic influence of increased fibrinogen and C-reactive protein levels in unstable coronary artery disease. FRISC Study Group. Fragmin during Instability in Coronary Artery Disease. *Circulation* 1997; **96**:4204–10.

22. Biasucci LM, Liuzzo G, Fantuzzi G, Caligiuri G, Rebuzzi AG, Ginnetti F, *et al.* Increasing levels of interleukin (IL)-1Ra and IL-6 during the first 2 days of hospitalization in unstable angina are associated with increased risk of in-hospital coronary events. *Circulation* 1999; **99**:2079–84.

23. Fragmin and Fast Revascularisation during InStability in Coronary Artery Disease Investigators. Invasive compared with non-invasive treatment in unstable coronary-artery disease: FRISC II prospective randomised multicentre study. *Lancet* 1999; **354**:708–15.

24. Wallentin L, Lagerqvist B, Husted S, Kontny F, Stahle E, Swahn E. Outcome at 1 year after an invasive compared with a non-invasive strategy in unstable coronary-artery disease: the FRISC II invasive randomised trial. FRISC II Investigators. Fast Revascularisation during Instability in Coronary Artery Disease. *Lancet* 2000; **356**:9–16.

25. Antiplatelet Trialists' Collaboration. Collaborative overview of randomised trials of antiplatelet therapy – I: Prevention of death, myocardial infarction, and stroke by prolonged antiplatelet therapy in various categories of patients. *BMJ* 1994; **308**:81–106.

26. Yusuf S, Zhao F, Mehta SR, Chrolavicius S, Tognoni G, Fox KA. Effects of clopidogrel in addition to aspirin in patients with acute coronary syndromes without ST-segment elevation. *N Engl J Med* 2001; **345**:494–502.

27. Klootwijk P, Meij S, Melkert R, Lenderink T, Simoons ML. Reduction of recurrent ischemia with abciximab during continuous ECG-ischemia monitoring in patients with unstable angina refractory to standard treatment (CAPTURE). *Circulation* 1998; **98**:1358–64.

28. FRISC Study Group. Low-molecular-weight heparin during instability in coronary artery disease, Fragmin during Instability in Coronary Artery Disease (FRISC) Study Group. *Lancet* 1996; **347**:561–8.

29. Yusuf S, Witte J, Friedman L. Overview of results of randomized trials in heart disease: unstable angina, heart failure, primary prevention with aspirin and risk factor modifications. *JAMA* 1988; **260**:2259–63.

30. Bertrand ME, Simoons ML, Fox KA, Wallentin LC, Hamm CW, McFadden E, *et al.* Management of acute coronary syndromes: acute coronary syndromes without persistent ST segment elevation; recommendations of the Task Force of the European Society of Cardiology. *Eur Heart J* 2000; **21**:1406–32.

31. Braunwald E, Antman EM, Beasley JW, Califf RM, Cheitlin MD, Hochman JS, *et al.* ACC/AHA guidelines for the management of patients with unstable angina and non-ST-segment elevation myocardial infarction. A report of the American College of Cardiology/American Heart Association Task Force on Practice Guidelines (Committee on the Management of Patients With Unstable Angina). *J Am Coll Cardiol* 2000; **36**:970–1062.

32. Norris RM, Caughey DE, Mercer CJ, Scott PJ. Prognosis after myocardial infarction. Six-year follow-up. *Br Heart J* 1974; **36**:786–90.

33. Kannel WB, Cupples LA. Silent myocardial infarction. Incidence, prevalence and prognostic significance. In: *Silent Myocardial Ischemia and Angina. Prevalence, Prognostic and Therapeutic Significance*, Singh BN (ed.). New York: Pergamon Press, 1988, 174–82.

34. O'Connor GT, Buring JE, Yusuf S, Goldhaber SZ, Olmstead EM, Paffenbarger RS Jr, *et al.* An overview of randomized trials of rehabilitation with exercise after myocardial infarction. *Circulation* 1989; **80**:234–44.

35. Van de Werf F, Ardissino D, Betriu A, Cokkinos DV, Falk E, Fox KA, *et al.* Management of acute myocardial infarction in patients presenting with ST-segment elevation. *Eur Heart J* 2003; **24**:28–66.

36. Ryan TJ, Antman EM, Brooks NH, Califf RM, Hillis LD, Hiratzka LF, *et al.* 1999 update: ACC/AHA Guidelines for the Management of Patients With Acute Myocardial Infarction: Executive Summary

and Recommendations: A report of the American College of Cardiology/American Heart Association Task Force on Practice Guidelines (Committee on Management of Acute Myocardial Infarction). *Circulation* 1999; **100**:1016–30.

37. Kannel WB, Thomas HE. Sudden coronary death: the Framingham study. *Ann NY Acad Sci* 1982; **382**:3.

38. The American Heart Association in collaboration with the International Liaison Committee on Resuscitation. Guidelines 2000 for Cardiopulmonary Resuscitation and Emergency Cardiovascular Care. Part 6: Advanced Cardiovascular Life Support: 7C: A guide to the International ACLS Algorithms. *Circulation* 2000; **102**(8 Suppl.): I142–57.

39. de Latorre F, Nolan J, Robertson C, Chamberlain D, Baskett P, European Resuscitation Council. European Resuscitation Council Guidelines 2000 for Adult Advanced Life Support. A statement from the Advanced Life Support Working Group (1) and approved by the Executive Committee of the European Resuscitation Council. *Resuscitation* 2001; **48**:211–21.

40. Cannon PJ, Connell PA, Stockley IH, Garner ST, Hampton JR. Prevalence of angina as assessed by a survey of prescriptions for nitrates. *Lancet* 1988; **1**:979–81.

41. Gandhi MM, Lampe FC, Wood DA. Incidence, clinical characteristics, and short-term prognosis of angina pectoris. *Br Heart J* 1995; **73**:193–8.

42. Maseri A. *Ischemic Heart Disease*. New York: Churchill Livingstone, 1995.

43. Cox J, Naylor CD. The Canadian Cardiovascular Society grading scale for angina pectoris: is it time for refinements? *Ann Intern Med* 1992; **117**:677–83.

44. Lee TH, Boucher CA. Noninvasive tests in patients with stable coronary artery disease. *N Engl J Med* 2001; **344**:1840–5.

45. Bruce RA. Exercise testing of patients with coronary heart disease. *Ann Clin Res* 1971; **3**:323–32.

46. Mark DB, Shaw L, Harrell FE Jr, Hlatky MA, Lee KL, Bengtson JR, *et al*. Prognostic value of a treadmill exercise score in outpatients with suspected coronary artery disease. *N Engl J Med* 1991; **325**:849–53.

47. Heidenreich PA, McDonald KM, Hastie T, Fadel B, Hagan V, Lee BK, *et al*. Meta-analysis of trials comparing beta-blockers, calcium antagonists, and nitrates for stable angina. *J Am Med Asoc* 1999; **281**:1927–36.

48. The West of Scotland Coronary Prevention Study Group. West of Scotland Coronary Prevention Study: identification of high-risk groups and comparison with other cardiovascular intervention trials. *Lancet* 1996; **348**:1339–42.

49. CAPRIE Steering Committee. A randomised, blinded, trial of clopidogrel versus aspirin in patients at risk of ischemic events (CAPRIE). *Lancet* 1996; **348**:1329–39.

50. Dagenais GR, Yusuf S, Bourassa MG, Yi Q, Bosch J, Lonn EM, *et al*. Effects of ramipril on coronary events in high-risk persons: results of the Heart Outcomes Prevention Evaluation Study. *Circulation* 2001; **104**:522–6.

51. Dugmore LD, Tipson RJ, Phillips MH, Flint EJ, Stentiford NH, Bone MF, *et al*. Changes in cardiorespiratory fitness, psychological wellbeing, quality of life, and vocational status following a 12 month cardiac exercise rehabilitation programme. *Heart* 1999; **81**:359–66.

52. Criteria Committee of the New York Heart Association. *Nomenclature and Criteria for Diagnosis of Diseases of the Heart and Great Vessels*, 7th edn. Boston: New York Heart Association/Little, Brown Co., 1973.

53. Wilson JR, Schwartz JS, Sutton MS, Ferraro N, Horowitz LN, Reichek N, *et al*. Prognosis in severe heart failure: relation to hemodynamic measurements and ventricular ectopic activity. *J Am Coll Cardiol* 1983; **2**:403–10.

54. Garg R, Yusuf S. Overview of randomized trials of angiotensin-converting enzyme inhibitors on mortality and morbidity in patients with heart failure. Collaborative Group on ACE Inhibitor Trials. *JAMA* 1995; **273**:1450–6.

55. Ghali JK, Cooper R, Ford E. Trends in hospitalization rates for heart failure in the United States, 1973–1986. Evidence for increasing population prevalence. *Arch Intern Med* 1990; **150**:769–73.

56. Wheeldon NM, MacDonald TM, Flucker CJ, McKendrick AD, McDevitt DG, Struthers AD. Echocardiography in chronic heart failure in the community. *Q J Med* 1993; **86**:17–23.

57. Smith WM. Epidemiology of congestive heart failure. *Am J Cardiol* 1985; **55**:3–8A.

58. Rodeheffer RJ, Jacobsen SJ, Gersh BJ, Kottke TE, McCann HA, Bailey KR, *et al*. The incidence and prevalence of congestive heart failure in Rochester, Minnesota. *Mayo Clin Proc* 1993; **68**:1143–50.

59. Cohn JN, Archibald DG, Ziesche S, Franciosa JA, Harston WE, Tristani FE, *et al*. Effect of vasodilator therapy on mortality in chronic congestive heart failure. Results of a Veterans Administration Cooperative Study. *N Engl J Med* 1986; **314**:1547–52.

60. The Task Force of the Working Group on Heart Failure of the European Society of Cardiology: the treatment of heart failure: guidelines. *Eur Heart J* 1997; **18**:736–53.

61. The Digitalis Investigation Group. The effect of digoxin on mortality and morbidity in patients with heart failure. *N Engl J Med* 1997; **336**:525–33.

62. Pitt B, Zannad F, Remme WJ, Cody R, Castaigne A, Perez A, *et al*. The effect of spironolactone on morbidity and mortality in patients with severe heart failure. Randomized Aldactone Evaluation Study Investigators. *N Engl J Med* 1999; **341**:709–17.

63. CIBIS II Investigators and Committees. The Cardiac Insufficiency Bisoprolol Study II (CIBIS-II): a randomised trial. *Lancet* 1999; **353**:9–13.

64. Packer M, Bristow MR, Cohn JN, Colucci WS, Fowler MB, Gilbert EM, *et al*. The effect of carvedilol on morbidity and mortality in patients with chronic heart failure. US Carvedilol Heart Failure Study Group. *N Engl J Med* 1996; **334**:1349–55.

65. Kron IL, Flanagan TL, Blackbourne LH, Schroeder RA, Nolan SP. Coronary revascularization rather than cardiac transplantation for chronic ischemic cardiomyopathy. *Ann Surg* 1989; **210**:348–52.

66. Kemp HG Jr, Vokonas PS, Cohn PF, Gorlin R. The anginal syndrome associated with normal coronary arteriograms. Report of a six year experience. *Am J Med* 1973; **54**:735–42.

67. Kaski JC, Valenzuela Garcia LF. Therapeutic options for the management of patients with cardiac syndrome X. *Eur Heart J* 2001; **22**:283–93.

68. Prinzmetal M, Kennamer R, Merliss R, Wada T, Bor N. Angina pectoris. I. A variant form of angina pectoris: preliminary report. *Am J Med* 1959; **27**:375–88.

5

Coronary angiography

RJ CHAMBERS AND MH AL-BUSTAMI

Detailed knowledge of the anatomy of the coronary arterial circulation and of the more common variants is an essential prerequisite for the diagnosis and treatment of all patients with known or suspected heart disease, whether this is related to the vessels themselves, the myocardium, the valves or the pericardium. Newer non-invasive techniques, including three-dimensional reconstruction of computerized tomography-acquired data and magnetic resonance imaging, are equally dependent on this awareness, and optimal results from both cardiological and surgical interventions can only be achieved using this knowledge.

NORMAL CORONARY ANATOMY

The coronary circulation consists of two main coronary arteries, which arise as the first branches from the proximal part of the ascending aorta, with subdivision into smaller vessels and capillaries within the myocardium. Venous drainage occurs into the coronary veins and then the coronary sinus, which subsequently drains into the right atrium.[1,2]

The two arteries are the right and left coronary arteries, the right vessel providing the arterial supply to the two right heart chambers, together with the inferior part of the interventricular septum and a variable part of the adjacent infero-lateral left ventricular free wall. By contrast, the left coronary artery supplies the left ventricle almost exclusively, including the septum, with the exception of very small vessels passing to the anterior right ventricular wall from the mid-section of the left anterior descending artery (Figure 5.1).

A numeric system for the identification of the major segments and branches of the coronary arterial tree is illustrated in Figure 5.2. The nomenclature was modified from the system used in the Coronary Artery Surgery Study (CASS), and used in the Bypass Angioplasty Revascularization (BARI).[3] By tradition, the coronary artery that gives rise to the posterior descending (also known as the posterior interventricular) artery is known as the dominant coronary artery; in approximately 85% of cases, the right coronary artery (RCA) is dominant. Thus, although the RCA is called the *dominant* vessel, this term defines a specific anatomical configuration, and the left coronary artery still provides 80% of blood supply to the left ventricle. In 8% of individuals, the posterior descending artery arises from the circumflex branch of the left coronary artery, called a left dominant coronary system. In the remaining 7%, the right and circumflex vessels both give rise to small vessels variably supplying different parts of the inferior septum, and this is termed a co-dominant or balanced coronary circulation.

Both coronary arteries arise from the aortic sinuses, the right from the right anterior sinus and the left from the left anterior sinus, with the remaining posterior non-coronary sinus lying inferior to the other two sinuses. Usually these vessels arise within the sinus, just below the sino-tubular junction, and midway between the commissures. Considerable variation occurs, however, even in the absence of other congenital variants, with the vessels occasionally arising above the level of the sino-tubular junction and sometimes close to one of the commissures, when these vessels will occasionally have an oblique course through the aortic wall, which has been associated with diffuse narrowing of this intramural segment.[3]

Rarely, an arc of tissue has been described along the superior margin of these arteries arising ectopically from the aortic root. Awareness of these variations is particularly important for the angiographer.

The main RCA passes from its origin in the right sinus of Valsalva anteriorly, to the right, and in a cephalad direction for a short distance to pass beneath the right atrial appendage, and then passes rightward directly into the right atrioventricular groove. The vessel then descends vertically within the atrioventricular groove towards the right or acute margin of the heart, and then curves round within the groove to reach the crux of the heart posteriorly, which represents the junction between the right and left atrioventricular rings and the interventricular septum. At this point, the artery divides into two branches, one

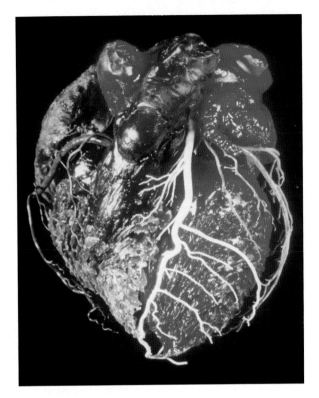

Figure 5.1 *Cast of heart chambers with coronary arteries showing anterior aspect of the heart. The right coronary artery (green) lies between the right atrium (purple) and right ventricle (blue), giving off the acute marginal branch before disappearing around the right margin of the heart to the back. The anterior descending artery (white) lies between the right ventricle (blue) and left ventricle (red), giving rise to septal branches between the ventricles and diagonal branches over the anterior aspect of the left ventricle. The circumflex artery (yellow) lies between the left atrium and left ventricle and gives rise to lateral branches over the left side of the left ventricle. Reproduced with permission from Clinical Cardiac Anatomy I: Allwork SP. Angiographic anatomy. In:* Slide Atlas of Cardiac Anatomy, *Vol. 7, Anderson RH, Becker AE (eds). London: Gower Medical Publishing Ltd, 1980, 75.*

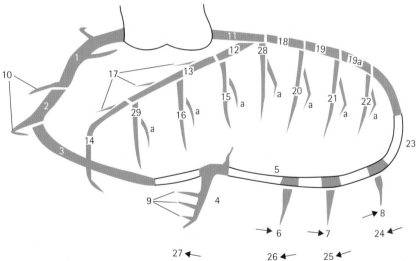

Figure 5.2 *The Bypass Angioplasty Revascularization Investigation coronary artery map. Right coronary artery: 1 = proximal; 2 = middle; 3 = distal; 4 = posterior descending; 5 = right postero-atrioventricular; 6 = first postero-lateral; 7 = second postero-lateral; 8 = third postero-lateral; 9 = inferior septal artery; 10 = acute marginal artery. Left coronay artery: 11 = left main; 12 = proximal left anterior descending; 13 = middle left anterior descending; 14 = distal left anterior descending; 15 = first diagonal; 15a = first diagonal branch; 16 = second diagonal; 16a = second diagonal branch; 17 = anterior septals; 18 = proximal circumflex; 19 = middle circumflex; 19a = distal circumflex; 20, 21, 22 = first, second and third obtuse marginal; 20a, 21a, 22a = first, second and third obtuse marginal branches; 23 = left atrioventricular; 24, 25, 26 = first, second and third postero-laterals; 27 = left posterior descending; 28 = ramus; 28a = ramus branch; 29 = third diagonal; 29a = third diagonal branch. (From: Protocol for the Bypass Angioplasty Revascularization Investigation.* Circulation *1991; 84[Suppl. V]:V1–27.)*

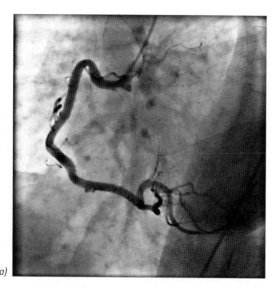
(a)

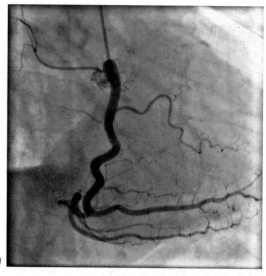
(b)

Figure 5.3 (a) The right coronary artery, LAO view. This view is interpreted as though the observer were looking at the heart from the apex towards the base. Characteristically, the right artery has a 'reversed D-shape'. The angiography catheter can be seen in the descending aorta on the right and helps orientation. (b) The right coronary artery, same patient as in (a), RAO view. This view is interpreted as though the observer were looking from the right anterior chest at the heart with the apex on the right and the atria towards the left. The main course of the right artery lies between the right atrium and right ventricle.

descending as the posterior interventricular (or posterior descending) artery for a variable distance towards the apex, and the second branch (left ventricular branch) continuing along the posterior left groove, taking an inverted U-shaped course to form a small loop. From the apex of this loop one or more small vessels arise to supply the atrioventricular node. The artery then divides into two or more branches (postero-lateral branches) to supply the adjacent infero-lateral left ventricular free wall (Figure 5.3).

For descriptive purposes, the RCA is arbitrarily divided into three segments. The proximal segment extends from the origin in the right aortic sinus to the beginning of the atrioventricular groove, and the middle segment of the vessel continues in the groove to the acute margin of the right ventricle. The distal third is the remainder of the vessel to the crux and beyond. The branches arising from each of these segments are fairly constant in their presence and distribution, although varying in size and sequence of origin, with the influence of dominance mainly confined to the distal third of the vessel.

The first branch from the proximal RCA in over 50% of cases is the branch to the right atrium and sinoatrial node, known as the sinoatrial node artery (see Figure 5.3b). This arises from the proximal third and passes cephalad beneath the right atrial appendage along the anterior wall of the right atrium to reach the interatrial septum, and then ascends to encircle the superior vena cava at the junction with the right atrium and to supply the sinoatrial node. A branch often extends to the crista

venticularis of the right ventricle from this point. This vessel arises from the RCA in the majority of cases, but arises from the proximal part of the main circumflex artery in 35% of cases.[5] The second branch arising from the RCA is the infundibular or conal branch. This may arise proximal to the sinoatrial branch, or may originate as an independent artery from the right aortic sinus in nearly 50% of cases. In this instance it is often not seen on the angiographic study due to its small size as an independent artery. Whichever the site of origin, the right conus branch passes anteriorly over the right ventricular outflow tract, which is also supplied by a conal branch from the proximal left anterior descending artery. The close proximity of the branches of these vessels provides a potential site for collateral flow in the event of obstructive coronary disease in the respective vessel of origin, and is known as the 'arc of Vieussens'.[6]

Beyond the origin of these two important branches (the sinoatrial nodal branch and the conal branch to the infundibulum) there is a variable number of relatively small vessels that arise from the mid-third of the main RCA and pass anteriorly to supply the free wall of the right ventricle. At the acute margin, a more constant and large right ventricular branch arises and passes along the acute margin of the right ventricle towards the apex. This acute marginal branch often reaches the apex, supplying the free wall of the right ventricle (Figure 5.4). When this vessel is large, the other right ventricular branches are reciprocally small, or even absent, and *vice versa*. Beyond the acute margin, the main RCA curves round in the atrioventricular

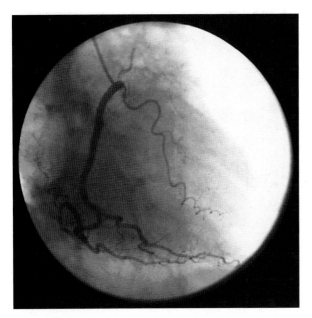

Figure 5.4 *Right coronary artery, RAO view. The conal branch is a narrow but extensive branch. There is a large acute marginal branch running to the apex. The posterior descending artery is of smaller caliber.*

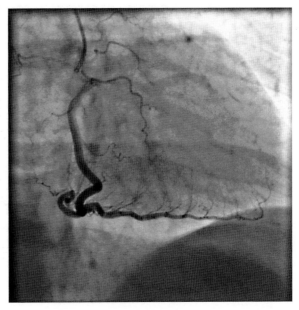

Figure 5.5 *Right coronary artery, RAO view. This late phase shows the posterior descending artery well with its inferior septal branches.*

groove to the crux, forming the third segment of the vessel. No constant large branches arise between the acute margin and the crux, which is identified by the inverted U-turn taken by the artery, and from the apex of which the branch to the atrioventricular node arises, together with a small vessel supplying the adjacent atrial wall.

Just beyond the U-turn, the RCA divides into two branches, one passing down towards the apex of the left ventricle along the inferior border of the interventricular septum, known as the posterior descending (or posterior interventricular) artery, providing blood supply to the inferior third of the septum. This vessel may also arise just before the U-turn (Figure 5.5). The second branch extends into the left atrioventricular groove for a short distance before dividing into a variable number and size of left ventricular branches supplying the infero-lateral wall of the adjacent left ventricle and the adjacent papillary muscle of the mitral valve.

The above configuration describes the anatomical pattern characteristic of the right dominant coronary artery, providing blood supply to the right atrium, right ventricle, including the right ventricular outflow tract, the sinus and atrioventricular nodes, the lower third of the interventricular septum, and the infero-lateral left ventricular free wall.

When the RCA is non-dominant, in 8% of cases, the continuation of the main vessel beyond the acute margin is absent, so that the vessel terminates in the mid-third, with numerous branches extending over the right ventricular

free wall. In this circumstance, the atrioventricular nodal artery arises from the continuation of the circumflex artery in the left atrioventricular groove, with the posterior descending artery progressing beyond this in a mirror-image configuration of the dominant RCA (Figure 5.6).

In the slightly less common co-dominant situation (approximately 7% of cases), the RCA and circumflex vessels continue to the crux, both often providing branches to the atrioventricular node, beyond which the vessels have a variable and individual course, either one, the other or both branches giving vessels to the interventricular septum, which may be small in calibre (Figure 5.7).

The appreciation of these varying anatomical configurations is important, and particularly relevant for the interventional cardiologist or cardiac surgeon, correlating the origin, size and distribution of vessels with their relative contribution to myocardial perfusion.

The left coronary artery arises from the left anterior sinus of Valsalva, as the left main trunk, which divides into two large vessels, the left anterior descending artery and the circumflex artery. The left anterior descending artery passes along the superior aspect of the interventricular septum, usually to the apex, and the circumflex artery lies in the left atrioventricular groove, curving round towards the crux laterally and then posteriorly for a varying distance. There is thus a reciprocal anatomical relationship between left and right coronary vessels. The left coronary artery extends along the superior aspect of the interventricular septum (as the left anterior

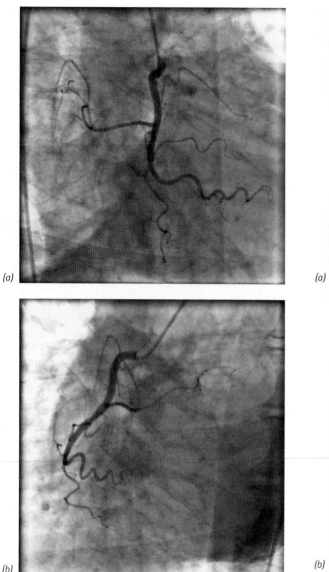

(a)

(b)

Figure 5.6 (a) A non-dominant right coronary artery, RAO view.
(b) The same artery as in (a) in LAO view.

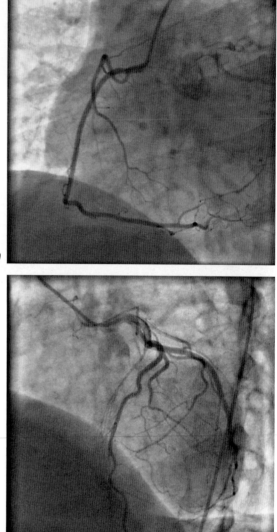

(a)

(b)

Figure 5.7 (a) A co-dominant right coronary artery, LAO view.
(b) The co-dominant left artery of the same patient as in (a),
LAO view. The position of the angiography catheter within
the descending aorta helps to orientate the observer.
Circumflex vessels are closest to the descending aorta and
vertebral column.

descending artery) and around the left atrioventricular
sulcus, surrounding the mitral annulus (as the circumflex artery). The RCA passes round the right atrioventricular sulcus adjacent to the tricuspid annulus and then
provides the posterior interventricular branch along the
inferior aspect of the interventricular septum.

The left main trunk is variable in length, from a few
millimetres to approximately 4 cm, and lies between the
pulmonary arterial trunk and the left atrial appendage as
it passes to the left atrioventricular sulcus. Usually there
are no branches arising from this vessel, although, rarely,
small left atrial and the sinoatrial branches have been
described to arise from it.[1]

The left main trunk is absent in approximately 1% of
cases, so that the anterior descending and circumflex

vessels then arise independently from the left coronary
sinus. The main trunk bifurcates into the left anterior
descending and circumflex vessels (Figure 5.8), although
in about 30% of cases subdivision into three instead of
two branches results in a third vessel (variously called the
'ramus intermedius', intermediate or isolated marginal
artery), which arises between the two major vessels and
extends over the high lateral left ventricular free wall
(Figure 5.9).

The anterior descending artery arises at an acute
angle from the main trunk and passes in the anterior
interventricular sulcus towards the apex of the left

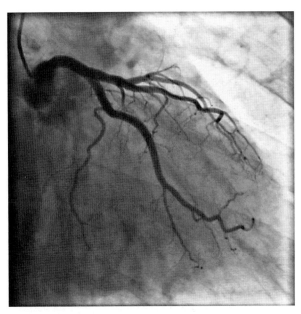

Figure 5.8 *The left coronary artery, RAO view. The left main artery divides into a relatively short anterior descending artery with a large diagonal branch, and a large circumflex artery, which soon becomes a large obtuse marginal artery leaving a small-lumen true circumflex artery.*

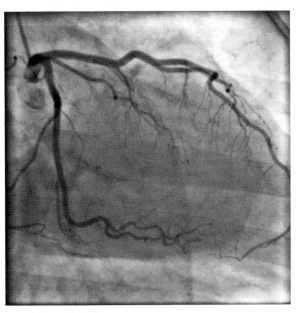

Figure 5.9 *Left coronary artery, RAO view. Between the anterior descending artery and the circumflex, there is a third vessel (intermediate or ramus intermedius), which in this case is relatively small.*

ventricle. Two sets of branches arise from the left anterior descending artery. Diagonal branches arise from the left margin of the vessel and extend over the antero-lateral left ventricular wall. The first diagonal artery is the most constant, often arising proximally near the origin of the

left anterior descending artery and, together with a variable number of subsequent diagonal branches, supplies the obtuse margin of the left ventricle. The second group of vessels is the septal arteries, which pass vertically into the septum as intramyocardial branches. The first septal artery is large, usually arising just beyond the origin of the left anterior descending artery and supplying vascularity to the conducting system, and may rarely arise from the first diagonal artery, while smaller septal branches arise throughout the length of the left anterior descending artery. The left anterior descending artery itself often extends round the apex, supplying the distal inferior left ventricular wall. Small right ventricular branches arise from the proximal anterior descending and extend rightward to supply the right ventricular outflow tract, and provide a potential pathway for collateral supply to the anterior descending in the presence of more proximal obstruction to flow (Figure 5.10).

As with other major coronary vessels, the left anterior descending runs in a sub-epicardial position, but a segment of the artery may descend into the myocardium for a short distance before emerging to its usual position. This is known as myocardial bridging, and is important to recognize because an error in vessel identification can be made, particularly during surgical procedures.[7] Alternatively, a small segment of vessel may lie beneath a muscle or fibrous band. These anatomic variations may produce vessel narrowing or obliteration during ventricular systole, with normal caliber in diastole. In the majority of cases, this is a benign occurrence, because the majority of blood flow occurs in diastole.[8] The first septal artery shows similar systolic compression in hypertrophic cardiomyopathy, but this also occurs in the normal ventricle.

The circumflex artery is a continuation of the left main trunk, passing beneath the left atrial appendage to emerge in the left atrioventricular sulcus, curving round the outer margin of the mitral annulus and terminating before reaching the crux. The branches of this artery are the obtuse marginal vessels, which extend anteriorly to supply the lateral and postero-lateral left ventricular wall. As noted previously, the first marginal vessel may arise as a trifurcation of the left main trunk, and is then identified as the intermediate or isolated marginal artery. In the event that the left coronary artery is dominant, the circumflex vessel extends to the crux, supplying the atrioventricular nodal artery, and then descends to the apex as the posterior interventricular artery, with blood supply to the inferior third of the septum. In the co-dominant situation, both the right and left circumflex vessels reach the crux from their respective atrioventricular sulci, and variably provide branches to the atrioventricular node and posterior interventricular regions, although these are often of small caliber.

As indicated previously, atrial branches also arise from the proximal circumflex artery. The branch to the

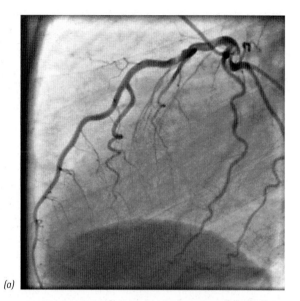

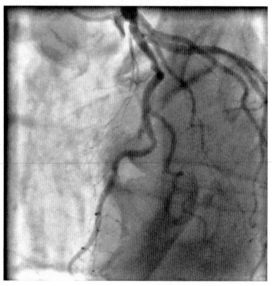

Figure 5.10 *(a) Left coronary artery, LAO view. The septal arteries are clearly visible and help to identify the anterior descending artery. Two large diagonal vessels are present and there is a small right ventricular branch. This patient has a large intermediate artery extending well towards the apex. (b) Left coronary artery, same patient as in (a), LAO view with cranial elevation. The anterior descending artery is mildly diseased and the two diagonal arteries are well seen. The first septal perforator arises near its origin. The intermediate artery overlaps the circumflex.*

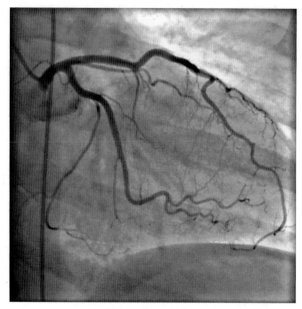

Figure 5.11 *Left coronary artery, RAO view. A large obtuse marginal branch of the circumflex leaves a relatively narrow true circumflex artery running in the atrioventricular groove.*

Successful therapeutic options are dependent on correct interpretation of these myriad variances in normal coronary vasculature and the associated area of myocardial perfusion.

Coronary veins

Knowledge of the coronary venous system is required for safe positioning of endocardial pacemaker and defibrillator leads, and for the interpretation of unfamiliar or unusual appearances seen on coronary angiograms.[9]

Following flow through the myocardial capillaries, venous channels return blood via the cardiac veins and the coronary sinus to the right atrium, or via smaller Thebesian connections directly into the atria or ventricles.

The anterior interventricular vein accompanies the anterior descending artery, with diagonal veins joining it as the vessel passes towards the left atrioventricular groove to become the great cardiac vein. This passes round the groove with adjoining marginal and oblique branches from the left ventricular free wall, and then passes as the coronary sinus to drain into the right atrium, the sinus orifice lying slightly caudal and posterior to the tricuspid orifice. The posterior ventricular vein joins the sinus a short distance from its orifice.

An alternative route for venous drainage is provided by the Thebesian veins, which are very small veins draining directly into the cardiac chambers, more commonly on the interatrial and interventricular septa,

sinoatrial node arises from the circumflex artery in 35% of cases, and a second atrial branch supplies the lateral wall of the left atrium (Figures 5.11, 5.12 and 5.13).

Appreciation and understanding of the details and multiple variations in coronary artery anatomy continue to be of prime importance for the successful analysis of both normal and particularly abnormal coronary vessels.

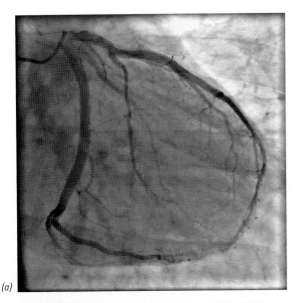

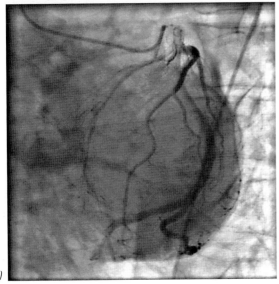

Figure 5.12 *(a) Left coronary artery, RAO view. This is a dominant left system with a large circumflex artery giving rise to postero-lateral and posterior descending branches. (b) Left coronary artery, same patient as in (a), LAO view, late phase. The dominant circumflex artery is well seen, with the large postero-lateral branch and posterior descending artery. The anterior descending artery opacification has almost cleared, and an unusually large diagonal artery can be seen running parallel to the anterior descending artery and giving off lateral branches.*

especially on the right side, and related to the papillary muscles on the left side. These are not commonly visualized during routine coronary angiography, but are frequently seen with a wedged right coronary injection, and in either situation awareness of the nature of this appearance and differentiation from thrombus vascularity are essential. Rarely, absence of the coronary sinus has been described.

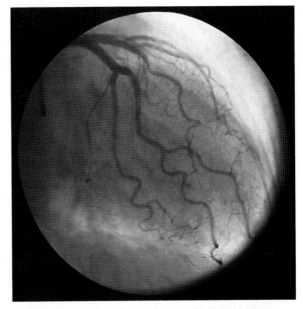

Figure 5.13 *Left coronary artery, RAO view. Although not a dominant left system, this circumflex artery gives large lateral branches that vascularize much of the left aspect of the left ventricular free wall.*

CORONARY ANOMALIES

Congenital coronary artery anomalies vary in reported incidence, but are present in 1% of adults undergoing coronary angiography and in 0.3% of autopsies.[10] The majority of variants are benign and unassociated with clinical symptoms, but knowledge of their appearance is essential for the correct interpretation of coronary angiograms, and for distinguishing anomalies that may be associated with significant morbidity or mortality. In these rare cases, the symptom may be angina, or there may be evidence of ischemia, heart failure or myocardial infarction. Sudden death may occur, especially in the young, when it is usually related to sports activities.

Classification[11] into three groups is as follows:

- anomalies of origin
- anomalies of course
- anomalies of termination.

Anomalies of origin

As previously indicated, the RCA usually arises from the right anterior sinus of Valsalva, the left coronary artery from the left sinus, with no vessel arising from the right posterior sinus. Variations in the height of the origin with respect to the sino-tubular ring have also been noted. Multiple sites of origin for the RCA are common, with the conus branch arising separately from the right sinus in up to 50% of cases. A separate origin of the left anterior

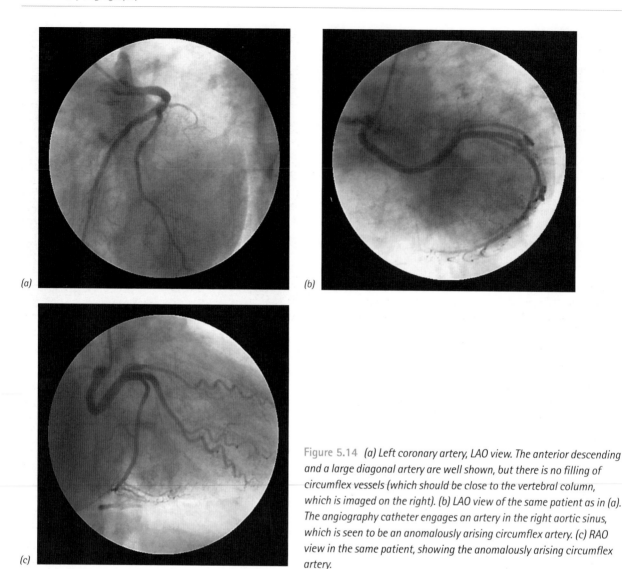

(a)

(b)

(c)

Figure 5.14 *(a) Left coronary artery, LAO view. The anterior descending and a large diagonal artery are well shown, but there is no filling of circumflex vessels (which should be close to the vertebral column, which is imaged on the right). (b) LAO view of the same patient as in (a). The angiography catheter engages an artery in the right aortic sinus, which is seen to be an anomalously arising circumflex artery. (c) RAO view in the same patient, showing the anomalously arising circumflex artery.*

descending and circumflex vessels from the left sinus with absence of the left main trunk occurs in 2% of cases. An anomalous site of origin may be from the opposite aortic sinus, the non-coronary sinus, the pulmonary artery or even from systemic vessels, and both coronary vessels may arise together from a single coronary ostium.

When both right and left coronary arteries arise from the left aortic sinus, there are usually no abnormal hemodynamic sequelae. When both vessels arise from the right sinus, myocardial ischemia or sudden death may result, as compression of the left coronary artery occurs (particularly on sudden exertion) as it passes between the aorta and the main pulmonary artery. The presence of this anomaly may be difficult to detect on angiography, and other imaging methods using contrast-enhanced computerized tomography or magnetic resonance imaging may be useful. Alternatively, the left coronary artery may pass anterior or posterior to the pulmonary artery, as a more benign variation in course.

The commonest anomaly related to a single coronary vessel is the origin of the circumflex artery from the proximal RCA, or from a separate orifice in the right aortic sinus (Figure 5.14). The left anterior descending artery may also arise from the right sinus, although this is more common in congenital heart disease, particularly tetralogy of Fallot. Awareness of this variant is important for the surgeon when these patients undergo surgical correction, because the anterior descending artery passes over the right ventricular outflow tract and is therefore vulnerable.

The right or the left coronary artery may arise from the posterior non-coronary sinus, although this also occurs more frequently in congenital heart disease, particularly complete transposition of the great vessels.

A single coronary artery may arise, either from the right or the left coronary sinus, with variable course of the alternate vessel anterior to, between or posterior to the great vessels. Several classifications have been described, notably that of Lipton.[12] This may be the cause of symptoms in young patients, particularly with passage of one of the vessels between the aorta and pulmonary artery. Rarely, one or both coronary arteries arise from the pulmonary artery, resulting in death in early infancy when the left artery is involved, but with improved survival with a left-to-right shunt to the main pulmonary artery when the right arises from this site.

Variations in course

These are of particular importance with regard to the anterior descending taking an intramyocardial route, and awareness of the several variations of anterior descending duplication is important for correct identification at surgery. The anterior descending may divide proximally or more distally, with one segment supplying the first septal and diagonal vessels, and the second segment passing more distally to extend to the apex. These multiple variations have surgical implications, because the incorrect vessel may be bypassed. It is also important to differentiate between a diagonal vessel running parallel to the anterior descending artery and the anterior descending artery itself (see Figure 5.12b).[13]

Anomalies of termination

The main anomaly in this group is the presence of coronary artery fistulae, with 60% of cases involving entry of the RCA into the right ventricle or, less frequently, into the right atrium or pulmonary artery.[14] The fistula commonly ends in an aneurysm just before the point of entry, plus or minus a relative stenosis at the entry site, thus significantly reducing the size of the potential shunt. Clinical presentation and physical findings depend on the size of the shunt and the site of entry. Fistulae involving the left coronary artery usually drain into left heart chambers, rarely the coronary sinus, and may be associated with cardiac murmurs, cardiomegaly and calcification of coronary vessels (Figure 5.15).

Thebesian vein drainage has been previously mentioned; other rare connections sporadically reported in the literature include extracardiac connections between coronary arteries and bronchial and other pulmonary vessels.[15]

CORONARY ANGIOGRAPHY

Coronary artery anatomy in a symptomatic patient is currently determined by coronary angiography, with alternative methods of investigation now being developed, particularly magnetic resonance angiography (MRA) and multislice computerized tomography (MSCT).

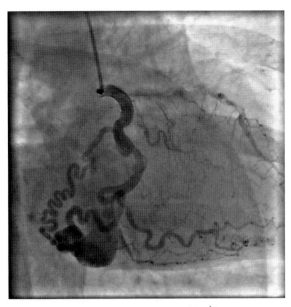

Figure 5.15 *Left coronary injection, RAO view. There is a fistula of circumflex artery draining into the coronary sinus.*

In the supine position, arterial access is achieved percutaneously using a preformed catheter varying in size between 4 and 8 French caliber (Judkin's technique). The catheter is inserted via the right or left femoral artery and advanced through the abdominal and thoracic aorta to a position just above the aortic valve, where the tip is inserted into the right or left coronary orifice. If femoral access is not available, the radial or brachial route is used. Arteriotomy via the brachial artery, pioneered by Sones, is now rarely performed. Manual or, infrequently, automated intracoronary injection of 4–10 mL of radio-opaque contrast is accompanied by simultaneous imaging of the opacified coronary vessels, with concurrent hemodynamic monitoring.

The position of the heart within the anterior left chest and the myriad variations in coronary artery anatomy necessitate several separate injections into the coronary arteries in different spatial projections for complete evaluation. Current technology enables the x-ray tube and the image intensifier, which are diagonally opposite one another, mounted on a C-arm with the intensifier above the patient, to be rotated around the patient in the axial plane, producing right anterior oblique (RAO), left anterior oblique (LAO) and transverse projections, the last-mentioned providing right or left lateral images at 90° (Figure 5.16). In any of these positions, the image intensifier can additionally be skewed towards the head (cranial) or feet (caudal), so producing the combined complex angulations required to show details of the coronary arterial tree. The speed of rotation of the C-arm supporting the x-ray apparatus is now sufficiently rapid to allow a comprehensive study to be performed

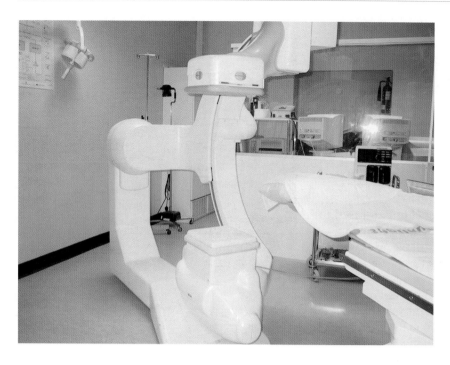

Figure 5.16 *The image intensifier (above) and the x-ray tube (below) are mounted opposite one another on a C-arm.*

in a short time, without the need for the more cumbersome bi-plane equipment, which can provide simultaneous imaging in two projections with each injection.

In routine practice, a universal protocol of views is taken, with each patient treated individually by the operator, who may decide to take additional views to overcome foreshortening and overlapping or to view a particular eccentric lesion in another plane.

The routine protocol performed in our laboratories is as follows.

Left coronary artery

1 Right anterior oblique (RAO)
   - Shallow 10° RAO with 20° caudal (Figure 5.17): provides an excellent view of the left main bifurcation, proximal left anterior descending (LAD) and proximal to middle circumflex.
   - Shallow 10° RAO with 25–40° cranial (Figure 5.18): provides a good view of the middle and distal LAD without overlap of diagonal and septal branches.
2 Left anterior oblique (LAO)
   - 30–60° LAO 15–30° cranial (Figure 5.19): provides good visualization of left main and proximal LAD, diagonals and ramus intermedius.
   - 40–60° LAO 10–20° caudal, spider view (Figure 5.20): visualization of left main, ramus intermedius, proximal LAD, and proximal circumflex.
3 Left lateral (Figure 5.21)
   - Proximal circumflex and improved LAD, and left internal thoracic artery insertion into LAD.

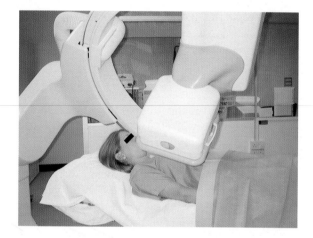

Figure 5.17 *RAO: shallow 10° RAO with 20° caudal angulation.*

Right coronary artery

1 Left anterior oblique (LAO) (Figure 5.22)
   - Proximal and middle RCA.
2 Right anterior oblique (RAO) (Figure 5.23)
   - Middle RCA.

Left ventricle

1 Right anterior oblique (RAO)
   - 30° RAO: provides profile view of left ventricle in longitudinal axis, showing anterior, apical and inferior margins, and profile view of mitral valve. Avoids superimposition of left ventricle on spine.

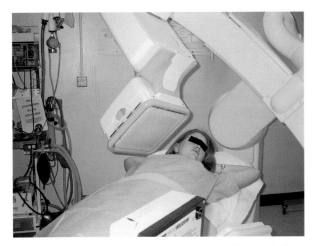

Figure 5.18 *RAO: shallow 10° RAO with 25° cranial angulation.*

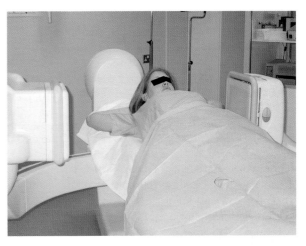

Figure 5.21 *Left lateral.*

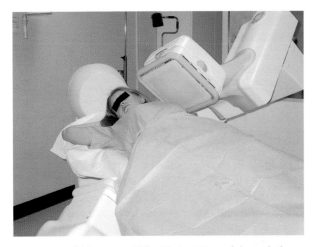

Figure 5.19 *LAO: 30–60° LAO with 15–30° cranial angulation.*

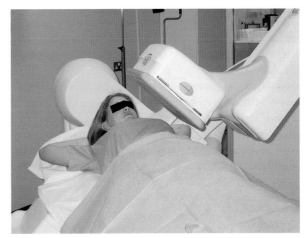

Figure 5.22 *LAO.*

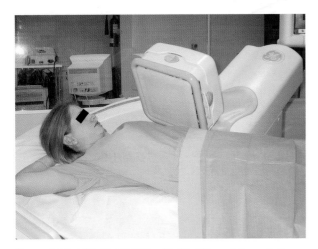

Figure 5.20 *LAO: 40–60° LAO with 10–20° caudal angulation (spider view).*

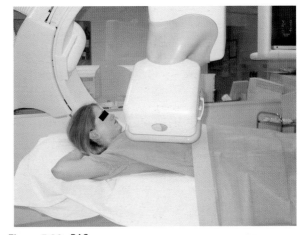

Figure 5.23 *RAO.*

2 Left anterior oblique (LAO)
   • 60° LAO 20–30° cranial angulation: shows entire septum in profile, and lateral and posterior left ventricular wall. This angulation avoids foreshortening.

QUANTITATIVE CORONARY ANALYSIS

The eccentric appearance of many coronary artery lesions, together with the significant observer variability in the estimation of coronary lesion severity, have both encouraged the development and use of automated techniques for assessing lesion severity. Initially developed in 1977 for images acquired on cine film,[16] automated computer-assisted quantitative analytical systems are now available for immediate on-line use during the investigative procedure, and for later post-study analysis. Automated edge detection on digitally acquired images is used to calculate both percentage diameter and area reduction. The reference diameter is the non-tapering segment of the coronary catheter in use. This automated technique is particularly useful during angioplasty and other interventional procedures. Operator over-estimation of lesion severity, known to occur with visual interpretation, is thus avoided, and significant improvement in inter-observer consistency in interpretation has been demonstrated.[17] The functional significance of stenotic lesions can also be estimated using this software, with calculation of myocardial flow reserve (Figure 5.24).

VENTRICULOGRAPHY

Left ventriculography allows a qualitative analysis of both global and segmental systolic myocardial function by visual analysis of changes in cavitary dimensions during the cardiac cycle. The size and shape of the left ventricular outline in both systole and diastole provide information regarding the presence or absence of myocardial contraction, the features of an aneurysm and volume overloading. A decreased left ventricular volume may be noted, which could be associated with increased myocardial wall thickness or possibly the presence of intracavitary thrombus. Mitral valve assessment, including leaflet excursion, regurgitation, location of calcification and abnormalities of the subvalvar apparatus, can be made, together with septal mobility and integrity, and aortic valve abnormalities.

Angiographically, a pigtail catheter is positioned with the tip in the mid-left ventricular cavity, and imaging performed in the 30° RAO projection during automated contrast injection, which provides an outline of the left ventricular cavity in the longitudinal axis and an image of the mitral valve in profile. A 60° LAO projection with 20–30° cranial angulation is at right angles to the RAO view, and profiles the septum, lateral and posterior left ventricular wall, but is not performed during routine coronary angiography.

The segments of the left ventricle are defined in Figure 5.25, ten segments in all, and correlation between the anatomical distribution of the coronary arteries and the specific myocardial segment supplied by each vessel is important in the evaluation of myocardial ischemia.

Visual analysis to assess left ventricular ejection fraction can be made from the end-systolic and end-diastolic frames of a sinus beat, which may be normal (50–69%), hyperdynamic (>70%) or show mild hypokinesis (35–49%), moderate hypokinesis (20–34%) or severe hypokinesis (<20%).[18] Actual measurement of the global ejection fraction is made by subtraction of the end-diastolic and end-systolic left ventricular outlines, usually

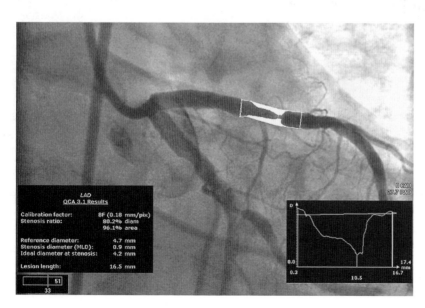

Figure 5.24 *Quantitative coronary analysis applied to lesion of anterior descending artery defines 80% loss of diameter (or 96% loss of lumen area) in a 16.5 mm long lesion.*

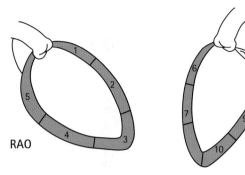

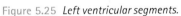

Figure 5.25 *Left ventricular segments.*

performed using automated software (Figure 5.26). Other methods of assessing global ejection fraction include echocardiography, radionuclide ventriculography and dynamic MRA, although these methods are not strictly comparable and give slightly differing values in the same patient.

Regional wall motion provides a more sensitive indicator of coronary artery abnormalities than global function, and automated software is now available defining abnormal areas of wall motion, classified as hypokinesis, akinesis and dyskinesis. Mitral regurgitation is assessed

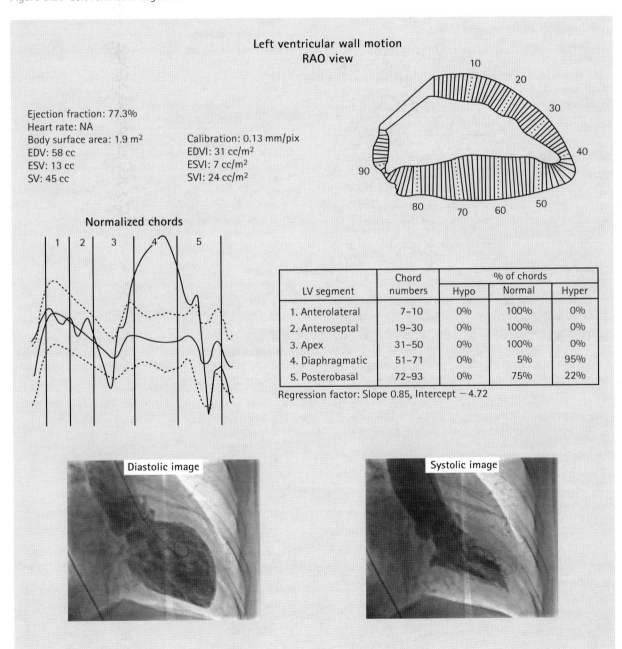

Figure 5.26 *End-diastolic and end-systolic frames of a normal ventricle with 77% ejection fraction captured for quantitative analysis.*

by observing contrast passing posteriorly across the mitral orifice during ventricular systole in sinus rhythm in the RAO projection, with severity estimated on a scale of 1 (mild) to 4 (severe). In the LAO projection, abnormalities of septal and lateral left ventricular wall motion are seen, and contrast passing across the septum in a rightward direction indicates the presence of a ventricular septal defect.

The change in appearance of the left ventriculogram in the RAO projection may be used to assess myocardial viability. During sinus rhythm, an ectopic beat is followed by a post-ectopic pause, and the subsequent sinus beat is potentiated in the presence of normal myocardium. This response may be observed in a segment previously showing impaired contraction, which indicates ischemia rather than infarction. Analysis of the left ventricular contraction response following the administration of various drugs has now been superseded in clinical practice by the thallium perfusion scan or dobutamine stress echo test.

The left ventriculogram is routinely performed before or immediately following coronary angiography, unless there is severe heart failure, significant elevation of the left ventricular end-diastolic pressure or aortic valve disease, particularly stenosis or the presence of a prosthetic valve precluding catheter access. Alternative methods of assessment of left ventricular function include two-dimensional echocardiography, magnetic resonance imaging and radio-isotope studies including positron emission tomography (PET).[19] The first two of these investigations have the added advantage of providing measurements of left ventricular wall thickness, not available with the angiographic study.

Right ventriculography is performed for the evaluation of congenital heart disease, and is therefore not part of the routine investigation of coronary artery abnormality, or of the routine assessment of the aortic or mitral valves.

KEY REFERENCES

Anderson RH, Becker AE (eds). *Cardiac Anatomy: An Integrated Text and Colour Atlas*. London: Gower Medical; Edinburgh, New York: Churchill Livingston, 1980.
A highly informative and unique pictorial atlas of coronary vessels showing their spatial relationship to cardiac structures.

Baim DS, Grossman W. *Grossman's Cardiac Catheterization, Angiography and Intervention*, 6th edn. Baltimore: Lippincott Williams and Wilkins, 2000.
For cardiac ventriculography and evaluation of cardiac function.

Kern ML. *The Cardiac Catheterization Handbook*, 3rd edn. St Louis, MI: Mosby, 1999.
Includes a clear diagrammatic description of the coronary vessels and their branches.

Nguyen TN, Saito S, Hu D, Dave V, Grines CL (eds). *Practical Handbook of Advanced Interventional Cardiology*. New York: Futura Publishing Company Inc., 2000.
Classification of coronary anomalies and angiographic projections of coronary vessels.

Scanlon PJ, Faxon DP, Audet A-M, Carabello B, Dehmer GJ, Eagle KA, *et al*. AAC/AHA Guidelines for Coronary Angiography. A Report of the American College of Cardiology/American Heart Association Task Force on Practice Guidelines (Committee on Coronary Angiography). *J Am Coll Cardiol* 1999; **33**: 1756–824.
A highly authoritative description of the indications for coronary angiography for all presentations of suspected coronary artery disease, together with a review of associated risks (549 references).

REFERENCES

1. Gray H, Williams PL, Bannister LH. *Gray's Anatomy: The Anatomical Basis of Medicine and Surgery*, 38th edn. New York: Churchill Livingstone, 1999.
2. von Luedinghausen, M. *The Clinical Anatomy of the Coronary Arteries*. Berlin, New York: Springer-Verlag, 2003.
3. Protocol for the Bypass Angioplasty Revascularization Investigation. *Circulation* 1991; **84** (Suppl. V):V1–27.
4. Taylor AJ, Farb A, Ferguson M, Virmani R. Myocardial infarction associated with physical exertion in a young man. *Circulation* 1997; **96**:3201–4.
5. Hutchinson MC. The study of atrial arteries in man. *J Anat* 1978; **125**:39–54.
6. Schlesinger MJ, Zoll PM, Wessler S. The conus artery: a third coronary artery. *Am Heart J* 1949; **38**:823–36.
7. Ge J, Erbel R, Rupprecht HJ, Koch L, Kearley P, Gorg G, *et al.* Comparison of intravascular ultrasound and angiography in the assessment of myocardial bridging. *Circulation* 1994; **89**:1725–32.
8. Yetman AT, McCrindle BW, MacDonald C, Freedom RM, Gow R. Myocardial bridging in children with hypertrophic cardiomyopathy – a risk factor for sudden death. *N Engl J Med* 1998; **339**:1201–9.
9. Spindola-Franco H, Eldh P, Adams DF, Abrams HL. Coronary vascular patterns during occlusion arteriography. *Radiology* 1975; **114**: 59–63.
10. Ogden JA. Congenital anomalies of the coronary arteries. *Am J Cardiol* 1970; **25**:474–9.
11. Greenberg MA, Fish BG, Spindola-Franco H. Congenital anomalies of the coronary arteries. Classification and significance. *Radiol Clin North Am* 1989; **27**: 1127–46.
12. Lipton MJ, Barry WH, Obrez I, Silverman JF, Wexler L. Isolated single coronary artery: diagnosis, angiographic classification, and clinical significance. *Radiology* 1979; **130**:39–47.
13. Spindola-Franco H, Grose R, Solomon N. Dual left anterior descending artery: angiographic description of important variants and surgical implications. *Am Heart J* 1983; **105**:445–55.
14. Neufeld H, Lester RG, Adam P Jr, Anderson RC, Lillehei CW, Edwards JE. Congenital communication of a coronary artery with a cardiac chamber or a pulmonary trunk ('coronary artery fistula'). *Circulation* 1961; **24**:171–9.

15. Smith SC, Adams DF, Herman MV, Paulin S. Coronary to bronchial anastomoses: an *in vivo* demonstration by selective coronary arteriography. *Radiology* 1972; **104**:289–90.

16. Brown BG, Bolson E, Frimer M, Dodge HT. Quantitative arteriography: estimation of dimensions, hemodynamic resistance, and atheroma mass of coronary artery lesions using the arteriogram and digital computation. *Circulation* 1977; **55**:329–37.

17. Danchin N, Juilliere Y, Foley D, Serruys PW. Visual versus quantitative assessment of the severity of coronary artery stenoses: can the angiographer's eye be re-educated? *Am Heart J* 1993; **126**:594–600.

18. Baim DS, Hillis LD. Cardiac ventriculography. In: *Grossman's Cardiac Catheterization, Angiography, and Intervention*, Baim DS, Grossman W (eds). Philadelphia: Lippincott Williams & Wilkins, 2000, 257–70.

19. Gambhir SS, Czernin J, Schwimmer J, Silverman DHS, Coleman RE, Phelps ME. A tabulated summary of the FDG PET literature. *J Nucl Med* 2001; **42** (Suppl.):70S.

6

Nuclear imaging in coronary artery disease

SL RAHMAN AND SR UNDERWOOD

Nuclear cardiology is an established subspeciality that has grown significantly in recent years because of developments in imaging hardware, software and tracers. Alongside these technical developments, there has been an increasing appreciation of the role that the functional information provided by nuclear techniques can play in clinical cardiology. This chapter covers the principles of nuclear cardiology and the most commonly used techniques, and reviews clinical applications, emphasizing the role and value of radionuclide myocardial perfusion imaging (MPI) in patient management.

TECHNIQUES

Radiopharmaceuticals

THALLIUM-201

Thallium-201 is the most commonly used radionuclide for myocardial perfusion studies. It decays by electron capture to mercury-201, emitting mainly x-rays of energy 67–82 keV (88% abundance) and gamma photons of 135 keV and 167 keV (12% abundance). It is administered intravenously as thallous chloride and the usual dose is 80–110 MBq (maximum 80 MBq in the UK). Following intravenous injection, approximately 88% is cleared from the blood after the first circulation,[1] with 4% of the injected dose localizing in the myocardium. The thallous ion is a monovalent cation similar in size to the hydrated potassium ion. Approximately 60% enters the cardiac myocytes using the sodium–potassium ATPase dependent exchange mechanism, and the remainder

enters passively along an electropotential gradient. The extraction efficiency is maintained under conditions of acidosis and hypoxia, and only when myocytes are irreversibly damaged is extraction reduced.[2] Distribution within the myocardium is proportional to perfusion over a wide range of values, although at high rates of flow, extraction may become rate limiting.[3,4]

Thallium is an excellent tracer of myocardial perfusion and it has been used clinically for more than two decades. It does, however, have limitations.

1 It has a relatively long physical half-life, which results in a high radiation burden for the patient. Eighty MBq delivers an effective dose of 18 mSv and this is of the same order as the radiation exposure during coronary angiography.
2 The relatively low injected dose results in a low signal to noise ratio and images can be suboptimal, especially in obese patients.
3 The relatively low energy emission leads to low resolution images and significant attenuation by soft tissue.

Technetium-99m compounds do not have these limitations and this has encouraged the development of such tracers.

TECHNETIUM-99M-LABELED TRACERS

Two technetium-labeled perfusion tracers are currently available commercially: Tc-99m-2-methoxy-isobutyl-isonitrile (MIBI) and Tc-99m-1,2-bis[bis(2-ethoxyethyl) phosphino] ethane (tetrofosmin). Tc-99m-MIBI is a cationic complex that diffuses passively through the capillary and cell membrane, although less readily than thallium, resulting in lower immediate extraction. Within the cell it is localized in the mitochondria, where it is trapped.[5] Clearance is ultimately through the liver and kidneys.

Tetrofosmin is also cleared rapidly from the blood and its myocardial uptake is similar to that of MIBI,[6] with approximately 1.2% of the administered dose taken up by the myocardium. Hepatic clearance is more rapid than that of MIBI, which allows image acquisition as early as 15 minutes after injection. The exact mechanism of uptake is unknown, but it is probably similar to that of MIBI, although with localization in the cytoplasm rather than the mitochondria.

POSITRON-EMITTING RADIOPHARMACEUTICALS

A number of positron-emitting radiopharmaceuticals can be used as tracers of myocardial perfusion. Oxygen-15-labeled water can be administered either intravenously or by inhalation of $^{15}CO_2$, with rapid transformation to water by carbonic anhydrase in the lungs. Mathematical modeling provides measurements of myocardial perfusion, although images of regional perfusion cannot be obtained directly because of blood pool activity. Cationic tracers such as nitrogen-13 ammonia (as $^{13}NH_4^+$), rubidium-82 and potassium-38 have also been used. Ammonia is trapped in the cell by incorporation into glutamine and the other cations enter by active transport. Kinetic models of these tracers have also been used to calculate myocardial perfusion.

Imaging protocols

IMAGING TECHNIQUES

Tomography is now almost universally used for MPI, although planar imaging is sometimes used with older equipment or if the patient is unable to lie still and flat for the duration of tomographic imaging. The best imaging protocol depends upon the tracer used, the dose given, the type of collimator and the number of heads of the camera. Typically, images are acquired over an arc of 180° from right anterior oblique to left posterior oblique using 64 projections of 25–30 seconds each for thallium and 20–25 seconds for technetium. These figures can be 5 seconds shorter using two heads at 90°. A high-resolution collimator is preferred if count rates permit, although a general purpose collimator may be needed for thallium.

THALLIUM

Thallium is usually given at peak exercise, with exercise continued for 2 minutes in order to maintain stable conditions over the period of extraction by the myocardium. Imaging starts within 5–10 minutes of injection and should be completed within 30 minutes. During this period the distribution of thallium within the myocardium is relatively fixed and the images reflect myocardial distribution at the time of injection. The thallium then exchanges with the extracellular and intravascular spaces and washes out of the myocardium at a slower rate in hypoperfused than in normally perfused myocardium. As a result, areas with decreased initial uptake appear to have a relative increase in uptake when imaged 2–4 hours later, a phenomenon known as redistribution. Comparison between the stress and redistribution images distinguishes between the reversible defect of inducible hypoperfusion and the fixed defect of myocardial necrosis, although in some cases redistribution may be incomplete at 4 hours. A second injection of thallium can then be given and re-injection images acquired for a more accurate assessment of myocardial viability.[7]

TECHNETIUM-LABELED TRACERS

Unlike thallium, MIBI and tetrofosmin are essentially fixed in the myocardium with no redistribution, and separate injections are given in order to assess stress and resting perfusion. The 6-hour half-life of technetium-99m means that the two studies should ideally be performed on separate days to allow for the decay of activity from the first injection. The 2-day protocol is performed with an initial stress study using 400 MBq of radiotracer, followed by a resting study on a different day using a similar dose. Imaging starts 30–60 minutes after injection. The two studies can be performed on the same day if a larger dose is given on the second occasion in order to swamp residual activity from the first injection, and some time is also allowed for the first injection to decay. The 1-day protocol typically uses 250 MBq at stress followed by 750 MBq at rest 4 hours later, although the reverse order can also be used. The order of studies depends to some extent on the indication for the study. When the diagnosis of ischemia is important, the stress study should be performed first to avoid reducing the contrast of a stress-induced defect by a previous normal resting study.[8] Conversely, if the problem is to detect viable myocardium and reversibility of a defect, perhaps in a patient with previous infarction, it is better to perform the rest study first. The radiation burden to the patient from 400 MBq of tracer is 5 mSv for MIBI and 4 mSv for tetrofosmin.

An important consequence of the lack of redistribution of the technetium-labeled tracers is that stress imaging can be delayed for some time after injection, and there is no need to inject close to the gamma camera. Injections can be given during treadmill exercise testing, in the catheter laboratory, or in the coronary care unit immediately before thrombolysis. In addition, because of the higher doses that can be used with technetium, ventricular function can be assessed either by first-pass imaging of the tracer as it passes through the central circulation or by ECG-gated acquisition of the myocardial perfusion images.

ECG–GATED MYOCARDIAL PERFUSION TOMOGRAPHY

The high count rate of the technetium tracers makes it possible to obtain ECG-gated images. The principles of acquisition are similar to those for equilibrium radionuclide ventriculography, although fewer frames are normally acquired in order to maximize counts in each frame: 8 to 16 frames are usual. Myocardial motion and thickening are normally assessed subjectively using gray scale images for motion and a color scale for thickening. Because of the relatively low spatial resolution, thickening is not assessed directly, but from myocardial count increases between diastole and systole. The relationship between myocardial counts and thickness arises from the partial volume effect, which leads to a reduction in counts from objects smaller than the resolution of the imaging system. As the myocardium thickens, the partial volume effect lessens and counts increase.

The simplest approach for measuring left ventricular ejection fraction (LVEF) from these images is to outline the endocardium manually in each slice and in each frame and to sum the areas of the ventricular cavity. This is too time-consuming for routine use, however, and it is rarely performed. Instead, automated algorithms have been developed to identify the endocardium and epicardium, and these provide relatively robust measurements, although LVEF is under-estimated if only eight frames are used. Absolute volumes are measured in the same way, although small volumes can be underestimated because of the low resolution of the images. Regional function also compares well with other techniques, although agreement is less good for patients with severe perfusion defects.[9]

Image interpretation

VISUAL ASSESSMENT

Myocardial perfusion and hence tracer distribution are uniform in normal myocardium (Figure 6.1). A regional defect indicates either reduced perfusion in viable myocardium or a reduced amount of viable myocardium, or a combination of both. If a stress defect returns to normal in the resting images, this indicates an inducible perfusion abnormality that is sometimes referred to as

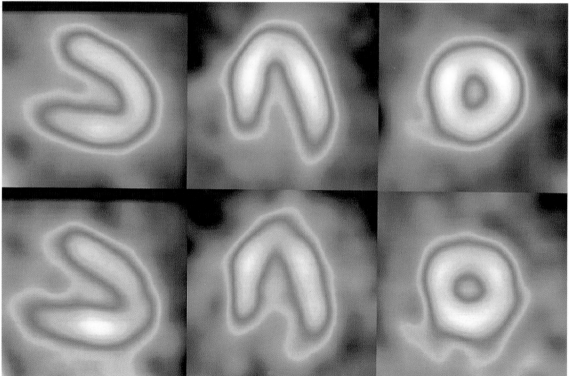

Figure 6.1 *Normal thallium myocardial perfusion tomograms in vertical long-axis (left), horizontal long-axis (center) and short-axis planes (right). Stress images (top) and redistribution (bottom). There is homogeneous uptake of tracer throughout the myocardium and hence no coronary obstruction.*

inducible ischemia. Strictly, the term 'ischemia' is incorrect since the image indicates heterogeneity of perfusion rather than an absolute reduction, but 'ischemia' is widely used shorthand. Areas of infarction show a defect in both stress and rest images, and the depth of the defect indicates the amount of myocardial loss (Figure 6.2). Ischemia can, of course, be superimposed upon partial thickness infarction and in this case a stress defect may be only partially reversible at rest.

Reverse redistribution is the term used to describe a defect in redistribution thallium images that is less apparent in the stress images. When the phenomenon is seen, it is often the result of artifact or other technical differences between images and in this case it is not, strictly speaking, reverse redistribution. When true reverse redistribution is seen, it is the result of rapid washout of tracer, as might occur in an area of partial thickness infarction supplied by a patent artery after angioplasty or thrombolysis.[10] It is not associated with future coronary events and it is not normally clinically significant. Sometimes, the phenomenon is seen in technetium images and in this case it is normally the result of artifact.

In addition to regional myocardial uptake, other features of the images are important. Ventricular dilatation is best judged from the planar images, although it is also apparent in the tomograms. Care must be taken in the tomograms not to be misled by technical factors as lower resolution images may give the impression of a smaller ventricle. Of particular significance is left ventricular dilatation in stress thallium images that is less marked on redistribution, since this implies extensive inducible ischemia and is associated with an adverse prognosis.[11]

The dilatation may be partly real, but it may also be the result of widespread sub-endocardial ischemia that simulates cavity enlargement. This explains why the phenomenon can also be seen in technetium images even though these may be acquired some time after stress, when the ventricle might be expected to have returned to its baseline size.

The normal right ventricular myocardium is much thinner than the left but it is not unusual to see right ventricular uptake. Hypertrophy in either ventricle can be seen as myocardial thickening and an increase in counts. When a relative defect is seen, care must be taken to distinguish between reduced uptake in an area of reduced perfusion and increased uptake in a neighboring area of hypertrophy. Because the myocardial images are not of high resolution, it is sometimes necessary to make this distinction only after echocardiography or magnetic resonance imaging has been used to define myocardial thickness.

Perfusion defects are not always the result of coronary artery disease. Abnormalities can be seen with coronary spasm, anomalous arteries, muscle bridges, small vessel disease as may occur in diabetes or syndrome X, the dilated and hypertrophic cardiomyopathies, hypertrophy caused by outflow obstruction or hypertension, infiltrative disorders such as sarcoidosis and amyloidosis, connective tissue disorders and conduction defects such as left bundle branch block. True perfusion defects must also be distinguished from artifact caused by motion and by attenuation. Attenuation can be seen as reduced counts in the inferior wall, often in slim males, or in the anterior wall, often from breast attenuation in females.

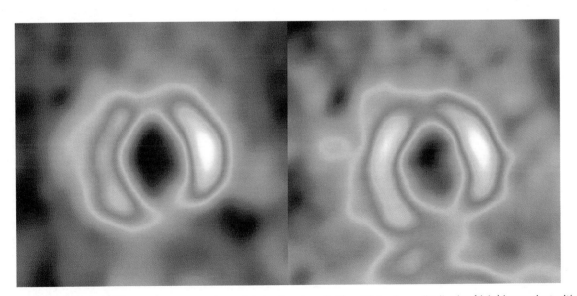

Figure 6.2 *Short-axis thallium-201 tomograms, immediately after stress (left) and following redistribution (right) in a patient with angina and previous inferior myocardial infarction. There is a reversible defect in the septum and a partially reversible defect in the anterior wall, which are both suggestive of inducible ischemia in the left anterior descending artery. In addition, there is a fixed defect in the inferior wall indicative of myocardial infarction.*

IMAGE QUANTIFICATION

Several methods have been used to quantify myocardial uptake, and these are all relative rather than absolute techniques in which uptake is expressed relative to the hottest voxel within the myocardium. The techniques include linear profiles, circumferential profiles[12] and analysis of count histograms, but a method that is popular for tomographic images is to display the whole myocardium as a polar map or 'bullseye' image.[13] Individual polar maps can be compared with a normal database and abnormalities detected automatically as areas with counts less than two standard deviations (or other threshold) from the mean. Polar maps with quantification are probably most helpful to assess the depth and extent of defects, but they should not be used in isolation. Most experienced nuclear cardiologists prefer to assess the presence of a defect from the tomograms initially and to use quantification to assess depth and extent of an abnormality. The polar map cannot distinguish true perfusion abnormality from artifact as the former can be mild and the latter can be profound.

Quantification is also used to assess uptake of thallium in the lungs and this is an important indicator of prognosis in patients with ischemic heart disease.[14] Lung uptake is determined by transit time, extraction efficiency and pulmonary capillary pressure, all of which can be abnormal if left ventricular function is impaired. Thus, the uptake is a reflection of impaired left ventricular function either at rest or induced by ischemia during exercise. It is expressed as a ratio between uptake in the lungs and the myocardium, even though myocardial uptake depends upon viability and perfusion. The measurements are made either from an initial anterior planar image or from the appropriate image of the tomographic acquisition, and a normal lung:heart ratio is less than 0.5.

Stress techniques

The response to stress is central to the assessment of most aspects of cardiovascular function. It is particularly important for coronary artery disease because resting coronary flow is normal until the luminal cross-sectional area of a coronary artery is reduced by approximately 85%, and resting ischemia only occurs when the artery is virtually occluded. Many investigations use some form of cardiovascular stress to highlight differences in the coronary flow reserve between arteries. Most of these induce myocardial ischemia by the manipulation of myocardial oxygen demand, but some, such as dipyridamole, have a primary action on myocardial perfusion. The most commonly used technique is dynamic exercise. This has the advantage that it is physiological and it mimics the stress that may provoke symptoms in patients with coronary artery disease. However, many patients with coronary artery disease are unable to exercise adequately because of vascular disease elsewhere or other physical or psychological problems. Pharmacological manipulation of myocardial perfusion and oxygen demand is therefore a valuable technique that is used increasingly.

ADENOSINE

Adenosine is a relatively specific coronary arteriolar dilator. Its main advantage is its very short plasma half-life of less than 10 seconds, which simplifies the control of plasma levels, increasing safety and reducing the duration of side effects. Although it is more expensive than dipyridamole, many centers use it in preference because of these advantages. An intravenous infusion of $140\,\mu g\,kg^{-1}\,min^{-1}$ causes maximal or near maximal hyperemia in 92% of patients, with mean coronary flow increasing by 4.4 times the resting value.[15] During the infusion there is a slight fall in blood pressure with an increase in heart rate, cardiac output and pulmonary capillary pressure. Adenosine is usually infused over 4–6 minutes with injection of radiotracer 2 minutes from the end. Its action as a vasodilator is more potent and consistent than that of dipyridamole, but side effects are more common, occurring in up to 80% of patients. Chest pain is provoked in nearly 40%,[16] but this does not necessarily imply myocardial ischemia because adenosine may cause chest pain even in normal volunteers. Headache and flushing are common and first-degree atrioventricular block occurs in 10%. Second-degree and third-degree atrioventricular block occurs in 4% and 1%, respectively. All of these side effects are short lived.

DOBUTAMINE

Patients with asthma or other causes of reversible airways obstruction are at risk of bronchospasm with either dipyridamole or adenosine and they are candidates for dobutamine. Dobutamine increases perfusion in normal myocardium approximately twofold (similar to dynamic exercise) by a combination of primary and secondary actions. It is a primary coronary vasodilator and in this sense it has a similar effect to adenosine. It also increases myocardial oxygen demand by increasing myocardial contractility, heart rate and blood pressure and this leads to a secondary increase in myocardial perfusion. Dobutamine has a short plasma half-life (90 seconds) and low arrhythmogenicity. It is normally infused into a peripheral vein, starting at $5\,\mu g\,kg^{-1}min^{-1}$ and increasing in increments of $5\,\mu g\,kg^{-1}min^{-1}$ to a maximum of 20 or $40\,\mu g\,kg^{-1}min^{-1}$, with stages lasting for 2–5 minutes to allow stabilization of the hemodynamic effect. Although in stress echocardiography atropine is also given if the heart rate response is inadequate, this is probably not necessary in perfusion imaging because of the primary vasodilator effect of dobutamine.

Dobutamine is safe in patients with coronary artery disease and serious complications are uncommon. The commonest complication that limits infusion is hypotension caused by peripheral vasodilatation. One-third of patients experience chest pain, and non-sustained ventricular tachycardia has been reported in approximately 4% of patients but without hemodynamic instability. Non-cardiac side effects are common but mild, usually skin tingling, heart pounding or flushing, and they are relieved within a few minutes of stopping the infusion. The positive inotropic and chronotropic effects of dobutamine make it unsuitable for patients with contraindications to dynamic exercise, most importantly aortic stenosis and unstable angina. The action of dobutamine is antagonized by beta-blockers and these should be discontinued at least 48 hours before the study, although recent studies have shown perfusion abnormalities even in patients on beta-blockade, probably because of the primary vasodilatation of dobutamine.

CHOICE OF STRESS TECHNIQUE

Dynamic exercise is the preferred technique for stressing patients in many centers, because it is familiar to physicians and patients and because the observations during exercise are an important part of clinical assessment. However, many patients attending for perfusion imaging have already had an exercise test, and the ease and reliability of the pharmacological techniques make them a better choice in this setting. Because it cannot always be predicted if a patient will not be able to exercise, even those without obvious restriction may benefit from pharmacological stress. It is also helpful in a busy stress schedule if the majority of patients undergo the same protocol, and adenosine infusion is the simplest and most widely applicable technique. A good case can therefore be made for using pharmacological stress as the default form of stress when information from dynamic exercise is not required.

The accuracy of the three forms of pharmacological stress is similar to that of dynamic exercise, with the sensitivity and specificity of dipyridamole for the detection of coronary artery disease being 89% and 78% respectively, adenosine 90% and 91%, and dobutamine 82% and 73%. The techniques are also equally successfully applied with thallium and with the technetium agents, although recent reports show that sensitivity with the technetium agents may be slightly less because of the more linear uptake characteristics of thallium.

It is also possible to combine stress techniques, and the commonest pairing is dynamic exercise with either adenosine or dipyridamole, which increases sensitivity for the detection of perfusion defects and also their conspicuity.[17] The addition of submaximal exercise has other benefits. It reduces the side effects caused by peripheral vasodilatation, it reduces the incidence of bradyarrhythmia, and it reduces splanchnic uptake of tracer, which can interfere with interpretation of the inferior wall when using the technetium tracers. For these reasons, our own routine form of stress is adenosine combined with exercise to 75 W on a bicycle ergometer, if tolerated.[18] In patients with contraindications to adenosine, such as asthma, we use dynamic exercise if possible and dobutamine if not. Patients with left bundle branch block, bifascicular block or paced rhythm receive adenosine without exercise in order to reduce the likelihood of visualizing perfusion defects related to the conduction abnormality rather than to coronary disease.

Myocardial metabolism

The myocardium has one of the highest energy demands of any tissue. It uses a variety of metabolic substrates, but under physiological conditions most of the energy required for contraction comes from the oxidation of free fatty acids. Glucose, lactate, pyruvate, ketone bodies and amino acids are also used, depending on availability, hormonal factors and myocardial oxygen demand. Under conditions of ischemia, oxidation of fatty acids is suppressed and there is increased glycolysis and glycogen breakdown. Imaging of myocardial metabolism therefore centers on fatty acids and glucose, which are mainly labeled with positron-emitting radionuclides. Qualitative imaging can be supplemented by quantitative analysis, although this requires knowledge of metabolic pathways and kinetics, and it is complicated sometimes by separation of the imaging radionuclide from the metabolic substrate or analog.

Glucose metabolism is most easily imaged using 2-fluoro-deoxyglucose (FDG) labeled with fluorine-18. It competes with glucose for transport into the cell and phosphorylation by the hexokinase reaction to FDG-6-phosphate, but it is not further metabolized and is trapped in the myocyte. The usual dose of F-18-FDG is 370 MBq and imaging is usually performed 40–60 minutes after intravenous injection. In order to maximize myocardial uptake, the FDG is normally given after an oral glucose load and, in patients with glucose intolerance or diabetes, it is also important to combine with glucose and insulin infusion: the 'euglycemic hyperinsulinemic clamp'. Despite this, the first-pass extraction fraction of FDG is low and variable but the cumulative uptake is 1–4% of the injected dose and is adequate for most studies.[19] Exogenous glucose utilization can be measured from the rate of supply and incorporation of FDG into the myocardium, correcting for the different rates of transport and phosphorylation of glucose and FDG.

A variety of fatty acids such as palmitic acid have been labeled with carbon-11, but their clinical use has been limited by complex kinetics and by back-diffusion of the unmetabolized tracer from the myocytes, which affects interpretation of the clearance phase. Acetate has also been proposed as a tracer of oxidative metabolism because it is metabolized by the tricarboxylic acid cycle. Its early rapid clearance from the myocardium is related to oxygen consumption and is only minimally influenced by the availability of other substrates.

Other fatty acids have been labeled with iodine-123 and these can be imaged using a conventional gamma camera. The straight chain fatty acids are metabolized by beta-oxidation and they are released rapidly from the myocardium, allowing fatty acid metabolism to be assessed by comparing initial uptake and the washout rates. Quantification, however, is complicated by decomposition of the molecule and by high background activity of free iodine. More accurate measurements can be achieved by adding a beta methyl branch to the chain, which leads to longer myocardial retention because of metabolic trapping. The most commonly used modified fatty acids are 15-(p-iodophenyl)-3-R,S-methyl pentadecanoic acid (BMIPP) and 15-(p-iodophenyl)-3,3-dimethyl pentadecanoic acid (DMIPP). Both have the potential to assess myocardial viability in patients with depressed ventricular function as well as stress-induced myocardial ischemia, although this requires combination with perfusion imaging (thallium or technetium perfusion tracers) to demonstrate mismatches of perfusion and metabolism. BMIPP images can also be gated, and this offers the prospect of simultaneous assessment of myocardial metabolism and function.

Neurotransmitter and receptor imaging

The sympathetic and parasympathetic nervous systems regulate heart rate and hemodynamics. Radiopharmaceuticals have been used to image the distribution of both presynaptic nerve terminals and post-synaptic receptors. False neurotransmitters such as ^{18}F-fluorometaraminol, ^{11}C-metahydroxyephedrine and ^{123}I-metaiodobenzylguanidine (MIBG) accumulate in the sympathetic nerve terminals because of their similarity to norepinephrine and their involvement in the norepinephrine reuptake mechanism and vesicular storage. Most experience has been gained with MIBG because iodine-123 and iodine-131 can be imaged using a conventional gamma camera. Abnormal innervation can be demonstrated in patients with ventricular arrhythmias and cardiomyopathies. Myocardial MIBG uptake in patients with congestive cardiac failure predicts medium-term survival,[20] and the rate of washout of MIBG predicts the response to beta-blockade.

Numerous beta-blockers have been labeled with positron-emitting tracers, the most promising being CGP-12177, which is hydrophilic. Labeled with carbon-11, it has been used to map functionally active myocardial beta-receptors in animals and in humans.

A satisfactory presynaptic parasympathetic tracer has not yet been developed, but muscarinic receptors can be imaged using methyl-quinuclidinyl benzylate (MQNB) labeled with carbon-11.

CLINICAL APPLICATIONS

Diagnosis of coronary artery disease

CHRONIC CHEST PAIN

A range of investigations is normally used in patients with suspected coronary artery disease, the simplest 'investigation' being the history. Typical angina is a good indicator of myocardial ischemia, and abolition of symptoms is the primary aim of treatment. However, symptoms can be indeterminate and they do not indicate the site or extent of ischemia. It is therefore often helpful to proceed to further investigations to aid the diagnosis and to guide future management. Radionuclide MPI is the only non-invasive and widely available method of assessing myocardial perfusion, and it therefore has an obvious role in this setting. Many studies have assessed the sensitivity and specificity of the technique for the detection of disease, the coronary arteriogram usually being used as the standard by which the accuracy of scintigraphy is judged. The wisdom of this approach can be debated, but at least the arteriogram provides a universal standard for coronary arterial anatomy, even if it is a less good standard by which to judge coronary arterial function. Published figures for sensitivity and specificity of MPI vary widely and they depend upon the population studied (sex, presenting symptoms, medication, presence of previous infarction, etc.), the imaging technique used (planar or tomographic, qualitative or quantitative analysis), and the experience of the center. Using modern techniques with tomographic imaging, good accuracy can be achieved, with sensitivity of 91% and specificity 89%.[21] This is significantly better than exercise electrocardiography, for which a large meta-analysis has shown sensitivity of 68% and specificity 77%.

It is reasonable to ask, therefore, whether radionuclide MPI should not replace exercise electrocardiography in patients with suspected coronary artery disease. Several factors militate against this. The most important is the relative availability of the two techniques, but radiation burden and cost are also relevant. Although the 1995 cost of MPI (£220) is higher than that of the exercise ECG (£70),[22] this is more than outweighed by its greater effectiveness. Studies of cost-effectiveness have shown significant advantages for strategies of investigation using MPI, with savings in total diagnostic and management costs over 2 years in the region of 20% in centers routinely using scintigraphy.[22]

Many centers use a staged approach, with the exercise ECG being the initial stress test and perfusion imaging next if the likelihood of disease is indeterminate after the exercise ECG, or if further information on myocardial perfusion is required to assist management decisions. Perfusion imaging should be the initial investigation in patients who are unlikely to exercise adequately, in women (because of the very high number of false-positive ECGs), and if the exercise ECG will be uninterpretable because of resting abnormalities such as left bundle branch block, pre-excitation, left ventricular hypertrophy or drug effects (Figure 6.3).

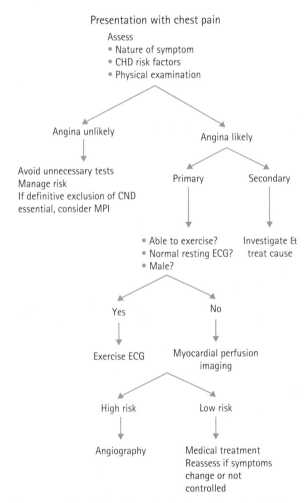

Figure 6.3 *Algorithm of investigation in stable angina. CHD, coronary heart disease; ECG, electrocardiogram; MPI, myocardial perfusion imaging. Reprinted from de Bono D. Investigation and management of stable angina: revised guidelines 1998. Joint Working Party of the British Cardiac Society and Royal College of Physicians of London.* Heart *1999; 81:546–55, with permission from BMJ Publishing Group.*

ACUTE CHEST PAIN

In general terms, nuclear techniques are less commonly used in patients presenting with acute chest pain, mainly because of the logistical problems of imaging in the emergency department or coronary care unit. Nonetheless, several centers have demonstrated the value of perfusion imaging in the acute setting, especially when the resting ECG is not diagnostic of myocardial ischemia.[23] The presence of a resting perfusion defect has a high positive predictive value for acute infarction in patients without previous infarction, particularly if it is associated with a wall motion abnormality on gated imaging, and these patients should be admitted to the coronary care unit. Conversely, a normal perfusion scan excludes acute infarction and suggests that exercise ECG or stress perfusion imaging should be the next diagnostic step. If the perfusion tracer is injected during chest pain, a normal perfusion scan excludes a cardiac cause and allows the patient to be discharged pending further investigation. An intriguing option in patients with acute chest pain that has settled is to use BMIPP, since fatty acid metabolism is reduced for some time even after acute ischemia has resolved. This 'metabolic memory' might allow diagnosis for up to 24 hours after ischemic chest pain and the theory is proven in principle, although it has not been widely applied.

Prognosis in coronary artery disease

Beyond diagnosis, the most valuable contribution that perfusion imaging can make to the management of known or suspected coronary artery disease is to assess the likelihood of a future coronary event such as myocardial infarction or coronary death. Prognosis is strongly influenced by the extent and severity of inducible perfusion abnormality and this can guide the need for invasive investigation and revascularization (Figures 6.4 and 6.5). Myocardial perfusion imaging is more powerful as an indicator of prognosis than clinical assessment, the exercise ECG and coronary angiography, and it provides incremental prognostic value even after the other tests have been performed.[24]

The most important variables that predict the likelihood of future events are the extent and depth of the inducible perfusion abnormality. The relative value of the fixed component of a stress defect is unclear, but it is likely that left ventricular function is the best indicator of prognosis in patients with predominantly fixed defects. Thus the patient with extensive ischemia is at high risk of a coronary event irrespective of the presence of infarction, and the patient without ischemia but with a fixed defect is only at risk if the defect leads to significantly impaired function. Additional markers of risk are increased lung uptake on stress thallium images (as this

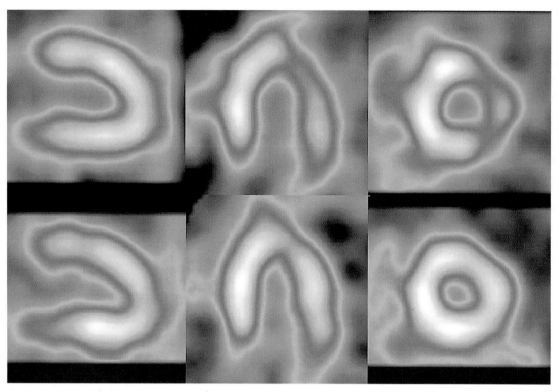

Figure 6.4 *Stress (top) and redistribution (bottom) thallium tomograms in the vertical long-axis (left), horizontal long-axis (center) and short-axis (right) planes in a patient with left circumflex stenosis. There is inducible ischemia of moderate extent and severity in the lateral wall, indicating a likelihood of future coronary events in the region of 10% per year.*

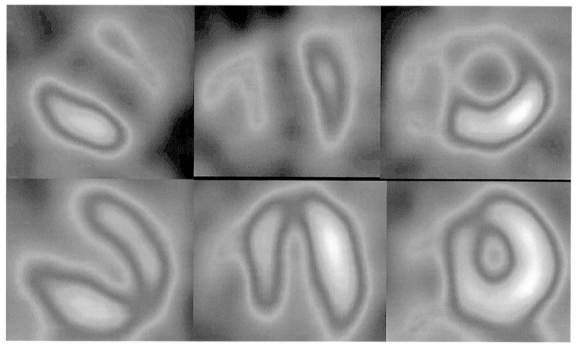

Figure 6.5 *Thallium tomograms in vertical long axis (left), horizontal long axis (center) and short axis (right) immediately after stress (top) and following re-injection of thallium at rest (bottom). There is severe and extensive inducible ischemia in most of the myocardium, sparing only the inferior wall. The appearances are characteristic of left main stem disease and indicate a likelihood of future coronary events in excess of 25% per year.*

indicates raised pulmonary capillary pressure either at rest or in response to stress) and ventricular dilatation that is greater in stress thallium images than at rest. Transient ischemic dilatation can also be seen with technetium imaging and it may be the result of extensive subendocardial ischemia giving the impression of cavity dilatation.

In patients with known or suspected coronary artery disease, a normal perfusion scan is very valuable because it indicates a likelihood of a coronary event of less than 1% per year, a rate that is lower than that in an asymptomatic population. Thus, whether minor coronary disease is present or not, further investigation can be avoided. This negative predictive value is independent of the type of imaging agent and technique, the method of stress, the population studied and the clinical setting.

PREOPERATIVE RISK ASSESSMENT

A common clinical problem is that of assessing cardiac risk in patients who require non-cardiac surgery. In this, as in other clinical settings, perfusion imaging provides useful prognostic information, although these patients are generally at low cardiac risk and the predictive value of a normal perfusion study is greater than that of an abnormal study. The decision on whether investigations for risk assessment are required should be based upon the urgency for surgery and its own cardiac risk, the risk factors of the individual, and his or her exercise tolerance. Patients with only minor clinical predictors (age > 70 years, abnormal resting ECG, history of stroke or hypertension) who are scheduled for a low-to-moderate-risk surgery are not at high risk and do not require further investigation. Patients with intermediate clinical predictors (mild angina, prior infarction, treated heart failure, or diabetes) or with minor predictors and impaired exercise tolerance need further assessment if they are to undergo moderate-risk or high-risk surgery. Patients at high clinical risk (recent infarction or unstable angina, decompensated heart failure, or significant arrhythmias) require investigation even for low-risk surgery.

For patients who are able to exercise, further investigation normally means exercise ECG, but if the resting ECG is abnormal or in patients who are unable to exercise, perfusion imaging should be used instead. If further testing suggests a low risk, surgery can proceed as planned. If it suggests a high risk, the need for revascularization is determined by the clinical setting. In general terms, revascularization should not be performed if it would not have been performed in the absence of surgery, since the risk of revascularization may still exceed the risk of the surgery. In patients at intermediate risk after further testing, the best strategy is uncertain, but aggressive medical management at the time of surgery rather than revascularization is preferred. This medical management involves rigorous control of pain, fluid balance and coagulation state after surgery, as well as preoperative beta-blockade and possible peroperative nitrate infusion.

Management of myocardial revascularization

Myocardial perfusion imaging can be valuable both before and after myocardial revascularization, either by angioplasty or bypass surgery. Neither procedure should be undertaken without objective evidence of ischemia, and perfusion imaging is often the most reliable way of obtaining this information and of ensuring that angioplasty is targeted at the culprit lesion. It has an excellent negative predictive value for predicting restenosis and clinical events after angioplasty, and this can be particularly helpful in patients with recurrent but atypical symptoms. Routine perfusion imaging after angioplasty in the absence of symptoms is not common, although it can sometimes be useful as a new baseline in case symptoms recur. It can, however, be justified routinely in patients with impaired left ventricular function, proximal left anterior descending and multivessel disease, suboptimal results of angioplasty, diabetes, and those with occupations requiring low coronary risk. If perfusion imaging is performed after angioplasty, it should ideally be performed later than 6 weeks since perfusion abnormalities can persist even with a good anatomical result. Possible exceptions to this are patients with high-risk anatomy who can benefit from earlier imaging.

As with angioplasty, patients who are asymptomatic after bypass surgery do not routinely undergo perfusion imaging, although it can be helpful as a baseline for future management as revascularization is not infrequently incomplete. More commonly, it is used for follow-up and it can be used roughly 5 years after surgery to guard against silent progression of prognostically important disease. Patients with symptoms after surgery may certainly benefit from perfusion imaging, and the algorithms to be used are very similar to those in the diagnostic setting.

Myocardial viability and hibernation

The term 'viable' is an umbrella term that includes several different subtypes of myocardium. One of these is hibernating myocardium, which is viable myocardium that is jeopardized by ischemia and that is akinetic. Hibernating myocardium has the potential to recover function after revascularization and hence it is important to detect hibernation in patients with ischemic left ventricular dysfunction. Failure to identify and rescue hibernating myocardium may lead to loss of viable myocytes, either by necrosis or apoptosis, deterioration of heart failure and death. A number of imaging techniques have been used to detect viable myocardium and to characterize it as hibernating.

POSITRON EMISSION TOMOGRAPHY

Positron-emitting radionuclides can be used to assess both myocardial perfusion and metabolism. The technique relies on the detection of reduced resting perfusion assessed by N-13 ammonia with normal or increased FDG uptake (perfusion–metabolism mismatch), as opposed to a matched reduction of perfusion and metabolism in fully infarcted myocardium or scar. The reported positive and negative accuracies for predicting recovery of regional function range from 72% to 95% and from 75% to 100%, respectively.[25–27] Mismatch also predicts improvement in global left ventricular function after revascularization.[28] Carbon-11 acetate has also been used to assess both oxidative metabolism and perfusion, with favorable results compared with ammonia and FDG imaging.

SINGLE PHOTON TRACERS

The disadvantage of positron emission tomography (PET) is that it is not widely available. Thallium is also a tracer of myocardial viability and perfusion and it has been widely used for identifying myocardial viability and hibernation. Because redistribution can be slow or incomplete in regions of reduced perfusion, the usual stress/redistribution protocol can underestimate myocardial viability and additional steps to ensure complete assessment of viability are required. These include late redistribution imaging at 8–72 hours after stress injection,[29] re-injection of tracer at rest after redistribution imaging,[7] and a resting injection on a separate day with both early and delayed imaging.[30]

In any of these viability images, the amount of viable myocardium is proportional to the amount of tracer uptake relative to a normal area. A common threshold for defining clinically significant viability is 50% of maximal uptake, although the best threshold may be higher. An important additional criterion is to require the presence of inducible ischemia before diagnosing hibernation as it is an ischemic syndrome (Figure 6.6).

MIBI and tetrofosmin have also been used for the detection of viable and hibernating myocardium. In theory, these tracers may underestimate viability in areas with reduced resting perfusion because they are combined tracers of viability and perfusion without the property of redistribution that allows viability to be assessed independently. Some studies have therefore found thallium to be better for the assessment of viability, but others have found them to be similar.[31,32] It does appear though that if the tracers are given under the cover of intravenous or sublingual nitrates, resting perfusion is improved and the technetium tracers are good markers of viability.[33] Other adjuncts such as glucose and insulin and D-ribose have been used and all three increase uptake in areas of previous infarction. Although the role of these agents has not been fully assessed, they are likely to improve sensitivity.

ECG-GATED PERFUSION IMAGING

An important problem in studies of hibernation is that viability and function are often assessed from different techniques, and it can be difficult to be sure that the same myocardial segment is being compared in each. Thus, the ideal technique should combine information on viability, perfusion and function in a single image, and ECG-gated technetium perfusion imaging is very helpful. This is our own initial technique in patients referred for the assessment of hibernation. Myocardial motion and thickening imaged by magnetic resonance imaging and gated perfusion imaging using both MIBI and tetrofosmin agree well. In regions of previous infarction with reduced tracer uptake, the assessment is more difficult, but this is not a major limitation since these areas contain little myocardium and will not benefit from revascularization.

OTHER NUCLEAR TECHNIQUES

Because PET is relatively expensive and less widely available than single-photon emission computed tomography (SPECT), alternative methods of imaging FDG are of interest. High-energy collimation on a conventional gamma camera is one alternative and the information provided is similar to that of PET.[34] Coincidence detection without collimation using a dual-headed gamma camera is another possibility, but to date this technique has not been assessed for hibernation.

Other metabolic tracers suitable for conventional cameras include ^{123}I-labeled fatty acids such as BMIPP combined with thallium or a technetium tracer for the assessment of perfusion.[35]

COMPARISON WITH FUNCTIONAL TECHNIQUES

In general terms, nuclear techniques are sensitive (average values between 86% and 91%) but not very specific (47–88%) for predicting recovery of segmental function after revascularization, and viable but akinetic segments defined in this way do not always improve. In contrast, functional techniques such as dobutamine echocardiography or magnetic resonance imaging are specific but less sensitive. However, the low specificity of the nuclear techniques may not be a limitation since factors other than improvement of segmental function may be important, such as protection against remodeling, necrosis or apoptosis. Certainly, the simple nuclear techniques have been shown to predict improvement of symptoms and medium-term outcome, and these are clearly more important parameters than segmental function.

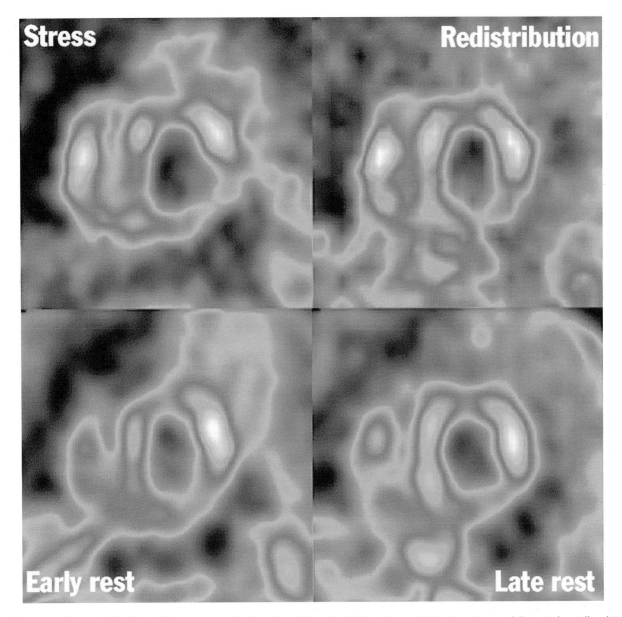

Stress

Redistribution

Early rest

Late rest

Figure 6.6 *Short-axis thallium-201 tomograms showing stress-induced perfusion abnormality in the septum and the anterior wall and a fixed defect in the infero-lateral wall in the conventional stress and redistribution images (top row). On a separate occasion, thallium was injected at rest with immediate and delayed imaging (bottom row). These images also show reduced perfusion in the septum and a fixed infero-lateral defect. MRI showed severe hypokinesis in most of the anterior wall and septum and akinesis in the infero-lateral wall. Thus, the antero-septal region is viable but ischemic and hypokinetic and it will recover function after revascularization. The infero-lateral wall is infarcted and it will not recover.*

KEY REFERENCES

American College of Physicians. Guidelines for assessing and managing the perioperative risk from coronary artery disease associated with major noncardiac surgery. *Ann Intern Med* 1997; **127**:309–12.
The most recent guidelines for coronary risk assessment before non-cardiac surgery. Nuclear cardiology techniques play an important role.

de Bono D. Investigation and management of stable angina: revised guidelines 1998. *Heart* 1999; **81**:546–55.
The most recent UK guidelines endorsed by the British Cardiac Society for the management of stable angina. Again, nuclear cardiology techniques play an important role.

Gibbons RJ, Chatterjee K, Daley J, Douglas JS, Fihn SD, Gardin JM, *et al.* ACC/AHA/ACP-ASIM guidelines for the management of patients with chronic stable angina: a report of the American College of Cardiology/

American Heart Association Task Force on Practice Guidelines. *J Am Coll Cardiol* 1999; **33**:2092–197.
The most recent US guidelines for the investigation and management of stable angina.

Skorton DJ, Schelbert HR, Wolf GL, Brundage BH (eds). *Cardiac Imaging. A Companion to Braunwald's Heart Disease*, 2nd edn. Philadelphia: W.B Saunders, 1996.
An important and comprehensive textbook covering the whole field of cardiac imaging.

Underwood SR. Myocardial perfusion imaging and pilot certification. *Eur Heart J Supplements* 1999; **1**(Suppl. D):D84–93.
A review of the assessment of prognosis using myocardial perfusion imaging. Although this is with special reference to assessment of risk in pilots, it contains the major references and other reviews of the risk assessment.

Wackers FJ TH, Soufer R, Zaret BL. Nuclear cardiology. In: *Heart Disease. A Text Book of Cardiovascular Medicine*, 5th edn, Braunwald E (ed.). Philadelphia: W.B Saunders, 1997, 273–316.
An important and lucid review of nuclear cardiology in general.

Zaret BL, Beller GA (eds). *Nuclear Cardiology, State of the Art and Future Direction*, 2nd edn. St Louis, MI: Mosby, 1999.
A major textbook on nuclear cardiology.

REFERENCES

1. Grunwald AM, Watson DD, Holzgrefe HH, Irving JF, Beller GA. Myocardial thallium-201 kinetics in normal and ischaemic myocardium. *Circulation* 1981; **64**:610–18.
2. Goldhaber SZ, Newell JB, Alpert NM, Andrews E, Pohost GM, Ingwall JS. Effects of ischemic-like insult on myocardial thallium-201 accumulation. *Circulation* 1983; **67**:778–86.
3. Goldhaber SZ, Newell JB, Ingwall JS, Pohost GM, Alpert NM, Fossel ET. Effects of reduced coronary flow on thallium-201 accumulation and release in an in vitro rat heart preparation. *Am J Cardiol* 1983; **51**:891–6.
4. Mueller TM, Marcus ML, Ehrhardt JC, Chandhuri T, Abboud FM. Limitations of thallium-201 myocardial perfusion scintigrams. *Circulation* 1976; **54**:640–6.
5. Li QS, Solot G, Frank TL, Wagner HNJ, Becker LC. Myocardial redistribution of technetium-99m-methoxyisobutyl isonitrile (SESTAMIBI). *J Nucl Med* 1990; **31**:1069–76.
6. Jain D, Wackers FJ, Mattera J, McMahon M, Sinusas AJ, Zaret BL. Biokinetics of technetium-99m-tetrofosmin: myocardial perfusion imaging agent: implications for a one-day imaging protocol. *J Nucl Med* 1993; **34**:1254–9.
7. Dilsizian V, Rocco TP, Freedman NMT, Leon MB, Bonow RO. Enhanced detection of ischemic but viable myocardium by the reinjection of thallium after stress-redistribution imaging. *N Engl J Med* 1990; **66**:394–9.
8. Heo J, Kegel J, Iskandrian AS, Cave V, Iskandrian BB. Comparison of same-day protocols using technetium-99m-sestamibi myocardial imaging. *J Nucl Med* 1992; **33**:186–91.
9. Anagnostopoulos C, Gunning MG, Pennell DJ, Laney R, Proukakis H, Underwood SR. Regional myocardial motion and thickening assessed at rest by ECG-gated 99m Tc-MIBI emission tomography and by magnetic resonance imaging. *Eur J Nucl Med* 1996; **23**:909–16.
10. Weiss AT, Maddahi J, Lew AS, Shah PK, Ganz W, Swan HT, et al. Reverse redistribution of thallium-201: a sign of nontransmural myocardial infarction with patency of the infarct-related coronary artery. *J Am Coll Cardiol* 1986; **7**:61–7.
11. Weiss AT, Berman DS, Lew AS, Nielsen J, Potkin B, Swan HJ, et al. Transient ischemic dilatation of the left ventricle on stress thallium-201 scintigraphy: a marker of severe and extensive coronary artery disease. *J Am Coll Cardiol* 1987; **9**:752–9.
12. Burow RD, Pond M, Schafer AW, Becker L. Circumferential profiles: a new method for computer analysis of thallium-201 myocardial perfusion images. *J Nucl Med* 1979; **20**:771–7.
13. Mahmarian JJ, Boyce TM, Goldberg RK, Cocanougher MK, Roberts R, Verani MS. Quantitative exercise thallium-201 single photon emission computed tomography for the enhanced diagnosis of ischemic heart disease. *J Am Coll Cardiol* 1990; **15**:318–29.
14. Gill JB, Ruddy TD, Newell JB, Finkelstein DM, Strauss HW, Boucher CA. Prognostic importance of thallium uptake by the lungs during exercise in coronary artery disease. *N Engl J Med* 1987; **317**:1486–9.
15. Wilson RF, Wyche K, Christensen BV, Zimmer S, Laxson DD. Effects of adenosine on human coronary arterial circulation. *Circulation* 1990; **82**:1595–606.
16. Verani MS, Mahmarian JJ, Hixson JB, Boyce TM, Staudacher RA. Diagnosis of coronary artery disease by controlled coronary vasodilation with adenosine and thallium-201 scintigraphy in patients unable to exercise. *Circulation* 1990; **82**:80–97.
17. Walker PR, James MA, Wilde RPH, Wood CH, Russell RJ. Dipyridamole combined with exercise for thallium myocardial imaging. *Br Heart J* 1986; **55**:321–9.
18. Pennell DJ, Mavrogeni SI, Forbat SM, Karwatowski SP, Underwood SR. Adenosine combined with dynamic exercise for myocardial perfusion imaging. *J Am Coll Cardiol* 1995; **25**:1300–9.
19. Ratib O, Phelps ME, Huang SC, Henze E, Selin CE, Schelbert HR. Positron tomography with deoxyglucose for estimating local myocardial glucose metabolism. *J Nucl Med* 1982; **23**:577–86.
20. Merlet P, Benvenuti C, Moyse D, Pouillart F, Dubois-Rande JL, Duval AM, et al. Prognostic value of MIBG imaging in idiopathic dilated cardiomyopathy. *J Nucl Med* 1999; **40**:917–23.
21. Maddahi J. Myocardial perfusion imaging for the detection and evaluation of coronary artery disease. In: *Cardiac Imaging. A Companion to Braunwald's Heart Disease*, 2nd edn, Skorton DJ, Schelbert HR, Wolf GL, Brundage BH (eds). Philadelphia: W.B. Saunders, 1996, 971–94.
22. Underwood SR, Godman B, Salyani S, Ogle JR, Ell PJ. Economics of myocardial perfusion imaging in Europe: the EMPIRE study. *Eur Heart J* 1999; **20**:157–66.
23. Kontos MC, Jesse RL, Schmidt KL, Ornato JP, Tatum JL. Value of acute rest sestamibi perfusion imaging for evaluation of patients admitted to the emergency department with chest pain. *J Am Coll Cardiol* 1997; **30**:976–82.
24. Marie PY, Danchin N, Durand JF, Feldmann L, Grentzinger A, Olivier P, et al. Long-term prediction of major ischemic events by exercise thallium-201 single-photon emission computed tomography. Incremental prognostic value compared with clinical, exercise testing, catheterization and radionuclide angiographic data. *J Am Coll Cardiol* 1995; **26**:879–86.
25. The Multicenter Postinfarction Research Group. Risk stratification and survival after acute myocardial infarction. *N Engl J Med* 1983; **309**:331–7.

26. Lucignani G, Paolini G, Landoni C, Zuccari M, Paganelli G, Galli L, *et al.* Presurgical identification of hibernating myocardium by combined use of technetium-99m hexokinase 2-methoxyisobutylisonitrile single photon emission tomography and fluorine-18 fluoro-2-deoxy-d-glucose positron emission tomography in patients with coronary artery disease. *Eur J Nucl Med* 1992; **19**:874–81.

27. Gropler RJ, Geltman EM, Sampathkumaran K, Perez JE, Schechtman KB, Conversano A, *et al.* Comparison of carbon-11-acetate with fluorine-18-fluorodeoxyglucose for delineating viable myocardium by positron emission tomography. *J Am Coll Cardiol* 1993; **122**:1587–97.

28. Tamaki N, Ohtani H, Yamashita K, Magata Y, Yonekura Y, Nohara R, *et al.* Metabolic activity in the areas of new fill-in after thallium-201 reinjection: comparison with positron emission tomography using fluorine-18-deoxyglucose. *J Nucl Med* 1991; **32**:673–8.

29. Tillisch JH, Brunken R, Marshall R, Schwaiger M, Mandelkern M, Phelps M, *et al.* Reversibility of cardiac wall motion abnormalities predicted by positron tomography. *N Eng J Med* 1986; **314**:884–8.

30. Kiat H, Berman DS, Maddahi J, De Yang L, Van Train K, Rozanski A, *et al.* Late reversibility of tomographic myocardial thallium-201 defects: an accurate marker of myocardial viability. *J Am Coll Cardiol* 1988; **12**:1456–63.

31. Gunning MG, Anagnostopoulos C, Knight CJ, Pepper J, Burman ED, Davies G, *et al.* Identification of hibernating myocardium. A comparison of Tl-201, Tc-99m tetrofosmin and dobutamine cine magnetic resonance imaging. *Circulation* 1998; **98**:1869–74.

32. Udelson JE, Coleman PS, Metherall J, Pandian NG, Gomez AR, Griffith JL, *et al.* Predicting recovery of severe regional ventricular dysfunction. Comparison of resting scintigraphy with ^{201}Tl and ^{99m}Tc-sestamibi. *Circulation* 1994; **89**:2552–61.

33. Bisi G, Sciagra R, Santoro GM, Rossi V, Fazzini PF. Technetium-99m-sestamibi imaging with nitrate infusion to detect viable hibernating myocardium and predict postrevascularisation recovery. *J Nucl Med* 1995; **36**:1994–2000.

34. Chen EQ, MacIntyre WJ, Go RT, Brunken RC, Saha GB, Wong CY, *et al.* Myocardial viability studies using fluorine-18-FDG SPECT: a comparison with fluorine-18-FDG PET. *J Nucl Med* 1997; **38**:582–6.

35. Ito T, Tanouchi J, Kato J, Morioka T, Nishino M, Iwai K, *et al.* Recovery of impaired left ventricular function in patients with acute myocardial infarction is predicted by the discordance in defect size on ^{123}I-BMIPP and ^{201}Tl SPET images. *Eur J Nucl Med* 1996; **23**:917–23.

7

Cardiovascular magnetic resonance in coronary artery disease

RAAD H MOHIADDIN

INTRODUCTION

The ideal imaging technique for assessing patients with coronary artery disease would be a safe, non-invasive, cheap and widely available method that is able simultaneously to assess coronary artery anatomy, myocardial function, perfusion and viability with 100% sensitivity and 100% specificity. Clearly, no such technique exists and the advantages/disadvantages of one method may be complemented by those of another. Therefore currently more than one method is used in the investigation of individual patients.

Cardiovascular magnetic resonance imaging (CMR, MRI) has well known and important clinical application in a number of cardiac conditions, particularly for the assessment of congenital heart disease and diseases of the aorta and pericardium, but only recently has it been possible to envisage significant applications in coronary artery disease.[1] Circumstances have changed because of the huge improvement in the technical capabilities of scanners, most notably in terms of speed of acquisition. These improvements have allowed coronary artery imaging, myocardial perfusion imaging and myocardial viability imaging, which were previously essentially impossible. The boost that this has given the field in general should not be underestimated, because perhaps 90% of clinical cardiology in the Western world revolves around coronary artery disease and any imaging technique without major application in this arena is likely to be doomed to playing understudy to echocardiography, nuclear cardiology and catheterization.

Cardiovascular magnetic resonance has now been accepted as the gold standard for non-invasive, accurate and reproducible assessment of cardiac mass and function. The interest in its use for myocardial viability, perfusion and coronary artery imaging is also growing rapidly as the hardware and expertise become widely available and the scans themselves become more cost-effective. This chapter reviews the established morphological role that CMR has in the assessment of ventricular function and then concentrates on the other areas where it is enabling advances in stress imaging, coronary artery imaging, myocardial perfusion imaging, myocardial viability imaging and cardiac magnetic resonance spectroscopy (MRS).

PHYSICAL PRINCIPLES

Nuclear magnetization

Understanding the basic principles and details of MRI is invaluable in appreciating the capabilities of the technique, and these have been well described many times.[2]

Most magnetic resonance studies are of the hydrogen nuclei (protons) in water. Protons spin on their axes and generate a tiny magnetic field and behave as a small magnet. They will align with an applied magnetic field and precess about the field in the same way that a spinning top precesses in a gravitational field (Figure 7.1). Applying radio waves at the resonant frequency, however, excites some protons to the higher energy anti-parallel orientation and these protons initially precess in phase together. The net effect is to rotate the net magnetization vector at an angle to the applied field, and this initial flip angle is determined by the amount of energy applied. After absorption of energy, the net magnetization vector precesses and relaxes back to its equilibrium position, tracing out a spiral. The rates at which the net magnetization parallel and perpendicular to the applied field return to equilibrium after a disturbance are called the longitudinal (T_1) and transverse relaxation times (T_2) respectively. They depend upon the fluctuating magnetic fields experienced by the nuclei, and hence upon their biochemical and biophysical environment.

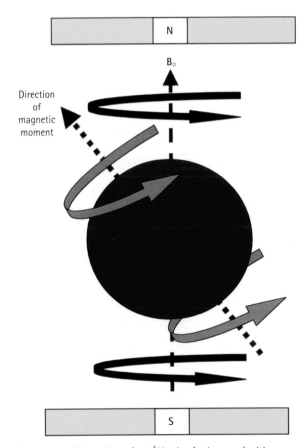

Figure 7.1 *Orientation of net ^1H spins (red arrows) with the main magnetic field (B_0). The angular momentum and the magnetic dipole moment of the ^1H nucleus result in a precession (black arrows) around the axis of the magnetic field.*

Magnetic resonance imaging

Conventional magnetic resonance images show the amplitude of the emitted magnetic resonance signal at each point in the imaging plane. The signal is stimulated and localized by pulses of radiofrequency energy and magnetic field gradients superimposed upon the main field. A common combination of pulses (or sequence) is the spin echo sequence in which signal from moving blood is lost, so it appears black, in contrast to other tissues which give some signal and appear increasing shades of grey. The signal strength, and hence the contrast in the images, depends partly upon proton density and upon the relaxation times of the nuclei.

Another common sequence is the gradient echo sequence, in which blood gives high signal and appears white, except where it is turbulent, when it can lose signal. A modification of gradient echo imaging can measure flow by encoding velocity in the phase of the magnetic resonance signal. A map of the phase of the signal rather than the amplitude then becomes a velocity map, and the images show velocity in any chosen plane.

Contrast agent

The most widely used magnetic resonance contrast agents are paramagnetic compounds that influence the relaxation times (T_1, T_2) of tissues with which they have close contact. Gadolinium (Gd) is a particularly powerful paramagnetic substance because of the seven unpaired electrons in its atom's outer shell. When Gd is complexed with ligands, such as diethylenetriaminepentaacetic acid (DTPA), it loses its natural toxicity. It has been used clinically for many years, mainly for the assessment of myocardial perfusion, contrast-enhanced magnetic resonance angiography, improved demarcation of normal and infarcted myocardium, delineation of the area at risk after acute coronary occlusion, and assessment of cardiac tumors.

ASSESSMENT OF CARDIAC FUNCTION

Heart failure

Coronary artery disease is the leading cause of heart failure in the Western world. Left ventricular dysfunction is an important prognostic determinant, and markers of impairment such as ejection fraction, end-diastolic volume (EDV), end-diastolic pressure, exercise capacity and symptom profile are all predictors of outcome.[3,4] There have been significant developments in pharmacological agents available for the treatment of heart failure. At the same time, both surgical and anesthetic techniques for coronary artery bypass surgery have improved. However, the decision to revascularize must be tempered with consideration of the appreciable perioperative mortality in patients with impaired left ventricular function. Therefore there is an important role for imaging techniques that differentiate viable tissue from myocardial scar, as this moderates the clinical strategy in such cases.

Assessment of cardiac function by CMR has some advantages over other techniques such as echocardiography and radionuclide ventriculography, namely the ability to provide accurate and reproducible tomographic static and dynamic images of high spatial and temporal resolution in any desired plane without exposure to ionizing radiation or limitation by acoustic access. Comparisons between CMR and the more established techniques are now being reported. Whereas the mean value in a study population of a parameter such as ejection fraction is similar between techniques, there is very considerable scatter of results. This is due to the variations in accuracy and other technical factors, and suggests that the results between techniques are not directly comparable.[5]

Assessment of global function

There are several approaches to the assessment of cardiac function with CMR. A simple semi-qualitative assessment may be made using cine CMR in the vertical and horizontal long axes (Figure 7.2). These views allow direct visualization of global and regional cardiac function in

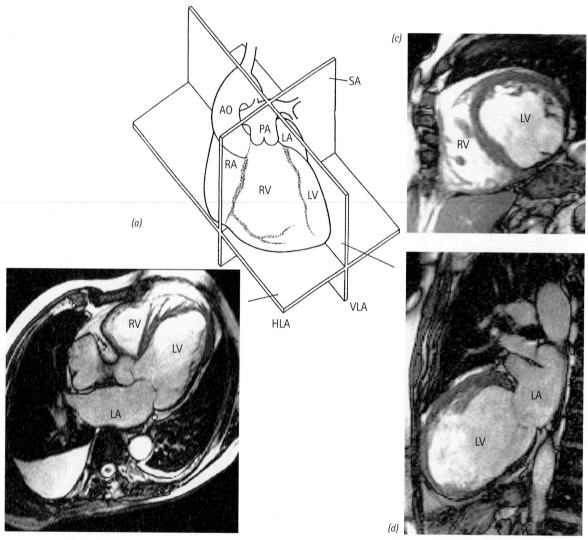

Figure 7.2 (a) Schematic representation of the standard oblique imaging planes of the left ventricle. (b), (c) and (d) Diastolic frames selected from complete cine study in the corresponding planes shown in (a) acquired in a patient with heart failure, following infero-lateral transmural infarction, and extensive left ventricular remodeling. The infero-lateral wall is thin and the ventricular geometry is asymmetric. HLA, horizontal long axis; VLA, vertical long axis; SA, short axis; LV, left ventricle; LA, left atrium; RV, right ventricle; RA, right atrium; AO, aorta; PA, pulmonary artery.

similar orientations obtainable with echocardiography (Figure 7.3). As with two-dimensional echocardiography, EDV and end-systolic volume (ESV) may be calculated using the area–length method.[6] Although simple and time-efficient, these methods rely on the geometric assumption that the left ventricle may be represented as an ellipsoid shape, which is not the case in patients with morphologically distorted left ventricle as a result of infarction. In order to capitalize on the strengths of CMR, quantitative methods are preferred. The most important CMR approach for assessment of cardiac function is by calculating the EDV and ESV from a stack of contiguous short axis slices encompassing the entire left and right ventricles in a three-dimensional fashion (Simpson's method, Figure 7.4). Endocardial border contours are traced on the diastolic and systolic images and the ventricular volumes (diastolic and systolic is equal to the sum of all the endocardial areas of the diastolic and systolic images respectively) multiplied by slice thickness. From EDV and ESV, the stroke volume (SV) and

ejection fraction (EF) is calculated:[7]

$$SV = EDV - ESV \quad EF = SV/EDV$$

The ventricular mass may be calculated by tracing the epicardial borders in diastole, applying Simpson's rule to obtain epicardial volume, and then subtraction of the EDV from this to give volume of the myocardium. Multiplication of this value by the specific gravity of muscle (1.05 g/mL) yields the myocardial mass.[8,9]

Assessment of regional function

Muscle thinning, myocardial rupture and aneurysm formation due to myocardial infarction are readily recognized by CMR (Figure 7.5), and previous infarction can be detected and quantified by the presence and extent of thinning[10] and wall motion abnormality. Cine CMR sequences allow qualitative assessment of regional function in a manner similar to echocardiography but without

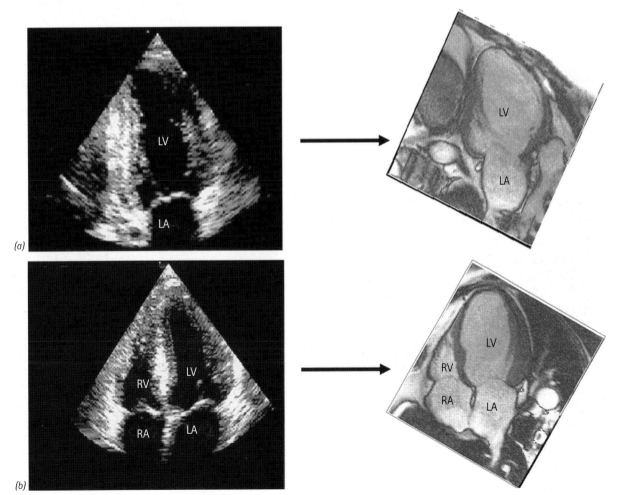

(a)

(b)

Figure 7.3 *Two-dimensional echocardiography of the vertical (a) and horizontal (b) long-axis views and the corresponding CMR images in a patient with antero-septal transmural infarction, and left ventricular remodeling. LV, left ventricle; LA, left atrium; RV, right ventricle; RA, right atrium.*

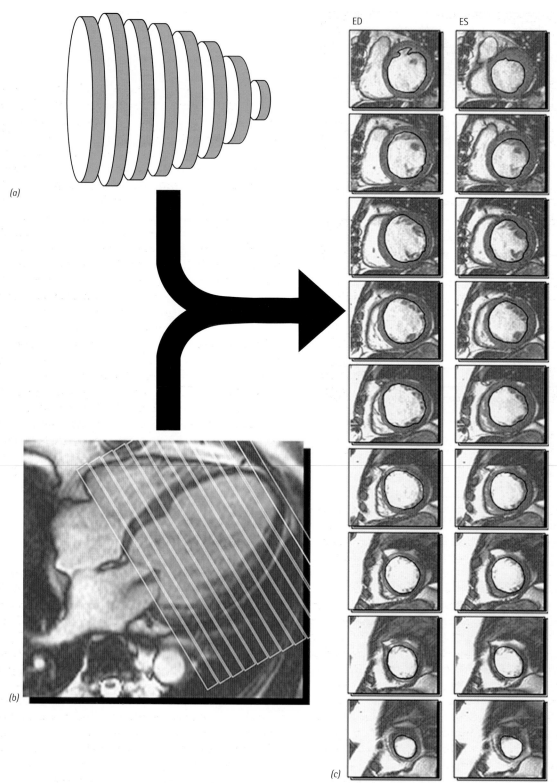

Figure 7.4 *Calculation of left ventricular volumes using a stack of contiguous short-axis slices (a, b and c) according to Simpson's method. ED, end-diastolic images; ES, end-systolic images. The epicardial borders (outer black) are defined on the end-diastolic images, and the endocardial borders (inner black) are defined on both the end-diastolic and end-systolic images. This allows accurate measurement of the area of blood pool and myocardium for each short-axis slice, and subsequently calculation of ventricular volumes and mass. The process is easily extended to calculate the same parameters for the right ventricle.*

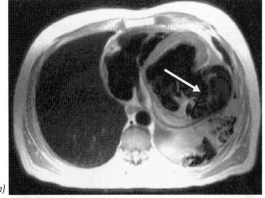

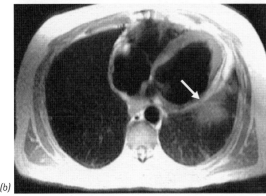

Figure 7.5 *Spin-echo images in transverse plane in a patient with large false left ventricular aneurysm, complicating transmural lateral wall infarction, acquired (a) before and (b) after surgical resection and patch closure.*

the limitations of acoustic windows. Wall motion analysis can be performed at rest, with low-dose dobutamine (beta agonists) for detection of viable myocardium[11] (Figure 7.6) and high-dose dobutamine for the detection of ischemia.[12] Several methods also exist for quantitative assessment of wall motion and wall thickening based on cine CMR. However, all of these methods require a degree of manual interaction, and in reality myocardial dynamics are more complicated than simple myocardial thickening and the two-dimensional model commonly used. Myocardial tagging offers a method for quantification of regional wall motion and myocardial strain.[13,14] In this technique, a grid of lines is physically placed in the heart at end-diastole, for example a short axis slice (Figure 7.7). The distortion of this grid during the cardiac cycle may be studied using a sophisticated computer analysis to derive quantitative measurements of intrinsic myocardial mechanics by tracking the motion of the points of intersection of the tagging lines. Myocardial motion can also be quantified using CMR velocity mapping.[15] Both myocardial tagging and velocity mapping are now being used with dobutamine stress to demonstrate localized dynamics of both normal and dysfunctional myocardium in patients with reversible ischemia.

CORONARY ARTERY IMAGING

Magnetic resonance coronary angiography

Since the late 1950s and early 1960s, invasive coronary angiography has been the gold standard for the diagnosis of coronary artery disease.[16,17] However, it does have a major complication rate of between 0.3 and 1.1%[18,19] and is expensive. The search for an alternative non-invasive diagnostic examination has stimulated research into magnetic resonance coronary angiography (MRCA). Substantial improvement in imaging of native coronary arteries only came with the development of much faster imaging, which allowed data acquisition within the period of a breath-hold, which significantly reduced artifact from respiratory motion. The technique currently most widely used is segmented k-space gradient echo imaging,[20] but other ultrafast techniques (spiral and rectilinear echo planar imaging) have also been developed. MRCA can be performed using a two-dimensional (Figures 7.8 and 7.9, page 106) or a three-dimensional approach (Figure 7.10, page 106). There are clear advantages to the development of three-dimensional techniques for MRCA, because the acquisition could be standardized for later interrogation in reformatted planes as required by the investigator. However, blurring from breathing was a problem for early studies,[21] although special breathing techniques[22] and the use of navigator echo imaging have helped, with patient feedback[23] or direct respiratory compensation.[24] The following paragraphs review the current clinical applications of MRCA.

CURRENT CLINICAL UTILITY OF MRCA

Magnetic resonance coronary angiography has already proven itself useful in a number of clinical areas, despite its lower resolution compared with x-ray angiography and the well-described limitations of the current techniques. These areas are imaging of anomalous coronary arteries (Figure 7.11, page 107), assessment of patency of the infarct-related artery, and vein graft patency imaging (Figure 7.12, page 108). The clinical significance of anomalous coronary arteries depends upon their proximal anatomical route, and so MRCA can contribute valuable information as to the diagnosis and significance of such anomalies.[25,26] In patients with myocardial infarction, patency of the infarct-related artery significantly improves short-term left ventricular function, reducing morbidity and mortality, and also appears to be associated with a better long-term outcome.[27] Recent results of vein graft patency imaging have been excellent, with both anatomical and flow imaging being used to detect patency and establish graft function through resting flow.[28,29] Complications following coronary graft surgery, for example hemopericardium (Figure

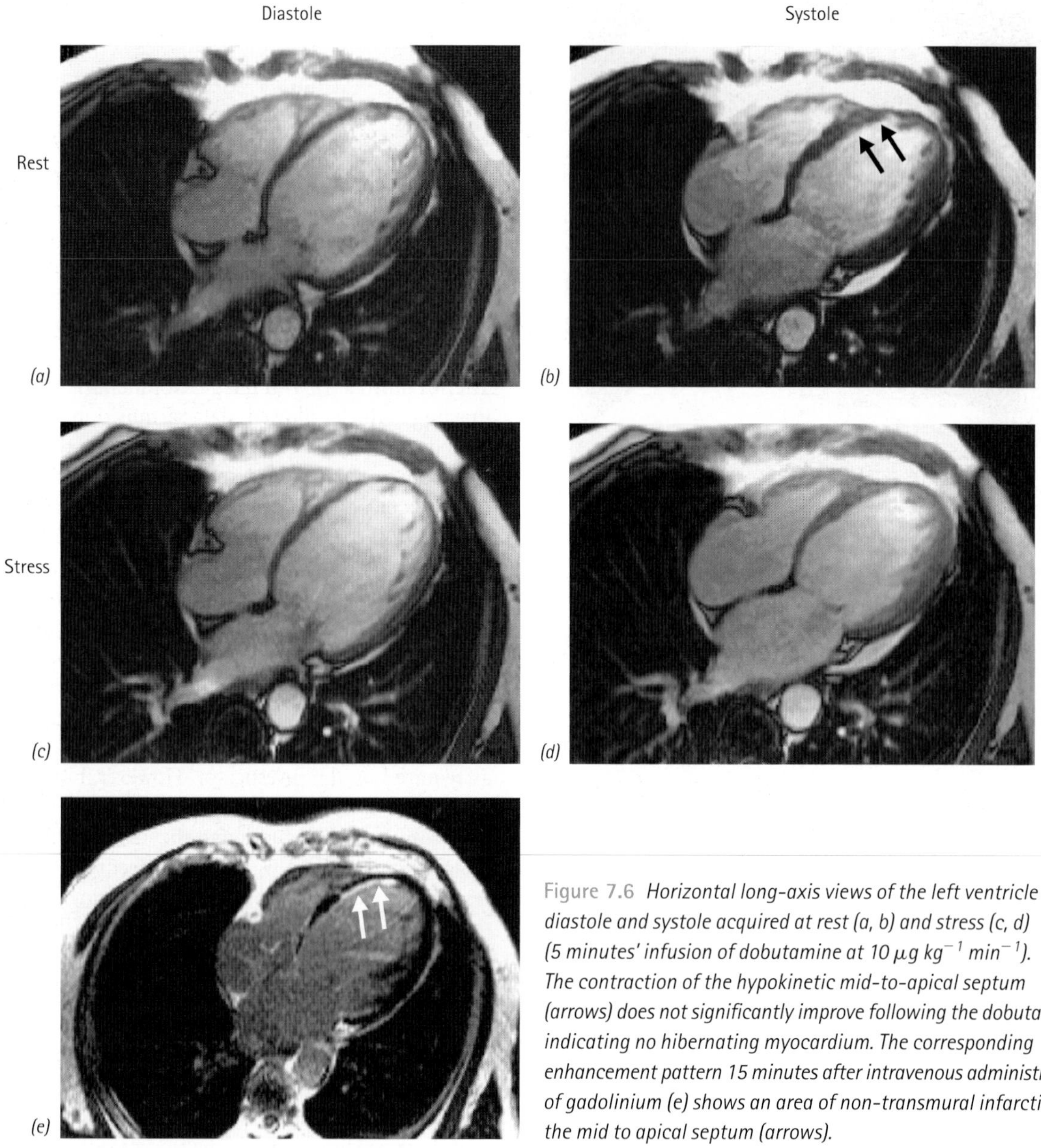

Diastole   Systole

Rest

(a)

(b)

Stress

(c)

(d)

(e)

Figure 7.6 *Horizontal long-axis views of the left ventricle in diastole and systole acquired at rest (a, b) and stress (c, d) (5 minutes' infusion of dobutamine at 10 μg kg^{-1} min^{-1}). The contraction of the hypokinetic mid-to-apical septum (arrows) does not significantly improve following the dobutamine, indicating no hibernating myocardium. The corresponding enhancement pattern 15 minutes after intravenous administration of gadolinium (e) shows an area of non-transmural infarction of the mid to apical septum (arrows).*

7.13, page 108) and coronary artery bypass graft aneurysm (Figure 7.14, page 109), are readily detectable by CMR.[30]

CLINICAL RESULTS USING MRCA TO DETECT CORONARY ARTERY STENOSIS

The feasibility of detecting coronary artery stenosis by MRCA was first shown in 1993, with results in 39 patients with a double-blind comparison of MRCA and x-ray contrast angiography.[31] The study group included 29 patients (74%) with coronary artery disease with a total of 52 hemodynamically significant stenoses (diameter stenosis >50%). The results demonstrated a high correlation between the two imaging methods.

Duerinckx[32] found a lower sensitivity in a second double-blind trial of 17 patients with significant stenosis (>50%). In our own experience, a comparative study primarily designed to investigate stenosis characteristics looked at 39 patients with known coronary artery disease.[33] MRCA detected 47 of the 55 stenoses that had been demonstrated at x-ray contrast angiography, giving an overall sensitivity of 85%, a result that was intermediate between those of the previous two studies (see Figure 7.9). Coronary arterial wall plaque imaging has been reported[34] (Figure 7.15, page 109) using new imaging techniques, and further work in this area is awaited with great interest. This advance may allow studies of plaque progression and regression to be planned *in vivo* in humans.

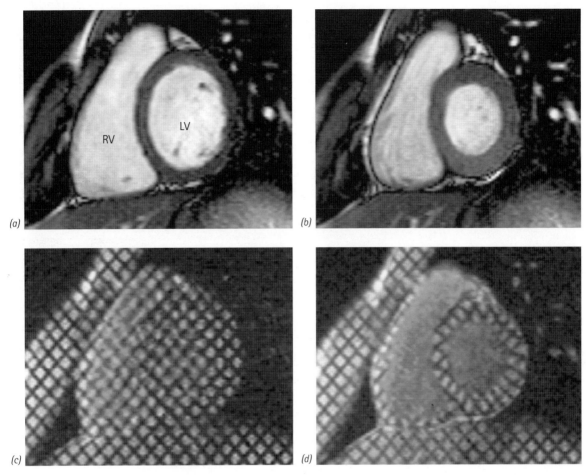

Figure 7.7 *Diastolic (a) and mid-systolic (b) images in the short-axis plane of the left ventricle of a healthy heart and the corresponding CMR tagging images (c and d). In this technique, a grid of low-signal tagging lines is placed in the myocardium at end-diastole to form a latticework of regular-shaped squares (as seen on the end-diastolic image before contraction and on the liver and chest wall). Deformation of the lines is followed during the cardiac cycle (as seen on the mid-systolic image). Deformation of the lines towards the blood caused by myocardial contraction is seen as curvature of the lines towards the center of the blood pool, and the circumferential shortening is seen as bunching of the lines. Thus the squares become distorted, thinned rectangles during contraction. Quantification is performed by mapping the tag line intersection points, which allows myocardial strain analysis. This has the advantage of being an objective and quantifiable measure of contractility, which is not dependent on endocardial excursion. RV, right ventricle; LV, left ventricle.*

Measurement of coronary blood flow

Measurement of coronary blood flow by CMR is of considerable clinical interest, as it offers the possibility of developing new, non-invasive methods for measuring coronary flow reserve and assessing velocity changes at the site of stenosis in order to measure stenosis severity.[35,36] Work on coronary flow and flow reserve in animals has shown that CMR yields results closely comparable with those of ultrasound. The partial volume effects of flow measurement in small vessels must also be considered; studies suggest that 3–5 pixels across the diameter of the vessel are necessary for accurate measurements. Correction for the effects of myocardial velocity

on the measurements must also be made for any instantaneous measurement of blood velocity. Although other techniques of flow measurement have been described for the coronary arteries, they are less easy to implement clinically.

MYOCARDIAL PERFUSION IMAGING

Magnetic resonance imaging using magnetic resonance contrast agents can assess myocardial perfusion.[37] At present, most paramagnetic contrast agents diffuse into the extracellular space and redistribute extremely

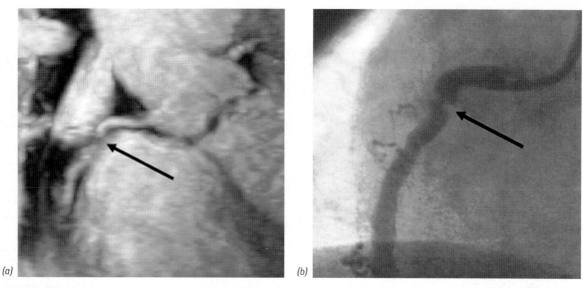

Figure 7.8 *Breath-hold two-dimensional coronary MRA (a) and corresponding x-ray angiography (b) in a patient with right coronary artery disease. Coronary MRA shows good agreement with x-ray angiography.*

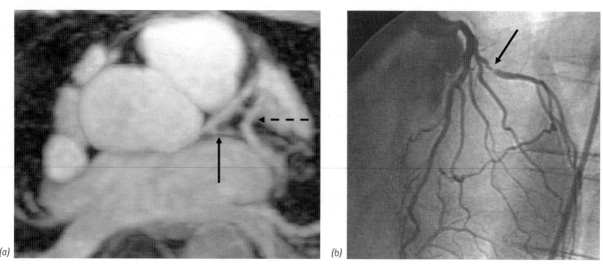

Figure 7.9 *Breath-hold two-dimensional coronary MRA (a) and corresponding x-ray angiography (b) in a patient with left circumflex coronary artery disease (solid arrow). Coronary MRA shows good agreement with x-ray angiography. The coronary vein is also seen (dotted arrow).*

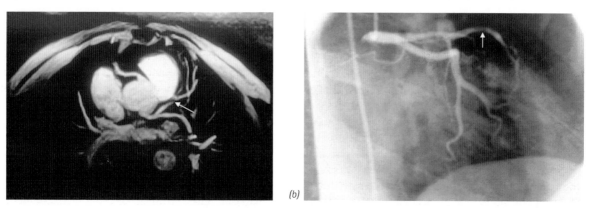

Figure 7.10 *Three-dimensional contrast-enhanced coronary MRA (a) and corresponding x-ray angiography (b) in a patient with left anterior descending coronary artery disease. Coronary MRA shows good agreement with x-ray angiographic disease. (Courtesy of Dr Debiao Li, PhD, Northwestern University, Chicago, USA.)*

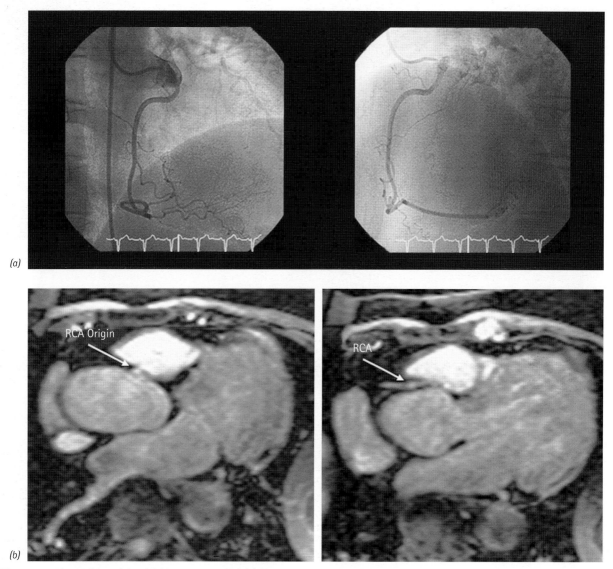

Figure 7.11 *Anomalous origin of right coronary artery. (a) Contrast x-ray angiographic right and left anterior oblique views of the right coronary artery (RCA). Abnormality is not apparent. (b) Transverse MR images of the origin and proximal course of the right coronary artery in the same patient. Note vessel origin at the left coronary cusp, and proximal course between the aortic root and pulmonary trunk. The proximal portion of this anomalous artery is potentially vulnerable to great artery compression, which can result in sudden death.*

rapidly, making it necessary to image their effect on the myocardium during their first pass in order to determine perfusion (Figure 7.16, page 110). Fast or ultrafast MRI is required for a complete image to be acquired in a single R–R interval. Gd-DTPA is the most commonly used contrast agent and is considered very safe. In low doses, it mainly shortens T_1 relaxation time, which increases signals in a dose-dependent fashion.

Myocardium perfused by a diseased vessel shows lower peak signal intensity and rate of signal increase, and longer time to reach peak.[38] Revascularization has been shown to reduce this, and to increase the peak signal intensity and slope. Pharmacological stress with dipyridamole or adenosine allows calculation of myocardial perfusion reserve, with results comparable to those of nuclear imaging techniques. At this time, CMR offers the highest resolution perfusion images available *in vivo* with sub-endocardial resolution easily achievable, and further technical improvements are expected.

Clinical studies of myocardial perfusion imaging

Reduced signal intensity has been demonstrated in areas of myocardium supplied by arteries with >70–80% stenosis when compared with areas supplied by non-stenosed arteries in the same patient, and in myocardium

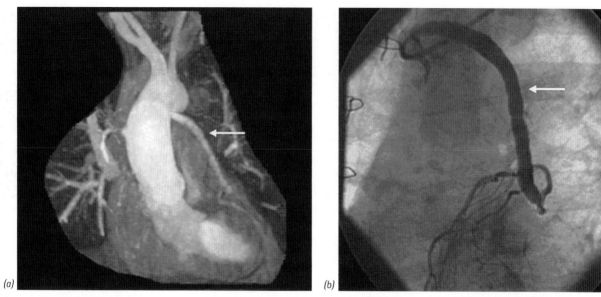

Figure 7.12 *(a) Gadolinium-enhanced three-dimensional breath-hold (maximum intensity projection, MIP) of a patent vein graft to the left anterior descending artery. (b) X-ray angiography of the same graft showing irregular luminal borders and no tight stenosis.*

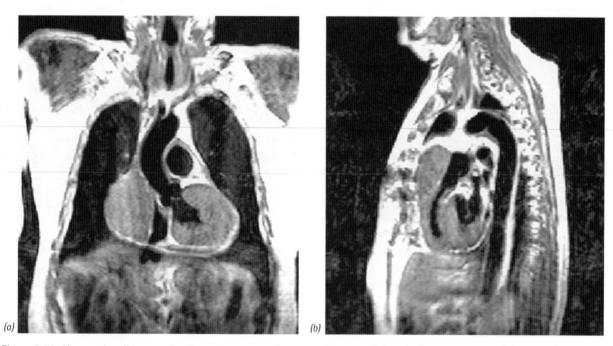

Figure 7.13 *Hemopericardium complicating coronary artery bypass graft surgery. Spin-echo images in coronal (a) and sagittal (b) planes show a large clot in the pericardial space compressing the right atrium and right ventricular outflow tract.*

from normal controls.[39] This is because of a reduced concentration of contrast agent in the vascular bed affected by the coronary stenosis or occlusion, findings that have been demonstrated both at rest and after pharmacological stress with dipyridamole or adenosine. The CMR results correlated well with dipyridamole stress thallium-201 (^{201}Tl) scintigraphy and coronary angiograms. When compared with exercise thallium-201 scintigraphy and coronary angiography, the sensitivity,

specificity and diagnostic accuracy of magnetic resonance myocardial perfusion imaging for the detection of ischemic regions were 65%, 76% and 74%, respectively.[40]

ASSESSMENT OF MYOCARDIAL VIABILITY

Patients with impaired left ventricular function have a poor prognosis. Those with three-vessel coronary artery

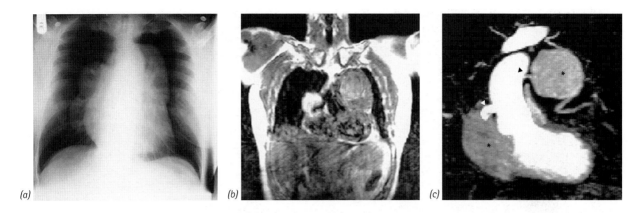

Figure 7.14 *Aneurysms of coronary bypass grafts. Chest roentgenogram (a), coronal spin-echo image (b), and maximal intensity projection image of contrast-enhanced MR coronary angiography (c). In (a), note bulges on the right and left cardiac borders. The spin-echo image shows two vascular masses at these sites. Bright signal within the masses on the spin-echo image represents slow-flowing blood and mural thrombus. CE-MRA shows the origins (arrowheads) of the bypass grafts and the aneurysms (asterisks). Permission is required from* Circulation 2000; *102:3148.*

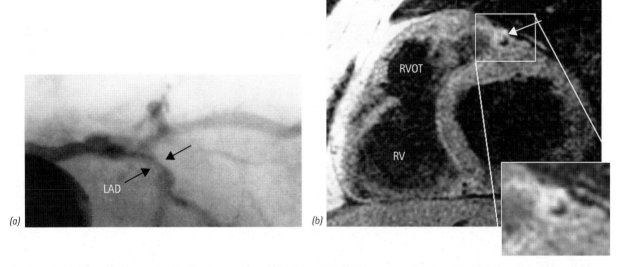

Figure 7.15 *(a) X-ray angiography showing luminal narrowing (arrow) in the LAD and (b) Turbo-spin echo image showing eccentric atheromatous plaque at the site of the narrowing (arrow). LAD, left anterior descending; RV, right ventricle; RVOT, right ventricular outflow tract. Reproduced from* Circulation 2000; *102:506.*

disease who successfully undergo revascularization have a better outlook but their perioperative risk is high. Viable, underperfused myocardium improves function following revascularization, and the preoperative identification of this 'hibernating myocardium' helps select those patients most likely to benefit from surgery. A simple definition for 'hibernation' is: viable, hypocontractile myocardium (supplied by a coronary vessel with a flow-limiting stenosis) that improves function following revascularization. From the clinical perspective, it is the identification of myocardial hibernation rather than viability that is important, because the implication is that restoring blood supply to this muscle will lead to a recovery of function. Considerable attention has been paid recently

to the potential of CMR to directly image myocardial infarction. In distinguishing myocardial tissue characteristics, myocardial fibrosis and scarring or necrosis and edema can be visualized, with transmural resolution providing a description of the extent, nature and location of myocardial damage and the extent of sub-endocardial infarction and residual myocardial viability.

Late myocardial enhancement with Gd–DTPA

The latest work in this area has concentrated on delayed myocardial enhancement patterns after intravenous injection of the contrast agent gadolinium.[41] The attractions

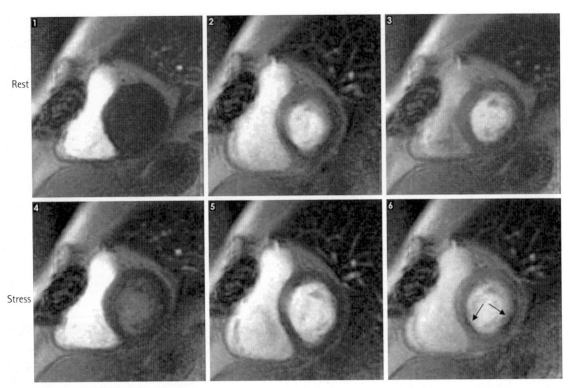

Figure 7.16 *Myocardial perfusion imaging in a patient with angiographically proven occluded native coronary arteries, patent LIMA graft to rather diffusely diseased LAD. Patent SVG to LCx territory. Good RIMA graft to posterior descending artery. The figure shows a selection of temporally resolved short-axis fast gradient-echo images (with saturation recovery prepulses to null tissue) acquired serially every heart beat at rest and following stress (adenosine infusion at 140 μg kg^{-1} min^{-1}) during first-pass infusion of gadolinium. Note the passage of contrast from the right ventricle to the left ventricle. There is sub-endocardial hypoperfusion at stress (arrows), indicating myocardial ischemia. For abbreviations, see text.*

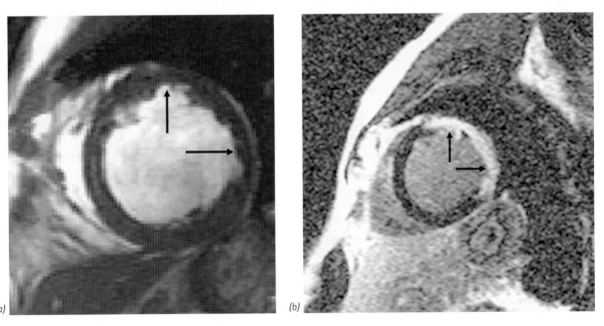

(a)

(b)

Figure 7.17 *Myocardial viability can be determined using the enhancement pattern approximately ≈ 15 minutes after intravenous administration of gadolinium. (a) An end-diastolic frame from cine gradient echo acquisition in the short axis of the left ventricle where the blood pool is bright. (b) The viability image in the same plane, where normal myocardium is black and infarcted myocardium is brightly enhanced (arrows).*

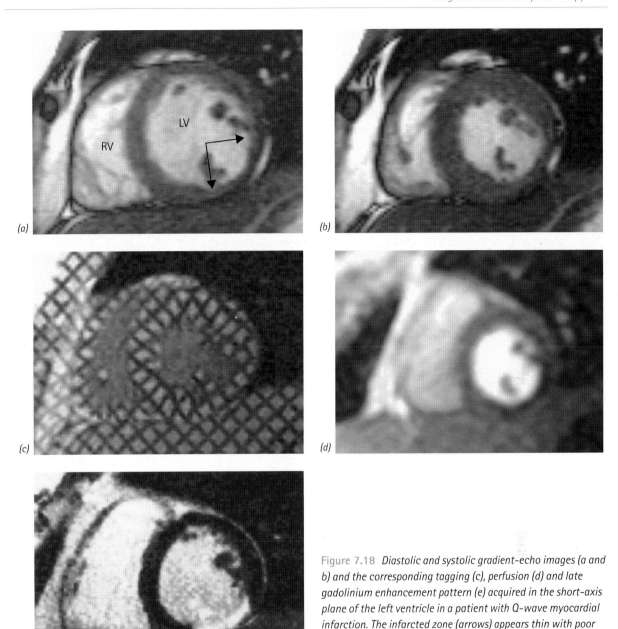

Figure 7.18 *Diastolic and systolic gradient-echo images (a and b) and the corresponding tagging (c), perfusion (d) and late gadolinium enhancement pattern (e) acquired in the short-axis plane of the left ventricle in a patient with Q-wave myocardial infarction. The infarcted zone (arrows) appears thin with poor contraction on cine imaging and myocardial tagging. There is a perfusion defect and transmural myocardial infarction in the infero-lateral wall. RV, right ventricle; LV, left ventricle.*

of this technique are the high image quality, simplicity of interpretation and high resolution allowing clear depiction of the transmural extent of necrosis and scar (Figures 7.17 and 7.18). In both acute and chronic infarction, the region of hyper-enhancement is very similar in size to the area of irreversible injury, whilst non-enhancement regions are viable.[42] Thus a combination of contrast-enhanced CMR and cine CMR in the same planes can be used to distinguish between myocardial scar (hyper-enhanced with reduced contractile dysfunction), hibernating myocardium (not hyper-enhanced but with reduced contractile dysfunction) and normal myocardium (not hyper-enhanced and with normal function). The technique has already been shown to predict recovery of function after revascularization according to the transmural extent of scar.[43]

MAGNETIC RESONANCE SPECTROSCOPY

Magnetic resonance imaging provides little information about cellular metabolism other than that reflected in measurements of more global parameters, such as T_1 or

T_2. MRS is capable of giving such valuable information in a non-destructive and non-invasive manner. The technique involves observing a single nuclear species in different environments within a homogeneous magnetic field. To obtain spectra instead of images, frequency variations in the magnetic resonance signal are used, known as chemical shift information. Thus, spatial encoding of the signal can no longer be performed by activating the frequency-encoding gradient, and different methods of spatial localization are required for clinical spectroscopy.[44]

Magnetic resonance spectroscopy is unique in its ability to study *in-vivo* cardiac metabolism non-invasively. It measures metabolites that play a key role in the myocardial energy supply, otherwise known as the cardiac high-energy phosphate metabolism. Myocardial adenosine triphosphate (ATP) and phosphocreatinine (PCr) can be measured by phosphorus (^{31}P) MRS, while the total creatinine pool can be measured with water-suppressed proton (^{1}H) MRS. ATP is the sole substrate for all energy-consuming reactions in the cell, while PCr acts as an energy reservoir and may serve as an energy transport molecule (Figure 7.19). MRS is still primarily a research tool and has no impact on clinical cardiology practice.

Applications of cardiac MRS

The normal human myocardial PCr:ATP ratio, measured by MRS, is approximately 1.8, but this is reduced in patients with dilated cardiomyopathy and the reduction correlates well with the clinical severity of the heart failure (New York Heart Association class).[45] Evaluation of the myocardial PCr:ATP ratio may therefore play a role in the evaluation of energetic effects of various forms of therapy. The PCr:ATP ratio may also have a prognostic value regarding the survival rate of patients with heart failure. Reduction of the PCr:ATP ratio was shown to correlate with left ventricular end-diastolic pressure and wall stress.

Magnetic resonance spectroscopy has great potential in the evaluation of coronary artery disease if the necessary technical developments required to improve the spatial and temporal resolutions of the technique can be achieved. A decrease in PCr and an increase in inorganic phosphate are among the very earliest metabolic responses to myocardial ischemia, and MRS can monitor these. Akinetic myocardium can be viable (hibernating or stunned) or non-viable (scarred); viable myocardium recovers contractile function after revascularization. Non-viable myocardium contains little ATP, whereas ATP levels in viable myocardium remain close to normal.

SAFETY

There are no known hazards associated with exposure to the level of radiofrequency radiation and magnetic fields

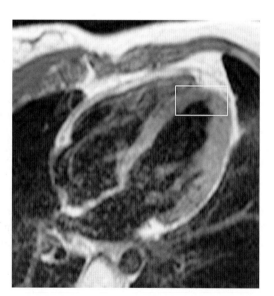
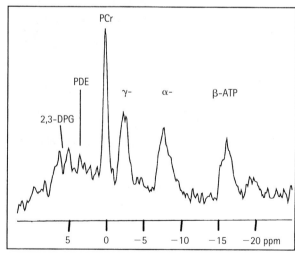

Figure 7.19 *Cardiac ^{31}P-MR spectrum (right panel) and corresponding spectroscopic voxel (left panel) of a healthy human volunteer. The spectrum shows resonances for the major high-energy phosphate metabolites in heart, ATP (three ^{31}P-atoms, thus, three resonances; the direct energy source for myofibrillar contraction) and phosphocreatine (PCr; the major energy storage compound in heart). In addition, resonances for phosphodiesters (PDE; mainly membrane phospholipids) and 2,3-diphosphoglycerate (DPG; resulting from blood contamination) are seen. Typically, spectra are quantified using the area ratio of PCr and ATP (PCr:ATP ratio), which is an index of the energetic state of the heart. (Courtesy of Dr S Neubauer, University of Oxford.)*

used in whole-body MRI. The absorption of radiowaves generates heat, but this does not produce significant heating *in vivo*. The rapidly changing magnetic field gradients induce currents in the body, but these are small. Absolute contraindications are few, but patients with pacemakers and defibrillators should not be scanned because of the effect of the magnetic field upon the electronics and because of the theoretical possibility of inducing currents in the pacing lead, which might cause arrhythmias. Cochleal implants and certain types of cerebral aneurysm clips should also not be scanned. Scanning patients with sternal wires is safe and the associated signal loss is localized to an area anterior to the heart, which rarely interferes with image analysis. All prosthetic valves are compatible with MRI, and scanning of patients with intracoronary stents is also safe. The confines of the magnet cause 4% of patients some anxiety, but the use of anxiolytics with reassurance can reduce this rate to 1%.

CONCLUSION

There is an opportunity for CMR to play a major role in the assessment of coronary artery disease using the techniques outlined in this chapter. A considerable amount of development work remains before clinical applications are likely to become mainstream in clinical cardiology, but there is great hope that the quantitative aspects of CMR combined with its versatility and safety will help it emerge into the fiercely competitive arena currently dominated by echocardiography, nuclear cardiology and catheterization. Only CMR can be considered as a likely technique to challenge all these alternatives.

ACKNOWLEDGMENTS

The author acknowledges his colleagues at the Cardiovascular Magnetic Resonance Unit, Royal Brompton Hospital. In particular, he thanks Dr Nick Bunce MD, Dr Kim Rajappan MD, Dr Andrew Elkington MD and Dr Peter Gatehouse PhD for various contributions.

KEY REFERENCES

Kim WY, Danias PG, Stuber M, Flamm SD, Plein S, Nagel E, *et al.* Coronary magnetic resonance angiography for the detection of coronary stenoses. *N Engl J Med* 2001; **345**:1863–9.
This is a prospective, multicenter study investigating the accuracy of coronary magnetic resonance angiography acquired during free breathing in patients with suspected coronary disease before elective x-ray coronary angiography, in which the results of the two diagnostic procedures were compared. Among patients referred for their first x-ray coronary angiogram, three-dimensional coronary magnetic resonance angiography allows for the accurate detection of coronary artery disease of the proximal and middle segments. This non-invasive approach reliably identifies (or rules out) left main coronary artery or three-vessel disease.

Kim RJ, Wu E, Rafael A, Chen EL, Parker MA, Simonetti O, *et al.* The use of contrast-enhanced magnetic resonance imaging to identify reversible myocardial dysfunction. *N Engl J Med* 2000; **343**:1445–53.
Contrast-enhanced MRI was used to predict whether regions of abnormal ventricular contraction will improve after revascularization in patients with coronary artery disease. Fifty patients with ventricular dysfunction before they underwent surgical or percutaneous revascularization were studied. The transmural extent of hyper-enhanced regions was postulated to represent the transmural extent of non-viable myocardium. The extent of regional contractility at the same locations was determined by cine MRI before and after revascularization in 41 patients. The authors showed that reversible myocardial dysfunction can be identified by contrast-enhanced MRI before coronary revascularization. The percentage of the left ventricle that was both dysfunctional and not hyper-enhanced before revascularization was strongly related to the degree of improvement in the global mean wall motion score and the ejection fraction after revascularization.

Klein C, Nekolla SG, Bengel FM, Momose M, Sammer A, Haas F, *et al.* Assessment of myocardial viability with contrast-enhanced magnetic resonance imaging: comparison with positron emission tomography. *Circulation* 2002; **105**:162–7.
MRI hyper-enhancement as a marker of myocardial scar was shown to agree closely with positron emission tomography (PET) data. Although hyper-enhancement correlated with areas of decreased flow and metabolism, it seems to identify scar tissue more frequently than PET, reflecting the higher spatial resolution. Additional functional studies after revascularization are required to define the significance of small islands of scar detected by MRI.

Mohiaddin RH (ed.) *Introduction to Cardiovascular MRI.* London: Current Medical Literature, 2002.
This book provides a concise and up-to-date guide to the basic concepts behind cardiovascular magnetic resonance (CMR), the uses of CMR in current cardiological practice, and the future possibilities of this technique.

Schwitter J, Nanz D, Kneifel S, Bertschinger K, Buchi M, Knusel PR, *et al.* Assessment of myocardial perfusion in coronary artery disease by magnetic resonance. A comparison with positron emission tomography and coronary angiography. *Circulation* 2001; **103**:2230–35.

Forty-eight patients and 18 healthy subjects were studied. Each subject underwent stress perfusion CMR (using dipyridamole), using a hybrid echo planar imaging sequence. The signal intensity upslope as a measure of myocardial perfusion was calculated in 32 segments for each individual (eight segments per short axis slice, four short axis slices per patient). Each subject also underwent a PET scan and coronary angiography. In comparison to PET, perfusion CMR had a sensitivity and specificity of 91% and 94%, respectively, for the detection of coronary artery disease. In comparison to coronary angiography, perfusion CMR had a sensitivity and specificity of 87% and 85%, respectively, for the detection of coronary artery disease.

REFERENCES

1. Task Force of the European Society of Cardiologists in collaboration with the Association of European Paediatric Cardiologists. The clinical role of magnetic resonance in cardiovascular diseases. *Eur Heart J* 1998; **19**:19–39.
2. Axel L. Physics and technology of cardiovascular MR imaging. *Cardiol Clin* 1998; **16**:125–33.
3. Cohn JN, Johnson GR, Shabeti R, Loeb H, Tristani F, Rector T, *et al.* Ejection fraction, peak exercise oxygen consumption, cardiothoracic ratio, ventricular arrhythmias and plasma norepinephrine as determinants of prognosis in heart failure. *Circulation* 1993; **87**:VI5–16.
4. Parameshwar J, Keegan J, Sparrow J, Sutton GC, Poole-Wilson PA. Predictors of prognosis in severe heart failure. *Am Heart J* 1992; **123**:421–6.
5. Bellenger NG, Burgess M, Ray SG, Lahiri A, Coats AJ, Cleland JG, *et al.*, on behalf of the CHRISTMAS Steering Committee and Investigators. Comparison of left ventricular ejection fraction and volumes in heart failure by two-dimensional echocardiography, radionuclide ventriculography and cardiovascular magnetic resonance: are they interchangeable? *Eur Heart J* 2000; **21**:1387–96.
6. Underwood SR, Gill CRW, Firmin DN, Klipstein RH, Mohiaddin RH, Rees RS, *et al.* Left ventricular volume measured rapidly by oblique magnetic resonance imaging. *Br Heart J* 1988; **60**:188–95.
7. Sakuma H, Globits S, Bourne MW, Shimakawa A, Foo TK, Higgins CB. Improved reproducibility in measuring LV volumes and mass using multicoil breath-hold cine MR imaging. *J Magn Reson Imaging* 1996; **6**:124–7.
8. Eichstädt HW, Felix R, Langer M, Gutmann ML, Dougherty FC, Huben HJ, *et al.* Use of nuclear magnetic resonance imaging to show regression of hypertrophy with ramipril treatment. *Am J Cardiol* 1987; **59**:98–103D.
9. Bottini PB, Carr AA, Prisant M, Flickinger FW, Allison JD, Gottdiener JS. Magnetic resonance imaging compared to echocardiography to assess left ventricular mass in the hypertensive patient. *Am J Hypertens* 1995; **8**:221–8.
10. Akins AW, Hill JA, Sievers KW, Conti CR. Assessment of left ventricular wall thickness in healed myocardial infarction by magnetic resonance imaging. *Am J Cardiol* 1987; **59**:24–8.
11. Baer FM, Voth E, Schneider CA, Theissen P, Schicha H, Sechtem U. Comparison of low dose dobutamine gradient echo magnetic resonance imaging and positron emission tomography with fluorodeoxyglucose in patients with chronic coronary artery disease. A functional and morphological approach to the detection of residual myocardial viability. *Circulation* 1995; **91**:1006–15.
12. Nagel E, Lehmkuhl HB, Bocksch W, Klein C, Vogel U, Frantz E, *et al.* Noninvasive diagnosis of ischemia induced wall motion abnormalities with the use of high dose dobutamine stress MRI. Comparison with dobutamine stress echocardiography. *Circulation* 1999; **99**:763–70.
13. Clark NR, Reichek N, Bergey P, Hoffman EA, Brownson D, Palmon L, *et al.* Circumferential myocardial shortening in the normal human left ventricle. *Circulation* 1991; **84**:67–74.
14. Rogers WJ, Shapiro EP, Weiss JL, Buchalter MB, Rademakers FE, Weisfeldt ML, *et al.* Quantification of and correction for left ventricular systolic longaxis shortening by magnetic resonance tissue tagging and slice isolation. *Circulation* 1991; **84**:721–31.
15. Karwatowski SP, Mohiaddin RH, Yang GZ, Firmin DN, Underwood SR, Longmore DB. Noninvasive assessment of regional left ventricular long axis motion using magnetic resonance velocity mapping in normal subjects. *J Magn Reson Imaging* 1994; **4**:151–5.
16. Sones FM. Acquired heart disease: symposium on present and future of cineangiography. *Am J Cardiol* 1959; **3**:710.
17. Judkins MP. Selective coronary arteriography. A percutaneous transfemoral technique. *Radiology* 1967; **89**:815–24.
18. Karnegis JN, Heinz J. The risk of diagnostic cardiovascular catheterization. *Am Heart J* 1979; **97**(3):291–7.
19. Gersh BJ, Kronmal RA, Frye RL, Schaff HV, Ryan TJ, Gosselin AJ, *et al.* Coronary arteriography and coronary artery bypass surgery: morbidity and mortality in patients 65 years or older. A report from the Coronary Artery Surgery Study. *Circulation* 1983; **67**(3):483–91.
20. Manning WJ, Li W, Edelman RR. A preliminary report comparing magnetic resonance coronary angiography with conventional angiography. *N Engl J Med* 1993; **328**:828–32.
21. Li D, Paschal CB, Haacke EM, Adler LP. Coronary arteries: three-dimensional MR imaging with fat saturation and magnetisation transfer contrast. *Radiology* 1993; **187**:401–6.
22. Doyle M, Scheidegger MB, de Graaf RG, Vermeulen J, Pohost GM. Coronary artery imaging in multiple 1-sec breath holds. *Magn Reson Imaging* 1993; **11**:3–6.
23. Wang Y, Grimm RC, Rossman PJ, Debbins JP, Riederer SJ, Ehman RL. 3D coronary MR angiography in multiple breath-holds using a respiratory feedback monitor. *Magn Reson Med* 1995; **34**:11–16.
24. Post JC, van Rossum AC, Hofman MBM, Valk J, Visser CA. Three-dimensional respiratory gated MR angiography of coronary arteries: comparison with conventional coronary angiography. *Am J Roentgenol* 1996; **166**:1399–404.
25. Post JC, van Rossum AC, Bronzwaer JG, *et al.* Magnetic resonance angiography of anomalous coronary arteries. A new gold standard for delineating the proximal course? *Circulation* 1995; **92**:3163–71.
26. McConnell MV, Ganz P, Selwyn AP, Edelman RR, Manning WJ. Identification of anomalous coronary arteries and their anatomic course by magnetic resonance coronary angiography. *Circulation* 1995; **92**:3158–62.
27. Hundley WG, Clarke GD, Landau C, Lange RA, Willard JE, Hillis LD, *et al.* Noninvasive determination of infarct artery patency by magnetic resonance angiography. *Circulation* 1995; **91**:1347–53.
28. Galjee MA, van Rossum AC, Doesburg T, van Eenige M, Visser CA. Value of magnetic resonance imaging in assessing patency and function of coronary artery bypass grafts. *Circulation* 1996; **93**:660–6.
29. Hoogendoorn LI, Pattynama PM, Buis B, van der Geest RJ, van der Wall EE, de Roos A. Noninvasive evaluation of aortocoronary bypass grafts with magnetic resonance flow mapping. *Am J Cardiol* 1995; **75**:845–8.
30. Bunce NH, Mohiaddin RH, Dahdal MD, Gibbs S, Pennell DJ. Contrast-enhanced MRA of coronary artery bypass graft aneurysm. *Circulation* 2000; **102**:3148.

31. Manning WJ, Li W, Edelman RR. A preliminary report comparing magnetic resonance coronary angiography with conventional angiography. *N Engl J Med* 1993; **328**:828–32.

32. Duerinckx A, Urman M. Two-dimensional coronary MR angiography: analysis of initial clinical results. *Radiology* 1994; **193**:731–8.

33. Pennell DJ, Bogren HG, Keegan J, Firmin DN, Underwood SR. Assessment of coronary artery stenosis by magnetic resonance imaging. *Heart* 1996; **75**:127–33.

34. Fayad ZA, Fuster V, Fallon JT, Jayasundera T, Worthley SG, Helft G, *et al.* Noninvasive *in vivo* human coronary artery lumen and wall imaging using black blood magnetic resonance imaging. *Circulation* 2000; **102**:506–10.

35. Clarke GD, Eckels R, Chaney C, Smith D, Dittrich J, Hundley WG, *et al.* Measurement of absolute epicardial coronary artery flow and flow reserve with breath-hold cine phase-contrast magnetic resonance imaging. *Circulation* 1995; **91**:2627–34.

36. Sakuma H, Blake LM, Amidon TM, O'Sullivan M, Szolar DH, Furber AP, *et al.* Coronary flow reserve: non-invasive measurement in humans with breath-hold velocity encoded cine MR imaging. *Radiology* 1996; **198**:745–50.

37. Wilke N, Simm C, Zhang J, Ellermann J, Ya X, Merkle H, *et al.* Contrast-enhanced first pass myocardial perfusion imaging: correlation between myocardial blood flow in dogs at rest and during hyperemia. *Magn Reson Med* 1993; **29**: 485–97.

38. Manning WJ, Atkinson DJ, Grossman W, Paulin S, Edelman RR. First-pass nuclear magnetic resonance imaging studies using gadolinium-DTPA in patients with coronary artery disease. *J Am Coll Cardiol* 1991; **18**:959–65.

39. Schaefer S, van Tyen R, Saloner D. Evaluation of myocardial perfusion abnormalities with gadolinium-enhanced snapshot MR imaging in humans. *Radiology* 1992; **185**:795–801.

40. Eichenberger AC, Schuiki E, Kochli VD, Amann FW, McKinnon GC, von Schulthess GK. Ischemic heart disease: assessment with gadolinium-enhanced ultrafast MR imaging and dipyridamole stress. *J Magn Reson Imaging* 1994; **4**:425–31.

41. Kim RJ, Fieno DS, Parrish TB, Harris K, Chen EL, Simonetti O, *et al.* Relationship of MRI delayed contrast enhancement to irreversible injury, infarct age, and contractile function. *Circulation* 1999; **100**:1992–2002.

42. Wu E, Judd RM, Vargas JD, Klocke FJ, Bonow RO, Kim RJ. Visualisation of presence, location, and transmural extent of healed Q-wave and non-Q-wave myocardial infarction. *Lancet* 2001; **357**:21–8.

43. Kim RJ, Wu E, Rafael A, Chen EL, Parker MA, Simonetti O, *et al.* The use of contrast-enhanced magnetic resonance imaging to identify reversible myocardial dysfunction. *N Engl J Med* 2000; **343**:1445–53.

44. Bottomley PA. MR spectroscopy of the human heart: the status and the challenges. *Radiology* 1994; **191**:594.

45. Neubauer S, Krahe T, Schindler R, Horn M, Hillenbrand H, Entzeroth C, *et al.* ^{31}P magnetic resonance spectroscopy in dilated cardiomyopathy and coronary artery disease: altered cardiac high-energy phosphate metabolism in heart failure. *Circulation* 1992; **86**:1810–18.

8

Percutaneous coronary intervention

ALI DENKTAS, MANDEEP SINGH AND DAVID R HOLMES JR

The field of interventional cardiology has evolved rapidly since its introduction in 1977. This evolution has been triggered by the rapid changes in technology, the ever-widening patient and lesion selection criteria, and the increasing experience of interventional cardiologists. All of these facets have resulted in a dramatic increase in the number and improved outcome of percutaneous coronary interventions (PCI). PCI has now become the most widely performed coronary revascularization procedure.

TECHNOLOGICAL CHANGES

There have been rapid changes in technology. Some of these changes have resulted in mainstream products, whereas others have resulted in niche devices. In addition, there has been a change in the frequency with which these devices have been used, as new devices have supplanted older ones.

The introduction of a series of debulking catheters was the first dramatic change in technology after conventional angioplasty. Initially, directional coronary atherectomy (DCA) was introduced in an attempt to make PCI more reliable, more reproducible and safer by minimizing the barotrauma associated with balloon dilatation.[1–3] This particular device also offered the opportunity of obtaining tissue for assessing the underlying pathophysiology of patients undergoing treatment. In addition, the initial angiographic results were improved compared with conventional balloon angioplasty. It was therefore felt that restenosis rates might be lower with DCA. This led to several randomized clinical trials involving patients with *de novo* coronary lesions as well as vein graft disease.[1–3] The majority of these trials were performed while the techniques were still evolving, and before the need for adjunctive dilatation and optimal debulking was recognized. The results of these trials indicated that the technique was difficult, complication rates (particularly post-procedural enzyme elevation) were increased with atherectomy, and restenosis rates were not significantly improved. Subsequent randomized clinical trials using more optimal techniques have documented improved clinical outcome.[4,5] However, the rigid, bulky design of DCA devices and the introduction of stent implantation resulted in a dramatic reduction in the use of DCA. In the National Heart, Lung, and Blood Institute (NHLBI) Dynamic Registry over 2 years (1997–1998), <1% of procedures involved DCA. Currently, there are many institutions that have no experience with the technique. Recently, a new-generation DCA has been introduced that is considerably more flexible and smaller; this may provide an impetus for a resurgence of interest.

At the present time, DCA may still be useful in debulking large bifurcation lesions, in treating ostial lesions that are not calcified, particularly the right coronary artery and the left anterior descending, and in some patients prior to stent implantation to facilitate optimal stent expansion. Randomized trials of debulking prior to stent implantation will have a major impact on device utilization.

ROTATIONAL ATHERECTOMY

Rotational atherectomy (RA) has become a niche technique. It relies on differential plaque abrasion and ablation, in which non-elastic tissue (calcified lesion) is ablated during device passage while more normal tissue is deflected. The device is more complicated to use than conventional balloon angioplasty because of the potential for 'no' or 'slow' reflow due to excessive particulate load resulting in distal embolization or spasm. Although RA does improve procedural outcome compared with balloon dilatation, particularly in patients with severe calcification, it does not appear to reduce restenosis in *de novo* lesions.[6–8] The strategy of adjunctive stent implantation after RA has also been studied and again has not been shown to improve outcome compared with stent implantation alone.[9] Finally, RA has been studied in the setting of treatment for in-stent restenosis (ISR) for debulking the lesions. The results of two randomized trials have provided conflicting data. The first of these, the Randomized Trial of Rotational Atherectomy Versus Balloon Angioplasty for In-Stent Restenosis (ROSTER), was a single-center trial comparing 75 patients undergoing percutaneous transluminal coronary angioplasty (PTCA) with 75 patients undergoing RA and found clinical restenosis rates of 20% versus 43% ($P = 0.01$), respectively.[10] These findings were supported by registry data suggesting improved 1-year outcomes for RA compared with PTCA and satisfactory outcomes in patients with proximal left anterior descending lesions treated with RA with adjunctive intravascular ultrasound. However, the Angioplasty Versus Rotational Atherectomy for Treatment of In-Stent Restenosis Trial (ARTIST) demonstrated the opposite effect. For patients with diffuse ISR (10–50 mm length), 146 patients undergoing PTCA had an angiographic restenosis rate of 51.2%, compared with 152 patients undergoing RA with a restenosis rate of 64.8% ($P = 0.04$).[11]

At the present time, RA is indicated in lesions that appear unlikely to respond well to balloon dilatation or to stent implantation. These would include heavily calcified lesions, ostial lesions, selected ostial bifurcation lesions and lesions that are excessively fibrotic and unable to be well dilated using conventional balloon angioplasty. In the last group of patients, if balloon dilatation does not fully open the arterial segment to be treated, stent implantation will also yield suboptimal results. If failure to dilate is the result of heavy calcification, RA will be very useful. Finally, RA may still be used for debulking ISR prior to definitive treatment either with vascular brachytherapy or some other approach. It will not, however, result in improved restenosis rates. There are some lesion types where RA should be avoided, including eccentric lesions, bends that have the potential for perforation, lesions with dissection and those with significant thrombus burden.

LASER ANGIOPLASTY

There was substantial interest in Excimer laser angioplasty during the early and mid-1990s. This approach was thought to have the potential to ablate tissues safely, thereby giving a more satisfactory initial result and potentially decreasing subsequent restenosis. Randomized trials failed to document the widespread utility of this approach.[12–14] This, plus economic considerations related to the cost of the units, led to them never being widely used. An important technique that was tested involved the use of a laser wire for chronic total occlusions. The technique was studied in several registries and some patients were identified in whom chronic total occlusions were treatable only with a laser guidewire. There was, however, a high incidence of perforation (asymptomatic, or resulting in tamponade), and the product has been abandoned by the sponsors.

At the present time, laser angioplasty is performed infrequently. It may be used to debulk ISR before definitive therapy,[15] or if a chronic total occlusion can be passed with a guidewire but no balloon catheter can follow. In the latter setting, laser may improve the ability to access the distal bed with a definitive treatment device.

CORONARY STENT IMPLANTATION

The most important advance in interventional cardiology after the initial introduction of balloon angioplasty was the widespread acceptance of coronary stent implantation.

Stents

Stents have revolutionized the field of interventional cardiology. They have now been studied exhaustively in multicenter randomized clinical trials, in a variety of patient subsets. Stents are effective for the treatment of acute or threatened closure after attempted balloon dilatation and in the reduction of angiographic and clinical restenosis.[16,17] With the introduction of stents, the need for emergency coronary bypass graft surgery for failed PCI has declined to a level of approximately 0.4%.[18] Currently, stents are used in approximately 80–90% of all patients undergoing PCI. The first-generation stents were rigid and inflexible and were used for large proximal coronary arteries. The latest generation of stents are much improved and can be delivered to most vascular territories.

There are still areas of concern with stent implantation, including:

- subacute stent thrombosis,
- in-stent restenosis,
- side branch access in bifurcation lesions.

The current dual antiplatelet therapy with aspirin and thienopyridine (ticlopidine or clopidogrel) has reduced the risk of subacute stent thrombosis to less than 1%. The major risk for complication is within the first 2 weeks of stent deployment. The predictors for this complication include the use of multiple stents, dissection and minimal diameter after stent deployment.[19] In a consecutive series of 827 patients from the Mayo Clinic, subacute closure was seen in 0.7%.[20] The major limitation of thienopyridine use from a cardiac surgical standpoint is the increased perioperative bleeding risk. Some surgeons will defer any elective procedure as long as the patient is on a thienopyridine. The use of stents is known to reduce the risk of restenosis. However, they do not eliminate it. Depending upon stent length, vessel size and the presence or absence of diabetes mellitus, ISR rates vary widely from 5–10% up to 40–45%. This ISR may be difficult to treat. Newer strategies to treat ISR include vascular brachytherapy with beta or gamma radiation.[21–23] The use of gamma radiation reduced ISR from 76% to 36% in diabetics ($P = 0.002$). However, there are still some patients who do not respond and who have recurrent resistant ISR.[23]

With stents, there are also some concerns about side branch access and the treatment of a bifurcation lesion. When stents are placed, they have the potential of covering side branches. If these are significant in size (>2.0 mm) and are unprotected, there is a risk of myocardial infarction. Strategies for dealing with bifurcation lesions have been developed. At the present time, however, they are still associated with high restenosis

rates if two stents are deployed, one in each of the branches.[24]

A recent development is the testing of drug-coated stents, including Rapamycin™ and Paclitaxel™.[25,26] Sirolimus is a naturally occurring compound derived from the streptomyces fungus and stimulates p27[kip1] levels causing cyclin-Cdk complex inhibition and cell cycle arrest. The recently reported Rapamycin-eluting Versus Plain Polymer Stents (RAVEL) trial randomized 238 patients to a sirolimus-coated stent or conventional stent for *de novo* coronary lesions and found a zero restenosis rate in the sirolimus group (vs 26%, $P < 0.0001$), clearly a finding with huge implications.[27] Similarly, Paclitaxel, a naturally occurring compound from the Pacific yew tree with potent antiproliferative effects thought to be due to an alteration in microtubular function, has shown promising early results in 14 patients stented with a Paclitaxel-derivative-impregnated sleeve incorporated into a stent design. Both agents have now proceeded to clinical trials.[28,29] Longer term follow-up is needed to address late clinical and angiographic outcomes.

Newer devices

CUTTING BALLOON

Fibrotic and ostial lesions remain a challenge. A relatively new balloon approach involves the use of a balloon with surgical microblades, which are longitudinally fixed to the balloon surface (Figure 8.1). Although the device is somewhat rigid by virtue of its design, it has been used with increasing frequency for ostial location stenoses, ISR, small vessel disease, and for some calcified lesions. The effect of the cutting balloon on subsequent restenosis varies in different series.[30–33] It has the advantage that it gives excellent initial angiography findings, even in fibrotic lesions, and facilitates adjunctive therapy such as stent placement. It is less complex to use than RA and accordingly its use has increased. Adjunctive therapy for

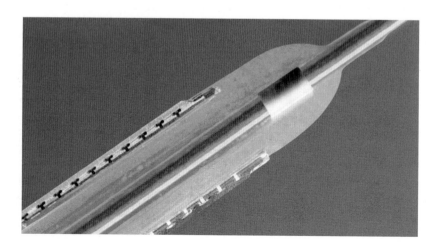

Figure 8.1 *The cutting balloon is useful for fibrotic or ostial lesions.*

cutting balloon procedures is similar to that for conventional angioplasty.

DISTAL PROTECTION DEVICES

The potential for distal embolization of thrombus or atheromatous material during PCI has received increasing attention over the past few years. In some patients, the distal embolization results in procedural myocardial infarction, which is particularly a problem in vein graft interventions or patients presenting with myocardial infarction. In other patients, it results in diminished flow to the distal vascular bed.

There are two broad groups of devices:

1 those that occlude the distal vessel and allow for aspiration of material, and
2 filters that allow continued flow during the procedure and then filter removal for the debris.

The only device that is approved is the PercuSurge™ guidewire, which is a distal protection device with an occlusion balloon. It is approved for use in the treatment of vein graft disease. The SAFER Trial utilized the PercuSurge™ device in 801 patients with vein graft disease.[34] There was a 42% reduction in major adverse coronary event rate (MACE) at 30 days with the use of the PercuSurge™ device (9.6% with vs 16.5% without, $P = 0.004$). The system was associated with significantly less 'no-reflow', which was independent of the use of glycoprotein IIb/IIIa inhibitors.

ADJUNCTIVE PHARMACOLOGICAL THERAPY

In addition to changing device technology, there have been major changes in adjunctive medical therapy. These changes have also improved the outcomes in multiple patient subsets.

Initially, ticlopidine was used for the prevention of subacute stent thrombosis. However, because of the potential for thrombotic thrombocytopenic purpura and the slow onset of action, the drug of choice is now clopidogrel, which is better tolerated, more effective and has rapid onset of action.[35] Typically, a loading dose of 300 mg is administered once the decision has been made to intervene and then the drug is continued for at least 30 days post-procedure. In patients being treated with vascular brachytherapy and in some patients with acute coronary syndromes, dual antiplatelet treatment is continued beyond 30 days (up to 6–9 months). There has been concern about increased bleeding in patients treated with clopidogrel and aspirin: an increase in minor bleeding was reported in the CAPRIE and CURE trials.[36,37] Some cardiovascular surgeons are reluctant to operate on patients if they are on clopidogrel; other surgeons are more sanguine. The issue is likely to become more significant following the publication of the CURE Trial, which documented improved outcome in patients treated with longer term clopidogrel, as a result of which more patients are being treated long-term with dual therapy.[37] If dual antiplatelet therapy is used, the dose of aspirin should be decreased to 75–80 mg.

IIB/IIIA AGENTS

An extensive literature has developed around the glycoprotein IIb/IIIa receptor inhibitors. They have been studied in multiple randomized clinical trials in patients with acute ischemic syndromes treated medically, and in patients undergoing PCI.[38] The most benefit demonstrated with the use of IIb/IIIa inhibitors is in a setting of PCI,[38] particularly in the highest risk patients, for example those with unstable angina and elevated baseline biomarker, those with diabetes and those with highest risk lesions. PCI of diseased vein grafts does not seem to benefit from the concomitant use of IIb/IIIa inhibitors.[39,40] In patients who undergo PCI while on IIb/IIIa and who require emergency coronary artery bypass grafting (CABG), outcome has been shown not to be adversely affected by the use of these powerful antiplatelet drugs. However, increased need for red blood cell and platelet transfusion due to bleeding or thrombocytopenia has been reported.[41,42]

PERCUTANEOUS CORONARY INTERVENTION (PCI) VERSUS CORONARY BYPASS GRAFT SURGERY

This has been the subject of considerable debate and study. It is complex and must take into consideration several important factors:

- What technology was available during trial performance – for example, were the PCI patients treated with conventional angioplasty or stent implantation and were surgical patients treated with multiple arterial grafts versus vein conduits and were off-pump procedures performed?
- Was equal revascularization required for each randomized limb (or was significant disparity in the anticipated extent of revascularization between the groups accepted)?
- What endpoints were compared (single or composite), and how were they defined (e.g. 'neurocognitive events' or simply 'stroke')? This has major implications for interpretation of the trial findings.
- What patient populations were included; for example one, two or three vessel disease, presence or absence of left ventricular dysfunction, or diabetes mellitus?

Another important issue is the generalizability of the trial to larger, non-randomized patient population groups.

Cardiac death or MI at 1 year

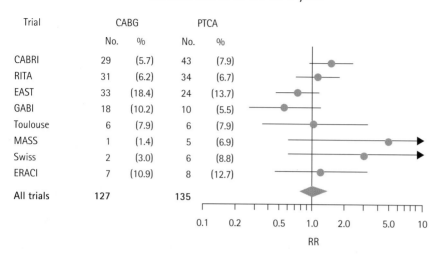

Trial	CABG		PTCA	
	No.	%	No.	%
CABRI	29	(5.7)	43	(7.9)
RITA	31	(6.2)	34	(6.7)
EAST	33	(18.4)	24	(13.7)
GABI	18	(10.2)	10	(5.5)
Toulouse	6	(7.9)	6	(7.9)
MASS	1	(1.4)	5	(6.9)
Swiss	2	(3.0)	6	(8.8)
ERACI	7	(10.9)	8	(12.7)
All trials	127		135	

Figure 8.2 Relative risk of cardiac death or myocardial infarction (MI) at 1 year in patients randomized to either surgery or percutaneous intervention. Reprinted from Lancet *1995; 346:1184–9, with permission.[43]*

Angina pectoris (⩾CCS 2) at 1 year

⩾2 angina at 1 year

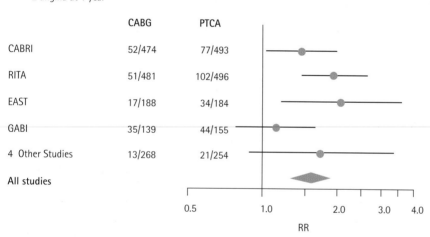

	CABG	PTCA
CABRI	52/474	77/493
RITA	51/481	102/496
EAST	17/188	34/184
GABI	35/139	44/155
4 Other Studies	13/268	21/254
All studies		

Figure 8.3 Effect of surgery versus percutaneous intervention on anginal status at 1 year. Reprinted from Lancet *1995; 346:1184–9, with permission.[43]*

In some of the early trials, only a small percentage of patients screened were felt to be suitable for randomization.

A final issue, which is the most important, relates to patient expectations concerning the outcome of treatment. For some patients, the goal is to avoid surgery unless absolutely necessary, whereas for others the goal is to avoid any need for repeat procedures. Obviously, the course of therapy recommended and chosen by each of these individual patients will be different.

A meta-analysis of the early randomized trials of coronary bypass surgery versus conventional PTCA evaluated the outcome in 3371 patients deemed suitable for either treatment option, with a mean follow-up of 2.7 years.[43] There was no difference in the combined primary endpoint of cardiac death and myocardial infarction between the two groups (Figure 8.2). Patients with PCI had more angina (Figure 8.3). As might be expected, there was a greater need for repeat procedures in the PCI

group for restenosis (33.7% vs 3.3%). The largest study was the BARI Trial with approximately 1800 patients. Overall, there was no difference in death/infarction at 5 years.[44] However, an important subgroup was identified: in those patients with diabetes mellitus, survival was improved in the surgical group.

In the recent Arterial Revascularization Therapy Study (ARTS), 1205 patients with either stable or unstable angina or silent myocardial ischemia and multivessel coronary artery disease were randomized to either coronary bypass graft surgery or angioplasty with a stent.[45] Eligibility criteria included the need for revascularization of at least two vessels. The primary endpoint was freedom from major adverse cardiac and cerebrovascular events at 1 year. Secondary endpoints included repeat revascularization, cost, angina status and quality of life. Ninety-nine percent of patients randomly assigned to stenting (593 patients) and 96% of those randomly assigned to surgery

Table 8.1 *Clinical endpoints at 1 year, in descending order of severity*[a]

| Variable | Worst event[b] | | All events[c] | | |
	Stenting group (n = 600)	Surgery group (n = 605)	Stenting group (n = 600)	Surgery group (n = 605)	Relative risk (95% CI)
Death	15 (2.5)	17 (2.8)	15 (2.5)	17 (2.8)	0.89 (0.45–1.77)
Cerebrovascular accident[d]	9 (1.5)	12 (2.0)	10 (1.7)	13 (2.1)	0.78 (0.34–1.76)
Myocardial infarction	32 (5.3)	24 (4.0)	37 (6.2)	29 (4.8)	1.29 (0.80–2.06)
Q-wave	28 (4.7)	22 (3.6)	32 (5.3)	26 (4.3)	1.24 (0.75–2.06)
Non-Q-wave	4 (0.7)	2 (0.3)	5 (0.8)	3 (0.5)	1.68 (0.40–7.00)
Repeated revascularization	101 (16.8)	21 (3.5)	126 (21.0)	23 (3.8)	5.52 (3.59–8.49)
CABG	28 (4.7)	3 (0.5)	40 (6.7)	4 (0.7)	10.08 (3.63–28.01)
PTCA	73 (12.2)	18 (3.0)	94 (15.7)	20 (3.3)	4.74 (2.96–7.58)
Event-free survival[e]	443 (73.8)	531 (87.8)	–	–	–
Any event	157 (26.2)	74 (12.2)	–	–	2.14 (1.66–2.75)

[a]One patient in the stenting group had a myocardial infarction while on the waiting list for the procedure; in the surgery group, three patients died while on the waiting list, one patient had a cerebrovascular accident, and four patients had myocardial infarctions. CI denotes confidence interval; CABG, coronary artery bypass grafting; PTCA, percutaneous transluminal coronary angioplasty.

[b]If a patient required repeated angioplasty and later required coronary artery bypass grafting, only the worst event (CABG) was counted as an event.

[c]If a patient required repeated angioplasty and later required coronary artery bypass grafting, the total count for 'CABG' and 'PTCA' at 365 days would reflect both events, not just the worst that occurred, but the count for the general variable 'Repeated revascularization' would reflect only one event.

[d]In the stenting group, five cerebrovascular accidents were thrombotic, one was hemorrhagic, and the nature of the other five is unknown.

[e]$P < 0.001$ by the Wilcoxon rank-sum test.

Figures in parentheses are percentages. Adapted from Serruys *et al.*[45]

(579 patients) received the assigned treatment. Each group had a mean of 2.8 lesions per patient.

Amongst patients randomly assigned to stent implantation, there was a high incidence of subacute closure. This occurred in 1.1% of the stented lesions and 2.8% of the patients, which is substantially higher than expected. The 1-year status in terms of clinical endpoints can be seen in Table 8.1. Freedom from death, cerebral vascular accident and myocardial infarction was very similar, at 90.7% in the stent group and 91.2% in the surgical group. The relative risk was 1.07 (95% confidence interval of 0.75–1.52). There was an increased need for repeat revascularization in the stent group (16.8%) versus the surgical group (3.5%). Accordingly, survival free from major adverse cardiac and cerebrovascular events and repeat revascularization was less in the stent group, at 73.8% versus 87.8% in the surgical group.

As previously mentioned, costs were a secondary endpoint and were significantly greater in the surgical group due to differences in the duration of the procedures and the length of hospital stay. This initial difference was reduced at 1 year but still favored stenting. Another important endpoint was that of procedural myocardial infarction. Creatinine kinase more than five times the upper limit of normal was found in 12.6% of the surgical patients and in only 6.2% of the stent group patients ($P < 0.001$).

The immediate results of PCI in the subset of patients undergoing multivessel angioplasty are improving steadily. The need for repeat revascularization in the earlier multivessel angioplasty versus surgery trials was 34%, and in the latest ARTS Trial it was 17%. The hard endpoints of death and myocardial infarction were not different. The increase in the incidence of repeat revascularization during the first year of follow-up probably represents ISR. Longer term follow-up would highlight the time-dependent attrition of the vein grafts. The widespread use of Rapamycin™-coated stents would further improve the outcome of patients treated with stenting. At the present time, patients who could have either stent implantation or surgery can be reassured that there is no significant difference in the risk of death and myocardial infarction unless they are diabetic. However, patients treated with stent implantation have a greater likelihood of requiring repeat revascularization at 1 year.

KEY REFERENCES

Baim DS, Wahr D, George B, Leon MB, Greenberg J, Cutlip DE, *et al.* Randomized trial of a distal embolic protection device during percutaneous intervention of saphenous vein aorto-coronary bypass grafts. *Circulation* 2002; **105**:1285–90.

The randomized trial that identified a predicate device for the treatment of vein graft disease.

Bhatt DL, Bertrand ME, Berger PB, L'Allier PL, Moussa I, Moses JW, *et al.* Meta-analysis of randomized and registry comparison of ticlopidine with clopidogrel after stenting. *J Am Coll Cardiol* 2002; **39**:9–14.

A fundamental change has been the introduction and widespread use of thienopyridine medications for the prevention of subacute stent closure. This article supports the use of clopidogrel, with fewer side effects.

Bhatt DL, Topol EJ. Current role of platelet glycoprotein IIb/IIIa inhibitors in acute coronary syndromes. *JAMA* 2000; **284**:1549–58.

The addition of platelet glycoprotein IIb/IIIa inhibitor has dramatically changed the medical therapy as well as the interventional therapy for patients with acute coronary syndromes.

Morice MC, Serruys PW, Sousa JE, Fajadet J, Ban Hayashi E, Perin M, *et al.* Randomized study with the Sirolimus coated Bx velocity balloon expandable stent in the treatment of patients with de novo native coronary artery lesions. *N Engl J Med* 2002; **346**:1773–80.

A pivotal study – the first publication of a completed randomized clinical trial of a drug-eluting stent documenting no restenosis.

Serruys PW, Unger F, Sousa JE, *et al.* Comparison of coronary artery bypass surgery and stenting for the treatment of multivessel disease. *N Engl J Med* 2001; **334**: 1117–24.

A multicenter randomized trial that extends prior observations and studies stenting versus surgery for multivessel disease. It documents marked improvement in outcome of patients treated with stents compared to earlier studies of patients treated with conventional PTCA.

REFERENCES

1. Holmes DR Jr, Garratt KN, Topol EJ. Coronary Angioplasty Versus Excisional Atherectomy Trial: CAVEAT. *Int J Cardiol* 1992; 35:143–6.
2. Elliott JM, Berdan LG, Holmes DR, Isner JM, King SB, Keeler GP, *et al.* One-year follow-up in the Coronary Angioplasty Versus Excisional Atherectomy Trial (CAVEAT I). *Circulation* 1995; 91:2158–66.
3. Lefkovits J, Holmes DR, Califf RM, Safian RD, Pieper K, Keeler GP, *et al.* Predictors and sequelae of distal embolization during saphenous vein graft intervention from the CAVEAT-II trial. Coronary Angioplasty Versus Excisional Atherectomy Trial. *Circulation* 1995; 92:734–40.
4. Baim DS, Cutlip DE, Sharma SK, Kalon KLH, Fortuna R, Schreiber TL, *et al.* Final results of the Balloon vs Optimal Atherectomy Trial (BOAT). *Circulation* 1998; 97:322–31.
5. Simonton CA, Leon MB, Baim DS, Hinohara T, Kent KM, Bersin RM, *et al.* Optimal directional coronary atherectomy: final results of the Optimal Atherectomy Restenosis Study (OARS). *Circulation* 1998; 97:332–9.
6. Stertzer SH, Rosenblum J, Shaw RE, Sugeng I, Hidalgo B, Ryan C, *et al.* Coronary rotational ablation: initial experience in 302 procedures. *J Am Coll Cardiol* 1993; 21:287–95.
7. Warth DC, Leon MB, O'Neill W, Zacca N, Powssar NL, Buchbinder M. Rotational atherectomy multicenter registry: acute results, complications and 6-month angiographic follow-up in 709 patients. *J Am Coll Cardiol* 1994; 24:641–8.
8. Guerin Y, Spaulding C, Desnos M, Funck F, Rahal S, Py A, *et al.* Rotational atherectomy with adjunctive balloon angioplasty versus conventional percutaneous transluminal coronary angioplasty in type B2 lesions: results of a randomized study. *Am Heart J* 1996; 131:879–83.
9. Dietz U, Rupprecht HJ, Ekinci O, Dill T, Erbel R, Kuck KH, *et al.* Angiographic analysis of immediate and long-term results of PTCR vs. PTCA in complex lesions (COBRA study). *Catheter Cardiovasc Interv* 2001; 53:359–67.
10. Sharma SK, Kini AS, King T, Reich D, Marmur JD. Randomized trial of Rotational Atherectomy versus Balloon Angioplasty for Diffuse In-stent Restenosis. (ROSTER): final results (Abstract). *Circulation* 2000; 102:II730.
11. vom Dahl J, Dietz U, Haager PK, Silber S, Niccoli L, Buettner HJ, *et al.* Rotational atherectomy does not reduce recurrent in-stent restenosis: results of the Angioplasty versus Rotational Atherectomy for Treatment of Diffuse In-stent Restenosis Trial (ARTIST). *Circulation* 2002; 105:583–8.
12. Reifart N, Vandormael M, Krajcar M, Gohring S, Preusler W, Schwarz F, *et al.* Randomized comparison of angioplasty of complex coronary lesions at a single center. Excimer Laser, Rotational Atherectomy, and Balloon Angioplasty Comparison (ERBAC) Study. *Circulation* 1997; 96:91–8.
13. Stone GW, de Marchena E, Dageforde D, Foschi A, Muhlestein JB, McIvor M, *et al.* Prospective, randomized, multicenter comparison of laser-facilitated balloon angioplasty versus stand-alone balloon angioplasty in patients with obstructive coronary artery disease. The Laser Angioplasty Versus Angioplasty (LAVA) Trial Investigators. *J Am Coll Cardiol* 1997; 30:1714–21.
14. Appelman YE, Piek JJ, Strikwerda S, Tijssen JG, de Feyter PJ, David GK, *et al.* Randomized trial of excimer laser angioplasty versus balloon angioplasty for treatment of obstructive coronary artery disease. *Lancet* 1996; 347:79–84.
15. Mehran R, Dangas G, Mintz GS, Waksman R, Abizaid A, Satler LF, *et al.* Treatment of in-stent restenosis with excimer laser coronary angioplasty versus rotational atherectomy: comparative mechanisms and results. *Circulation* 2000; 101: 2484–9.
16. Fischman DL, Leon MB, Baim DS, Schatz RA, Savage MP, Penn I, *et al.* A randomized comparison of coronary in-stent placement and balloon angioplasty in the treatment of coronary artery disease. Stent Restenosis Study Investigators. *N Engl J Med* 1994; 331:496–501.
17. Serruys PW, de Jaegere P, Kiemeneij F, Macaya C, Rutsch W, Heyndrickx G, *et al.* A comparison of balloon-expandable-stent implantation with balloon angioplasty in patients with coronary artery disease. Benestent Study Group. *N Engl J Med* 1994; 331:489–95.
18. Hasdai D, Berger PB, Bell MR, Rihal CS, Garratt KN, Holmes DR Jr. The changing face of coronary interventional practice. The Mayo Clinic experience. *Arch Intern Med* 1997; 157:677–82.
19. Cutlip DE, Baim, DS, Ho KK, Popma JJ, Lansky AJ, Cohen DJ, *et al.* Stent thrombosis in the modern era: a pooled analysis of multicenter coronary stent clinical trials. *Circulation* 2001; 103:1967–71.

20. Berger PB, Bell MR, Hasdai D, Grill DE, Melby S, Holmes DR. Safety and efficacy of ticlopidine for only 2 weeks after successful intracoronary stent placement. *Circulation* 1999; **99**:248–53.

21. Waksman R, White RL, Chan RC, Bass BG, Geirlach L, Mintz GS, *et al*. Intracoronary gamma-radiation therapy after angioplasty inhibits recurrence in patients with in-stent restenosis. *Circulation* 2000; **101**:2165–71.

22. Waksman R, Bhargava B, White L, Chan RC, Mehran R, Lansky AJ, *et al*. Intracoronary beta-radiation therapy inhibits recurrence of in-stent restenosis. *Circulation* 2000; **101**:1895–8.

23. Leon MB, Teirstein PS, Moses JW, Tripuraneni P, Lansky AJ, Jani S, *et al*. Localized intracoronary gamma-radiation therapy to inhibit the recurrence of restenosis after stenting. *N Engl J Med* 2001; **344**:250–6.

24. Al Suwaidi J, Berger PB, Rihal CS, Garratt KN, Bell MR, Ting HH, *et al*. Immediate and long-term outcome of intracoronary stent implantation for true bifurcation lesions. *J Am Coll Cardiol* 2000; **35**:929–36.

25. Sousa JE, Costa MA, Abizaid A, Abizaid AS, Feres F, Pinto IMF, *et al*. Lack of neointimal proliferation after implantation of sirolimus-coated stents in human coronary arteries: a quantitative coronary angiography and three-dimensional intravascular ultrasound study. *Circulation* 2001; **103**:192–5.

26. Sousa JE, Cost MA, Abizaid AC, Rensing BJ, Abizaid AS, Tanajura LF, *et al*. Sustained suppression of neointimal proliferation by sirolimus-eluting stents: one-year angiographic and intravascular ultrasound follow-up. *Circulation* 2001; **104**:2007–11.

27. Sousa JE, Morice M-C, Serruys PW. The RAVEL study: a randomized study with the sirolimus coated BX Velocity balloon-expandable stent in the treatment of patients with de novo native coronary artery lesions (Abstract). *Circulation* 2001; **104**:II462.

28. Grube E, Silber SM, Hauptmann KE. Prospective, randomized, double-blind comparison of Nirx™ stents coated with paclitaxel in a polymer carrier in de-novo coronary lesions compared with uncoated controls (Abstract). *Circulation* 2001; **104**:II463.

29. Park S-J, Shim WH, Ho DS, Raizner AE, Park SW, Kim JJ, *et al*. The clinical effectiveness of paclitaxel-coated coronary stents for the reduction of restenosis in the ASPECT trial (Abstract). *Circulation* 2001; **104**:II464.

30. Adamiam M, Colombo A, Briguori C, Nishida T, Marsico F, Di Mario C, *et al*. Cutting balloon angioplasty for the treatment of in-stent restenosis: a matched comparison with rotational atherectomy, additional stent implantation and balloon angioplasty. *J Am Coll Cardiol* 2001; **38**:672–9.

31. Izumi M, Tsuchikane E, Funamoto M, Kobayashi T, Sumitsuji S, Otsuji S, *et al*. Final results of the CAPAS trial. *Am Heart J* 2001; **142**:782–9.

32. Ergene O, Seyithanoglu BY, Tastan A. Comparison of angiographic and clinical outcome after cutting balloon and conventional balloon angioplasty in vessels smaller than 3 mm in diameter: a randomized trial. *J Invas Cardiol* 1998; **10**:70–75.

33. Kondo T, Kawaguchi K, Awaji Y, Mochizuki M. Immediate and chronic results of cutting balloon angioplasty: a matched comparison with conventional angioplasty. *Clin Cardiol* 1997; **20**:459–63.

34. Baim DS, Wahr D, George B, Leon MB, Greenberg J, Cutlip DE, *et al*. Randomized trial of a distal embolic protection device during percutaneous intervention of saphenous vein aorto-coronary bypass grafts. *Circulation* 2002; **105**:1285–90.

35. Bhatt DL, Bertrand ME, Berger PB, L'Allier PL, Moussa I, Moses JW, *et al*. Meta-analysis of randomized and registry comparisons of ticlopidine with clopidogrel after stenting. *J Am Coll Cardiol* 2002; **39**:9–14.

36. Anonymous. A randomized, blinded, trial of Clopidogrel versus Aspirin in Patients at Risk of Ischemic Events (CAPRIE). CAPRIE Steering Committee. *Lancet* 1996; **348**:1329–39.

37. Yusuf S, Zhao F, Mehta SR, Chrolavicius S, Tognoni G, Fox KK. Effects of clopidogrel in addition to aspirin in patients with acute coronary syndromes without ST-segment elevation. *N Engl J Med* 2001; **345**:494–502.

38. Vorchheimer DA, Badimon JJ, Fuster V. Platelet glycoprotein IIb/IIIa receptor antagonists in cardiovascular disease. *JAMA* 1999; **281**:1407–14.

39. Singh M, Reeder GS, Ohman EM, Mathew V, Hillegass WB, Anderson RD, *et al*. Does the presence of thrombus seen on a coronary angiogram affect the outcome after percutaneous coronary angioplasty? An Angiographic Trials Pool data experience. *J Am Coll Cardiol* 2001; **38**:624–30.

40. Mathew V, Grill DE, Scott CG, Grantham JA, Ting HH, Garratt KN, *et al*. The influence of abciximab use on clinical outcome after aortocoronary vein graft interventions. *J Am Coll Cardiol* 1999; **34**:1163–9.

41. Singh M, Nuttall GA, Ballman KV, Mullany CJ, Berger PB, Holmes DR Jr, *et al*. Effect of abciximab on the outcome of emergency coronary artery bypass grafting after failed percutaneous coronary intervention. *Mayo Clin Proc* 2001; **76**:784–8.

42. Lincoff AM, LeNarz LA, Despotis GJ, Smith PK, Booth JE, Raymond RE, *et al*. Abciximab and bleeding during coronary surgery: results from the EPILOG and EPISTENT trials. Improved long-term outcome with abciximab IIb/IIIa blockade. Evaluation of platelet IIb/IIIa inhibition in stenting. *Ann Thorac Surg* 2000; **70**:516–26.

43. Pocock SJ, Henderson RA, Rickards AF, Hampton JR, King SB 3rd, Hamm CW, *et al*. Meta-analysis of randomized trials comparing coronary angioplasty with bypass surgery. *Lancet* 1995; **346**:1184–9.

44. Anonymous. Comparison of coronary bypass surgery with angioplasty in patients with multivessel disease. The Bypass Angioplasty Revascularization Investigation (BARI) Investigators. *N Engl J Med* 1996; **335**:217–25.

45. Serruys PW, Unger F, Sousa JE, Jatene A, Bonnier HJRM, Schonberger JPAM, *et al*. Comparison of coronary artery bypass surgery and stenting for the treatment of multivessel disease. *N Engl J Med* 2001; **344**:1117–24.

9

Indications for surgery in coronary artery disease

ERIC J DEVANEY, KIM A EAGLE AND RICHARD L PRAGER

INTRODUCTION

The goal of therapy for coronary artery disease is conceptually simple: to reduce any mismatch between myocardial oxygen supply and demand. The clinical application of this concept has undergone considerable evolution over the last several decades and currently encompasses three varied approaches:

1 medical therapy, which is directed at reducing demand with beta-blockade, preventing platelet deposition with aspirin or glycoprotein inhibitors, or initiating clot lysis with heparin or thrombolytics;
2 catheter-based interventional cardiology, which increases supply by means of coronary angioplasty or stenting;
3 surgical revascularization, which increases supply by augmenting coronary blood flow by the creation of alternative conduits to bypass fixed coronary stenoses or obstructions.

HISTORY

Most patients with coronary artery disease present with symptoms of angina. Initial surgical approaches to angina were indirect and included thyroidectomy for reduction of metabolic rate and sympathectomy to reduce symptoms by elimination of afferent input. Next, therapies were developed to increase collateral blood flow to the myocardium by the creation of pericardial adhesions or

omental transposition. The Vineberg procedure involved implantation of an internal mammary artery into the myocardium. Although there were earlier instances of bypass grafting, their true potential seems to have been missed, and the real credit for establishing coronary artery bypass as a legitimate therapy should be attributed to Rene Favaloro, who collaborated with Mason Sones at the Cleveland Clinic in the late 1960s. In the early years, the saphenous vein was the workhorse conduit, but the internal mammary artery subsequently assumed the predominant role due to its favorable long-term patency. Other arterial conduits have also evolved as excellent alternatives to veins.

Soon after its introduction, surgical therapy was shown to be very effective for the treatment of stable angina. The early success of surgical revascularization led to the development of several large trials to aid in defining the proper indications for surgery for patients with either stable angina or acute coronary syndromes.

STABLE ANGINA

Medical versus surgical therapy

A number of randomized trials were performed to clarify the indications for surgical therapy in the early years of coronary bypass. Various limitations in these trials have led to widespread criticism of their conclusions and subsequent application to current practice. The trials enrolled a patient population that was predominantly male and under 65 years of age. The patients were generally stable without significant co-morbidities. Medical therapy was not optimal by today's standard. Aspirin, beta-blockers, angiotensin-converting enzyme (ACE) inhibitors and lipid-lowering drugs were either not widely used or not available. Surgical technique was also quite primitive by comparison to currently available therapy. Arterial grafts were vastly underutilized, modern techniques of myocardial protection were not available and, again, optimal pharmacological postoperative management was not delivered. Despite these limitations, useful information can be derived from a careful analysis of the data, and the results of the three major randomized trials comparing medical and surgical treatment are summarized here.

The Veterans Administration (VA) Cooperative Study was a randomized, controlled trial comparing medical and surgical therapy for patients with stable angina and angiographically positive coronary artery disease.[1-7] Between 1970 and 1974, a total of 1015 patients were enrolled. The initial phase of the study lasted 2 years, during which time angiographic and surgical techniques were developed. The final phase of the study, lasting from 1972 to 1974, evaluated a cohort of 686 patients and represented the source of data for most of the published results from this trial. Patients were required to have had stable angina for at least 6 months and to have been treated medically for at least 3 months prior to enrollment. Criteria for exclusion were myocardial infarction within 6 months, refractory diastolic hypertension, presence of a left ventricular aneurysm, unstable angina, or uncompensated congestive heart failure.

Medical therapy included nitrates and beta-blockers. Surgical patients received an average of 2.0 grafts, which were generally reversed saphenous vein grafts (only 14 patients received internal mammary grafts). Operative mortality was 5.6% overall. Follow-up vein graft angiography was performed in 79% of surgical patients, revealing patency of 70% at 1 year (with 87% of patients having at least one patent graft) and 67% at 5 years. A total of 38% of patients in the medical group eventually 'crossed over' to surgery after a follow-up of 11 years. When the main cohort of patients was evaluated, a small but statistically significant difference in survival favoring surgery was noted at a follow-up of 7 years (77% vs 72%, $P = 0.04$). When analysis was extended to 11 years, this survival advantage was lost. When patients with left main disease were excluded from the analysis, no significant difference in survival was identified at any point in follow-up.

The main group of patients was stratified for further analysis. A tendency for improved survival in patients with three-vessel disease undergoing surgery was noted at 7 years (75% vs 63%, $P = 0.06$), but this difference did not reach statistical significance and, moreover, the difference diminished by 11 years. There was no advantage to surgery in subgroups with one-vessel or two-vessel disease. When patients with impaired ventricular function (ejection fraction (EF) <50%) were assessed, a significant survival benefit from surgery was found at 7 years (74% vs 63%, $P = 0.05$) but not at 11 years of follow-up. Patients with both ventricular dysfunction and three-vessel coronary disease showed an even greater survival benefit with surgery compared to medicine at 7 years (76% vs 52%, $P = 0.002$) and at 11 years (50% vs 38%, $P = 0.026$). One of the earliest results published from this trial involved the subgroup of patients with significant (>50%) left main coronary stenosis.[2] The survival advantage of the surgical group became apparent after only 2 years of follow-up, with 93% survival in the surgical group and 71% in the medical group. Survival at 4 years was 93% in the surgical group and 58% in the medical group.

Like the VA Cooperative Study, the European Coronary Surgery Study (ECSS) was designed to compare the medical and surgical treatment of patients with stable angina.[8,9] From 1973 to 1976, this study recruited 767 men under the age of 65 with stable mild or moderate angina of at least 3 months' duration, angiographically confirmed significant (>50%) stenoses in two or more major vessels, and normal ventricular function (EF >50%). Patients with medically refractory angina were excluded. Both groups received the optimal medical care available in that era. Within the surgical group, an average of 1.9 grafts were constructed in patients with two-vessel disease and 2.4 grafts in those with three-vessel disease. Operative mortality was 3.2%. Subsequent vein graft angiography revealed graft patency of 90% at 9 months and 77% between 9 and 18 months. A crossover to surgical therapy occurred in 24% of the medical patients by 5 years and in 36% by 12 years. For the entire group, a significant improvement in survival among patients treated surgically was found at the projected 5-year follow-up (92% vs 84%, $P = 0.0001$). This benefit tended to decrease over time, but remained significant at 12 years of follow-up (71% vs 67%, $P = 0.04$). Unlike the VA study, the ECSS could not demonstrate a statistically significant survival advantage for patients with left main disease undergoing surgery, although an absolute difference was measured. A number of subgroups were shown to have significant survival advantages with surgery, including patients with three-vessel disease, significant proximal left anterior descending (LAD) disease, ST-segment depression on preoperative exercise stress tests, and peripheral vascular disease. Also, angina was significantly decreased in the surgical patients at 5 years. Exercise performance was better in the surgical group, but this did not reach statistical significance. The benefit from surgery tended to be greatest at 5 years, declining over time, but persisting at 12 years for all the groups mentioned. This declining benefit has generally been attributed to vein graft atherosclerosis and progression of native coronary atherosclerosis. Older patients were shown to derive the greatest benefit.

The Coronary Artery Surgery Study (CASS) comprised a multicenter patient registry including a total of 24 959 patients who underwent coronary angiography during the years 1974 to 1979 at 15 participating centers. The majority of these patients underwent non-randomized therapy and this registry has provided a rich source of data for a number of longitudinal studies.[10–13] CASS also generated a randomized, controlled clinical trial comparing medical and surgical therapy for coronary artery disease.[14–19] From within the registry, patients with mild angina (CCS Class I and II) with or without evidence of prior myocardial infarction were recruited. Exclusion criteria included prior coronary artery bypass grafting (CABG), angina worse than Class II, unstable angina, New York Heart Association (NYHA) Class III or IV heart failure, or coexisting serious illness. Angiographic requirements were stenosis of at least 70% of a major vessel or at least 50% stenosis of the left main coronary artery. Patients with greater than 70% stenosis of the left main artery were excluded, as were patients with severe ventricular dysfunction (EF <35%), ventricular aneurysms, concomitant valvular disease or absent target vessels. Ultimately, from 1319 eligible patients, 780 were randomized to medical or surgical therapy. Medical therapy was limited to nitrates and beta-blockers. Crossover to surgical therapy occurred in 24% of medical patients by 5 years and in 40% by 10 years. In patients undergoing surgery, the operative mortality was 1.4% and perioperative myocardial infarction occurred in 6.4%. The average numbers of grafts in patients with one-vessel, two-vessel and three-vessel disease were 1.7, 2.7, and 3.4, respectively. Follow-up vein graft angiography was performed within 2 months and showed graft patency of 90%, with 97% of patients having at least one open graft. After 5 years, there were no significant differences in survival for the two treatment groups (95% for surgery and 92% for medicine). The incidence of non-fatal Q-wave myocardial infarction also did not significantly differ between the two groups (14% for surgery and 12% for medicine). Subgroups were analyzed according to number of diseased vessels and ejection fraction, and again no significant differences were detected at 5 years. When quality of life was assessed, however, the surgical subgroup was found to have a significant advantage, with decreased chest pain, fewer activity limitations, decreased use of anti-anginal medications and improved exercise tolerance. The randomized CASS cohort was followed over time and after 7 and 10 years there remained no significant survival differences between the surgical and medical groups. However, the subgroup of patients with a low ejection fraction (<50%) demonstrated a benefit with surgery, with survival of 84% versus 70% ($P = 0.01$) at 7 years and 79% versus 61% ($P = 0.01$) at 10 years; in patients with both three-vessel disease and low ejection fraction, the advantage was more pronounced, with survival of 88% versus 65% ($P = 0.009$) at 7 years and 75% versus 58% ($P = 0.08$) at 10 years. Analyses of the non-randomized CASS registries also showed a survival advantage of surgery in patients with left main equivalent disease (characterized by both proximal stenosis of the LAD and proximal stenosis of the circumflex) and in patients with three-vessel disease and concomitant severe angina.

Although these classic studies are generally considered obsolete, some general principles can be applied to current practice. The survival benefits of surgical therapy compared to medical therapy occur in patients with the most severe coronary disease and with the presence of ventricular dysfunction. Other benefits of surgery include improved quality of life.

Surgery versus percutaneous transluminal coronary angioplasty (PTCA)

Since its introduction by Gruentzig in 1977, coronary angioplasty has completely changed coronary revascularization by providing a less invasive approach. The adjunctive use of intracoronary stenting has further expanded the utility of this approach. As technology and experience have evolved, the indications for surgical versus interventional coronary revascularization have become increasingly difficult to define. In general, whereas interventional therapy is less invasive and requires shorter hospitalization, the disadvantages include restenosis and requisite re-intervention as well as less potential for complete revascularization. A number of studies have been completed comparing CABG and percutaneous coronary intervention (PCI) for both single and multivessel coronary artery disease, several of which are summarized here.

The Randomized Intervention Treatment of Angina (RITA) trial compared the effects of percutaneous transluminal coronary angioplasty (PTCA) and CABG in patients with single (45%) and multivessel (55%) coronary disease.[20–22] Patients with angina and angiographically demonstrable coronary disease in whom revascularization was indicated and could be achieved by either PTCA or CABG were eligible. Patients with left main disease were excluded. A total of 1011 patients were randomized for therapy at one of multiple centers in the UK. Patients were enrolled between 1988 and 1991 and the 6.5-year follow-up was reported in 1998. Stents were not used in any of the randomized procedures. An internal mammary graft was used in 74% of patients undergoing CABG. The operative mortality for surgical patients was quite low at 1.2%. The rate of emergency CABG for patients assigned to PTCA was 4.5%. The primary endpoint of death or non-fatal myocardial infarction was not significantly different between the groups (17% for PTCA and 16% for CABG). The rates of death alone and of non-fatal myocardial infarction alone were also similar. No differences in mortality or myocardial infarction were seen when patients were stratified based on single-vessel or multivessel disease. Differences in re-intervention rates were clearly demonstrated. A subsequent CABG was required in 26% of patients assigned to PTCA (compared to 3% for the CABG group), and repeat PTCA was required in 27% of PTCA patients (compared to 9% for CABG). Most re-interventions were required during the first year. Also, the incidence of angina was significantly higher in the PTCA patients (and tended to increase over time). Cost analysis at 5 years showed no difference between the two groups.

The Coronary Angioplasty versus Bypass Revascularization (CABRI) trial was a randomized, multinational European study comparing PTCA and CABG, which published its 1-year results in 1995.[23] Patients with symptomatic multivessel disease were screened. Patients with single-vessel or left main disease, ventricular dysfunction (EF <35%), congestive heart failure, recent myocardial infarction or prior cardiac intervention were excluded. A total of 1054 patients (only 15% of those eligible) were randomized. At 1 year, the rates of death (2.7% for CABG and 3.9% for PTCA) and non-fatal myocardial infarction (3.5% for CABG and 4.9 for PTCA) were not significantly different. The incidence of angina was significantly lower in surgical patients (10.1% vs 13.9%), as was the use of anti-anginal medications. The re-intervention rate was also significantly lower for the surgical patients (6.5% vs 33.6%, P <0.001).

The Medicine, Angioplasty, or Surgery Study (MASS) was a single-institution, Brazilian study that examined patients with isolated proximal LAD stenosis of 80% or greater.[24] Patients with unstable angina, prior myocardial infarction, congestive heart failure, left ventricular dysfunction or prior cardiac intervention were excluded. From 1988 to 1991, a total of 214 patients were randomized to one of the therapeutic groups. All surgical patients received an internal mammary graft. Stents were not used in the PTCA group. The primary endpoint examined was combined cardiac death, myocardial infarction or refractory angina requiring re-intervention (although multiple PTCAs were allowed in the PTCA group). At a mean follow-up of 3 years, the primary endpoint occurred in 3% of CABG patients, 24% of PTCA patients and 17% of medically treated patients. This benefit of surgery was statistically significant. When survival or rate of myocardial infarction was examined separately, no significant differences were observed. Follow-up angiography demonstrated graft patency in all but one of the surgical patients, and a 29% restenosis and 8% occlusion rate was found in the PTCA patients.

The German Angioplasty Bypass Surgery Investigation (GABI) was another randomized study comparing the efficacy of CABG with PTCA.[25] Patients with severe angina and multivessel disease were evaluated. Patients with left main disease, occluded vessels, recent myocardial infarction or prior cardiac intervention were excluded. A total of 359 patients were enrolled from eight sites during the years 1986 to 1991 and randomized to therapy. Patient characteristics included two-vessel disease in 80%, unstable angina in 15% and diabetes in about 12%. Only 37% of surgical patients received an internal mammary graft. Results after 1 year of follow-up were reported in 1994. The periprocedure rate of myocardial infarction was significantly greater in surgical patients (8.1% vs 2.3%, P = 0.02), although early mortality was similar in the two groups. At 1 year, there was a dramatically increased rate of re-intervention in the PTCA group (44% vs 6%, P <0.001). Although mortality was similar between the groups at 1 year, the cumulative rate of death or non-fatal myocardial infarction was significantly less in the PTCA group (6% vs 13.6%, P = 0.017). In this study, the incidence of angina at 1 year was similar in the two groups.

The Argentine Estudio Argentino de Angioplastia vs Cirugia (ERACI) study enrolled 127 patients with severe angina and multivessel disease to either PTCA or CABG during the years 1988 to 1990.[26,27] Patients with left main disease, occluded vessels, evolving myocardial infarction or severe ventricular dysfunction (EF <35%) were excluded. No stents were used in the PTCA group. An internal mammary graft was utilized in 76.5% of surgical patients. Three-year follow-up results were published in 1996. The composite freedom from death, Q-wave myocardial infarction, angina and repeat revascularization was significantly higher in the surgical group (77% vs 47%, P <0.001). Mortality alone was lower in the surgical patients but this was not statistically significant. The rate of Q-wave myocardial infarction alone was similar in the two groups. The incidence of re-intervention was lower in the CABG group (6.3% vs 37%, P <0.001). More surgical patients were found to be angina free (79% vs 57%, P <0.001). Cost analysis revealed that the expenses of treatment in the PTCA group were significantly less than in the CABG group.

The Emory Angioplasty Surgery Trial (EAST) examined patients with stable or unstable angina and documented multivessel disease.[28] Patients with chronically occluded vessels, marked ventricular dysfunction (EF < 25%), left main disease, myocardial infarction within 5 days or prior cardiac intervention were excluded. A total of 842 patients (47% of those who were eligible) were randomized to CABG or PTCA from 1987 to 1990. A primary endpoint of death, Q-wave myocardial infarction or large reversible ischemic defect on thallium scanning was assessed at a mean follow-up of 3 years, and the results were reported in 1994. The composite endpoint occurred at a similar rate in both groups (27.3% for CABG vs 28.8% for PTCA). The rate of death was also similar (6.2% for CABG vs 7.1% for PTCA). The rate of repeat revascularization was significantly less for the surgical group (a subsequent CABG or PTCA was required in 1% or 13% of patients in the CABG group and in 22% or 41% of patients in the PTCA group). The incidence of angina was also significantly lower in the surgical group (20% vs 12%), as was the use of anti-anginal medications. Although the cumulative incidence of myocardial infarction was not different between the two groups, the periprocedural rate of Q-wave myocardial infarction was higher in the surgical group (10.3% vs 3%).

Other small randomized trials, including the Swiss Lausanne trial and the French Monocentric (Toulouse) trial, have reported similar comparisons between CABG and PTCA. A meta-analysis of eight of these randomized trials has been performed and includes a total of 3371 randomized patients and a mean follow-up of 2.7 years.[29] Although there are a number of differences in trial design and heterogeneity of patient populations, several results are consistently demonstrated. For patients who are candidates for either strategy of revascularization, neither method is associated with a survival advantage. During follow-up, the incidence of angina and the need for re-intervention are higher in patients undergoing PTCA. Therefore the selection of therapy may be determined on the basis of availability, local expertise and patient as well as physician choice.

The largest randomized trial comparing PTCA and CABG is the Bypass Angioplasty Revascularization Investigation (BARI) study, which was initiated by the National Heart Lung and Blood Institute.[30,31] Patients with clinically severe angina or objective evidence of ischemia and documented multivessel coronary disease were assessed. Patients with unstable angina or acute myocardial infarction requiring emergency treatment were excluded, as were patients with left main disease (>50%). A total of 1829 patients (which represented 48% of those eligible) were randomized at multiple centers between 1988 and 1991 to CABG or PTCA. Patient characteristics included a mean age of 61 years, diabetes requiring treatment in 20%, three-vessel disease in 41%, unstable angina in 63%, ventricular dysfunction (EF < 50%) in about 22%, and women representing 26%. Multiple-outcome events were measured and analyzed at a mean follow-up of 5.4 years, and the results were reported in 1996. Stents were generally not used in the PTCA group. An internal mammary graft was placed in 91% of CABG patients. A total of 6.3% of patients in the PTCA group required emergency CABG. There was no difference in in-hospital mortality between the groups as a whole (1.3% for CABG and 1.1% for PTCA). The peri-procedure incidence of Q-wave myocardial infarction

was, however, greater in the surgical patients (4.6% vs 2.1%, P <0.01). At 5 years, survival in the two groups was similar (89.3% for CABG and 86.3% for PTCA), as was survival free from Q-wave myocardial infarction. The requirement for repeat revascularization was significantly reduced in the surgical group (8% vs 54%). By 5 years, 31% of PTCA patients crossed over and required surgery. Most revascularizations were required during the first year. One very important finding from the BARI trial was an increased survival at 5 years within the subgroup of treated diabetics undergoing surgery (80.6% vs 65.5%, P <0.003). This observation was not seen in previous trials, probably because of insufficient numbers of diabetics. Other subgroups stratified by severity of angina, ventricular dysfunction or number of diseased vessels showed no differences in survival with the two therapies. When cost analysis was performed, the early expense associated with surgery was ultimately offset by the repeat interventions required in the PTCA group, and at 5 years the costs in the two groups were similar. Quality of life analysis revealed a significant benefit for surgical patients during the first 3 years of follow-up, although return to employment was quicker in the PTCA patients.

The Duke University Medical Center database has been used to assess long-term survival benefits of medical therapy, PTCA and CABG in patients with coronary disease.[32] This database enrolled 9263 patients with single-vessel and multivessel coronary disease from 1984 to 1990 who underwent non-randomized therapy and were followed for an average of 5.3 years. Differences among treatment groups in baseline characteristics were adjusted by statistical methods to allow for comparison. The anatomic severity of coronary artery disease was found most accurately to define ultimate survival benefit. This study found that PTCA or surgery was associated with better survival than medical therapy for all levels of disease severity. All patients with single-vessel disease (except those with >95% proximal LAD disease) benefited most with PTCA. All patients with three-vessel disease and those with both two-vessel disease and >95% proximal LAD disease had a survival advantage with CABG. All other two-vessel disease patients and those with isolated >95% LAD stenosis had a similar benefit from PTCA and CABG. The greatest survival benefit was conferred upon patients with severe three-vessel disease undergoing CABG.

The comparison of surgical and catheter-based therapy remains a moving target as techniques evolve and new technology is introduced. PCI now encompasses intracoronary stents, the use of which has dramatically increased, with reports of fewer early complications and decreased late restenosis when compared to PTCA. The Argentine ERACI II study represents the largest randomized comparison of CABG and PCI employing stent implantation.[33] Symptomatic (severe stable angina, unstable angina and post-infarct angina) patients with multivessel disease were assessed. Patients with left main disease, myocardial infarction within 24 hours, prior cardiac intervention or more than two chronically occluded vessels were excluded. A total of 450 patients were randomized. In addition to stent use, PCI patients received a medical regimen including ticlopidine and glycoprotein IIb/IIIa inhibitors. An internal mammary graft was used in 88.5% of patients in the surgical group. Complete anatomic revascularization was more frequently achieved in the CABG group (85% vs 50%, $P = 0.002$), although thallium scintigraphy demonstrated comparable myocardial perfusion. At 30 days, mortality was significantly less in the PCI group (0.9% vs 4.8%, $P < 0.013$), as was the rate of non-fatal Q-wave myocardial infarction (0.9% vs 5.7%, $P < 0.013$). After an average follow-up of 18.5 months, survival remained significantly higher in the PCI group (96.9% vs 92.5%, $P < 0.017$), as did freedom from myocardial infarction (97.7% vs 93.7%, $P < 0.017$). In contrast, re-intervention was lower in the surgical group (4.8% vs 16.8%, $P < 0.001$). Event-free survival was similar in the two groups. Presumably due to the added expense of glycoprotein IIb/IIIa inhibitors and stent technology, 30-day costs were similar in the two groups. Longer term follow-up will be needed before clear conclusions can be drawn.

ACUTE CORONARY SYNDROMES

The acute coronary syndromes represent a spectrum of disease from unstable angina to non-Q-wave myocardial infarction to Q-wave myocardial infarction. Pathophysiologically, the acute coronary syndrome is generally associated with plaque rupture and subsequent deposition of a platelet-rich clot. Plaque instability is a generalized process, which may be related to an underlying inflammatory process or an inherent architectural predisposition. The clinical syndrome that develops is a measure of the severity and duration of plaque disruption, with unstable angina being the least severe, non-Q-wave myocardial infarction intermediate, and Q-wave myocardial infarction the most severe, leading to transmural infarction. More recently, acute coronary syndromes have been defined predominantly by the presence or absence of ST-segment elevation on the presenting electrocardiogram, and presence or absence of elevated cardiac biomarkers, particularly troponin I or T, and/or elevated CK-MB.

Unstable angina and non-Q-wave (or non-STE) myocardial infarction

Therapy for unstable angina was examined in a VA Cooperative Study that compared medical therapy to surgical therapy in a randomized fashion.[34–37] Patients under the age of 70 who presented with chest pain were screened for unstable angina. Those with an acute myocardial infarction, prior CABG, left main disease or ventricular dysfunction were excluded. Ultimately, 468 patients were randomized from 1976 to 1982. Among the surgical patients, the operative mortality was fairly high at 4.1%, and only one patient received an internal mammary graft. Follow-up angiography was performed 1 year postoperatively and demonstrated graft patency of about 75%. Medically treated patients crossed over to surgery at the rates of 34% at 2 years, 43% at 5 years and 50% at 10 years. A significantly higher periprocedural rate of myocardial infarction after CABG was found (11.7% vs 4.6% after PTCA, $P = 0.003$). Overall, no significant differences in survival or non-fatal myocardial infarction could be demonstrated during long-term follow-up. However, when the patients were stratified by ventricular function and severity of coronary disease, important differences were noted. Among patients with ventricular dysfunction (EF 30–58%), survival in the surgical group was significantly better at 5 years (86% vs 73%, $P = 0.03$), although this advantage was lost by 10 years. Similarly, among patients with three-vessel disease, a survival advantage was found for the surgical patients at 5 years (89% vs 76%, $P < 0.02$). Additionally, surgically treated patients experienced less angina, required fewer anti-anginal drugs and demonstrated improved exercise tolerance when compared to the patients undergoing medical therapy.

Only one randomized trial has been reported comparing CABG and PTCA in patients with unstable angina, although many trials (including those previously discussed) have included patients who presented with acute coronary syndromes. The AWESOME (Angina with Extremely Serious Operative Mortality Evaluation) trial is a VA Cooperative Study that enrolled patients with medically refractory angina and at least one of five risk factors, including prior heart surgery, myocardial infarction within 7 days, ventricular dysfunction (EF < 35%), age greater than 70 or requirement for an intra-aortic balloon pump for stabilization.[38–40] Stents and glycoprotein inhibitors were used increasingly in the PCI group as the study progressed. Enrollment from 1995 to 2000 resulted in a pool of 2431 eligible patients, from which 454 patients were randomized to CABG or PCI. Survival rates at 30 days, 6 months and 3 years were found to be equivalent for the two treatment groups, although at the later time points the need for repeat revascularization was significantly higher in the PCI group.

Much of the current debate surrounding the care of patients with acute coronary syndromes has revolved around the indications for and timing of revascularization (either PCI or CABG). Four major studies have examined strategies of aggressive early intervention versus a selective approach of revascularization for patients with unstable angina and non-Q-wave myocardial infarction.

The Thrombolysis in Myocardial Ischemia (TIMI) IIIB study examined early angiography and revascularization versus a conservative approach for patients with unstable angina or non-Q-wave myocardial infarction.[41] Patients randomized to a conservative approach were not denied invasive therapy, but it was given only in the event of a failure of medical therapy and, in fact, nearly 50% of these patients ultimately required revascularization. TIMI IIIB also evaluated the use of tissue plasminogen activator (TPA) versus placebo in patients in the conservative arm. Revascularization consisted of PTCA at the time of angiography or CABG for patients with left main disease (>50%), three-vessel disease with ventricular dysfunction (EF <40%) or failure of PTCA. Stents and glycoprotein inhibitors were not available. All patients received aspirin, heparin, nitrates, beta-blockers and calcium-channel blockers. A total of 1473 patients were randomized and the results at a follow-up of 6 weeks were reported in 1994. The composite rate of death, myocardial infarction or treatment failure was no different between the early invasive and conservative groups. The use of TPA was found to be detrimental, with a higher rate of myocardial infarction compared to placebo (7.4% vs 4.9%, $P = 0.04$), presumably due to the platelet-rich nature of the obstructive lesion in these patients.

Another study that pre-dated the use of stents and glycoprotein inhibitors was the VA Non-Q-Wave Infarction Strategies in Hospital (VANQWISH) trial, which randomized 920 patients with non-Q-wave myocardial infarction to early invasive versus conservative therapy.[42] Revascularization guidelines were similar to those in TIMI IIIB. Patients in the early invasive group fared poorly, with significantly higher rates of death and myocardial infarction at 30 days and 1 year. At 2 years, survival had equalized between the two groups. About half of all patients undergoing revascularization underwent CABG, and postoperative mortality in these patients was high at 7.7%.

The Scandinavian Fragmin and Fast Revascularization during Instability in Coronary Artery Disease (FRISC) II study also randomized patients to early invasive versus conservative therapy for unstable coronary artery disease.[43,44] All patients received an aggressive medical regimen including aspirin, beta-blockers, ACE inhibitors and statins. The long-term use of subcutaneous heparin was also examined in a blinded fashion. A total of 2267 patients were randomized between 1996 and 1998. Stents and glycoprotein inhibitors were used in the patients undergoing PCI. Revascularization was performed in 78% of the invasive patients (among whom 55% underwent PCI and 45% CABG) and in 37% of the conservative patients (of whom 49% underwent PCI and 51% CABG). In this study, CABG was indicated in patients

with three-vessel disease or left main disease. An internal mammary graft was used in 95% of surgical patients. Operative mortality was 2.1%. After 6 months, there was a significant decrease in the rate of myocardial infarction in the invasive group (9.4% vs 12.1%, $P = 0.03$) and a non-significant reduction in mortality (1.9% vs 2.9%, $P = 0.10$). Symptoms of angina and readmission rates were reduced by 50% in the invasive group. Patients who were at increased risk (characterized by elevated troponin level, ST-segment depression or persistent angina at rest) at admission received the greatest benefit with early invasive therapy.

The Treat Angina with Aggrastat and Determine Cost of Therapy with an Invasive or Conservative Strategy (TACTICS) – Thrombolysis in Myocardial Infarction (TIMI)-18 study enrolled 2220 patients with unstable angina or non-Q-wave myocardial infarction from 1997 to 1999.[45] Patients were randomized to early invasive versus conservative (selectively invasive) therapeutic regimens. All patients received optimal medical therapy with aspirin, heparin and glycoprotein inhibitors, and most were treated with long-term beta-blockers and statins. In the invasive group, 60% underwent revascularization (two-thirds having PCI and one-third CABG). By 6 months, 45% of the conservative patients required revascularization. A composite endpoint of death, myocardial infarction or rehospitalization was reached more frequently in the patients treated conservatively (19.4% vs 15.9%, $P = 0.025$) at 6 months. The rate of death or myocardial infarction was also higher in the conservative group (9.5% vs 7.3%, $P < 0.05$). Again, the benefits of early invasive therapy were greatest in patients presenting with unfavorable prognostic factors (echocardiographic changes or troponin elevations), whereas there was no advantage for an aggressive approach in patients presenting at low risk.

Q-wave myocardial infarction

The modern treatment of acute myocardial infarction is based upon the premise that early reperfusion of the infarct-related artery will reduce the extent of myocardial injury and thereby reduce morbidity and mortality. Controlled surgical reperfusion provides what is likely to be the best modality for the preservation of myocardium at risk; however, the expense and logistics involved in this approach make it unsuitable for general clinical application.[46] Instead, the use of intravenous thrombolytic agents has assumed a dominant role in the treatment of acute myocardial infarction, and a number of studies have documented its effectiveness.[47] Recent studies have suggested that aggressive early angiography and PCI is superior to thrombolytic therapy for 'high-risk' patients with acute myocardial infarction.[48] Generally, CABG is recommended in the face of an acute myocardial infarction for left main disease, severe three-vessel disease, or for mechanical complications of acute infarction (free wall rupture, ventricular septal defect, papillary muscle rupture). The operative mortality of CABG is thought to be excessive when performed during the first 48 hours after Q-wave myocardial infarction, but there seems to be little advantage to waiting for more than 2 days for 'cooling off' if CABG is indicated. There is clear evidence that operative mortality remains higher for patients who have had a recent myocardial infarction compared to those who have not.

Cardiogenic shock develops in 7–10% of cases of acute myocardial infarction. The mortality rate associated with cardiogenic shock is as high as 70–80%. The SHOCK (Should We Emergently Revascularize Occluded Coronaries for Cardiogenic Shock) trial was designed to assess the strategy of aggressive early revascularization for acute myocardial infarction complicated by cardiogenic shock.[49,50] A total of 302 patients were randomized to emergency revascularization or initial stabilization. Revascularization was performed by PCI (in 64%) or CABG (in 36%). No difference in mortality was noted at 30 days. At 6 months, however, mortality was significantly lower in the early intervention group (50.3% vs 63.1%, $P = 0.03$). There is clear room for improvement in the management of this patient population, in whom mechanical support and transplantation remain the mainstays of salvage therapy following revascularization.

SUMMARY

Surgical coronary revascularization reduces mortality in selected patients and relieves angina in most patients. The benefits of this therapy must be weighed against the morbidity and mortality associated with the operation. The randomized trials of medical versus surgical therapy have clearly defined patient groups in whom survival is enhanced following surgery: those with left main disease, three-vessel disease, two-vessel disease with proximal LAD stenosis, and advanced coronary disease with impaired ventricular function. Early vein graft stenosis and occlusion have previously limited the long-term benefits of CABG, but the increasing use of arterial conduits and the adjunctive use of platelet inhibitors and statins will probably improve the late results of surgery. PCI has emerged as an effective alternative to surgical revascularization for many patients, although restenosis remains a problem. Additional weaknesses of PCI include the management of patients with chronically occluded, diffusely diseased or tortuous vessels and patients with diabetes. New drug-coated stents offer promise to reduce restenosis, but percutaneous therapy will continue to be limited by its tendency to deal only with areas of most severe stenosis in the larger vessels. Despite a wealth of

data, the decision to recommend one therapy over another remains difficult and must be individualized. The most recent American College of Cardiology/American Heart Association Guidelines for CABG Surgery include current generally accepted indications for surgery, and these are summarized below.[51]

Indications for CABG in asymptomatic or mild angina

- Significant left main coronary artery stenosis.
- Left main equivalent: significant (>70%) stenosis of the proximal LAD and proximal left circumflex artery.
- Three-vessel disease.
- Proximal LAD stenosis with one-vessel or two-vessel disease.

Indications for CABG in stable angina

- Significant left main coronary artery stenosis.
- Left main equivalent.
- Three-vessel disease.
- Two-vessel disease with significant proximal LAD and either EF <50% or objective ischemia on non-invasive testing.
- One-vessel or two-vessel disease with a large area of viable myocardium.
- Medically refractory angina.

Indications for CABG in unstable angina or non-Q-wave myocardial infarction

- Significant left main coronary artery stenosis.
- Left main equivalent.
- Proximal LAD stenosis with one-vessel or two-vessel disease.
- Ongoing ischemia not responsive to maximal non-surgical therapy.

Indications for CABG in Q-wave myocardial infarction

- Ongoing ischemia not responsive to maximal non-surgical therapy.
- Mechanical complications of acute myocardial infarction.

FUTURE DIRECTIONS

As the understanding of the biology of coronary ischemia continues to increase and studies of interventional approaches and pharmacological alterations enhance our knowledge and therapeutic abilities, technical advances continue to evolve, challenging current approaches. The evolution of 'off-pump' or beating-heart coronary revascularization has stimulated re-review of the potential deleterious effects of cardiopulmonary bypass and influenced the approach to operative revascularization, potentially enhancing the safety of operative revascularization in the elderly cohort, those patients with significant non-dialysis renal dysfunction and those with atheromatous aortic changes.[52] The expansion of the beating-heart approach to all CABG patients remains unsupported by long-term data and this will continue to be an area for future investigation, clarification and technological advancement.[53,54]

Less invasive approaches in all surgical disciplines have advanced over the last 15 years, and operative procedures in cardiac surgery have been influenced as well. Minimal incisions for direct revascularization continue to be utilized (MIDCAB) and adjunctive robotic assistance is evolving in coronary procedures with internal mammary harvest techniques and planned revascularization approaches.

The challenges created by robotic devices without tactile feedback will need to be measured against the efficient, open operative procedure, CABG, with or without cardiopulmonary bypass. All of these techniques may stimulate further study of the efficiency of combined interventional and operative revascularization, the 'hybrid approach', and the subset of patients who potentially benefit from this combined approach.

Finally, approaches to enhancing the efficiency and safety of cardiopulmonary bypass continue, and should improve the overall safety of the system.

Tremendous advances have occurred in operative myocardial revascularization since its inception in the 1960s, and one need only recall a sentence from Paul Dudley White's textbook *Heart Disease*, published in 1932, to realize the phenomenal knowledge that has evolved in the last 70 years: 'there is no specific treatment for coronary disease unless it is due to syphilis, a rare cause'.[55] With this historical reference, the perspective becomes clearer and the advances to date even more spectacular, allowing one to anticipate ongoing dramatic, exciting advances in the operative treatment of coronary artery disease in the coming years.

KEY REFERENCES

Eagle KA, Guyton RA, Davidoff R, Ewy GA, Fonger J, Gardner TJ, *et al.* ACC/AHA Guidelines for Coronary Artery Bypass Graft Surgery: A Report of the American College of Cardiology/American Heart Association Task Force on Practice Guidelines (Committee to Revise the 1991 Guidelines for Coronary Artery Bypass Graft Surgery). American College of Cardiology/ American Heart Association. *J Am Coll Cardiol* 1999; **34**(4):1262–347.
Comprehensive, authoritative overview of current coronary surgical practice with recommended indications for surgery.

Hlatky MA, Rogers WJ, Johnstone I, Boothroyd D, Brooks MM, Pitt B, *et al.* Medical care costs and quality of life after randomization to coronary angioplasty or coronary bypass surgery. Bypass Angioplasty Revascularization Investigation (BARI) Investigators. *N Engl J Med* 1997; **336**(2):92–9.
One of a number of reports from this large randomized trial of surgery and angioplasty that have added to understanding of the role of surgery.

Jones RH, Kesler K, Phillips HR 3rd, Mark DB, Smith PK, Nelson CL, *et al.* Long-term survival benefits of coronary artery bypass grafting and percutaneous transluminal angioplasty in patients with coronary artery disease. *J Thorac Cardiovasc Surg* 1996; **111**(5): 1013–25.
The Duke University Medical Center database has been an important source of evidence for supporting current recommendations for surgery, angioplasty or medical therapy relevant to current practice.

Myers WO, Schaff HV, Gersh BJ, Fisher LD; Kosinski AS, Mock MB, *et al.* Improved survival of surgically treated patients with triple vessel coronary artery disease and severe angina pectoris. A report from the Coronary Artery Surgery Study (CASS) registry. *J Thorac Cardiovasc Surg* 1989; **97**(4):487–95.
One of many authoritative reports from this large American study that contributes to the evidence base underpinning current recommendations for coronary artery surgery.

Varnauskas E. Twelve-year follow-up of survival in the randomized European Coronary Surgery Study. *N Engl J Med* 1988; **319**(6):332–7.
Long-term outcome of the European contribution to defining the role of surgery in coronary disease. Despite developments in medical and surgical practice, this study still has lessons relevant to current practice.

REFERENCES

1. Anonymous. Eleven-year survival in the Veterans Administration randomized trial of coronary bypass surgery for stable angina. The Veterans Administration Coronary Artery Bypass Surgery Cooperative Study Group. *N Engl J Med* 1984; **311**:1333–9.

2. Takaro T, Hultgren HN, Lipton MJ, Detre KM. The VA cooperative randomized study of surgery for coronary arterial occlusive disease II. Subgroup with significant left main lesions. *Circulation* 1976; **54**(6 Suppl.):III107–17.

3. Takaro T, Peduzzi P, Detre KM, Hultgren HN, Murphy ML, van der Bel-Kahn J, *et al.* Survival in subgroups of patients with left main

coronary artery disease. Veterans Administration Cooperative Study of Surgery for Coronary Arterial Occlusive Disease. *Circulation* 1982; **66**:14–22.

4. Murphy ML, Hultgren HN, Detre K, Thomsen J, Takaro T. Treatment of chronic stable angina. A preliminary report of survival data of the randomized Veterans Administration Cooperative Study. *N Engl J Med* 1977; **297**:621–7.

5. Bonow RO, Kent KM, Rosing DR, Lan KK, Lakatos E, Borer JS, *et al.* Exercise-induced ischemia in mildly symptomatic patients with coronary-artery disease and preserved left ventricular function. Identification of subgroups at risk of death during medical therapy. *N Engl J Med* 1984; **311**:1339–45.

6. Detre K, Peduzzi P, Murphy M, Hultgren H, Thomsen J, Oberman A, *et al.* Effect of bypass surgery on survival in patients in low- and high-risk subgroups delineated by the use of simple clinical variables. *Circulation* 1981; **63**:1329–38.

7. Detre KM, Takaro T, Hultgren H, Peduzzi P. Long-term mortality and morbidity results of the Veterans Administration randomized trial of coronary artery bypass surgery. *Circulation* 1985; **72**(6 Pt 2):V84–9.

8. Anonymous. Long-term results of prospective randomised study of coronary artery bypass surgery in stable angina pectoris. European Coronary Surgery Study Group. *Lancet* 1982; **2**:1173–80.

9. Varnauskas E. Twelve-year follow-up of survival in the randomized European Coronary Surgery Study. *N Engl J Med* 1988; **319**:332–7.

10. Taylor HA, Deumite NJ, Chaitman BR, Davis KB, Killip T, Rogers WJ. Asymptomatic left main coronary artery disease in the Coronary Artery Surgery Study (CASS) registry. *Circulation* 1989; **79**:1171–9.

11. Myers WO, Schaff HV, Gersh BJ, Fisher LD, Kosinski AS, Mock MB, *et al.* Improved survival of surgically treated patients with triple vessel coronary artery disease and severe angina pectoris. A report from the Coronary Artery Surgery Study (CASS) registry. *J Thorac Cardiovasc Surg* 1989; **97**:487–95.

12. Bell MR, Gersh BJ, Schaff HV, Holmes DR, Jr., Fisher LD, Alderman EL, *et al.* Effect of completeness of revascularization on long-term outcome of patients with three-vessel disease undergoing coronary artery bypass surgery. A report from the Coronary Artery Surgery Study (CASS) Registry. *Circulation* 1992; **86**:446–57.

13. Chaitman BR, Davis KB, Kaiser GC, Mudd G, Wiens RD, Ng GS, *et al.* The role of coronary bypass surgery for 'left main equivalent' coronary disease: the Coronary Artery Surgery Study registry. *Circulation* 1986; **74**(5 Pt 2):III17–25.

14. Alderman EL, Bourassa MG, Cohen LS, Davis KB, Kaiser GG, Killip T, *et al.* Ten-year follow-up of survival and myocardial infarction in the randomized Coronary Artery Surgery Study. *Circulation* 1990; **82**:1629–46.

15. Anonymous. Coronary Artery Surgery Study (CASS): a randomized trial of coronary artery bypass surgery. Quality of life in patients randomly assigned to treatment groups. *Circulation* 1983; **68**:951–60.

16. Anonymous. Coronary Artery Surgery Study (CASS): a randomized trial of coronary artery bypass surgery. Survival data. *Circulation* 1983; **68**:939–50.

17. Anonymous. Myocardial infarction and mortality in the Coronary Artery Surgery Study (CASS) randomized trial. *N Engl J Med* 1984; **310**:750–8.

18. Passamani E, Davis KB, Gillespie MJ, Killip T. A randomized trial of coronary artery bypass surgery. Survival of patients with a low ejection fraction. *N Engl J Med* 1985; **312**:1665–71.

19. Rogers WJ, Coggin CJ, Gersh BJ, Fisher LD, Myers WO, Oberman A, *et al.* Ten-year follow-up of quality of life in patients randomized to receive medical therapy or coronary artery bypass graft surgery. The Coronary Artery Surgery Study (CASS). *Circulation* 1990; **82**:1647–58.

20. Anonymous. Coronary angioplasty versus coronary artery bypass surgery: the Randomized Intervention Treatment of Angina (RITA) trial. *Lancet* 1993; **341**:573–80.

21. Henderson RA. The Randomised Intervention Treatment of Angina (RITA) Trial protocol: a long term study of coronary angioplasty and coronary artery bypass surgery in patients with angina. *Br Heart J* 1989; **62**:411–14.

22. Henderson RA, Pocock SJ, Sharp SJ, Nanchahal K, Sculpher MJ, Buxton MJ, *et al.* Long-term results of RITA-1 trial: clinical and cost comparisons of coronary angioplasty and coronary-artery bypass grafting. Randomised Intervention Treatment of Angina. *Lancet* 1998; **352**:1419–25.

23. Anonymous. First-year results of CABRI (Coronary Angioplasty versus Bypass Revascularisation Investigation). CABRI Trial Participants. *Lancet* 1995; **346**:1179–84.

24. Hueb WA, Bellotti G, de Oliveira SA, Arie S, de Albuquerque CP, Jatene AD, *et al.* The Medicine, Angioplasty or Surgery Study (MASS): a prospective, randomized trial of medical therapy, balloon angioplasty or bypass surgery for single proximal left anterior descending artery stenoses. *J Am Coll Cardiol* 1995; **26**:1600–5.

25. Hamm CW, Reimers J, Ischinger T, Rupprecht HJ, Berger J, Bleifeld W. A randomized study of coronary angioplasty compared with bypass surgery in patients with symptomatic multivessel coronary disease. German Angioplasty Bypass Surgery Investigation (GABI). *N Engl J Med* 1994; **331**:1037–43.

26. Rodriguez A, Boullon F, Perez-Balino N, Paviotti C, Liprandi MI, Palacios IF. Argentine Randomized Trial of Percutaneous Transluminal Coronary Angioplasty Versus Coronary Artery Bypass Surgery in Multivessel Disease (ERACI): in-hospital results and 1-year follow-up. ERACI Group. *J Am Coll Cardiol* 1993; **22**:1060–7.

27. Rodriguez A, Mele E, Peyregne E, Bullon F, Perez-Balino N, Liprandi MI, *et al.* Three-year follow-up of the Argentine Randomized Trial of Percutaneous Transluminal Coronary Angioplasty Versus Coronary Artery Bypass Surgery in Multivessel Disease (ERACI). *J Am Coll Cardiol* 1996; **27**:1178–84.

28. King SB 3rd, Lembo NJ, Weintraub WS, Kosinski AS, Barnhart HX, Kutner MH, *et al.* A randomized trial comparing coronary angioplasty with coronary bypass surgery. Emory Angioplasty versus Surgery Trial (EAST). *N Engl J Med* 1994; **331**:1044–50.

29. Pocock SJ, Henderson RA, Rickards AF, Hampton JR, King SB, 3rd, Hamm CW, *et al.* Meta-analysis of randomized trials comparing coronary angioplasty with bypass surgery. *Lancet* 1995; **346**:1184–9.

30. Hlatky MA, Rogers WJ, Johnstone I, Boothroyd D, Brooks MM, Pitt B, *et al.* Medical care costs and quality of life after randomization to coronary angioplasty or coronary bypass surgery. Bypass Angioplasty Revascularization Investigation (BARI) Investigators. *N Engl J Med* 1997; **336**:92–9.

31. Anonymous. Comparison of coronary bypass surgery with angioplasty in patients with multivessel disease. The Bypass Angioplasty Revascularization Investigation (BARI) Investigators. *N Engl J Med* 1996; **335**:217–25.

32. Jones RH, Kesler K, Phillips HR 3rd, Mark DB, Smith PK, Nelson CL, *et al.* Long-term survival benefits of coronary artery bypass grafting and percutaneous transluminal angioplasty in patients with coronary artery disease. *J Thorac Cardiovasc Surg* 1996; **111**:1013–25.

33. Rodriguez A, Bernardi V, Navia J, Baldi J, Grinfeld L, Martinez J, *et al.* Argentine Randomized Study: Coronary Angioplasty with Stenting versus Coronary Bypass Surgery in patients with Multiple-Vessel Disease (ERACI II): 30-day and 1-year follow-up results. ERACI II Investigators. *J Am Coll Cardiol* 2001; **37**:51–8.

34. Booth DC, Deupree RH, Hultgren HN, DeMaria AN, Scott SM, Luchi RJ. Quality of life after bypass surgery for unstable angina.

5-year follow-up results of a Veterans Affairs Cooperative Study. *Circulation* 1991; **83**:87–95.

35. Scott SM, Deupree RH, Sharma GV, Luchi RJ. VA Study of Unstable Angina. 10-year results show duration of surgical advantage for patients with impaired ejection fraction. *Circulation* 1994; **90**(5 Pt 2):II120–3.

36. Luchi RJ, Scott SM, Deupree RH. Comparison of medical and surgical treatment for unstable angina pectoris. Results of a Veterans Administration Cooperative Study. *N Engl J Med* 1987; **316**:977–84.

37. Parisi AF, Khuri S, Deupree RH, Sharma GV, Scott SM, Luchi RJ. Medical compared with surgical management of unstable angina. 5-year mortality and morbidity in the Veterans Administration Study. *Circulation* 1989; **80**:1176–89.

38. Morrison DA, Sethi G, Sacks J, Grover F, Sedlis S, Esposito R, *et al.* A multicenter, randomized trial of percutaneous coronary intervention versus bypass surgery in high-risk unstable angina patients. The AWESOME (Veterans Affairs Cooperative Study #385, Angina with Extremely Serious Operative Mortality Evaluation) investigators from the Cooperative Studies Program of the Department of Veterans Affairs. *Control Clin Trials* 1999; **20**:601–19.

39. Morrison DA, Sethi G, Sacks J, Henderson W, Grover F, Sedlis S, *et al.* Percutaneous coronary intervention versus coronary artery bypass graft surgery for patients with medically refractory myocardial ischemia and risk factors for adverse outcomes with bypass: a multicenter, randomized trial. Investigators of the Department of Veterans Affairs Cooperative Study #385, the Angina With Extremely Serious Operative Mortality Evaluation (AWESOME). *J Am Coll Cardiol* 2001; **38**:143–9.

40. Morrison DA, Sethi G, Sacks J, Henderson W, Grover F, Sedlis S, *et al.* Percutaneous coronary intervention versus coronary bypass graft surgery for patients with medically refractory myocardial ischemia and risk factors for adverse outcomes with bypass: The VA AWESOME multicenter registry: comparison with the randomized clinical trial. *J Am Coll Cardiol* 2002; **39**:266–73.

41. Anonymous. The effects of tissue plasminogen activator, streptokinase, or both on coronary-artery patency, ventricular function, and survival after acute myocardial infarction. The GUSTO Angiographic Investigators. *N Engl J Med* 1993; **329**:1615–22.

42. Boden WE, O'Rourke RA, Crawford MH, Blaustein AS, Deedwania PC, Zoble RG, *et al.* Outcomes in patients with acute non-Q-wave myocardial infarction randomly assigned to an invasive as compared with a conservative management strategy. Veterans Affairs Non-Q-Wave Infarction Strategies in Hospital (VANQWISH) Trial Investigators. *N Engl J Med* 1998; **338**:1785–92.

43. Anonymous. Invasive compared with non-invasive treatment in unstable coronary-artery disease: FRISC II prospective randomized multicentre study. FRagmin and Fast Revascularisation during InStability in Coronary Artery Disease Investigators. *Lancet* 1999; **354**:708–15.

44. Anonymous. Long-term low-molecular-mass heparin in unstable coronary-artery disease: FRISC II prospective randomized multicentre study. FRagmin and Fast Revascularization during InStability in Coronary Artery Disease Investigators. *Lancet* 1999; **354**:701–7.

45. Cannon CP, Weintraub WS, Demopoulos LA, Vicari R, Frey MJ, Lakkis N, *et al.* Comparison of early invasive and conservative strategies in patients with unstable coronary syndromes treated with the glycoprotein IIb/IIIa inhibitor tirofiban. *N Engl J Med* 2001; **344**:1879–87.

46. Allen BS, Buckberg GD, Fontan FM, Kirsh MM, Popoff G, Beyersdorf F, *et al.* Superiority of controlled surgical reperfusion versus percutaneous transluminal coronary angioplasty in acute coronary occlusion. *J Thorac Cardiovasc Surg* 1993; **105**:864–79; discussion 879–84.

47. Anonymous. Indications for fibrinolytic therapy in suspected acute myocardial infarction: collaborative overview of early mortality and major morbidity results from all randomized trials of more than 1000 patients. Fibrinolytic Therapy Trialists' (FTT) Collaborative Group. *Lancet* 1994; **343**:311–22.

48. Anonymous. A clinical trial comparing primary coronary angioplasty with tissue plasminogen activator for acute myocardial infarction. The Global Use of Strategies to Open Occluded Coronary Arteries in Acute Coronary Syndromes (GUSTO IIb) Angioplasty Substudy Investigators. *N Engl J Med* 1997; **336**:1621–8.

49. Hochman JS, Sleeper LA, Webb JG, Sanborn TA, White HD, Talley JD, *et al.* Early revascularization in acute myocardial infarction complicated by cardiogenic shock. SHOCK Investigators. Should we emergently revascularize occluded coronaries for cardiogenic shock. *N Engl J Med* 1999; **341**:625–34.

50. Menon V, Slater JN, White HD, Sleeper LA, Cocke T, Hochman JS. Acute myocardial infarction complicated by systemic hypoperfusion without hypotension: report of the SHOCK trial registry. *Am J Med* 2000; **108**:374–80.

51. Eagle KA, Guyton RA, Davidoff R, Ewy GA, Fonger J, Gardner TJ, *et al.* ACC/AHA Guidelines for Coronary Artery Bypass Graft Surgery: A Report of the American College of Cardiology/American Heart Association Task Force on Practice Guidelines (Committee to Revise the 1991 Guidelines for Coronary Artery Bypass Graft Surgery). American College of Cardiology/American Heart Association. *J Am Coll Cardiol* 1999; **34**:1262–347.

52. VanDijk D, Jansen E, Hijman R, Nierich AP, Diephuis JC, Moons KG, *et al.* Cognitive outcome after off-pump and on-pump coronary artery bypass graft surgery. *JAMA* 2002; **287**:1405–12.

53. Jegaden O, Mikaeloff P. Off-pump coronary artery bypass surgery. The beginning of the end? *Eur J Cardiothoracic Surg* 2001; **19**:237–8.

54. Cooley D. Con Beating heart surgery for coronary revascularization: Is it the most important development since the introduction of the heart–lung machine? *Ann Thorac Surg* 2000; **70**:1779–81.

55. White PD. In: *Heart Disease.* New York: The Macmillan Co., 1932, 424.

10

Anesthetic and perioperative management in coronary surgery

MICHAEL J HIGGINS AND STEPHEN HICKEY

GENERAL PRINCIPLES

In the absence of anesthesia, major surgery would be an horrific psychological trespass. Further, it would generate extreme adverse sympathetic responses, with tachycardia, increased peripheral vascular resistance, hypertension and hugely increased cardiac work. The main aims of anesthesia are to negate these effects. In addition, mechanical ventilation of the lungs allows respiration to continue efficiently despite the disruption caused by sternotomy. Maintenance of a physically stable surgical field is aided by suppression of diaphragmatic or other unwanted movements. The anesthetist must also compensate for other actual or potential physiological insults such as blood loss, electrolyte and acid–base abnormalities and the effects of the drugs that have been given, and assist in minimizing the mortality and morbidity associated with coronary surgery.

Suppression of awareness

The mental processes underlying general anesthesia remain ill-understood. Unlike physiological sleep, there is probably no universal underlying process. Rather, the condition reflects a set of superficially similar effects produced through various mechanisms by different 'anesthetic' drugs.[1,2] The key common element is the reversible dose-related suppression of the neuronal information processing that underlies conscious awareness. Suppression of awareness is not, however, an obligatory part of all anesthetic techniques for major surgery. For instance, provided the patient is mentally prepared, many types of major operation can be carried out satisfactorily on conscious patients using spinal or epidural anesthesia. However, in the presence of a vertical sternotomy, even when complete afferent blockade through a thoracic epidural catheter forms a major part of the technique, there is a requirement for mechanical ventilation, which, in practice, necessitates general anesthesia.

The adverse effects of unintentional (as opposed to planned) overt awareness during surgery include serious long-term psychological morbidity.[3,4] Experimental paradigms have also demonstrated the phenomenon of subliminal awareness (implicit memory) where there is no conscious recall of events but it is suggested that patients can meaningfully but unconsciously process, for example, auditory information presented during surgical anesthesia.[5] The potential consequences of this kind of cognitive processing remain unknown.

In the past, cardiac surgery has been considered an area of relatively high risk for awareness during anesthesia.[6-8] A number of factors have contributed to this, including a fashion for using high-dose opioids as the sole sedative agent, the pharmacokinetic uncertainties introduced by cardiopulmonary bypass and hypothermia, lack of normal hemodynamic responses during bypass, and a desire to avoid the adverse hemodynamic effects of anesthetic drugs. Appreciation of the issues, modern balanced anesthetic techniques, better pharmacokinetic understanding and the ready availability of techniques for continuous drug delivery may prevent the problem.[9] There is currently no well-validated monitor that satisfactorily measures cerebral information processing, although efforts are being made in this direction.

Autonomic and cardiovascular effects

In addition to producing oblivion, anesthetic drugs blunt the acute autonomic responses to noxious stimulation in a dose-related fashion. All anesthetic drugs (inhalational and intravenous) also have direct cardiovascular effects. Although there is some quantitative variation between individual drugs, they all decrease blood pressure in a concentration-related fashion, mainly by peripheral vasodilatation (decreased preload and afterload), but also by a varying degree of negative cardiac inotropy.

An important aim of anesthesia for the cardiovascular system is to maintain a beneficial balance between energy supply and demand in the cardiac muscle throughout the operation. Normally, myocardial perfusion, particularly of the left ventricle, occurs largely in diastole. Decreased diastolic arterial pressure, decreased diastolic time and increased cardiac wall pressure all decrease cardiac muscle perfusion. Increased heart rate, which decreases the relative length of diastole compared to systole, adversely affects the balance between supply and demand by increasing the rate of cardiac work while decreasing the time available for cardiac muscle perfusion.

In practice, the anesthetist must continuously balance the actions of the anesthetic and other cardiovascular-active drugs with appropriate intravascular fluid administration against the fluctuating consequences of the ongoing surgery, avoiding hypotension, hypertension, tachycardia, excessive bradycardia, dysrhythmias and low cardiac output states.

PREOPERATIVE ASSESSMENT AND OPTIMIZATION

Patients presenting for surgery have already been through a selection process that should ensure an expectation of benefit from the operation. In addition, their co-morbidity should have been quantified, any unexplained signs and symptoms (such as unexpected anemia) investigated and any modifiable factors optimized. Coexisting conditions may present specific management problems. Often, however, the mechanisms linking specific preoperative diagnoses and postoperative outcome are complex and only partially understood. This is the case, for example, with the increased mortality associated with diabetes or

chronic renal impairment.[10–12] In addition to general morbidity, there may be conditions, such as drug allergies or anticipated difficulties with endotracheal intubation, which present a problem only in the specific context of an anesthetic. Patients will be on a range of medications. The effects and potential interactions of these with perioperative pathophysiology must be understood and optimal perioperative drug administration regimens developed.

Finally, it is useful for the anesthetist to assess the precise pattern of the patient's cardiac disease. This will have implications for the likely margins of safety in the face of the impending physiological challenge. It will inform the ongoing management of cardiovascular changes once anesthesia and surgery are underway, and it may directly influence the anesthetic plan of action, for instance in determining what monitoring is instituted at the start of anesthesia. Of particular interest are the anatomical distribution of the coronary artery disease, the degree of left ventricular impairment, the presence or absence of left ventricular hypertrophy, the cardiac rhythm and the presence or absence of associated valvular dysfunction. Patients with symptomatic coronary artery disease have limited ability to increase myocardial blood flow in the face of increased energy demand. They have smaller margins of safety in the face of decreased perfusion pressure or the decreased diastolic time associated with increased heart rate. Inadequate myocardial perfusion may lead to ventricular dysfunction or arrhythmia, which in turn worsens myocardial perfusion and starts a rapidly deteriorating vicious circle. Patients with left main stem disease (or equivalent) are likely to be particularly vulnerable. Patients with left ventricular hypertrophy are particularly vulnerable to sub-endocardial ischemia and to the loss of the atrial contribution to ventricular filling should atrial fibrillation occur. Impaired left ventricular function is associated with increased operative mortality[13] and may be an indication for invasive monitoring of cardiac output and left heart filling pressures, particularly after cardiopulmonary bypass.

Some important coexisting conditions

DIABETES

The incidence of diabetes mellitus in the patients undergoing coronary surgery in the US is almost 30%, based on the Society of Thoracic Surgeons comprehensive database.[14] This includes diabetics controlled by diet alone. Patients with diabetes have an approximately twofold early mortality and reduced long-term survival after coronary artery surgery.[10,11] Diabetic patients have an increased risk of important postoperative complications, including deep sternal wound infection and major neurological abnormality.[15,16]

There is evidence that the incidence of infective complications, including deep sternal infections, is reduced if diabetic patients are managed on continuous intravenous insulin perioperatively.[17] This includes type II diabetics (who are not normally dependent on insulin). In this (non-randomized) study,[17] blood glucose was controlled to below $11.1 \, \text{mmol L}^{-1}$ in the treatment group. Insulin treatment (glucose/insulin infusion for 24 hours followed by intermittent subcutaneous insulin) has also been shown to decrease mortality following myocardial infarction in patients with diabetes. The effect was particularly marked in type II diabetics not normally dependent on insulin. This suggests that insulin therapy might be beneficial in the context of myocardial damage.[18]

There has been concern that the sulphanylurea group of oral hypoglycemic drugs might increase the vulnerability of the myocardium to ischemia–reperfusion injury. Studies have shown increased mortality in sulphonylurea-treated diabetics undergoing coronary angioplasty.[19,20] The effect could be related to the action of these drugs in preventing the protective effect of myocardial ischemic preconditioning.[21] In turn, this may be due to their antagonism at K_{ATP} channels, although the concentration of sulphonylureas required to act at cardiac and vascular K_{ATP} channels is very much higher than that required to promote insulin release from the pancreas.

It is not known whether treatment with sulphonylureas is associated with adverse outcomes in patients undergoing coronary artery surgery. Almassi and Warltier have published reassuring data from the Society of Thoracic Surgeons database. Data were available on 636 826 patients undergoing coronary artery bypass grafting (CABG) from 1994 to 1997. In these patients, mortality was 2.90% for non-diabetics, 5.01% for insulin-treated, 3.54% for oral hypoglycemic-treated, and 3.96% for diet/no treatment groups. The rate of perioperative myocardial infarction was similar for all groups (1.42% non-diabetics, 1.31% insulin treated, 1.25% oral hypoglycemic treated, and 1.30% diet/no control group).[14] It may be that omitting sulphanylurea drugs on the day of surgery, as would be standard practice, is enough to allow plasma concentrations to fall sufficiently to prevent adverse effects on the myocardium.

The authors' current practice for the management of patients with diabetes mellitus is to continue hypoglycemic agents (including insulin) and normal diet on the day before surgery. Oral hypoglycemic agents and subcutaneous insulin are omitted on the day of surgery, blood glucose is measured, and an insulin infusion is started to maintain blood glucose in the range 6–$10 \, \text{mmol L}^{-1}$. The insulin is delivered from a dedicated syringe driver ($50 \, \text{mL}$ syringe containing insulin 1 unit mL^{-1}). Patients for morning surgery are fasted from midnight; patients for afternoon surgery may have an early, light ('tea and toast') breakfast, allowing at least

4 hours fasting before surgery. While waiting for surgery, blood glucose concentrations must be re-measured at 1–2-hourly intervals, depending on the absolute value and the rate of any changes. Blood glucose concentrations below $4.0 \, \text{mmol L}^{-1}$ should be treated with intravenous dextrose. It is important to realize that the amount of insulin required to maintain a given blood glucose varies markedly amongst patients, and at different times in a given patient. Insulin regimens must therefore have built-in flexibility. A typical regimen starting with an infusion of 1 unit h^{-1} when the blood glucose is in the range 8.3–$11.1 \, \text{mmol L}^{-1}$ is given by Furnary and colleagues.[17]

There is some recent evidence that tighter control of blood glucose may provide further benefits. In a large randomized study[22] in a surgical intensive care population that comprised 62% postoperative cardiac surgery patients, intensive care mortality was decreased by more than 30% when blood glucose was strictly controlled to between 4.4 and $6.1 \, \text{mmol L}^{-1}$ compared with 'conventional control' to a target of between 10 and $11.1 \, \text{mmol L}^{-1}$. The effect applied to both diabetics and non-diabetics. Benefit was seen in all patient subgroups, including the cardiac surgical patients. It was only apparent, however, in patients requiring more than 5 days of intensive care. The potential disadvantage is an increased risk of hypoglycemia.

A question currently unanswered is whether it is beneficial to start intravenous glucose administration along with insulin as soon as fasting commences on the morning of surgery. At physiological concentrations, insulin achieves its main hypoglycemic effect by reducing glucose production by the liver rather than increasing glucose uptake by other tissues.[23] This would suggest that providing additional glucose is illogical, a view currently favored by the authors. There is some circumstantial evidence, however, for the converse view,[24,25] particularly if the regimen involves achieving supraphysiological concentrations of insulin, as is the case with 'GIK' – glucose–insulin–potassium regimens.[25]

CHRONIC OBSTRUCTIVE PULMONARY DISEASE

Many patients presenting for coronary artery bypass surgery have chronic obstructive pulmonary disease (COPD) because of the common causal link with smoking.

The primary feature of COPD is irreversible pulmonary airflow limitation. Other features include chronic cough, dyspnea, sputum production and wheeze. Tobacco smoking is the main risk factor for COPD, although not all smokers develop COPD and some patients with COPD are lifelong non-smokers. The diagnosis will encompass most patients with chronic bronchitis and emphysema and a proportion of patients with longstanding asthma. Precise definitions of the condition vary, particularly in terms of quantifying airflow limitation and reversibility, and disease severity.[26]

Spirometry is the main tool used for the quantification of airflow limitation and hence is important in the diagnosis and severity classification of COPD. The presence or absence of airflow limitation is usually defined in terms of the FEV_1:FVC ratio, where FEV_1 is the forced expiratory volume in 1 second and FVC the forced vital capacity. The US National Heart, Lung, and Blood Institute/ World Health Organization Global Initiative for Chronic Obstructive Lung Disease (GOLD)[27] defines significant airflow limitation as post-bronchodilator FEV_1:FVC <70%. Disease severity is then stratified in terms of the FEV_1, although the relationship between symptom severity and objectively measured airflow limitation is quite variable. GOLD criteria for mild, moderate and severe (Stage 1, 2 and 3) COPD are $FEV_1 \geqslant 80\%$ predicted, 30–80% predicted, and <30% predicted, respectively.

The general course of COPD is usually inexorably progressive. Severe COPD is associated with the development of respiratory failure and cor pulmonale (right heart failure). Respiratory failure is defined by blood gas abnormalities. Hypoxemia (arterial PO_2 <8.0 kPa at sea level) occurs first. Hypercapnia (arterial PCO_2 >6.7 kPa) often develops later. Superimposed upon the underlying chronic condition, patients are subject to a variable pattern of acute exacerbations, often associated with respiratory infection.

The main long-term treatments for COPD are smoking cessation, bronchodilator therapy, glucocorticosteroid inhalation (not systemic steroid therapy), exercise training and, for some patients with respiratory failure, regular long-term oxygen therapy for >15 hours a day.

Patents with COPD who undergo coronary surgery are at increased risk of postoperative pulmonary and other complications, including prolonged postoperative ventilation, and both early and late mortality.[28–31] In a large observational study,[31] an FEV_1 of less than 1.25 L, which would place most patients at least well down in the moderate category, was associated with an approximately threefold increase in operative mortality on univariate analysis. Mortality increased at lower values of FEV_1, with a sharp increase at the lowest values.

Patients with mild to moderate COPD may undergo coronary surgery with an acceptable increase in risk. If there is any evidence of acute respiratory infection or exacerbation, surgery should be postponed for treatment of the lung disease. Evidence of any acute exacerbation should be sought in the history and examination, and would include an increase in dyspnea, sputum volume or sputum purulence. Treatment may include increased bronchodilator therapy and systemic steroids.[27] An increase in sputum volume or purulence, particularly in association with fever, suggests bacterial infection, which should be treated with antibiotics.

Postoperatively, the authors' practice is to extubate and mobilize patients with uncomplicated COPD as early as possible. Physiotherapy is aimed at promoting deep breathing and coughing. Meticulous attention to pain relief is important so that breathing and coughing are not inhibited. Regular non-steroidal analgesic therapy may be beneficial if there is no contraindication. (A tendency to wheeze is not in itself a contraindication to these drugs, although they may precipitate bronchospasm in a small set of susceptible patients.) Intraoperative and postoperative thoracic epidural anesthesia using a local anesthetic has been shown to reduce postoperative pulmonary complications in a general (non-COPD) population of patients undergoing coronary surgery.[32] The potential benefits of this technique may not be realizable when it is used sporadically rather than as part of a regular program.

There is little published evidence to guide the decision to offer coronary artery surgery to patients with severe COPD. Each patient must be assessed individually. The severity of each disease, the contribution of each to reduced quality of life, the expected benefit from coronary artery surgery, the natural history of the pulmonary disease and the presence of other risk factors must all be taken into account. Operative mortality is likely to be high but is hard to quantify. At least one small case-control study has included some patients with hypoxemia in the COPD group. There was a 16-month mortality of 5/37, compared to 0/37 in the control group.[28] Amongst the survivors, improvement in the self-reported quality of life after surgery was much less for the patients with COPD.

It may be helpful to involve the anesthetist and possibly a respiratory physician early in the decision process for these patients. Ongoing treatment should be optimized. If adjustments are necessary, for instance to steroid therapy or for the addition of exercise training, it may take several weeks for the benefits to accrue and be assessed.

Patients with COPD who are still smoking at assessment for coronary surgery should be unequivocally advised to stop. One group has reported that the incidence of postoperative respiratory complications might be higher in patients who stop smoking during a 2–6-week window preoperatively compared to those who continue to smoke.[33] However, this applies to respiratory complications only. There are advantageous effects on the cardiovascular system which suggest that a period of abstinence of even 12–24 hours preoperatively is of value.[34]

CEREBROVASCULAR DISEASE

There is an increased incidence of cerebrovascular disease in patients presenting for coronary artery surgery because of the shared underlying pathology. The incidence of significant (>50%) carotid stenosis in the coronary surgery population is around 10–20%.[35–37] The presence of significant carotid stenosis increases the risk of stroke or other serious adverse neurological outcome associated with undergoing cardiac surgery.[35,37,38]

The American National Institute of Neurological Diseases and the American Heart Association have produced evidence-based guidelines for the treatment of significant carotid stenosis by carotid endarterectomy, stratified according to the associated surgical risk of death and stroke.[39,40] It is widely accepted that significant symptomatic carotid stenosis is a clear indication for carotid endarterectomy. Surgery for even severe (>80%) *asymptomatic* carotid stenosis has remained controversial.[41] However, coronary artery disease increases the mortality and cardiac morbidity associated with carotid endarterectomy.[42–44]

Current practice varies amongst institutions and amongst individual surgeons.[45,46] The American College of Cardiology/American Heart Association (ACC/AHA) guidelines for coronary artery surgery state that 'current tactics are best left to local team policies and preferences based on careful examination of team outcomes'. The authors suggest that when the procedure is staged, and the urgency of the coronary surgery permits, carotid endarterectomy should be performed first, between 1 and 5 days before coronary surgery.[47] One study, quoted in the guidelines, included a group of patients with unstable coronary disease and asymptomatic carotid lesions. The patients were randomized to a combined procedure or to coronary surgery first. There was a significantly higher incidence of stroke in the patients who had their carotid endarterectomies performed after the coronary surgery. However, virtually all the strokes occurred in patients who had an interval of less than 2 weeks between operations. The incidence of stroke in patients who had carotid surgery more than 2 weeks after coronary surgery was very low (1/46).[48]

Patients with unstable coronary syndromes have an ongoing inflammatory response. Patients who have undergone procedures utilizing cardiopulmonary bypass and, to a lesser extent, other forms of surgery have a systemic inflammatory response that is associated with a prothrombotic state for several days after surgery. Clinically silent brain damage may occur in association with coronary or carotid surgery. The acute pathophysiology of central nervous system damage, from whatever cause, is complex. It involves inflammatory and other mechanisms that blend into resolution and repair over a time course of days to weeks. Given these considerations, there is a good argument that time intervals longer than a few days should be allowed for proper healing between staged operations. There are no good clinical outcome studies to guide this decision, however.

Given current uncertainties, we would advocate that, whatever staging plan is adopted, carotid endarterectomy should only be carried out if it is indicated in its own right, i.e. independently of the necessity for cardiac surgery.

OTHER MAJOR SURGERY

Mortality and cardiac morbidity associated with non-cardiac major surgery, including vascular, thoracic, abdominal and major head and neck surgery, are increased two- to threefold in patients with significant coronary artery disease.[49,50] This increased risk is attenuated by prior CABG.[49] For this reason, patients requiring major surgery who would also benefit from coronary artery bypass surgery should have the coronary surgery performed first, if at all possible. However, the indications for coronary artery surgery are not changed by the need to undergo other surgery, and there is currently no evidence that prophylactic coronary artery surgery is beneficial in these circumstances unless it is indicated in its own right.

CHRONIC RENAL IMPAIRMENT

Coronary surgery may result in a significant insult to renal function. A large multicenter observational study found an incidence of postoperative renal dysfunction of 7.7% in 2222 coronary surgery patients.[51] Renal dysfunction was defined as postoperative serum creatinine of $177\,\mu mol\,L^{-1}$ or greater coupled with a perioperative rise of $62\,\mu mol\,L^{-1}$ or greater. Not surprisingly, patients with preoperative renal impairment were at greater risk of postoperative renal dysfunction. Preoperative creatinine concentrations of between 124 (approximately the upper limit of the normal range) and $177\,\mu mol\,L^{-1}$ were associated with a three-fold risk for postoperative renal dysfunction. Patients who already had a serum creatinine greater than $177\,\mu mol\,L^{-1}$ or were on renal replacement therapy preoperatively were excluded from this study. Other preoperative risk factors for postoperative renal dysfunction were age, congestive heart failure, previous coronary artery surgery, and type 1 diabetes or a serum glucose level above $16.6\,mmol\,L^{-1}$.

Overall, 1.4% of this study population required postoperative renal replacement therapy. This is similar to the 0.9% of 34 874 coronary artery surgery patients without pre-existing end-stage renal failure reported in another large multicenter study.[52] Again, any degree of preoperative renal impairment was linearly related to the risk of requiring postoperative renal replacement therapy. The development of postoperative renal dysfunction, short of requiring renal replacement therapy, is associated with increased postoperative mortality.[51] The need for postoperative renal replacement therapy is associated with an early mortality rate of more than 60%.[51,52] However, this may not be a direct consequence of compromised or absent renal function, as the severity of renal dysfunction probably tends to reflect the degree of failure in other organ systems.

Preoperative renal impairment, as defined by a raised plasma creatinine, is associated with an increase in operative mortality that may be several times baseline.[53,54] Coronary surgery, however, may be carried out with acceptable mortality even in patients on preoperative renal replacement therapy. Hosoda and colleagues, for instance, describe a series of 45 consecutive patients with no in-hospital mortality.[12]

Unfortunately, there is currently no useful pharmacological prophylaxis against acute renal damage. The risk of renal insult must be minimized by avoiding renal hypoperfusion secondary to low blood pressure, intravascular hypovolemia or low cardiac output. Meticulous attention must be paid to these imperatives in high-risk patients. Prolonged fluid deprivation due to preoperative fasting should be avoided and, if a wait of more than 4 hours is anticipated, a saline infusion should be started. During and after surgery, a pulmonary artery catheter, particularly one that measures continuous cardiac output or mixed venous oxygen saturation, is helpful. The development of oliguria postoperatively must be addressed in terms of the underlying causes, rather than with diuretic therapy. Great care must be taken with the administration of potentially nephrotoxic drugs such as aminoglycoside antibiotics. Non-steroidal anti-inflammatory analgesics should be avoided.

Ongoing drug therapy

As a general rule, drugs for most pre-existing conditions and most cardiovascular drugs, including calcium-channel antagonists, nitrates and vasodilators, should be continued up to the time of surgery. Doses due on the day of operation should *not* be withheld because the patient is 'fasting' before surgery. Medications should be restarted as soon as possible after surgery. It may be necessary to substitute parenteral preparations or alternatives in patients who do not make an early return to oral intake. Drugs given for the control of angina may no longer be required after successful revascularization and can be stopped. However, this does not apply to β-adrenergic receptor blockers or drugs given primarily for hypertension. Important exceptions to the general rule, and areas where there may be controversy, are discussed below. (Hypoglycemic agents have already been discussed in relation to the management of patients with diabetes.)

DRUGS WHICH MODIFY THROMBOTIC/HEMOSTATIC FUNCTION

Aspirin

Aspirin irreversibly inhibits cyclo-oxygenase which contributes to normal platelet function. Platelets cannot synthesize new stocks of this enzyme. Exposure to aspirin thus affects platelet function for the life of the platelet. Patients who take aspirin until the day of surgery are at increased risk of allogenic blood transfusion, delayed chest closure and early reopening for bleeding.[55] In accordance with the ACC/AHA guidelines,[47] we currently stop aspirin therapy 7 days preoperatively in patients with stable angina. However, it has been argued that an aspirin-free period of 3 days may be adequate.[56] In addition, a large retrospective case-control study has found decreased mortality in patients who took aspirin within 7 days of surgery compared with those who did not.[57] Possible confounding factors in this study include postoperative commencement or restoration of aspirin therapy, about which no information is provided.

Aspirin significantly reduces vein graft closure provided it is given within 24 hours after operation. The benefits are clear cut and the ACC/AHA Task Force on Practice Guidelines suggest that fail-safe mechanisms should exist to ensure the early (within hours of operation) re-institution of aspirin therapy.[47] Aspirin may be given by suppository or nasogastric tube to patients not yet able to swallow. In patients with true aspirin intolerance, an alternative form of antiplatelet therapy such as clopidogrel should be given instead.

Clopidogrel

Like aspirin, clopidogrel affects platelet function for the life of the individual platelet. It acts by inhibiting ADP-induced platelet aggregation, and is therefore synergistic in its action with aspirin. The optimal treatment-free period preoperatively for clopidogrel has not been determined. A pragmatic approach is to adopt the same policy as with aspirin and stop administration 7 days before surgery. In a prospective observational study of 247 patients undergoing CABG, Yende and Wunderink noted that treatment with clopidogrel in addition to aspirin during any of the 5 days before surgery was associated with a five-fold increase in risk of re-exploration for bleeding.[58]

Platelet glycoprotein (GP) IIb/IIIa antagonists

Three intravenous GP IIb/IIIa antagonists have received approval for use in the UK and USA – abciximab, eptifibatide and tirofiban – with several oral agents undergoing evaluation. Although platelet activation can be stimulated by a number of agonists, adhesion and aggregation are highly dependent on GP IIb/IIIa receptors. Unbound abciximab has a plasma half-life of only 10–15 minutes, but once bound to the receptors its effect is markedly prolonged, with platelet inhibition of 50–60% remaining 24 hours after stopping its infusion. Eptifibatide and tirofiban have much shorter duration of action, with platelet aggregation returning to normal within 4 hours of stopping the drug.

The perioperative management of patients receiving GP IIb/IIIa antagonists has been reviewed, with strategies to reduce the risk of hemorrhage suggested.[59] The authors suggest that if the patient's condition permits, surgery should be delayed for at least 12 hours after discontinuation of abciximab. The role of prophylactic platelet transfusion is controversial: however, given the short plasma half-life of abciximab, platelets can be given in the knowledge that little of the drug will be available to inhibit their function (although some redistribution of the drug will take place). A reduced heparin dose is required to achieve the usual target-activated clotting time, with Kereiakes noting a total of only 2000–4000 units needed to reach an activated clotting time of 400 seconds in some patients.[60] As there are many factors affecting activated clotting time, we would adopt the policy of Levy, who has suggested that standard heparin doses should be given, ideally with actual heparin levels measured at point of care as a guide to dosing.[61] It is also suggested that antifibrinolytic therapy, such as aprotinin, be given before cardiopulmonary bypass, and that an 'off-pump' approach be considered.[55]

DRUGS WHICH MODIFY CARDIOVASCULAR FUNCTION

Angiotensin–converting enzyme (ACE) inhibitors and angiotensin II (AII) receptor antagonists

As well as inhibiting AII formation, ACE inhibitors attenuate the breakdown of bradykinin, which probably contributes substantially to their hypotensive effects.[62,63]

The induction of anesthesia can lead to significant hypotension in patients who have received ACE inhibitors and AII antagonists until the day of surgery. This has led to the suggestion that these drugs be withdrawn before surgery.[64,65] ACE inhibitors have also been implicated in the etiology of the low systemic vascular resistance syndrome after cardiopulmonary bypass, and have been associated with the need for increased vasopressor use after cardiopulmonary bypass.[66,67] Hypotension associated with ACE inhibitors may be refractory to treatment with standard adrenergic agonists, in which case a vasopressin agonist might be effective.[68]

The adverse effect of ACE inhibitors and AII antagonists on arterial pressure seems to be clear cut. However, there may beneficial effects of renin–angiotensin system antagonism on certain regional circulations. The clinical relevance of these is difficult to assess. Captopril, given just before surgery, has been shown to lessen the reduction in renal plasma flow and in glomerular filtration rate normally observed during cardiopulmonary bypass.[69] Some evidence exists to suggest that renin–angiotensin system antagonism may improve splanchnic circulation. It has also been suggested that treatment with an intravenous ACE inhibitor (enalaprilat) before commencing cardiopulmonary bypass may provide myocardial protection in patients undergoing coronary surgery.[70]

In concert with many other clinicians, we currently aim to withdraw ACE inhibitors and AII antagonists for at least 24 hours preoperatively. However, this is an area of active debate, and recommendations may well change. It has already been suggested that withdrawal of ACE inhibitors before cardiac surgery leads to more hypertension in the early postoperative period.[71] The authors concluded that 'omitting ACE inhibitors before surgery did not have sufficient advantage to be recommended routinely'.

Dupuis has highlighted the changes in recommendations regarding the preoperative use of β-blockers over the years. In 1972 it was suggested that propranolol (the only β-blocker available at the time) should be discontinued 2 weeks before surgery because of its potential myocardial depressant effect: it is now suggested that continuing β-blockers throughout the perioperative period may be associated with improved outcome. With regard to AII antagonists, he suggests that anesthetists 'adapt their anesthesia plan' rather than discontinue an efficacious chronic therapy.[72]

Nicorandil

Nicorandil is a nitrate derivative and an ATP-sensitive potassium (K_{ATP}) channel opener. Its effects include reductions in preload, afterload and cardiac contractility. Despite its smooth muscle relaxing properties, there are to date no data to suggest that it may cause unwanted hypotension perioperatively. Indeed, there is growing evidence that nicorandil administered intraoperatively may have myocardial protective properties, by a mechanism similar to that of ischemic preconditioning.[73,74] Kaneko and colleagues demonstrated a marked, dose-dependent, prophylactic effect of intravenous nicorandil on intraoperative myocardial ischemia in patients undergoing non-cardiac surgery who had at least two risk factors for ischemic heart disease.[75] The applicability of these studies may be limited by the local availability of nicorandil for injection. However, in patients already on treatment with nicorandil, it should be continued right up to the time of surgery.

β–Adrenergic receptor blockers

Patients on treatment with β-blockers should continue to take them right up to the time of surgery in order to prevent the possibility of rebound hypertension and to attenuate the adverse sympathetic responses to endotracheal intubation and surgery. β-Blockade should be re-instituted as soon as possible after surgery, i.e. as soon as the patient is cardiovascularly stable without inotropic support.

Withdrawal of β-blockers in the perioperative period is associated with a twofold increase in the incidence of atrial fibrillation after CABG, and a two- to threefold increase in the incidence of stroke. The peak incidence of new atrial fibrillation occurs in the second or third postoperative day. A recent observational study shows a marked reduction of stroke and coma (odds ratio 0.43) associated with perioperative β-blocker administration in 2575 consecutive coronary surgery patients.[76] If β-blockers are neuroprotective, it is not clear whether or not this effect is completely accounted for by their action in decreasing atrial fibrillation.

Strong consideration should be given to starting β-blockade in patients who are not being treated with β-blockade when they present for surgery, and who have no contraindications to their administration. Ideally, β-blockers should be started at least 3 days preoperatively. Currently, 'preoperative or early postoperative administration of β-blockers is considered standard therapy to prevent atrial fibrillation after coronary bypass surgery'.[47]

The preoperative visit: premedication

Many patients have specific fears about anesthesia, compounding their general worries about such major surgery. Anxiety may be intense enough to precipitate angina. Good communication at this stage should reduce anxiety as well as being necessary for developing informed consent.[77]

The practice of pharmacological 'premedication' arose historically because induction of anesthesia by inhalation of ether or chloroform could be performed more smoothly in patients who were already sedated and medicated with an anti-sialogogue. Premedication has become one of the rituals of general anesthesia, although the original indications have long disappeared. However, there is a good rationale for prescribing anxiolytics, starting the night before coronary artery surgery and repeated on the day of operation, to prevent anxiety-induced ischemia. Oral benzodiazepines are particularly useful and safe, with a slow onset of action and high therapeutic index.

In many centers it is customary to prescribe precautionary supplemental oxygen with sedative premedication. Anesthetists may also prescribe drugs to promote gastric emptying and decrease acidity. This is to increase the margins of safety against lung injury by aspiration of gastric contents when the airway is unprotected at induction of anesthesia. Although a good argument may be made for this practice, there is a lack of supporting outcome data.[78,79]

ANESTHETIC MONITORING EQUIPMENT

A large number of monitoring devices is used to gather data about patients and their care during surgery and recovery. It is important to consider how these data are used. An individual piece of information or an individual device is usually neither absolutely required nor completely redundant. Rather, each piece of information is integrated with every other to inform a judgment of the patient's current condition. The clearer the picture, the easier it is to make the correct therapeutic manipulations.

Some of the most useful monitoring techniques in anesthesia for major surgery and intensive care are associated with the possibility of causing important harm. Over a large number of uses, these harms are real and measurable. Monitoring has no intrinsic therapeutic benefit. In instituting these techniques, we thus start off burdened with negative equity in the cost–benefit balance. Any benefit to the patient arises from the managements we make as a result of our increased knowledge. Similarly, inappropriate therapy as a result of misinterpretation or failure to recognize the limitations of the monitoring device leads to additional harm.

The Association of Anaesthetists of Great Britain and Ireland and the American Society of Anesthesiologists (among others) have produced guidelines on a minimum monitoring set to be used for all patients undergoing general anesthesia.[80,81] This minimum is the starting point (although few would consider it sufficient without further addition) for monitoring patients undergoing coronary revascularization.

Continuous electrocardiogram

In patients undergoing coronary artery surgery, the electrocardiogram (ECG) can provide information on heart rate, rhythm, conduction, ischemia and the effect of cardioplegia solution. A single rhythm strip is not acceptable as the only form of ECG monitoring in coronary surgery patients. Most modern intraoperative monitoring devices allow the continual display of at least two and often three or more ECG leads. While lead II is accepted as providing good information on basic rhythm, in isolation it has a low sensitivity in detecting ST segment changes. Combining it with a lateral chest lead or leads will increase the sensitivity of ST segment change detection from around 33% to about 80%.[82] Modern machines will measure ST segment changes automatically and display trends over time. It is important to remember that the ECG is particularly susceptible to interference from electrodiathermy: examination of the arterial pressure waveform will help determine whether any perceived arrhythmias are real or artifactual.

Arterial pressure

All patients undergoing cardiac surgery need to have their arterial pressure measured via an indwelling intra-arterial catheter. This allows the beat-by-beat measurement of systolic, diastolic and mean arterial pressures. Examination of the trace will provide immediate information on the effect of arrhythmias. In addition, the rate of rise of pressure gives some information on myocardial contractility. For convenience, the usual site of measurement is the radial artery, although it must first be ascertained whether the surgeon is planning to harvest the chosen radial artery as a conduit. Other commonly used sites are the brachial and femoral arteries.

The effectiveness of the ulnar artery in providing an adequate blood supply to the hand can be tested using the modified Allen test[83] before cannulating the radial artery.

Although the radial artery remains a safe and popular site for intra-arterial cannulation, its trustworthiness has been questioned. Stern and colleagues demonstrated that radial systolic (and often radial mean) pressures were lower relative to aortic pressure after cardiopulmonary bypass in all 18 patients that they studied.[84] In 13 patients, the differences were large enough to be of clinical concern (12–32 mmHg), and persisted for up to an hour after cardiopulmonary bypass. The authors speculated that this was due to lowered forearm vascular resistance associated with warming at the end of cardiopulmonary bypass.

All direct pressure monitoring systems are prone to artifact caused by loose connections, air bubble entrapment, over-damping and under-damping, and drifting of the baseline. All of these problems must be excluded at the start of monitoring, and should be considered when a sudden change in pressure is observed that does not fit in with other clinical signs. A reproducible zero point must be identified and adhered to whenever the operating table or the patient is moved.

Pulse oximetry

Pulse oximeters measure oxyhemoglobin as a percentage of total hemoglobin. They also measure heart rate. In addition, most pulse oximeters also provide a visual display of the pulse waveform. They cannot differentiate between oxyhemoglobin and methemoglobin, which is of importance in patients receiving nitric oxide. (They similarly fail to distinguish carboxyhemoglobin from oxyhemoglobin, although this is of less relevance in the cardiac patient.) False-positive information (i.e. reading a normal saturation in the presence of arterial hypoxemia) is therefore possible with pulse oximeters, but rare. False-negative information is a much more common finding. The performance of oximeters is significantly impaired by poor peripheral circulation, a common feature after hypothermic cardiopulmonary bypass. However, a low saturation should never be assumed to be due to poor perfusion and should always prompt the clinician to measure an arterial blood gas. Pulse oximeters depend on the phasic light absorption that occurs as a result of vessel pulsatility and are therefore of no use during non-pulsatile cardiopulmonary bypass.

Capnography

The measurement of expired CO_2 in the anesthetic breathing circuit is essential initially to confirm the correct placement of the endotracheal tube, and subsequently to monitor the adequacy of ventilation. Usually, the value of arterial PCO_2 ($PaCO_2$) and the CO_2 measured in expired gas at the end of expiration (the end-tidal (ET) CO_2) are close to each other and the latter mirrors changes in the former. However, an increase in $PaCO_2$–$ETCO_2$ will occur when alveolar units with a high dead space are underperfused and the transfer of CO_2 from the pulmonary capillaries to the alveoli is reduced. This situation may arise from low cardiac output, excessive lung inflation (high positive end-expiratory pressure – PEEP), and high physiological dead space (for example in COPD).

Inspired oxygen, end-tidal anesthetic agent and ventilator function

In addition to expired CO_2, the fraction of O_2 in the inspired gas mixture must be measured in order to allow the clinician to relate oxygen saturation levels and PaO_2 to the FiO_2, to prevent the possibility of administering a hypoxic mixture to the patient, and to reduce the likelihood of oxygen toxicity. If the patient is anesthetized using a volatile anesthetic agent, the end-tidal agent concentration should be measured and displayed to allow the anesthetist to deliver the required concentration. A disconnect alarm must be fitted into the system to alert the anesthetist immediately should any loss of pressure suggesting failure to ventilate the patient's lungs occur. Mechanical ventilators should incorporate airway pressure measurement, which is usually displayed continuously during the ventilatory cycle. Additionally, they will measure gas flow in the breathing system and display some combination of tidal volume, minute volume and respiratory rate.

Temperature

Patients undergoing coronary revascularization may be deliberately cooled or develop hypothermia unintentionally. The most appropriate site to measure the core temperature remains unknown, although tympanic membrane temperature appears to be an accurate reflection of brain temperature. The nasopharynx is commonly used during surgery and is convenient. Rectal temperature is considered to be intermediate between core and peripheral temperatures. Bladder temperature correlates with pulmonary artery temperature when the urine output is high, and with rectal temperature when it is low.

Central venous pressure

Central venous access is required preoperatively in patients undergoing CABG surgery to provide a secure route for the administration of vasoactive drugs, which may include resuscitation drugs. There is therefore no debate about the safety and efficacy of central venous catheterization, as there is with pulmonary artery catheterization (see below). There does, however, remain the question of how the pressure measured in the central veins relates to the patient's intravascular volume status, and to the preload of the left ventricle. Interpretation of the central venous pressure (CVP) must be made with a knowledge of the patient's ventricular and heart valve function. As with invasive arterial pressure monitoring, a reproducible zero point must be identified and adhered to. Examination of the CVP trend provides more relevant information than any single pressure measurement, especially if this is done during a particular therapeutic maneuver. Additional useful information can be obtained from the CVP waveform.[85]

Pulmonary artery catheterization

Clinical assessment of the circulation has important limitations.[86,87] In patients with circulatory dysfunction, it is helpful to have additional, objective, measurements of filling pressures and cardiac output. In most instances this will mean inserting a pulmonary artery catheter.

The American Society of Anesthesiologists Task Force on Pulmonary Artery Catheterization suggests that a pulmonary artery catheter should be considered for perioperative monitoring in appropriate circumstances.[88] However, concerns have arisen as to the efficacy and safety of pulmonary artery catheters. Some authorities have suggested a moratorium on their use until an appropriately designed, randomized clinical trial of pulmonary artery catheter use in critically ill patients is undertaken.[89]

A distinction can be drawn between the use of the pulmonary artery catheter in the acute setting of coronary surgery and its use in the general (non-cardiac) intensive care setting. The use of the pulmonary artery catheter to assess and guide therapy in the cardiac surgery patient is

more like the cardiologist's use of the pulmonary artery catheter to perform a 'right heart catheterization' than the intensivist's use in the management of the multi-organ failure, critically ill patient. Hemodynamic changes in the cardiac surgery patient can occur over a time frame of minutes rather than tens of hours or days. Left and right, systolic and diastolic ventricular dysfunction can occur together or separately against a background of variable peripheral circulatory dysfunction. The need for trials in elective, low-risk (ejection fraction >50%) coronary surgical patients has, however, been recognized, although this is not a straightforward undertaking.[90]

Stocking and Lake conclude that the role of the pulmonary artery catheter is in transition, but given its multiple capabilities and its (qualified) support by a number of societies, it will probably remain 'a vital tool in the clinician's armamentarium'.[91] One of the few indisputable facts concerning its use is that, in the mid-1990s, 1–2 million were placed annually in the US, at an estimated cost of $2 billion.[92]

Pulmonary artery catheters provide direct continuous measurement of pulmonary artery pressures and CVPs.

Table 10.1 *Normal hemodynamic values*

Right atrial pressure (mean)	0–8 mmHg
Right ventricular pressure (systolic/diastolic)	25/0–4 mmHg
Pulmonary artery pressure (systolic/diastolic/mean)	25/12/16 mmHg
Pulmonary artery occlusion pressure (mean)	8–12 mmHg
Left atrial pressure (mean)	8–12 mmHg
Left ventricular pressure: (systolic/diastolic)	120/8–12 mmHg
Cardiac index[a]	2.5–3.5 L min^{-1} m^{-2}
Systemic vascular resistance[b]	900–1500 dyn s cm^{-5} (12–18 Wood units)
Systemic vascular resistance index[c]	1700–2600 dyn s cm^{-5} m^2 (20–32 Wood units m^2)
Pulmonary vascular resistance[d]	40–100 dyn s cm^{-5} (0.5–1.5 Wood units)
Pulmonary vascular resistance index[e]	70–180 dyn s cm^{-5} m^2 (0.8–2.3 Wood units m^2)

[a]$Ci = CO.BSA^{-1}$.
[b]$SVR = (BP - RAP).CO^{-1}$.
[c]$SVRI = (BP - RAP).Ci^{-1}$.
[d]$PVR = (PAP - PAOP).CO^{-1}$.
[e]$PVRI = (PAP - PAOP).Ci^{-1}$.
Abbreviations: Ci, cardiac index; CO, cardiac output; BSA, body surface area; SVR, systemic vascular resistance; BP, mean systemic blood pressure; RAP, mean right atrial pressure; SVRI, systemic vascular resistance index; PVR, pulmonary vascular resistance; PAP, mean pulmonary artery pressure; PAOP, mean pulmonary artery occlusion pressure; PVRI, pulmonary vascular resistance index.

Pulmonary artery occlusion pressure provides an estimate of left atrial pressure. Interpretation of the pulmonary artery occlusion pressure must be made with knowledge of potential sources of error and artifact. It is necessary to have a good understanding of the pathophysiological implications of the measurements. Pulmonary artery catheters can be used to measure cardiac output intermittently by the bolus thermodilution method. Modern catheters are available that measure and display cardiac output continuously and automatically. They are based on the thermodilution principle or on the rate of heat energy transfer from a heat exchanger on the catheter. The latest systems have a temporal resolution of tens of seconds. Some pulmonary artery catheters also incorporate an oximeter, which allows continuous monitoring of mixed venous oxygen saturation in the pulmonary artery. Some normal hemodynamic values are given in Table 10.1. Potential problems arising from pulmonary artery catheters include arrhythmias, catheter knotting, infection and pulmonary artery rupture. A more detailed discussion of the principles and intricacies of pulmonary artery catheter use can be found in recent reviews.[93,94]

Non-invasive cardiac output monitoring

Some of the controversies referred to above have led to a resurgence of interest in non-invasive measurement of cardiac output.[95] Currently, there are four techniques that can measure the cardiac output non-invasively:

1 Doppler ultrasound,[96]
2 partial CO_2 rebreathing,[97]
3 thoracic bioimpedance,[98]
4 pulse contour analysis.[99,100]

In addition to being non-invasive, the ideal cardiac output monitor should be accurate, reliable, continuous and convenient. Currently, no systems based on the above techniques have been shown to meet these criteria well enough to become widely adopted in clinical practice, although one pair of commentators has said of the PulseCO system of arterial waveform contour analysis (LiDCO Ltd, London, UK) that 'fully non-invasive cardiac output monitoring from arterial pressure could at last be in sight'.[101]

The Doppler principle also allows cardiac output measurement with transesophageal echocardiography (TEE). This has the advantage over simpler Doppler systems in allowing direct measurement of the cross-sectional area of the structure across which the flow is being measured (e.g. the aortic valve) rather than using a fixed estimated value in the calculation. Excellent agreement with cardiac output measured by thermodilution has been described.[102]

Transesophageal echocardiography

The American Society of Anesthesiologists and the Society of Cardiovascular Anesthesiologists Task Force on Transesophageal Echocardiography have produced guidelines for the use of TEE backed by category of evidence base.[103] While the routine use of TEE for the detection of myocardial ischemia is a category two indication, its use in evaluating the patient with severe hemodynamic upset is backed by category one evidence. TEE allows assessment of the dynamic anatomy of the heart. Its usefulness is dependent on the skill and experience of the operator, both in acquiring and, even more so, in interpreting the images. It can be used to assess global ventricular function (left and right), volume status, regional wall motion abnormality and valve function in quantifiable detail. It can be used to estimate cardiac output as described above. It is useful in the diagnosis of pericardial effusion and tamponade. TEE (in combination with epiaortic scanning) has a particular role in the detection of aortic atheroma.[104]

Neuromonitoring

Neurological monitoring may be undertaken for two reasons: to warn of actual or impending central nervous system damage, and to assess the adequacy of anesthesia.

With regard to the first indication, Edmonds, in a recent review,[105] suggested that neuromonitoring is infrequently employed because the general belief is that it 'only serves to document disaster, not prevent injury'. However, he suggests that the insight gained from continuous monitoring with, for example, transcranial Doppler can lead to the adoption of surgical and cardiopulmonary bypass techniques that may reduce the overall potential for injury. An 'emboli reduction programme', guided by transcranial Doppler monitoring, has been suggested as being at least partly responsible for one group's low (0.4%) incidence of new neurological deficit after coronary surgery.[106]

With regard to the second indication, there is considerable interest currently in the measurement of anesthesia-induced hypnosis, or 'depth of anesthesia'. Virtually all major manufacturers of anesthesia monitoring equipment are introducing devices for quantifying changes in cerebrocortical excitability. The two main surrogates of anesthesia-induced hypnosis are the auditory evoked potential,[107] and the bispectral index.[108] Both techniques are interesting, but have yet to prove their widespread practical worth. Neither technique has been comprehensively validated as a measure of the effects of different pharmacological methods of anesthesia on cognitive information processing.

INDUCTION OF ANESTHESIA

Choice of agents and techniques

There is currently no good evidence that the use of any single pharmacological recipe or specific technique to provide anesthesia results in superior outcomes for the patient in terms of mortality or overall morbidity. *How* the anesthetic drugs are used, in their moment-to-moment administration and combination, seems, in the current state of knowledge, as important as *which* drugs are used.

There is some limited evidence of discrete advantageous effects associated with particular drugs or techniques. Examples are the lower instance of supraventricular arrhythmias associated with the use of local anesthetics to provide anesthesia and continuing analgesia via thoracic epidural catheters,[32] and the possible direct cardioprotective action of anesthetic vapors such as isoflurane.[109]

Opioids are useful. They are not classified as anesthetic drugs because they do not reliably suppress conscious awareness, even at very high doses.[8] However, they are extremely effective at attenuating the acute autonomic responses to surgery with little direct cardiovascular depression (although some opioids such as morphine tend to cause hypotension by releasing histamine). The ultra-short-acting opioid remifentanil[110] has an effective half-life of less than 5 minutes, which allows very high concentrations to be used intraoperatively without post-operative respiratory depression. Such short-acting drugs can be used with particular flexibility and control when they are delivered by target-controlled infusion devices. Target-controlled infusion devices (e.g. the Diprifusor™) have an incorporated drug-specific pharmacokinetic model. Using this, they can automatically adjust infusion rate to maintain a target drug concentration in the plasma. After the pump has been programmed with the patient's details, a plasma drug concentration is specified and can be maintained or varied at will, with the infusion device continually and automatically making the appropriate adjustments to drug delivery rate.

Conduct of induction

Induction is a relatively hazardous time. The physiological state of the patient is changing rapidly over tens of seconds and there is great potential for things to go awry. Induction of anesthesia must take place in a quiet and relaxed environment. In the UK, many anesthetists prefer to use a separate anesthetic room for this reason. ECG monitoring and pulse oximetry must be in place, and

direct arterial blood pressure monitoring should be established under local anesthesia before general anesthesia is induced. Capnography should be available to confirm endotracheal tube placement.[80] The authors use target-controlled propofol infusion with fentanyl or remifentanil infusion, rather than bolus injections, for induction of anesthesia. This gives a gentle, controlled onset of anesthesia. Changes in blood pressure occur relatively gradually and predictably. Hypotension may be easily controlled with small doses of a vasopressor and fluid administration.

Occasionally, it may be necessary to anesthetize an emergency patient with incompletely controlled heart failure. These patients are likely to be dependent on a large intrinsic sympathetic drive to maintain their blood pressure. A low-dose infusion of epinephrine, or norepinephrine started at the same time as the propofol infusion and titrated appropriately, may be useful in avoiding precipitous hypotension, as this intrinsic drive is suppressed by the anesthetic. The epinephrine or norepinephrine can often be discontinued once surgical stimulation starts and the patient stabilizes in the new state.

Many anesthetists site central venous lines and pulmonary artery catheters after the patient is anesthetized, as this is more pleasant for the patient and provides the anesthetist with ideal conditions for the procedure. Some prefer to insert these lines under local anesthesia before induction, particularly in high-risk patients. The latter practice allows the anesthetist to concentrate completely on the patient's physiological responses once the anesthetic is underway without the distraction of what will occasionally turn out to be a difficult technical procedure.

Strict asepsis is important during the insertion of central lines. We do not routinely site pulmonary artery catheters at induction in low-risk patients with good or only mildly impaired ventricular function, but we have a low threshold for inserting them should problems develop at a later stage, after bypass or in the postoperative recovery area. We preferably use pulmonary artery catheters that measure and display cardiac output and mixed venous oxygen saturation continuously. Bladder catheterization for the drainage and measurement of urine is also undertaken with careful sterile and atraumatic technique at this time.

Intravenous antibiotic for prophylaxis against wound infection (e.g. a cephalosporin such as cefuroxime) should be given when the patient arrives for induction. Antibiotic prophylaxis is reviewed in the ACC/AHA guidelines for coronary artery bypass surgery.[47] Antibiotic prophylaxis is effective in substantially reducing the risk of postoperative infection,[111] but timing is important to achieve adequate tissue concentrations at the time of the skin incision. Incorporating antibiotic administration into the routine of anesthetic induction should avoid errors of omission and ensure the dose is administered within the optimal 30–60 minutes before the surgical skin incision.

MAINTENANCE OF ANESTHESIA

There still persists, mostly amongst non-anesthetists, a perception of anesthesia as an intrinsically dangerous state. In fact, the state of being anesthetized is generally a beneficial one for patients with coronary artery and other heart disease. Modern anesthesia is essentially the institution of intensive care. Metabolic demands are reduced by sedation and neuromuscular blockade. The work of breathing is removed. Cardiac afterload is reduced by arterial vasodilatation. Blood pressure is monitored continuously in real time with a resolution of less than one heartbeat. Vascular tone, cardiac preload, heart rate and, if necessary, cardiac inotropy may largely be manipulated separately and predictably by fluid administration and a range of well-understood drugs. These advantages may be particularly apparent in sicker patients with less physiological reserve. This perspective is important because it implies that, except in the case of specific difficulty, there is rarely an urgency to rush onto bypass after induction of anesthesia. The perceived danger of prolonging the anesthetic, for example, should not influence the decision about whether or not to use an internal mammary artery in a sick or elderly patient.[112]

The authors prefer to maintain anesthesia using a mixture of low-dose target-controlled propofol (continued from induction), isoflurane vapor (for its potential cardioprotective properties) and fentanyl or remifentanil. Hypertension in response to surgical stimulation can often be managed by increasing the concentration of anesthetic drugs or opioids, although vasodilators such as glyceryl trinitrate or sodium nitroprusside may sometimes be required in addition. β-Blockers, particularly esmolol, may be useful for controlling tachycardia. Esmolol is a relatively β-1-selective adrenergic antagonist with a short half-life, of about 9 minutes, which makes it easy and safe to titrate to effect.[113] Hypotension may require small doses of vasopressor and/or intravascular volume expansion with fluid transfusion (crystalloid or colloid) to counteract the venodilatation produced by the anesthetic agents. Note that excessive hemodilution will result in a low hematocrit after the start of cardiopulmonary bypass.

Vigilance should be maintained for new signs of myocardial ischemia such as ST-segment depression or ventricular wall motion abnormality if a TEE probe is in place. If new signs of ischemia appear, the underlying cause should be sought and addressed, for instance by raising perfusion pressure or decreasing heart rate or

excessive afterload. Glyceryl trinitrate may be useful as an effective coronary vasodilator.

Cardiopulmonary bypass

The purpose of cardiopulmonary bypass in coronary artery surgery is to allow physical manipulation of the heart without compromising the circulation and to provide a still, potentially bloodless field for fashioning the distal anastomoses. During bypass, support of the systemic circulation is taken over by the bypass machine. Blood leaves the venous side of the circulation (usually from the right atrium or venae cavae) to enter a reservoir in the bypass machine. It is then pumped through a heat exchanger, through a gas exchanger where it is oxygenated and carbon dioxide diffuses out, and back into the arterial side of the circulation (usually into the ascending aorta). While the distal anastomoses are being performed, the coronary arteries may be isolated from the systemic circulation by an occluding clamp across the ascending aorta between the heart and the inflow from the pump. This will also prevent blood flow through the left heart chambers and therefore through the right heart and pulmonary circulation.

During bypass, the perfusionist may control the rate of blood flow into the patient via the arterial pump, the rate of venous drainage from the patient, the temperature of the blood, the composition and flow rate of the fresh gas flow to the oxygenator, and the degree of suction on additional drainage lines from the patient. In addition, drugs and fluids may be added to the blood in the venous pump reservoir.

Recommendations have been made for minimal standards of monitoring and alarms to be used during cardiopulmonary bypass.[114] These include the statement that 'Safe conduct of cardiopulmonary bypass is a joint responsibility of surgeons, anesthetists and clinical perfusionists and requires a high level of communication between the team members'.[114] In the UK, it has been recommended that a suitably qualified anesthetist be present in the operating room at all times during cardiopulmonary bypass.[80,114] During bypass, blood gas (oxygen and carbon dioxide) partial pressures, serum potassium concentration, acid–base status and hemoglobin or hematocrit must be measured at regular intervals (approximately every 15 minutes, according to local protocol). Guidelines for the conduct of cardiopulmonary bypass have been published by the American Society of Extra-Corporeal Technology.[115]

Before cannulation for cardiopulmonary bypass, the patient must be adequately anticoagulated with heparin. A protocol should be in place to ensure that cardiopulmonary bypass is not commenced until the patient is adequately heparinized. An initial dose of $3\,\mathrm{mg\,kg^{-1}}$

(1 mg = 100 units) will usually raise the activated clotting time (ACT) above 480 seconds. If not, further heparin is given until the ACT is above this time. The ACT should be maintained above 480 seconds by giving further heparin as required. In our institution, the pump-priming solution contains an additional 80 mg (8000 units) of heparin, which provides a safeguard against a drop in heparin concentration as a result of hemodilution at the start of bypass and against falling heparin concentration should there be a delay between giving the heparin and starting bypass.

Continued anesthesia during cardiopulmonary bypass may be provided by continuous intravenous infusion of anesthetic drugs (e.g. propofol) or by anesthetic vapors such as isoflurane in the oxygenator fresh gas flow, in addition to other agents such as opioids and benzodiazepines. Cardiovascular signs of anesthetic adequacy are lost when on bypass, and it is important to ensure that plasma concentrations of anesthetic drugs remain high enough to prevent awareness. The authors use concentrations of anesthetic agents during bypass similar to those that were found to be adequate in the pre-bypass period. Note that the plasma concentrations of some drugs such as fentanyl are markedly reduced by cardiopulmonary bypass, and supplementation will be necessary to achieve plasma concentrations similar to those existing before bypass.[116]

A detailed consideration of the many issues concerning the conduct and effects of cardiopulmonary bypass is well beyond the scope of this chapter, but it is worth addressing briefly some important points.

A range of acceptable target values for some important variables is given in Table 10.2.

During cardiopulmonary bypass, the patient may be cooled, usually to between 28 °C and 32 °C, as a partial safeguard against inadequate or unphysiological perfusion of vital organs, especially the brain. The overall advantages of cooling are not clear cut and are the subject of current debate (see, e.g., Arrowsmith and colleagues[117]). The current trend is towards only mild hypothermia (32 °C).

In the past there has been a debate as to the correct method of maintaining acid–base balance during hypothermic bypass. Carbon dioxide is more soluble in cold blood. This means that the partial pressure of carbon dioxide ($PaCO_2$ – a measure of the gas's tendency to escape from solution) is lower for a given molecular concentration of the gas. Similarly, water is less dissociated at lower temperatures, so the hydrogen ion concentration that represents acid–base neutrality is lower. To maintain unchanging values of $PaCO_2$ and hydrogen ion concentration, or pH, as the patient's blood cools, the concentration of CO_2 must be increased (by adding CO_2 to the oxygenator fresh gas flow). The CO_2 acidifies the blood according to the Henderson–Hasselbalch

Table 10.2 *Indicative normal values during cardiopulmonary bypass*

Pump flow rate	
37 °C	2.4 × BSA L min^{-1}
30 °C	1.8 × BSA L min^{-1}
25 °C	1.2 × BSA L min^{-1}
PaO_2	13.6–25 kPa
SVO_2	>60%
$PaCO_2$	4.7–6.0 kPa
Potassium concentration	4.0–6.0 mmol L^{-1}
Hydrogen ion concentration	35–45 nmol L^{-1}
ACT	>480 s
Perfusion pressure	50–80 mmHg
Hemoglobin concentration	70–100 g L^{-1}

BSA, body surface area (m^2) = height (cm)$^{0.725}$ × weight (kg)$^{0.429}$ × 71.84 × 10^{-4}.
Abbreviations: PaO_2, inline or systemic partial pressure arterial oxygen; $PaCO_2$, systemic arterial partial pressure carbon dioxide; SVO_2, inline mixed venous oxygen saturation; ACT, activated clotting time; perfusion pressure = mean arterial pressure − central venous pressure.

equation, which holds true at different temperatures. This is called pH-stat management.

It is now clear, in the cold patient, that the physiological effects of CO_2 such as cerebral vasodilatation are related to the molecular concentration of the gas, not to the partial pressure. Furthermore, there are good theoretical reasons for maintaining a normal acid–base balance (rather than an unchanged hydrogen ion concentration). Normal molecular concentration of CO_2 and normal acid–base balance may be achieved by adjusting CO_2 such that the $PaCO_2$ and pH are normal when the sample is measured at 37 °C, irrespective of the temperature of the patient. This is called alpha-stat management (from constant protonation of alpha-imidazole buffering groups). Alpha-stat acid–base management is the appropriate acid–base management strategy unless it is deliberately intended to cause hypercarbia. (Hypercarbia may be beneficial, for instance, before total circulatory arrest in children.[118])

Cardiopulmonary bypass necessitates significant hemodilution because of the additional volume of the artificial circuit. Unless red cells are added, this produces acute anemia without blood loss. We aim to keep the blood hemoglobin concentration above 70 g L^{-1} (equivalent to a hematocrit of about 21%) by adding concentrated red blood cells if necessary. A recent retrospective observational study of 6980 consecutive coronary graft patients showed a linear increase in in-hospital mortality as the lowest on-pump hematocrit fell below 23%,[119] with a doubling of mortality associated with hematocrits below 19%. Although the association is not necessarily causal, it seems prudent to avoid very low hematocrits.

Table 10.3 *Typical pump prime as used at the authors' institution*

Heparin	8000 units
Potassium chloride	15 mmol
Sodium bicarbonate	50 mmol
Mannitol	10 g
Cefuroxime[a]	750 mg
Aprotinin[b]	2 million units
Hartmann's solution	To a total prime volume of 1800 mL

[a]Erythromycin 1 g substituted if known sensitivity to cefuroxime.
[b]Optional.

The constituents of our normal pump prime are given in Table 10.3.

Cardiopulmonary bypass causes a clinically important deficit in hemostasis. This occurs secondary to complex effects on the coagulation cascade, increased fibrinolysis and a qualititative and quantitative platelet deficit.[120] Inextricably bound up with the effects on hemostasis is the initiation of a systemic inflammatory response and then, in the hours and days after bypass, a prothrombotic state.[121] For most patients, these changes have only minor clinical importance, but for a substantial minority they lead to significant organ complications and occasionally even death. Effective pharmacological prophylaxis against the effects of bypass on hemostasis is possible with antifibrinolytic agents such as aprotinin and tranexamic acid.[122]

Aprotinin, a serine protease inhibitor, has a wide spectrum of effects in addition to plasmin inhibition. It helps to preserve platelet function during cardiopulmonary bypass and at higher concentrations has anti-inflammatory effects, which may be beneficial. Many surgeons and anesthetists (including ourselves) now use such agents routinely, but there is still concern about potential adverse side effects such as vein graft thrombosis and anaphylactoid reactions. It is a moderately expensive drug. A single dose of aprotinin of 2 million kallikrein inhibitor units, added to the pump prime before the extracorporeal circuit is connected to the patient, is effective in reducing postoperative blood loss and decreasing exposure to allogenic blood.[123] It is financially efficient, even in straightforward 'low-risk' patients. There is no convincing evidence that the practice has any deleterious effects on postoperative cardiac outcomes.

The authors have adopted a policy of using 'pump-prime' aprotinin for routine, low-risk patients in whom there is no contraindication (known aprotinin sensitivity or previous exposure within 6 months[124]), and 'full-dose' aprotinin for patients who are either at high risk of excessive bleeding or whose general condition is so compromised that bleeding complications might have important

direct adverse effects on outcome. 'Full-dose' aprotinin comprises a 2 million unit loading dose, a continuous infusion of 0.5 million units per hour throughout surgery, and 2 million units in the pump-prime fluid. Recent national Scottish guidelines on perioperative blood transfusion recommend that prophylactic 'full-dose' aprotinin or tranexamic acid should be given to patients undergoing cardiac surgery that carries a high risk of transfusion, including repeat cardiac operations and patients on preoperative aspirin up to the time of surgery.[125] However, they do not recommend aprotinin for low-risk primary coronary artery surgery.

If aprotinin is used, it is important to use a kaolin-based ACT rather than one with celite activator, as aprotinin artifactually prolongs celite-activated clotting times, and inadequate heparinization may ensue.

Separation from bypass

After completion of graft anastomoses, the patient can be weaned from the bypass machine. The patient should be normothermic, have a normal hydrogen ion concentration and a potassium concentration in the upper part of the normal range. The heart must be beating, ideally in sinus rhythm. DC shock should be used to try to convert new atrial fibrillation or flutter. Very slow heart rates (less than about 60 beats min^{-1}) may allow the heart to distend unduly and be a cause of hypotension. Either epicardial pacing or an isoprenaline infusion can be used to increase the heart rate. Dual chamber (atrioventricular) pacing gives flexibility and allows preservation of the atrial contribution to ventricular filling. This may be particularly useful if the left ventricle is hypertrophied, as it may have reduced compliance after bypass. The lungs should be gently expanded and ventilation commenced.

The importance of good communication at this time between surgeon, anesthetist and perfusionist cannot be overstated. Each must know exactly what the others are doing and what role each expects the others to play. Separation from bypass involves gently decreasing forward flow from the pump while optimizing intravascular volume. It is particularly important not to let the heart become over-distended by over-filling at this time and in the vulnerable minutes after bypass. In our practice, this initial process is orchestrated by the surgeon, who must be aware of any drugs the patient is given by the anesthetist. In some institutions, this process will be managed by the anesthetist. The important thing is clarity about who is doing what.

Pharmacological support of the heart and circulation may be necessary during and immediately following separation from bypass. The heart at this time may be suffering a degree of functional contractile impairment as a result of ischemia and reperfusion. In addition, there may be a background of systemic vasodilatation due to the inflammatory endothelial activation engendered by the cardiopulmonary bypass process. As is a common theme, good studies showing the effect of different strategies on important clinically relevant endpoints are lacking. However, there is much known that is useful and it is important to take a rational approach.

In the majority of patients with some mild cardiac stunning and mild to moderate circulatory dysfunction, it is probably not important which drugs are chosen to achieve the desired goals, although the worse the cardio-circulatory dysfunction, the less the margin for error. Blood pressure must be raised to the level at which cardiac perfusion is not compromised, and cardiac output must be adequate to support the other organs. It is important to avoid a vicious circle of increasingly inadequate cardiac performance secondary to inadequate cardiac perfusion. In our practice, low doses of dopamine (1–$8\,\mu g\,kg^{-1}\,min^{-1}$) or epinephrine (starting at about $0.03\,\mu g\,kg^{-1}\,min^{-1}$) and/or vasopressors (e.g. small boluses of metaraminol) are commonly employed. If the problem is clearly predominantly peripheral vasodilatation, a norepinephrine infusion (starting at about $0.03\,\mu g\,kg^{-1}\,min^{-1}$ and adjusted appropriately) is the drug of choice. Excessive systemic resistance, however, increases cardiac work, shifts the balance towards cardiac (particularly endocardial) ischemia and may be the limiting factor in an inadequate cardiac output. Attention to detail, anticipation and early intervention are important.

With good myocardial protection and satisfactory revascularization, many patients will separate from the pump and rapidly achieve a good circulation, given careful attention to intravascular filling, without the need for any specific pharmacological intervention.

Once hemodynamic stability has been secured, residual heparin is neutralized with enough protamine to return the ACT to the normal control value. One milligram of protamine will neutralize 1 mg (100 units) of heparin. Protamine should be injected slowly over several minutes to prevent or minimize hypotension as a result of peripheral vasodilatation. Rarely, it may cause a rise in pulmonary vascular resistance.

Beating-heart surgery

Coronary artery surgery may be performed without the use of cardiopulmonary bypass, thereby avoiding the complications associated with its use. In 'off-pump' surgery, the heart must continue to support the circulation during the operation. Compromise to cardiac function arises from two sources.

1 Native coronary blood flow is compromised in the vessel being operated on whilst the anastomosis is being performed: this may be minimized by the use of intracoronary shunts.
2 Physical manipulation of the heart is required to gain access, particularly for grafts to the circumflex artery: hemodynamic instability arises from physical distortion of the cardiac chambers, ischemia and arrhythmias.

There is no clear consensus on optimal monitoring during off-pump surgery.[126] Clearly, direct arterial pressure monitoring is crucial. Pulmonary artery catheterization is not mandatory. A pulmonary artery catheter with the capacity for continuous mixed venous oxygen saturation, however, will provide a rapidly responsive proxy measure of cardiac output. Direct continuous cardiac output measurement based on continuous thermodilution has too slow a response time to be useful. Maintained mixed venous oxygen saturation is reassuring in the face of a decreased arterial pressure. Conversely, a decrease in mixed venous oxygen saturation, particularly in conjunction with hypotension, provides an early indication that all is not well. Transesophageal echo may provide useful information. Mid-esophageal views can be obtained even when the heart is lifted from the pericardial cavity for circumflex grafting. Transient regional wall abnormalities during surgery are very common, but new abnormalities that persist at the end of surgery suggest inadequate revascularization.

Hemodynamic problems may be minimized by lifting the heart in stages, with small rests for recovery in between. Right heart outflow obstruction is the main factor causing reduced cardiac output when the heart is lifted for circumflex grafting. This may be partially compensated for by increasing right heart filling. Head-down tilt, fluid transfusion and small doses of vasopressor, such as metaraminol or phenylephrine, may all therefore be helpful. Occasionally an inotrope may be necessary.

Particular care is required to minimize heat loss, as these patients cannot be rewarmed in the absence of an extracorporeal circuit with heat exchanger. Techniques for mimimizing heat loss have been described.[127]

If good surgical conditions cannot be maintained, or serious hemodynamic instability occurs and cannot be immediately corrected, it may be necessary to institute cardiopulmonary bypass. We prefer to have patients fully heparinized for off-pump surgery, as this allows prompt institution of cardiopulmonary bypass. Lesser degrees of heparinization (to an activated clotting time of >250 seconds) are acceptable, although in this case further heparinization will be necessary if cardiopulmonary bypass is required. In addition to its relevance for cardiopulmonary bypass, systemic heparinization is prophylactic against thrombus formation should coronary flow be occluded or compromised during grafting. Full cardiopulmonary bypass facilities must be standing by and available during off-pump surgery.

TRANSFER TO THE INTENSIVE CARE AREA: THE IMMEDIATE POSTOPERATIVE PERIOD

There should be a seamless continuance of care between the end of the operation in the operating room and the early postoperative period in the intensive care or recovery unit. The patient must be stable before being moved from the operating theatre. Monitoring must be continuous.

The first few hours after surgery are a key time in patient management. Developing problems must be identified early and appropriate interventions made. Arterial blood gas tension, acid–base status, concentration of blood hemoglobin and glucose, and serum potassium should be measured when the patient enters the postoperative care area and then re-measured as clinically indicated. A chest x-ray at this time will confirm the correct placement of the endotracheal tube, central lines and drains, normal lung expansion, and the absence of significant pleural effusions, and is useful for comparison if the patient's condition deteriorates later.

Arterial blood pressure, CVP, electrocardiogram, pulse oximetry, temperature, urine output and mediastinal/pleural drainage should be monitored continuously. Cardiac output and/or mixed venous oxygen saturation may or may not be measured directly in routine cases, but the adequacy of the cardiac output must always be constantly assessed. This requires integrating information from urine output measurements, core and peripheral temperature measurements and their rate of change, clinical examination of peripheral perfusion, and acid–base status. Low cardiac output causes cold ($<30\,^\circ$C), pale, mottled or cyanosed peripheries with poor capillary refill, associated with failure to re-warm (normally $0.5–1\,^\circ$C per hour), acidosis and oliguria. Blood pressure alone is a poor guide to cardiac output.

In recent years there has been a move away from a prolonged period of mechanical ventilation after cardiac surgery. The policy of deliberately aiming to extubate patients within 4 hours or so after the end of surgery has become known as 'fast tracking'. Whether or not there is a formal policy of fast tracking, the aim should be to keep each patient intubated for only as long as they continue to derive therapeutic benefit. This judgment is made easier by a precise understanding of exactly what therapeutic support endotracheal intubation and positive pressure ventilation provide. There are five elements associated with the process:

1 the ability reliably to deliver a known high concentration of oxygen,
2 maintenance of a clear protected airway,
3 the ability to provide some or all of the mechanical work of breathing,
4 the ability to compensate for absent or diminished respiratory drive,
5 the ability to maintain PEEP.

A requirement for any or all of these elements may exist in the early postoperative period. Modern ventilators allow the different elements to be separated, for instance pressure-support ventilation allows patients to set their own respiratory rate and the proportion of breathing work contributed by the machine may be adjusted by varying the support pressure.

Patients are likely to have a depressed respiratory drive for a time after surgery, depending on the amount of opioid they have received. Similarly, they will probably have a depressed level of consciousness, with impaired ability to maintain and protect their airway. With modern anesthetic drugs and techniques, it is possible to reduce this time to as short as a few minutes after the end of surgery. In practice, unless there is a deliberate policy to achieve such a rapid wake-up time as part of an aggressive fast-tracking protocol, this phase may last up to several hours.

If patients have been cooled on bypass, they are likely to be hypothermic immediately postoperatively. Poorly perfused tissues such as fat are usually not re-warmed fully by the end of bypass, causing an 'after drop' in body temperature as heat slowly redistributes. Patients should continue with positive pressure ventilation until they have completed re-warming. This is because the physiological response to reduced core temperature is shivering. Anesthetic drugs prevent shivering, but as the concentration of anesthetic drugs falls, hypothalamic mechanisms recover, first increasing muscle tone, then switching on vigorous shivering. The increased respiratory work of performing the extra gas exchange associated with this additional metabolic load may be considerable, particularly if the lungs are stiff. In turn, this increased respiratory work imposes a considerable extra cardiac burden in addition to the relatively huge workload directly associated with servicing the shivering muscles. To compound the insult further, the hypothalamic set point – the temperature the hypothalamus regards as 'normal' – may be raised postoperatively because of inflammatory processes triggered by cardiopulmonary bypass, causing the hypothalamus to drive the body into a temporary pyrexia. Metabolic acidosis and hypoxemia may ensue. Relieving a substantial part of the work of breathing during postoperative re-warming will mitigate the effects of shivering.

Shivering may also be decreased or abolished with boluses of intravenous pethidine (25 mg)[128] or by increasing continuous sedation with propofol back towards anesthetic levels. Muscle relaxants are an effective treatment. However, the possibility of psychological morbidity associated with awareness under anesthesia must be remembered. Muscle relaxants must never be given to a patient who may be conscious or is likely to become conscious while the muscle relaxant is still acting.

Gas exchange is likely to be impaired postoperatively as a result of atelectasis and raised lung water secondary to inflammatory endothelial injury or raised left heart filling pressures.

Once patients are warm, adequately oxygenated (arterial oxygen saturation 95% or above on an inspired oxygen concentration of 50% or less), breathing comfortably with minimal mechanical support, with a stable arterial carbon dioxide concentration in the normal range or only slightly elevated, and awake enough to maintain their airway, the endotracheal tube may be removed. Our routine is to establish patients on pressure support ventilation as soon as they regain an adequate respiratory drive, while maintaining mechanical support until they are fully re-warmed. Ongoing sedation, usually with continuous propofol infusion, is used if necessary during re-warming. The endotracheal tube should not be removed if there is a significant likelihood of the patient requiring early re-thoracotomy, for example because of ongoing bleeding.

Careful attention must be paid to intravascular fluid balance during the first postoperative hours. The commonest cause of hypotension in this period is relative hypovolemia. There is an increase in venous capacity associated with re-warming. At the same time, the patient is likely to be undergoing a brisk diuresis, particularly if the osmotic diuretic mannitol has been added to the pump-prime. There will probably be an ongoing loss of fluid from the intravascular to the extravascular space as a result of capillary leak caused by the inflammatory endothelial injury. Finally, there may be significant ongoing blood loss.

The need for substantial cardiovascular support, even the presence of an intraortic balloon pump, is not an absolute indication for maintaining endotracheal intubation. However, the work of breathing, which may be substantial, and the extra cardiac workload associated with it, is an important consideration in such circumstances. Furthermore, if there is any suggestion of delirium or restlessness, it may be necessary to keep such a patient unconscious.

Good pain relief is vital. Pain retards deep breathing and coughing, which are key factors in returning the lungs to normal and preventing further respiratory complications. It inhibits general mobilization and makes patients miserable. The principles of good postoperative pain relief are well established. They include regular (and therefore preventative) analgesia, a proactive approach by nursing staff to seek out inadequate analgesia, and a graded step-down approach as analgesic requirements diminish. These must be incorporated into a formal protocol. After the first few hours during which intravenous morphine is given as required, we move to a protocol that allows for frequent doses of subcutaneous morphine on a background of regular oral paracetamol. Additional regular non-steroidal anti-inflammatory analgesics (such as diclofenac sodium) are useful if there are no contraindications such as peptic ulceration or renal impairment. It is particularly important to be wary of acute postoperative renal impairment if non-steroidal analgesics are used.

In summary, anesthetic management is an integral part of preoperative assessment, the revascularization process itself, and the recovery phase. Recent changes in surgical techniques have necessitated modifications in some aspects of anesthetic technique,[127,129,130] and similarly advances in perioperative monitoring and anesthesia have enabled coronary surgery to be successfully undertaken in the elderly or those with advanced disease or morbidity, emphasizing the interdependence of surgery and anesthesia in the management of coronary artery disease.

KEY REFERENCES

Marino P. *The ICU Book*, 2nd edn. Philadelphia: Lippincott Williams & Wilkins, 1997.
A useful, practical handbook of intensive care. A single-author text strong on pathophysiological principles. It is aimed at the general intensivist but has considerable relevance to many aspects of the perioperative and postoperative care of cardiac surgical patients.

Reich DL, Konstadt SN, Kaplan JA (eds). *Cardiac Anesthesia*, 4th edn. Philadelphia: W.B. Saunders, 1999.
An authoritative and detailed account of cardiac anesthesia and perioperative care. A good reference book.

Thomas SJ (ed.). *Manual of Cardiac Anesthesia*, 3rd edn. New York: Churchill Livingstone, 2002.
A useful, succinct, physiologically based introduction.

REFERENCES

1. Antkowiak B. How do general anaesthetics work? *Naturwissenschaften* 2001; **88**:201–13.
2. Collins JG, Kendig JJ, Mason P. Anesthetic actions within the spinal cord: contributions to the state of general anesthesia. *Trends Neurosci* 1995; **18**:549–53.
3. Lennmarken C, Bildfors K, Enlund G, Samuelsson P, Sandin R. Victims of awareness. *Acta Anaesthesiol Scand* 2002; **46**:229–31.
4. Blacher RS. On awakening paralyzed during surgery. A syndrome of traumatic neurosis. *JAMA* 1975; **234**:67–8.
5. Ghoneim MM, Block RI. Learning and memory during general anesthesia: an update. *Anesthesiology* 1997; **87**:387–410.
6. Phillips AA, McLean RF, Devitt JH, Harrington EM. Recall of intraoperative events after general anaesthesia and cardiopulmonary bypass. *Can J Anaesth* 1993; **40**:922–6.

7. Ranta S, Jussila J, Hynynen M. Recall of awareness during cardiac anaesthesia: influence of feedback information to the anaesthesiologist. *Acta Anaesthesiol Scand* 1996; **40**:554–60.

8. Goldman L, Shah MV, Hebden MW. Memory of cardiac anaesthesia. Psychological sequelae in cardiac patients of intra-operative suggestion and operating room conversation. *Anaesthesia* 1987; **42**:596–603.

9. Dowd NP, Cheng DC, Karski JM, Wong DT, Munro JA, Sandler AN. Intraoperative awareness in fast-track cardiac anesthesia. *Anesthesiology* 1998; **89**:1068–73.

10. Thourani VH, Weintraub WS, Stein B, Gebhart SS, Craver JM, Jones EL, *et al.* Influence of diabetes mellitus on early and late outcome after coronary artery bypass grafting. *Ann Thorac Surg* 1999; **67**:1045–52.

11. Herlitz J, Wognsen GB, Karlson BW, Sjoland H, Karlsson T, Caidahl K, *et al.* Mortality, mode of death and risk indicators for death during 5 years after coronary artery bypass grafting among patients with and without a history of diabetes mellitus. *Coron Artery Dis* 2000; **11**:339–46.

12. Hosoda Y, Yamamoto T, Takazawa K, Yamasaki M, Yamamoto S, Hayashi I, *et al.* Coronary artery bypass grafting in patients on chronic hemodialysis: surgical outcome in diabetic nephropathy versus nondiabetic nephropathy patients. *Ann Thorac Surg* 2001; **71**:543–8.

13. Jones RH, Hannan EL, Hammermeister KE, Delong ER, O'Connor GT, Luepker RV, *et al.* Identification of preoperative variables needed for risk adjustment of short-term mortality after coronary artery bypass graft surgery. The Working Group Panel on the Cooperative CABG Database Project. *J Am Coll Cardiol* 1996; **28**:1478–87.

14. Almassi GH, Warltier D. Oral hypoglycemic agents in coronary artery bypass grafting. *Ann Thorac Surg* 2001; **71**:2086.

15. Trick WE, Scheckler WE, Tokars JI, Jones KC, Reppen ML, Smith EM, *et al.* Modifiable risk factors associated with deep sternal site infection after coronary artery bypass grafting. *J Thorac Cardiovasc Surg* 2000; **119**:108–14.

16. Roach GW, Kanchuger M, Mangano CM, Newman M, Nussmeier N, Wolman R, *et al.* Adverse cerebral outcomes after coronary bypass surgery. Multicenter Study of Perioperative Ischemia Research Group and the Ischemia Research and Education Foundation Investigators. *N Engl J Med* 1996; **335**:1857–63.

17. Furnary AP, Zerr KJ, Grunkemeier GL, Starr A. Continuous insulin infusion reduces the incidence of deep sternal wound infection in diabetic patients after cardiac surgical procedures. *Ann Thorac Surg* 1999; **67**:352–60.

18. Malmberg K. Prospective randomised study of intensive insulin treatment on long term survival after acute myocardial infarction in patients with diabetes mellitus. *BMJ* 1997; **314**:1512–15.

19. Garratt KN, Brady PA, Hassinger NL, Grill DE, Terzic A, Holmes DR Jr. Sulfonylurea drugs increase early mortality in patients with diabetes mellitus after direct angioplasty for acute myocardial infarction. *J Am Coll Cardiol* 1999; **33**:119–24.

20. O'Keefe JH, Blackstone EH, Sergeant P, McCallister BD. The optimal mode of coronary revascularization for diabetics. A risk-adjusted long-term study comparing coronary angioplasty and coronary bypass surgery. *Eur Heart J* 1998; **19**:1696–703.

21. Tomai F, Crea F, Gaspardone A, Versaci F, De Paulis R, Penta DP, *et al.* Ischemic preconditioning during coronary angioplasty is prevented by glibenclamide, a selective ATP-sensitive K$^+$ channel blocker. *Circulation* 1994; **90**:700–5.

22. Van den Berghe G, Wouters P, Weekers F, Verwaest C, Bruyninckx F, Schetz M, *et al.* Intensive insulin therapy in critically ill patients. *N Engl J Med* 2001; **345**:1359–418.

23. Sonksen P, Sonksen J. Insulin: understanding its action in health and disease. *Br J Anaesth* 2000; **85**:69–79.

24. Ljungqvist O, Thorell A, Gutniak M, Haggmark T, Efendic S. Glucose infusion instead of preoperative fasting reduces post-operative insulin resistance. *J Am Coll Surg* 1994; **178**:329–36.

25. Lazar HL, Chipkin S, Philippides G, Bao Y, Apstein C. Glucose–insulin–potassium solutions improve outcomes in diabetics who have coronary artery operations. *Ann Thorac Surg* 2000; **70**:1445–50.

26. Mannino DM. COPD: epidemiology, prevalence, morbidity and mortality, and disease heterogeneity. [Review – 41 refs]. *Chest* 2002; **121**:121–6S.

27. NHLBI/WHO Workshop Report. Global strategy for the diagnosis, management and prevention of chronic obstructive pulmonary disease. www.goldcopd.com: 2002.

28. Cohen A, Katz M, Katz R, Hauptman E, Schachner A. Chronic obstructive pulmonary disease in patients undergoing coronary artery bypass grafting. *J Thorac Cardiovasc Surg* 1995; **109**:574–81.

29. Canver CC, Nichols RD, Kroncke GM. Influence of age-specific lung function on survival after coronary bypass. *Ann Thorac Surg* 1998; **66**:144–7.

30. Thompson MJ, Elton RA, Mankad PA, Campanella C, Walker WS, Sang CT, *et al.* Prediction of requirement for, and outcome of, prolonged mechanical ventilation following cardiac surgery. *Cardiovasc Surg* 1997; **5**:376–81.

31. Grover FL, Hammermeister KE, Burchfiel C. Initial report of the Veterans Administration Preoperative Risk Assessment Study for Cardiac Surgery. *Ann Thorac Surg* 1990; **50**:12–26.

32. Scott NB, Turfrey DJ, Ray DA, Nzewi O, Sutcliffe NP, Lal AB, *et al.* A prospective randomized study of the potential benefits of thoracic epidural anesthesia and analgesia in patients undergoing coronary artery bypass grafting. *Anesthes Analg* 2001; **93**:528–35.

33. Warner MA, Offord KP, Warner ME, Lennon RL, Conover MA, Jansson-Schumacher U. Role of preoperative cessation of smoking and other factors in postoperative pulmonary complications: a blinded prospective study of coronary artery bypass patients. *Mayo Clin Proc* 1989; **64**:609–16.

34. Akrawi W, Benumof JL. A pathophysiological basis for informed preoperative smoking cessation counseling. *J Cardiothorac Vasc Anesthes* 1997; **11**:629–40.

35. Schwartz LB, Bridgman AH, Kieffer RW, Wilcox RA, McCann RL, Tawil MP, *et al.* Asymptomatic carotid artery stenosis and stroke in patients undergoing cardiopulmonary bypass. *J Vasc Surg* 1995; **21**:146–53.

36. Berens ES, Kouchoukos NT, Murphy SF, Wareing TH. Preoperative carotid artery screening in elderly patients undergoing cardiac surgery. *J Vasc Surg* 1992; **15**:313–21.

37. Faggioli GL, Curl GR, Ricotta JJ. The role of carotid screening before coronary artery bypass. *J Vasc Surg* 1990; **12**:724–9.

38. Salasidis GC, Latter DA, Steinmetz OK, Blair JF, Graham AM. Carotid artery duplex scanning in preoperative assessment for coronary artery revascularization: the association between peripheral vascular disease, carotid artery stenosis, and stroke. *J Vasc Surg* 1995; **21**:154–60.

39. Biller J, Feinberg WM, Castaldo JE, Whittemore AD, Harbaugh RE, Dempsey RJ, *et al.* Guidelines for carotid endarterectomy: a statement for healthcare professionals from a Special Writing Group of the Stroke Council, American Heart Association. [Review – 79 refs]. *Circulation* 1998; **97**:501–9.

40. Moore WS, Barnett HJ, Beebe HG, Bernstein EF, Brener BJ, Brott T, *et al.* Guidelines for carotid endarterectomy. A multidisciplinary consensus statement from the ad hoc Committee, American Heart Association. [Review – 174 refs]. *Stroke* 1995; **26**:188–201.

41. Sacco RL. Clinical practice. Extracranial carotid stenosis. *N Engl J Med* 2001; **345**:1113–18.

42. Hertzer NR, Arison R. Cumulative stroke and survival ten years after carotid endarterectomy. *J Vasc Surg* 1985; **2**:661–8.

43. Hertzer NR, Lees CD. Fatal myocardial infarction following carotid endarterectomy: three hundred and thirty-five patients followed 6–11 years after operation. *Ann Surg* 1981; **194**:212–18.

44. Ennix CLJ, Lawrie GM, Morris GCJ, Crawford ES, Howell JF, Reardon MJ, *et al.* Improved results of carotid endarterectomy in patients with symptomatic coronary disease: an analysis of 1,546 consecutive carotid operations. *Stroke* 1979; **10**:122–5.

45. Antunes PE, Anacleto G, de Oliveira JM, Eugenio L, Antunes MJ. Staged carotid and coronary surgery for concomitant carotid and coronary artery disease. *Eur J Cardiothorac Surg* 2002; **21**:181–6.

46. Zacharias A, Schwann TA, Riordan CJ, Clark PM, Martinez B, Durham SJ, *et al.* Operative and 5-year outcomes of combined carotid and coronary revascularization: review of a large contemporary experience. *Ann Thorac Surg* 2002; **73**:491–7.

47. Eagle KA, Guyton RA, Davidoff R, Ewy GA, Fonger J, Gardner TJ, *et al.* ACC/AHA Guidelines for Coronary Artery Bypass Graft Surgery: a report of the American College of Cardiology/American Heart Association Task Force on Practice Guidelines (Committee to Revise the 1991 Guidelines for Coronary Artery Bypass Graft Surgery). American College of Cardiology/American Heart Association. *J Am Coll Cardiol* 1999; **34**:1262–347.

48. Hertzer NR, Loop FD, Beven EG, O'Hara PJ, Krajewski LP. Surgical staging for simultaneous coronary and carotid disease: a study including prospective randomization. *J Vasc Surg* 1989; **9**:455–63.

49. Eagle KA, Rihal CS, Mickel MC, Holmes DR, Foster ED, Gersh BJ. Cardiac risk of noncardiac surgery: influence of coronary disease and type of surgery in 3368 operations. CASS Investigators and University of Michigan Heart Care Program. Coronary Artery Surgery Study. *Circulation* 1997; **96**:1882–7.

50. Lee TH, Marcantonio ER, Mangione CM, Thomas EJ, Polanczyk CA, Cook EF, *et al.* Derivation and prospective validation of a simple index for prediction of cardiac risk of major noncardiac surgery. *Circulation* 1999; **100**:1043–9.

51. Mangano CM, Diamondstone LS, Ramsay JG, Aggarwal A, Herskowitz A, Mangano DT. Renal dysfunction after myocardial revascularization: risk factors, adverse outcomes, and hospital resource utilization. The Multicenter Study of Perioperative Ischemia Research Group. *Ann Intern Med* 1998; **128**:194–203.

52. Chertow GM, Lazarus JM, Christiansen CL, Cook EF, Hammermeister KE, Grover F, *et al.* Preoperative renal risk stratification. *Circulation* 1997; **95**:878–84.

53. Weerasinghe A, Hornick P, Smith P, Taylor K, Ratnatunga C. Coronary artery bypass grafting in non-dialysis-dependent mild-to-moderate renal dysfunction. *J Thorac Cardiovasc Surg* 2001; **121**:1083–9.

54. Anderson RJ, O'Brien M, MaWhinney S, VillaNueva CB, Moritz TE, Sethi GK, *et al.* Renal failure predisposes patients to adverse outcome after coronary artery bypass surgery. VA Cooperative Study #5. *Kidney Int* 1999; **55**:1057–62.

55. Sethi GK, Copeland JG, Goldman S, Moritz T, Zadina K, Henderson WG. Implications of preoperative administration of aspirin in patients undergoing coronary artery bypass grafting. Department of Veterans Affairs Cooperative Study on Antiplatelet Therapy. *J Am Coll Cardiol* 1990; **15**:15–20.

56. Weightman WM, Gibbs NM, Weidmann CR, Newman MA, Grey DE, Sheminant MR, *et al.* The effect of preoperative aspirin-free interval on red blood cell transfusion requirements in cardiac surgical patients. *J Cardiothorac Vasc Anesth* 2002; **16**:54–8.

57. Dacey LJ, Munoz JJ, Johnson ER, Leavitt BJ, Maloney CT, Morton JR, *et al.* Effect of preoperative aspirin use on mortality in coronary artery bypass grafting patients. *Ann Thorac Surg* 2000; **70**:1986–90.

58. Yende S, Wunderink RG. Effect of clopidogrel on bleeding after coronary artery bypass surgery. *Crit Care Med* 2001; **29**:2271–5.

59. Sreeram GM, Sharma AD, Slaughter TF. Platelet glycoprotein IIb/IIIa antagonists: perioperative implications. *J Cardiothorac Vasc Anesth* 2001; **15**:237–40.

60. Kereiakes DJ. Prophylactic platelet transfusion in abciximab-treated patients requiring emergency coronary artery bypass graft surgery. *Am J Cardiol* 1998; **81**:373.

61. Levy JH. Pharmacologic preservation of the hemostatic system during cardiac surgery. *Ann Thorac Surg* 2001; **72**:S1814–20.

62. Kiowski W, Linder L, Kleinbloesem C, van Brummelen P, Buhler FR. Blood pressure control by the renin–angiotensin system in normotensive subjects. Assessment by angiotensin converting enzyme and renin inhibition. *Circulation* 1992; **85**:1–8.

63. Russell RM, Jones RM. Postoperative hypotension associated with enalapril. *Anaesthesia* 1989; **44**:837–8.

64. Coriat P, Richer C, Douraki T, Gomez C, Hendricks K, Giudicelli JF, *et al.* Influence of chronic angiotensin-converting enzyme inhibition on anesthetic induction. *Anesthesiology* 1994; **81**:299–307.

65. Bertrand M, Godet G, Meersschaert K, Brun L, Salcedo E, Coriat P. Should the angiotensin II antagonists be discontinued before surgery? *Anesth Analg* 2001; **92**:26–30.

66. Carrel T, Englberger L, Mohacsi P, Neidhart P, Schmidli J. Low systemic vascular resistance after cardiopulmonary bypass: incidence, etiology, and clinical importance. *J Card Surg* 2000; **15**:347–53.

67. Tuman KJ, McCarthy RJ, O'Connor CJ, Holm WE, Ivankovich AD. Angiotensin-converting enzyme inhibitors increase vasoconstrictor requirements after cardiopulmonary bypass. *Anesth Analg* 1995; **80**:473–9.

68. Brabant SM, Eyraud D, Bertrand M, Coriat P. Refractory hypotension after induction of anesthesia in a patient chronically treated with angiotensin receptor antagonists. *Anesth Analg* 1999; **89**:887–8.

69. Colson P, Ribstein J, Mimran A, Grolleau D, Chaptal PA, Roquefeuil B. Effect of angiotensin converting enzyme inhibition on blood pressure and renal function during open heart surgery. *Anesthesiology* 1990; **72**:23–7.

70. Boldt J, Rothe G, Schindler E, Doll C, Gorlach G, Hempelmann G. Can clonidine, enoximone, and enalaprilat help to protect the myocardium against ischaemia in cardiac surgery? *Heart* 1996; **76**:207–13.

71. Pigott DW, Nagle C, Allman K, Westaby S, Evans RD. Effect of omitting regular ACE inhibitor medication before cardiac surgery on haemodynamic variables and vasoactive drug requirements. *Br J Anaesth* 1999; **83**:715–20.

72. Dupuis JY. Against the discontinuation of angiotensin II antagonists before surgery. *Anesth Analg* 2001; **92**:1616–17.

73. Hayashi Y, Sawa Y, Ohtake S, Nishimura M, Ichikawa H, Matsuda H. Controlled nicorandil administration for myocardial protection during coronary artery bypass grafting under cardiopulmonary bypass. *J Cardiovasc Pharmacol* 2001; **38**:21–8.

74. Li Y, Iguchi A, Tsuru Y, Nakame T, Satou K, Tabayashi K. Nicorandil pretreatment and improved myocardial protection during cold blood cardioplegia. *Jpn J Thorac Cardiovasc Surg* 2000; **48**:24–9.

75. Kaneko T, Saito Y, Hikawa Y, Yasuda K, Makita K. Dose-dependent prophylactic effect of nicorandil, an ATP-sensitive potassium channel opener, on intra-operative myocardial ischaemia in patients undergoing major abdominal surgery. *Br J Anaesth* 2001; **86**:332–7.

76. Amory DW, Grigore A, Amory JK, Gerhardt MA, White WD, Smith PK, *et al.* Neuroprotection is associated with beta-adrenergic receptor antagonists during cardiac surgery: evidence from 2575 patients. *J Cardiothorac Vasc Anesth* 2002; **16**:270–7.

77. Klafta JM, Roizen MF. Current understanding of patients' attitudes toward and preparation for anesthesia: a review. *Anesth Analg* 1996; **83**:1314–21.

78. Ng A, Smith G. Gastroesophageal reflux and aspiration of gastric contents in anesthetic practice. *Anesth Analg* 2001; **93**:494–513.

79. Engelhardt T, Webster NR. Pulmonary aspiration of gastric contents in anaesthesia. *Br J Anaesth* 1999; **83**:453–60.

80. Anonymous. *Recommendations for Standards of Monitoring during Anaesthesia and Recovery.* London: Association of Anaesthetists of Great Britain and Ireland, 2000.

81. Anonymous. *Standards for Basic Anesthetic Monitoring.* The American Society of Anesthesiologists, 1998, www.asahq.org.

82. London MJ, Hollenberg M, Wong MG, Levenson L, Tubau JF, Browner W, *et al.* Intraoperative myocardial ischemia: localization by continuous 12-lead electrocardiography. *Anesthesiology* 1988; **69**:232–41.

83. Fuhrman TM, Pippin WD, Talmage LA, Reilley TE. Evaluation of collateral circulation of the hand. *J Clin Monitor* 1992; **8**:28–32.

84. Stern DH, Gerson JI, Allen FB, Parker FB. Can we trust the radial artery pressure immediately following cardiopulmonary bypass? *Anesthesiology* 1985; **62**:557–61.

85. Mark JB. Central venous pressure monitoring: clinical insights beyond the numbers. *J Cardiothorac Vasc Anesth* 1991; **5**:163–73.

86. Ariza M, Gothard JW, Macnaughton P, Hooper J, Morgan CJ, Evans TW. Blood lactate and mixed venous–arterial PCO_2 gradient as indices of poor peripheral perfusion following cardiopulmonary bypass surgery. *Intensive Care Med* 1991; **17**:320–4.

87. Bailey JM, Levy JH, Kopel MA, Tobia V, Grabenkort WR. Relationship between clinical evaluation of peripheral perfusion and global hemodynamics in adults after cardiac surgery. *Crit Care Med* 1990; **18**:1353–6.

88. Anonymous. Practice guidelines for pulmonary artery catheterization. A report by the American Society of Anesthesiologists Task Force on Pulmonary Artery Catheterization. *Anesthesiology* 1993; **78**:380–94.

89. Dalen JE, Bone RC. Is it time to pull the pulmonary artery catheter? *JAMA* 1996; **276**:916–18.

90. Bernard GR, Sopko G, Cerra F, Demling R, Edmunds H, Kaplan S, *et al.* Pulmonary artery catheterization and clinical outcomes: National Heart, Lung, and Blood Institute and Food and Drug Administration Workshop Report. Consensus Statement. *JAMA* 2000; **283**:2568–72.

91. Stocking JE, Lake CL. The role of the pulmonary artery catheter in the year 2000 and beyond. *J Cardiothorac Vasc Anesth* 2000; **14**:111–12.

92. Kefalides P. Pulmonary artery catheters on trial. *Ann Intern Med* 1998; **129**:170–2.

93. Cruz K, Franklin C. The pulmonary artery catheter: uses and controversies. *Crit Care Clin* 2001; **17**:271–91.

94. Rothenberg DM, Tuman KJ. Pulmonary artery catheter: what does the literature actually tell us? *Int Anesthesiol Clin* 2000; **38**:171–87.

95. Botero M, Lobato EB. Advances in noninvasive cardiac output monitoring: an update. *J Cardiothorac Vasc Anesth* 2001; **15**:631–40.

96. DiCorte CJ, Latham P, Greilich PE, Cooley MV, Grayburn PA, Jessen ME. Esophageal Doppler monitor determinations of cardiac output and preload during cardiac operations. *Ann Thorac Surg* 2000; **69**:1782–6.

97. Botero M, Hess P, Kirby D, Briesacher K, Gravenstein N, Lobato EB. Measurement of cardiac output during coronary artery bypass grafting: comparison of pulmonary artery catheter, noninvasive partial CO_2 rebreathing and direct aortic flow. *Anesth Analg* 2000; **90**:SCA87.

98. Perrino ACJ, Lippman A, Ariyan C, O'Connor TZ, Luther M. Intraoperative cardiac output monitoring: comparison of impedance cardiography and thermodilution. *J Cardiothorac Vasc Anesth* 1994; **8**:24–9.

99. Erlanger J, Hooker DR. An experimental study of blood-pressure and of pulse-pressure in man. *Johns Hopkins Hosp Rep* 1904; **12**:145–378.

100. Linton NW, Linton RA. Estimation of changes in cardiac output from the arterial blood pressure waveform in the upper limb. *Br J Anaesth* 2001; **86**:486–96.

101. van Lieshout JJ, Wesseling KH. Continuous cardiac output by pulse contour analysis? *Br J Anaesth* 2001; **86**:467–9.

102. Perrino AC, Harris SN, Luther MA. Intraoperative determination of cardiac output using multiplane transesophageal echocardiography: a comparison to thermodilution. *Anesthesiology* 1998; **89**:350–7.

103. Anonymous. Practice Guidelines for Perioperative Transesophageal Echocardiography. A Report by the American Society of Anesthesiologists and the Society of Cardiovascular Anesthesiologists Task Force on Transesophageal Echocardiography. *Anesthesiology* 1996; **84**:986–1006.

104. Konstadt SN, Reich DL, Kahn R, Viggiani RF. Transesophageal echocardiograpy can be used to screen for ascending aortic atherosclerosis. *Anesth Analg* 1995; **81**:225–8.

105. Edmonds HL Jr. Advances in neuromonitoring for cardiothoracic and vascular surgery. *J Cardiothorac Vasc Anesth* 2001; **15**:241–50.

106. Edmonds HL Jr, Toney KA, Thomas MH, Pollock SB Jr, Strickland TJ. Neuromonitoring cost–benefit for adult cardiac surgery. *Anesthesiology* 1997; **87**:A426.

107. Mantzaridis H, Kenny GN. Auditory evoked potential index: a quantitative measure of changes in auditory evoked potentials during general anaesthesia. *Anaesthesia* 1997; **52**:1030–6.

108. Rampil IJ. A primer for EEG signal processing in anesthesia. *Anesthesiology* 1998; **89**:980–1002.

109. Agnew NM, Pennefather SH, Russell GN. Isoflurane and coronary heart disease. *Anaesthesia* 2002; **57**:338–47.

110. Cohen J, Royston D. Remifentanil. *Curr Opin Crit Care* 2001; **7**:227–31.

111. Kreter B, Woods M. Antibiotic prophylaxis for cardiothoracic operations. Meta-analysis of thirty years of clinical trials. *J Thorac Cardiovasc Surg* 1992; **104**:590–9.

112. Leavitt BJ, O'Connor GT, Olmstead EM, Morton JR, Maloney CT, Dacey LJ, *et al.* Use of the internal mammary artery graft and in-hospital mortality and other adverse outcomes associated with coronary artery bypass surgery. *Circulation* 2001; **103**:507–12.

113. Barbier GH, Shettigar UR, Appunn DO. Clinical rationale for the use of an ultra-short acting beta-blocker: esmolol. *Int J Clin Pharmacol Ther* 1995; **33**:212–18.

114. Anonymous. *Recommendations for Standards of Monitoring and Alarms during Cardiopulmonary Bypass.* Society of Perfusionists of Great Britain and Ireland, Association of Cardiothoracic Anaesthetists, Society of Cardiothoracic Surgeons of Great Britain and Ireland, 2001, www.scts.org.

115. *AmSECT Guidelines for Perfusion Practice.* The American Society of Extracorporeal Technology, 1998, www.amsect.org.

116. Miller RS, Peterson GM, McLean S, Moller C. Effect of cardiopulmonary bypass on the plasma concentrations of fentanyl and alcuronium. *J Clin Pharm Ther* 1997; **22**:197–205.

117. Arrowsmith JE, Grocott HP, Reves JG, Newman MF. Central nervous system complications of cardiac surgery. *Br J Anaesth* 2000; **84**:378–93.

118. Pua HL, Bissonnette B. Cerebral physiology in paediatric cardiopulmonary bypass [Review – 83 refs]. *Can J Anaesth* 1998; **45**:960–78.

119. DeFoe GR, Ross CS, Olmstead EM, Surgenor SD, Fillinger MP, Groom RC, *et al.* Lowest hematocrit on bypass and adverse outcomes associated with coronary artery bypass grafting.

Northern New England Cardiovascular Disease Study Group. *Ann Thorac Surg* 2001; **71**:769–76.

120. Bevan DH. Cardiac bypass haemostasis: putting blood through the mill. *Br J Haematol* 1999; **104**:208–19.

121. Paparella D, Yau TM, Young E. Cardiopulmonary bypass induced inflammation: pathophysiology and treatment. An update. *Eur J Cardiothorac Surg* 2002; **21**:232–44.

122. Levi M, Cromheecke ME, de Jonge E, Prins MH, de Mol BJ, Briet E, *et al*. Pharmacological strategies to decrease excessive blood loss in cardiac surgery: a meta-analysis of clinically relevant endpoints. *Lancet* 1999; **354**:1940–7.

123. Lemmer JHJ, Dilling EW, Morton JR, Rich JB, Robicsek F, Bricker DL, *et al*. Aprotinin for primary coronary artery bypass grafting: a multicenter trial of three dose regimens. *Ann Thorac Surg* 1996; **62**:1659–67.

124. Dietrich W, Spath P, Ebell A, Richter JA. Prevalence of anaphylactic reactions to aprotinin: analysis of two hundred forty-eight reexposures to aprotinin in heart operations. *J Thorac Cardiovasc Surg* 1997; **113**:194–201.

125. *SIGN Guideline 54. Perioperative Blood Transfusion for Elective Surgery. A National Clinical Guideline.* Edinburgh: Scottish Intercollegiate Guidelines Network (www.sign.ac.uk), 2001.

126. Heames RM, Gill RS, Ohri SK, Hett DA. Off-pump coronary artery surgery. *Anaesthesia* 2002; **57**(7):676–85.

127. Resano FG, Stamou SC, Lowery RC, Corso PJ. Complete myocardial revascularization on the beating heart with epicardial stabilization: anesthetic considerations. *J Cardiothorac Vasc Anesth* 2000; **14**:534–9.

128. De Witte J, Sessler DI. Perioperative shivering: physiology and pharmacology [Review – 353 refs]. *Anesthesiology* 2002; **96**:467–84.

129. Nierich AP, Diephuis J, Jansen EW, Borst C, Knape JT. Heart displacement during off-pump CABG: how well is it tolerated? *Ann Thorac Surg* 2000; **70**:466–72.

130. Schaff HV. New surgical techniques: implications for the cardiac anesthesiologist: mini-thoracotomy for coronary revascularization without cardiopulmonary bypass. *J Cardiothorac Vasc Anesth* 1997; **11**:6–9.

11

Principles, evolution and techniques of coronary surgery

DAVID J WHEATLEY

THE PRINCIPLES OF CORONARY SURGERY

Successful surgery for coronary artery disease requires skill in the relevant surgical procedures. However, for surgery to be *rational* and *appropriate*, the surgeon must have a thorough understanding of the disease and its management. This includes knowledge of anatomical, physiological and pathological features, clinical manifestations, natural history, techniques for investigation, the role of all available therapeutic options, and measures for limiting disease progression. Surgery should be regarded as one of a number of potential options in a continuing, life-time management strategy, which may include modification of risk factors and lifestyle, pharmacological measures, and non-surgical intracoronary interventions.[1–4]

Coronary artery disease often exists for many years in the absence of symptoms, and is not commonly diagnosed at this stage. It may be discovered in the course of general health assessment or during investigation of valvular heart disease. Usually it comes to light with the onset of angina in its various clinical presentations, or it may present as myocardial infarction or infarct-related complications. Coronary artery bypass grafting has a potential role in all of these manifestations, though it is most commonly undertaken for chronic stable angina and acute coronary syndromes unresponsive to medical therapy. Other surgical procedures have a role (often in combination with bypass grafting) in the treatment of complications of myocardial infarction (rupture of ventricular septum or papillary muscle, left ventricular scar and aneurysm). Indications for surgery depend on many factors, including clinical presentation, the nature and extent of disease and the feasibility and likely outcome of alternative non-surgical interventions, as well as an assessment of risk and the anticipated result of surgery in the particular individual under consideration.

Coronary artery bypass surgery and percutaneous coronary interventions have the same aim – restoration of normal myocardial perfusion. The non-surgical catheter-based interventions achieve results by directly altering the morphology of obstructing atheromatous coronary lesions with percutaneously introduced endovascular devices such as balloons and stents. Surgery achieves its results by the insertion of bypass conduits during an operation in which the epicardial coronary arteries are exposed and conduits are inserted distal to atheromatous obstructions to provide an alternative route for blood to reach jeopardized myocardium. In general, although technological advances are expanding the role for percutaneous coronary interventions, extensive and complex coronary lesions are more appropriately managed with surgery.[4]

Coronary bypass grafting, in augmenting the perfusion of myocardium supplied by stenosed coronary arteries, mimics the effect of naturally occurring collateral vessels. Collateral vessels arise in response to regional ischemia resulting from severe coronary stenosis and form a connecting network of vessels between well-supplied coronary arteries, or even extracardiac sources, and severely stenosed coronary arteries. They are capable of providing a degree of protection against infarction and heart failure, and confer improved survival, though they may not be adequate to abolish angina.[5,6] Surgical bypass conduits are more efficient than natural collateral vessels as they are of relatively large caliber, have a direct course outside the myocardium and its compressive influence, arise from a copious source of arterial blood, and are directed to strategic sites of the surgeon's choice.

Although the principle of inserting conduits to conduct blood around obstructions in the coronary arteries is simple, in practice a number of issues arise that have direct relevance to the conduct of the operation. These concern:

- disease progression in grafted and ungrafted arteries following surgery,
- fate of the bypass conduits,
- degree of obstruction meriting bypass,
- location of obstructions suitable for bypass,
- caliber of vessel appropriate for bypass,
- extent of revascularization required,
- type of conduit,
- source of arterial inflow to the conduit,
- influence of left ventricular function on surgery,
- technique for establishing the surgical conditions for bypass grafting.

Following the pioneering work in the late 1960s on coronary artery bypass grafting by groups such as Favaloro and colleagues at the Cleveland Clinic[7] and Dudley Johnson in Milwaukee,[8] the technique was rapidly adopted by others. The fate of both the bypassed coronary arteries and the saphenous vein conduits used to bypass them soon attracted interest. Progression of disease in the coronary arteries and development of obstruction in the conduits were obvious potential limitations to the effectiveness of coronary bypass grafting.

Progression of disease in the coronary arteries

It had long been recognized that coronary atherosclerosis is a progressive condition; continued progression of disease was therefore only to be anticipated following bypass grafting. However, in the early 1970s, reports emerged raising concerns over the incidence of disease progression, particularly proximal to vein graft insertion.[9–12]

Contemporary experimental studies suggested explanations. Even with no proximal coronary occlusion, a venous bypass conduit to the distal artery could reduce flow in the proximal artery by 50%.[13] It was also shown that the proportions of flow in the graft and the bypassed artery depended on the ratio of graft to artery diameter, as well as on the degree of coronary obstruction.[14] Larger diameter bypass conduits carried a greater proportion of total flow (up to 95%) destined for the distal artery than smaller caliber grafts, even without coronary obstruction. These findings supported the concept of reduced coronary flow as a possible explanation of the high incidence of angiographically demonstrated coronary disease progression following bypass grafting.

It required observations over a longer period, however, to put the progression of disease in the coronary arteries into perspective. Bourassa and colleagues showed that during the first year after surgery only 9.5% of stenoses progressed in ungrafted arteries, compared with more than 50% in grafted arteries. However, in the grafted vessels there was little further progression, and by 5–7 years disease progression in ungrafted vessels had caught up with that in the grafted vessels.[15] This pattern persisted at 11 years.[16]

Two studies[17,18] of patients randomly allocated to medical or surgical treatment showed that progression of disease in ungrafted vessels and vessels distal to grafts in surgical patients was similar to that in medically treated patients. More progression of disease occurred proximal to graft insertion sites than in the same sites of medically treated patients,[18] a finding confirmed by a more recent report of the Coronary Artery Surgery Study (CASS) patients.[19] This later report also drew attention to the greater propensity for progression of severe, compared with mild lesions.

In summary, there is broad consensus that in arteries distal to bypass grafts (patent or occluded), and in unbypassed vessels in surgical patients, disease progression is similar following surgery to that of comparable disease in arteries of non-operated patients. Progression is most rapid in severe lesions – usually proceeding to occlusion – and slow or infrequent in mild lesions. The artery proximal to the insertion of a vein graft is prone to early occlusion, probably thrombotic in nature, due to alterations in flow. This may be responsible for some myocardial damage in the perioperative period. However, the early anxieties about accelerated coronary disease progression thwarting the efforts of the surgeon have proved largely unfounded.

Practical conclusions are that bypass grafting should be avoided for mild lesions (the conventional indication of 50% or greater loss of lumen is supported). Early use of antiplatelet agents may reduce the tendency for proximal arterial thrombosis, though this is as yet unproven. Most of the literature derives from patients having venous grafts; the problem of progressive disease in the coronary arteries may be less with arterial conduit use, possibly because of the generally smaller lumen of arterial conduits and their ability to regulate flow.[20–22] All studies are in agreement that the atherosclerotic process continues in the coronary arteries and leads to recurrent coronary events. This emphasizes the need for continued treatment following surgery to minimize disease progression.

Development of obstruction in the conduits

In view of its ready availability and abundance, together with the safety and ease of harvesting, by far the most commonly used conduit in coronary bypass surgery has been the autologous saphenous vein. The fate of these conduits has been extensively studied, particularly by the Cleveland Clinic group and the Montreal Heart Institute, and the subject has been well reviewed by Nwasokwa in 1995[23] and Motwani and Topol in 1998.[24] It is well established that saphenous veins, used as aortocoronary bypass conduits, have an increasing propensity to occlude over time.[16] Thrombosis, mainly in the first month, has been reported to account for occlusion of about 10% of saphenous vein grafts. Technical errors, major graft/ target size mismatch, poor graft flow due to small target vessels, poor run-off or competing flow from non-significantly stenosed grafted arteries are implicated. Intimal hyperplasia narrows most grafts over the next few months and years, and from about 5 years on, there is progressive atheromatous change in many vein grafts. By 10 years, 50% of vein grafts are believed to be occluded and most have some disease.[23–25] The atheroma of vein grafts is more malign than native coronary atheroma: it progresses more rapidly, is more diffusely located in the vein than atheroma in the coronary artery; it has little fibrous cap, is more friable and poses a greater risk of atheroembolism at re-operation than arterial atheroma. It is also more refractory to medical therapy when it causes unstable angina.[26]

The Cleveland Clinic group, in 1990, reported some 2500 patients who had undergone re-operation and showed that 'vein graft atherosclerosis is the leading cause of re-operation, more than progressive coronary atherosclerosis *per se*'.[27] Fitzgibbon and colleagues[28] showed 88% early vein graft patency, which had fallen to 75% at 5 years and 50% at 15 years or more. They showed that vein graft disease and occlusion were major determinants of re-operation and survival.

Much research has been aimed at ameliorating the problem of vein graft failure.[23,24] It is likely that measures to reduce injury to the vein at the time of surgery will help. Avoidance of direct handling, excessive distending pressure, ischemia, non-physiological perfusion, and possibly inclusion of surrounding tissues with the harvested vein have all been advocated to enhance patency.[23,24,29] Commencement of antiplatelet therapy (aspirin) within 48 hours, lipid-lowering drugs and avoidance of smoking have been shown to have a beneficial influence.[1] However, it is clear that the best way of avoiding the problem of vein graft disease is the use of arterial conduit alternatives wherever possible.

The Cleveland Clinic group[30] was the first to show that inclusion of at least one internal thoracic artery graft (usually to the left anterior descending artery) gave patients clinical benefit by 10 years – less recurrent angina, better survival, fewer hospitalizations for myocardial infarction or other coronary events – when compared with patients receiving saphenous vein grafts only. Similar evidence from the CASS registry shows survival benefit for those having internal thoracic artery grafting compared with those having only vein conduits.[31]

Encouraged by the clinical benefits of using the internal thoracic artery as one of the conduits for revascularization, as well as documented patency rates of 90% or better at 10 years,[24] many groups have developed the use of multiple arterial conduits. There are now numerous reports attesting to the excellent clinical outcomes achievable with multiple arterial bypass conduit use.[32–36]

Identification of appropriate coronary stenoses

In order to warrant bypassing, coronary obstructions should be of sufficient severity to produce a hemodynamic effect. This manifests as impairment of coronary flow under conditions of increased demand and results in myocardial ischemia (commonly reflected symptomatically as angina on effort). The degree of stenosis beyond which impairment of coronary flow reserve and reduction of distal coronary pressure become apparent is about 75% loss of cross-sectional area, or 50% loss of arterial diameter.[37] Stenoses of this severity or greater are often referred to as 'hemodynamically significant' or 'critical'. This degree of coronary stenosis is also recognized as being 'important' in the majority of randomized trials concerned with survival following coronary surgery[1] and is the basis of the definition of a significant stenosis in the Bypass Angioplasty Revascularization Investigation (BARI).[38]

Although the angiographic appearance (with or without calliper or computer-aided quantification) is the usual criterion for deciding the severity of a coronary stenosis, such an assessment may be difficult. Comparison with adjacent normal vessel is often not feasible, as clear-cut transition from diseased to disease-free artery is not always present. Suboptimal imaging, vessel overlap and complex lesion morphology are practical difficulties. Multiple angiographic views are helpful in assessment (Figure 11.1). The length, morphology, vascular tone and distending pressure of the stenosed segment influence the hemodynamic effect, as do the effects of coronary collateral vessels. These influences are impossible to assess from angiography alone.

For more accurate assessment of the importance of coronary lesions, it is now possible to use direct measures of physiological significance, such as distal pressure, flow velocity or coronary vasodilatory reserve at the time of angiography.[37,39–41] Further help can be obtained by

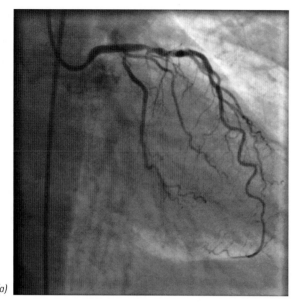
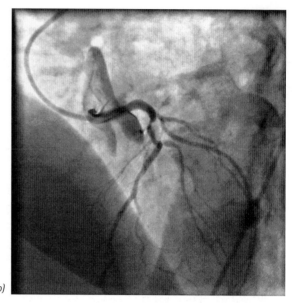

(a)   (b)

Figure 11.1 *(a) In this right anterior oblique view, stenosis is apparent in the proximal anterior descending artery but vessel overlap obscures detail. (b) In this cranio-caudal view, the proximal anterior descending artery is better seen and is about 90% stenosed. There is also severe stenosis at the origin of the large first diagonal branch.*

stress testing with electrocardiography, echocardiography or nuclear perfusion studies. However, in the majority of instances, where the clinical presentation suggests significant coronary obstructions, the surgical decisions about the need for bypass grafts are made primarily on the basis of angiographic appearances. Investigation of physiological impact, if any, of coronary disease is often reserved for those with atypical presentation or equivocal angiographic findings.

A pragmatic guide is to recommend bypassing coronary lesions resulting in loss of 50% or more of vessel diameter, provided that the vessel is of adequate size and distribution (Figure 11.2). If none of the major coronary arteries has a stenosis of 50% or more, bypass grafting is probably not indicated, unless radionuclide studies have shown perfusion deficits.

With stenosis equivalent to loss of 75–80% of diameter, there is impairment of coronary flow under resting conditions – clinically correlating with angina at rest (Figure 11.3). The totally occluded artery that has distal filling from collateral vessels provides least difficulty in making a decision for bypass grafting, as pressure in the distal artery beyond a complete obstruction is low, and natural collateral vessels are less effective than an appropriately placed surgical conduit (Figures 11.4 and 11.5).

The pressure gradient created by a critical coronary stenosis is necessary to ensure optimal flow in a bypass conduit. When there is a non-critical stenosis, there is insufficient pressure drop in the distal coronary artery to ensure good flow in a conduit, and poor flow is likely to result in graft occlusion.[24] Bypass of a less than critically

stenosed vessel in anticipation of subsequent progression of disease is therefore generally not advisable. The reported slow progression of mild lesions[42] and the propensity of vein grafts to accelerate proximal disease are further disincentives.

The best policy for lesions that are just below 50% stenosed, when other vessels have significant stenoses requiring surgery, is not entirely resolved. The influence of competing flow is unclear.[24] Cosgrove and colleagues reported on 92 patients (out of nearly 18 000 in their database) who had vessels with less than 50% stenosis bypassed. At an average of nearly 16 months, progression of disease had occurred in 63% of these arteries (compared with 20% of non-bypassed vessels), though patency of bypass grafts to these vessels was similar to that of grafts bypassing greater than 50% stenoses.[20] Cashin and colleagues[43] showed accelerated progression to affect not only severe lesions, but also lesions of less than 50% stenosis in bypassed arteries. Only 3% of non-bypassed minimally stenosed vessels showed disease progression, compared with 38% of bypassed vessels with similar stenosis. As a result, the authors cast doubt on the wisdom of bypassing lesions of less than 50% stenosis in the anticipation of disease progression.

There is also evidence to indicate that *conduit patency* may be adversely influenced when the degree of obstruction in the bypassed coronary artery is not severe.[24,44] Patency rates for radial artery bypass conduits have been reported to be lower when used to bypass less severely stenosed coronary arteries than when used for severely stenosed or occluded arteries.[45]

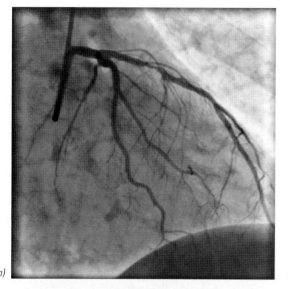

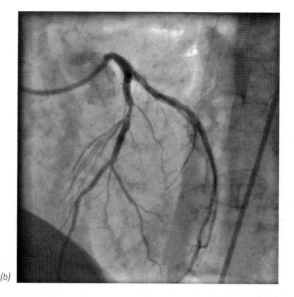

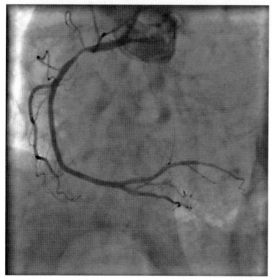

Figure 11.2 (a) Right anterior oblique view of the left coronary artery showing 75% stenosis of the proximal anterior descending artery, which has a good distal lumen for bypass. (b) In the same patient as in (a), the left anterior oblique view with cranio-caudal tilt shows >50% stenosis in the anterior descending artery. (c) The same patient's right coronary artery seen in left anterior oblique projection shows a proximal lesion of at least 50% stenosis.

Location of obstruction

For effective bypass, obstructions must be in proximal locations in the major epicardial coronary arteries or their larger branches. If the obstruction is distally located, there are often enough natural collateral vessels arising proximal to the stenosis to provide sufficient flow around the lesion to make bypass of the vessel unnecessary. Furthermore, the more distal the obstruction is, the smaller will be the amount of jeopardized myocardium and the narrower the caliber of artery to receive the conduit beyond the obstruction.

Caliber of target coronary artery

Coronary arteries distal to significant obstructions must be of adequate caliber and distribution to allow sufficient

flow through a bypass conduit to make a clinically significant impact on myocardial perfusion. Although arteries with a diameter of as little as 1 mm can be bypassed, the technical difficulties are increased, and arteries should ideally have a caliber of 1.5 mm diameter or more for reliably successful bypass. The BARI investigators defined a significant lesion as a stenosis of 50% loss of lumen diameter in a vessel of 1.5 mm or greater reference diameter.[38]

The exact site of bypass target in a vessel which has a significant stenosis is determined by a number of factors, including ease of access to the vessel, course of the planned conduit, state of the arterial wall at the proposed anastomosis site, as well as the size of the vessel. In a vessel of 1.5 mm or more in diameter, its territory of distribution (run-off) will generally ensure that flow in a bypass graft will be sufficient to avoid early graft closure. Graft flow measured at surgery has been shown to predict subsequent graft patency, flow over 30 mL min^{-1}

being necessary to maintain patency in vein grafts with any certainty. Vessels with a diameter of less than 1.5 mm have the disadvantage both of being technically more difficult to anastomose accurately and of carrying lower

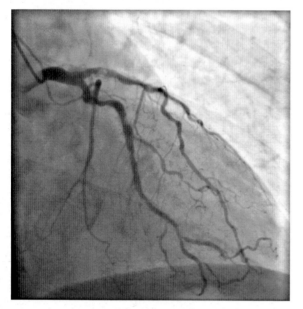

Figure 11.3 *This right anterior oblique view of the left coronary artery of a patient with rest pain and unstable angina shows severe stenosis (90%+) in the proximal anterior descending artery and a further severe stenosis in the large obtuse marginal branch of the circumflex artery.*

flow with smaller territory of supply, and with lower late patency for saphenous vein grafts to these vessels.[24] Vessels with a diameter of less than 1 mm are probably not practical coronary bypass targets, and are unlikely to perfuse clinically significant amounts of myocardium.

Target vessel size is estimated from the angiogram, where the angiography catheter and other coronary vessels provide guidance, and from observation of the vessel at surgery before it is opened. Comparison with graded coronary sizers helps, but the evaluation is sometimes difficult and subjective, and must be made in the overall context of the number, size and locality of other bypass targets. It is particularly important with vessels of small caliber to have a suitable bypass conduit – ideally, an internal thoracic artery or other arterial conduit, or a thin-walled vein. Major discrepancy between graft and coronary lumen or undue thickness of graft wall may make an effective anastomosis to a small-caliber distal vessel impossible.

When there is no obvious satisfactory target vessel, coronary endarterectomy may be a feasible option for making a large, severely diseased artery suitable for receiving a conduit, and will often allow sufficient run-off for a bypass graft to perfuse a clinically significant amount of myocardium and stay patent.

Extent of revascularization

Revascularization should be 'complete'. Many reports indicate that complete revascularization has a favorable

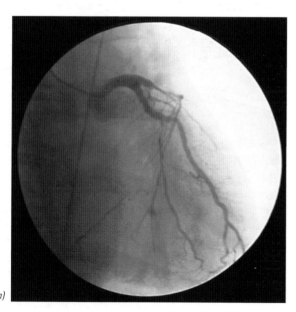

(a)

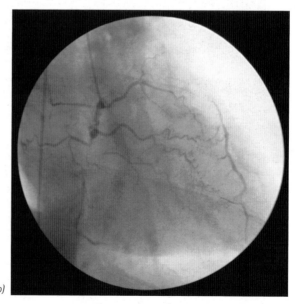

(b)

Figure 11.4 *(a) This right anterior oblique view of the left coronary artery shows a large obtuse marginal branch of circumflex but no filling of the anterior descending artery beyond the first septal branch. (b) In the same projection as in (a), the injection into the right coronary artery shows it to be totally occluded in its first third, but proximal collaterals from it fill the anterior descending artery, which is a good surgical target.*

influence on operative outcome, recurrent coronary events and survival.[46–52] As a result, surgeons may feel obliged to insert as many bypasses as feasible. However, the definition of 'complete' is not straightforward.[53] The commonest understanding of 'complete' revascularization appears to be that in which all diseased arterial systems (anterior descending, intermediate, circumflex and right) with a stenosis of 50% or greater loss of lumen diameter receive at least one graft.[46,54] A careful analysis of surgery and its results in 1507 patients from the randomized and registry arms of the BARI study[53] has suggested a survival *disadvantage* if more than one graft was inserted into a coronary system other than the anterior descending.

Thus, insertion of at least one bypass into the territory of the anterior descending, one into the intermediate artery (if present), one into the circumflex, and one into the right coronary artery would appear to be optimal practice for the commonly presenting 'three-vessel disease' patient. Given the need for reasonable target vessel size (1.5 mm diameter) and adequate distal run-off, it is uncommon to have more than five distal targets. Indeed, more than this number risks some of the grafts carrying too small a flow to remain patent, and the report from the BARI investigation[53] is a further disincentive to excessive surgical zeal. The commonest distal target sites are the mid or distal thirds of the anterior descending artery, one or more diagonal branches of the left anterior descending artery, the intermediate branch of a trifurcating left artery, one of the lateral (obtuse marginal) branches of the circumflex artery, the distal right or posterior descending artery, or the left ventricular branch of

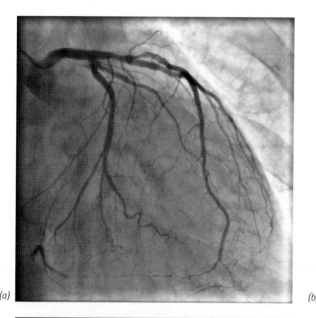

(a)

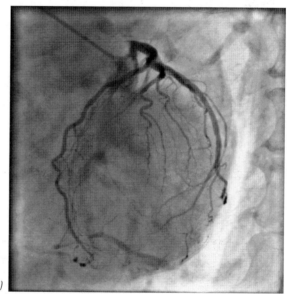

(b)

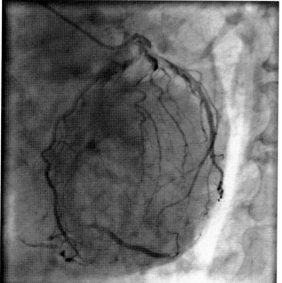

(c)

Figure 11.5 *(a) The right anterior oblique projection of this left coronary artery shows a high-grade obstruction in the proximal anterior descending artery and filling of the distal right artery in the region of the crus. (b) This left anterior oblique projection of the left coronary artery in the same patient as in (a) shows faint filling of a large left ventricular branch of the right artery – a good bypass target. (c) A later phase of the same projection as in (b) shows improved contrast in the left ventricular branch of the right coronary artery from late filling via collaterals, indicative of occlusion of the right artery.*

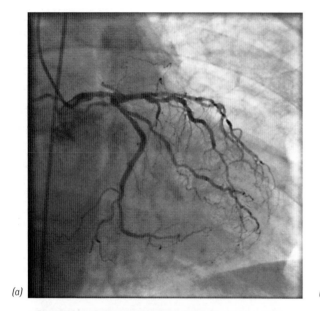

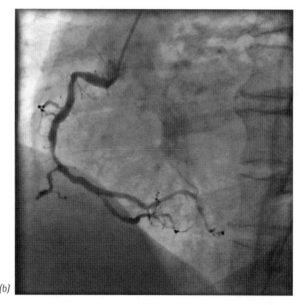

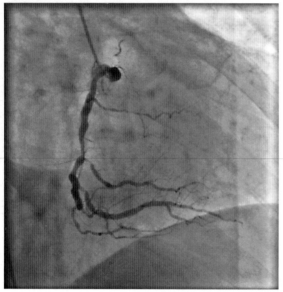

Figure 11.6 (a) Right anterior oblique view of left coronary artery showing 50% left main stenosis and stenoses of about 50% in the obtuse marginal branch of circumflex. This vessel, as well as the anterior descending artery, would be an appropriate bypass target. (b) The right coronary artery of the same patient as in (a) in left anterior oblique view shows a 75% mid–third lesion with less severe stenosis in the proximal third. (c) In the same patient, right anterior oblique view of the right artery shows severe stenosis at the origin of the posterior descending artery, which is a good bypass target.

the right artery (or a descending branch of this vessel) (Figures 11.6 and 11.7).

Choice of bypass conduit

Sufficient conduit vessel of suitable caliber and wall thickness must be available to permit construction of the planned bypasses. Although saphenous vein is still commonly used, arterial conduits should always be considered as a preferable alternative to vein grafts. The internal thoracic artery and the radial artery are usually very well suited for anastomosis to small-caliber coronary arteries.

For anterior descending artery bypass, the *pedicled (or in situ) left internal thoracic artery* (also known as the internal mammary artery), because of its appropriate

lumen size and wall thickness, anatomical proximity, direct course to the front of the heart (Figure 11.8) and well-documented long-term patency in this role, is the conduit of choice at all ages and for both elective and urgent surgery.[30,31,55–57]

If the lie of the vessels is appropriate (not too far apart), it is often possible to construct a sequential graft of the internal thoracic artery to a jeopardized diagonal artery (side-to-side) and the anterior descending artery (end-to-side) (Figure 11.9). This should not be done if the internal thoracic artery is of narrow caliber or if the diagonal artery is very diseased or large, when it would merit a separate graft. It should not be done if there is too great a separation between the targets, as this carries a risk of angulating and obstructing the internal thoracic artery at the side-to-side anastomosis.

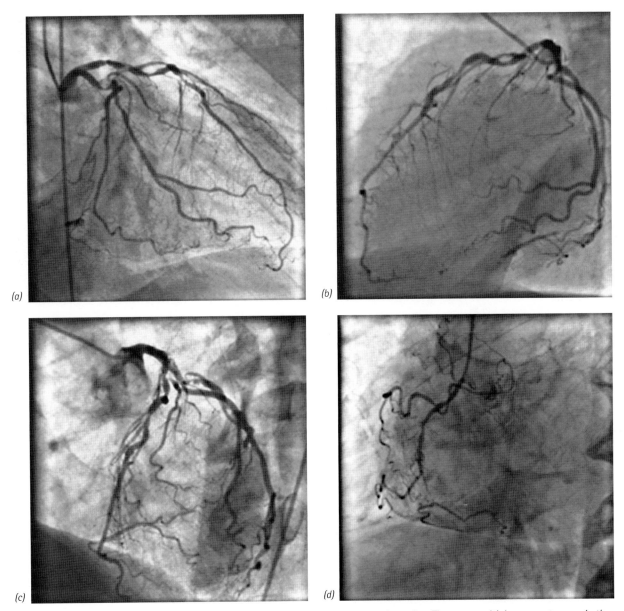

Figure 11.7 *(a) Right anterior oblique view of left artery from a patient with chronic angina. There are multiple severe stenoses in the first third of the anterior descending artery and a severe obstruction in the proximal circumflex artery, with further obstruction near the origin of its obtuse marginal branch. This branch and the anterior descending artery are good bypass targets. (b) Left lateral view of the left artery of the same patient as in (a) shows, in addition to the anterior descending and circumflex lesions, filling of a distal right artery by collaterals. (c) The left anterior oblique view of the same patient's left artery shows additional stenosis of the first diagonal artery at its origin, and the posterior descending and left ventricular branches of the right artery are filling by collaterals. (d) The left anterior oblique view of the right artery shows the anticipated total occlusion in the mid-third.*

There may be circumstances in which it is wiser to use the left internal thoracic artery as a free graft. When the left lung is emphysematous and likely to distort the graft, or if the artery is clearly not long enough to reach the intended anterior descending target, it should be detached and used as a free graft. Occasionally, when there is doubt about the adequacy of flow in the pedicled vessel, it may be wise to detach it and insert a small cannula into the proximal end to confirm flow through the artery. If there is proximal surgical injury or disease, the vessel should similarly be detached and the normal segment used as a free graft.

The *right internal thoracic artery* has more limited application as a pedicled graft. It is not often of large enough caliber to make it appropriate for the distal right coronary artery, and it may not be long enough to reach

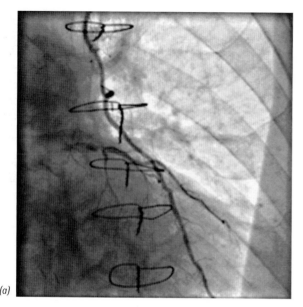
(a)

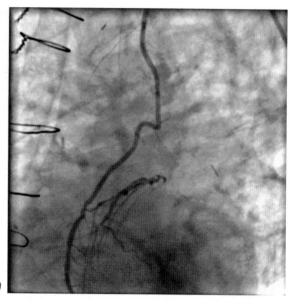
(b)

Figure 11.8 *(a) Postoperative angiogram showing the left internal thoracic artery feeding a similar caliber anterior descending artery. (b) Lateral view of the same patient as in (a) shows the relatively direct course of the internal thoracic artery to the anterior descending artery.*

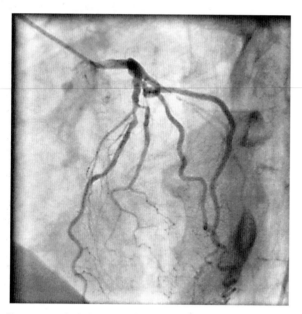

Figure 11.9 *Left anterior oblique view with cranio-caudal tilt shows at least 50% stenosis in the anterior descending artery just beyond the first septal branch and a 75% stenosis at the origin of the first diagonal branch. Sequential bypass of the first diagonal and the anterior descending artery with the internal thoracic artery would be feasible.*

the posterior descending artery. It can be routed posterior to the aorta through the transverse sinus to the lateral branches of the circumflex artery (with the small drawback of difficulty in accessing the conduit in the event

of a side branch bleeding). Some groups route the right internal thoracic artery across the midline to the anterior descending artery (leaving the pedicled left artery for other left-sided targets).

The right internal thoracic artery can be used as a free graft for most distal targets. The caliber of the internal thoracic artery makes it difficult to achieve a reliable graft to the aorta, and it is usually better anastomosed to another conduit. The proximal end can be anastomosed to the proximal left internal thoracic artery or to another free graft (venous or arterial).

The *radial artery* has become established as a good bypass conduit. Its lumen and wall thickness are ideal for most distal coronary targets, and its length gives versatility of use for any target or for sequential grafting. Though not as consistently satisfactory as the internal thoracic artery, it has shown good results, usually in combination with internal thoracic grafts.[45]

The *gastro-epiploic artery*, used as a pedicled graft, has established safety and efficacy for the revascularization of arteries on the inferior surface of the heart.[58] Other arterial grafts have less frequent application.

The *long saphenous vein* provides a reasonably satisfactory source of conduit in the absence of suitable arterial alternatives, though with recognized less satisfactory long-term patency (Figure 11.10). The mechanisms of the pathological changes and strategies for retarding or ameliorating vein graft disease are well described.[24]

There are patients in whom sufficient satisfactory conduit may not be available, especially in repeat operations where the best conduit vessels have already been

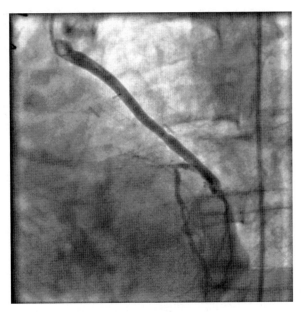

Figure 11.10 *Postoperative view of saphenous vein bypass conduit inserted into the obtuse marginal branch of a stenosed circumflex artery. The lumen size disparity is apparent.*

used. The lesser saphenous system and the cephalic veins may provide reasonable sources of conduit. Use of varicose venous conduit or conduit with major discrepancy in lumen from that of the bypassed vessel is likely to give a poor outcome. Although efforts are continuing to achieve a satisfactory prosthetic graft,[59] synthetic conduits generally remain unsatisfactory and are only used as a last resort for bypass to large coronary targets. Every effort should be made to obtain arterial conduit and use it in the most effective manner for the most important grafts. Sequential grafting may reduce the length of conduit required.[36,60–62]

Source of arterial inflow to the conduit

The left and right internal thoracic arteries and the gastro-epiploic artery are commonly used as pedicled grafts – their arterial inflow is left undisturbed, the graft is mobilized and side branches are divided, leaving the distal end for anastomosis to the target vessel. In the presence of extensive arterial disease, inflow into these arterial conduits may be impaired, and the conduit should then be detached for use as a free graft. Flow should be assessed prior to anastomosis, not only to exclude the possibility of vessel injury during mobilization, but also to confirm that inflow is adequate. This is done by allowing the distal divided end of the vessel to bleed into a container. A brisk flow is easy to recognize; a sluggish flow is often a matter for judgment. Systemic pressure and vessel caliber affect the flow rate and should be

considered in making a decision on flow adequacy – generally, anything less than $30\,\text{mL}\,\text{min}^{-1}$ should result in abandonment of the vessel as a pedicled conduit. Probing of the vessel runs a risk of injury and should not be done.

The anterior aspect of the ascending aorta is the commonest source of inflow into free grafts. When extensive atheroma of the ascending aorta is apparent at surgery, or where insufficient space is present for placing the proximal anastomoses, alternative strategies must be adopted. These include siting of proximal anastomoses on a single large venous graft, on a synthetic replacement of the ascending aorta, on the brachio-cephalic artery, or on a pedicled internal thoracic artery.

ALTERNATIVE OPTIONS FOR ISOLATED CORONARY OSTIAL STENOSIS

Occasionally, localized occlusion at the right or left coronary ostium, in the presence of an otherwise near-normal coronary system, can be managed by placement of a pericardial vein or arterial patch graft across the stenosed segment.[63–66] This is an uncommon approach and should be undertaken with care, and only if the ostial lesion is short and isolated.

Left ventricular function

Poor left ventricular function increases surgical risk.[1] However, when ischemic myocardium can be revascularized in patients with poor left ventricular function, the relative prognostic benefit, as compared with non-interventional strategies, is greater than for those with normal left ventricular function. Definition of the lower limit of impairment of left ventricular function compatible with satisfactory surgical outcome is not easy. In general, if angina, rather than breathlessness, is the predominant symptom, revascularization is worthwhile. If breathlessness predominates, a radionuclide study showing reversible ischemia in the territory of graftable coronary arteries increases the likelihood of revascularization being successful. The patient with a left ventriculogram showing severe generalized hypokinesia, and an ejection fraction below 20%, is usually not satisfactorily managed by surgical revascularization (Figures 11.11 and 11.12).

Technique for the provision of a suitable operating field

The achievement of a suitable, immobile, bloodless operating field for coronary artery bypass grafting traditionally requires a vertical sternotomy incision, cardiopulmonary bypass and cardiac arrest, each with inherent risks and drawbacks.[67–72] Attempts to minimize the injury of

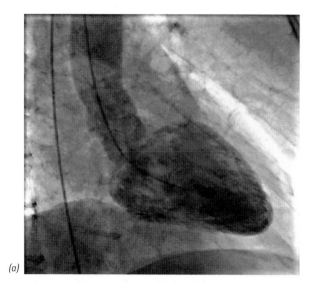 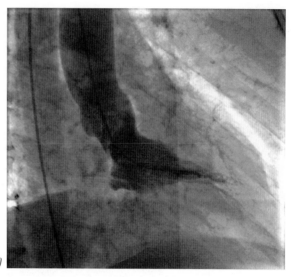

(a) (b)

Figure 11.11 *(a) Right anterior oblique view of left ventricle and ascending aorta, at end-diastole, showing normal contours. (b) The same view as in (a) at end-systole showing excellent left ventricular contraction of a normal ventricle.*

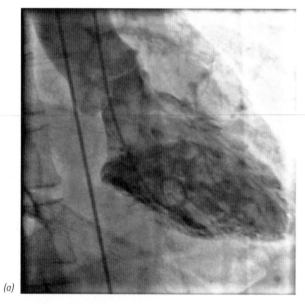 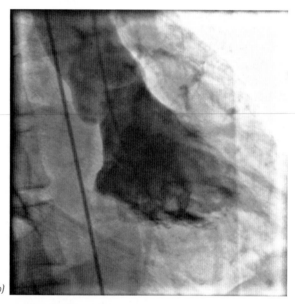

(a) (b)

Figure 11.12 *(a) Right anterior oblique view of left ventricle at end-diastole shows mild bulging of inferior margin, the site of previous infarction. (b) The same view as in (a) at end-systole shows increased volume with akinetic inferior margin in this moderately impaired left ventricle (ejection fraction 40%).*

access to the heart have stimulated minimally invasive approaches.[73,74] Efforts to avoid the damaging effects of cardiopulmonary bypass have resulted in 'beating-heart surgery'.[75–80] These approaches are continuing to evolve, and their respective roles are yet to be fully defined.[81]

Extensive or complex coronary procedures (grafts to multiple arteries, grafting to intramyocardial vessels, or endarterectomy) are probably more easily and satisfactorily achieved with cardiopulmonary bypass. There is

evidence that beating-heart surgery has advantages in traditionally 'high-risk' patients, though prospective randomized studies comparing the two approaches in high-risk patients are awaited.[75,82] Minimal access surgery usually implies beating-heart surgery for single-vessel disease. It has a limited role in view of the success of angioplasty and stenting in this setting, and its use is often dictated by personal experience and preference. There are particular instances when beating-heart surgery with limited cardiac access is advantageous – especially in repeat surgery when access to circumflex arteries is all that is required.

CONDUCT OF THE OPERATION UTILIZING CARDIOPULMONARY BYPASS

An experienced team will have little difficulty in planning the operation for the majority of patients, and most operations will follow a standard pattern. Many centers have an institutional policy reflecting surgical preference – such as favoring the use of cardiopulmonary bypass, or the use of 'beating-heart' techniques, the virtually exclusive use of arterial conduits, or the use of specific myocardial protective strategies. Given the complexity of inter-relating steps in treatment, it may well be that a number of different approaches will yield equally satisfactory results. To ensure that surgical practice is of a high standard, it is essential, therefore, for the surgical team to keep accurate data on its procedures and their outcomes, and to compare with outcomes from larger, regional or national cardiac surgical databases.

A number of factors influence the decisions about technique. Information from the history and clinical examination of the patient should be correlated with the angiographic demonstration of coronary stenoses in order to plan the surgical strategy. Such factors as previous coronary surgery, obesity, diabetes, emphysema, severe varicosities, and results of the modified Allen test[83,84] will influence the choice of conduit.

Accurate knowledge of the sites and severity of coronary obstructions as well as of the course, size and nature of the coronary arteries is fundamental to successful surgery. So important is this that having a display of the angiographic appearances, either in the form of angiographic images or annotated drawings or diagrams, in the operating room is strongly recommended. This practice is a good precaution against erroneous or inappropriate bypass graft placement. It should always be possible to correlate the angiographic findings with the operative appearances of the visible coronary tree with a high degree of confidence.

Positioning of the patient

For the usual sternotomy approach, the patient is positioned supine, with arms in the neutral position (between pronation and supination) at the sides. For radial artery harvesting, the appropriate arm (normally the non-dominant side) is positioned at right angles to the body with the arm supinated.

Important aspects of patient positioning are the avoidance of localized pressure (e.g. heels), care in support of the upper limbs to minimize peripheral nerve injury, and adequate restraint to allow movements necessary for gaining optimal surgical access. This applies particularly in beating-heart surgery, where positioning of the patient may be a means of maintaining cardiac output from the displaced heart.

Ensuring a sterile operating field

Basic surgical principles of aseptic operating room technique assume even greater importance when cardiopulmonary bypass is involved, with its multiple routes for bacterial ingress to the body, as well as its associated impaired immunological response. Preoperative clipping of excess hair from the planned operative fields and antiseptic skin washes precede skin preparation in the operating room. Aseptic techniques for the insertion of monitoring catheters, careful surgical draping and avoidance of contamination of the instruments or operative field are essential.

The prevalence of elderly or diabetic patients in current practice adds to the hazard of infection. The potential devascularization of tissues from electrocautery and internal thoracic artery mobilization, together with long periods of exposure of tissues to the atmosphere increase the infective risk. Prophylactic antibiotics should be viewed as a 'safety net', and not the primary strategy for ensuring recovery free from infection.

Access to the heart: sternotomy

The commonest approach to the heart for coronary surgery is by vertical sternotomy, particularly when cardiopulmonary bypass is used as an adjunct. (Minimal access incisions and lateral thoracotomy more often have a role in beating-heart procedures.) Important points in the technique of sternotomy are staying in the midline, avoiding excessive use of electrocautery, especially near skin and sternal edges, and minimizing the use of bone wax.

It is helpful to avoid incising into the xiphisternum and linea alba by cutting the lower end of the sternum to one side, particularly in obese patients. This restricts access somewhat, but reduces the risk of postoperative separation of the lower sternum. Use of clips, rather than electrocautery, when dividing internal thoracic artery branches during mobilization may reduce the risk of sternal devascularization.

If the patient has had a previous sternotomy, particular care is required to avoid damage to the underlying structures, which may include previously placed bypass conduits. Techniques and recommendations for safe reopening of the sternum are available.[85–90] Key points are division of the anterior and posterior sternal tables with an appropriate oscillating saw, elevation of the sternum during division of adhesions under vision, and wide mobilization prior to sternal spreading to prevent tearing of adherent structures.

Access to the ascending aorta and the heart is improved by pulling the pericardial edges toward the skin edges with sutures anchored through the subcutaneous tissue or wound towels. This maneuver creates a 'well' for containing cooling saline around the heart if topical cooling is part of myocardial protective strategy. This is particularly helpful when the pleural cavities are opened in the course of internal thoracic artery mobilization.

Once the heart is decompressed on cardiopulmonary bypass, access to the epicardial vessels becomes much easier, and it is not usually necessary to open the sternal retractor much more than 10–12 cm. Excessive spreading of the sternal retractor risks brachial plexus injury, costochondral dislocation, rib fractures and spraining of costo-vertebral joints – all contributors to postoperative pain and immobility.

Harvesting of conduits

INTERNAL THORACIC ARTERIES

Left internal thoracic artery preparation is common to most coronary operations. Following sternotomy, the left half of the sternum is retracted upwards using one of the specially designed retractors that are available for the purpose. Appropriate positioning of the table and use of a headlight and surgical loupes aid accurate dissection and mobilization.

The pleura is mobilized laterally to expose the internal thoracic artery, which is usually visible over at least two or three costal cartilages, and is identifiable by the prominent veins on either side. The overlying fascia provides a handle for gentle traction on the internal thoracic artery. The mediastinal fascia is incised medial to the internal thoracic artery and veins. The pedicle of artery, veins and related fat and muscle is dissected by carefully separating from the chest wall using blunt dissection and allowing the pedicle to fall away from the chest wall. This facilitates exposure of the intercostal branches. All branches are clipped with metal clips – one on the artery side and one on the chest wall side – and each branch is divided between the clips with scissors. Dissection is continued superiorly to the lower margin of the subclavian vein, and inferiorly to the major division of the internal thoracic artery into superior epigastric and musculophrenic branches, at about the level of the sixth interspace. Following mobilization of the pedicle a topical vasodilator may be applied, and the pedicle is not divided until required.

If both internal thoracic arteries are to be used, the retractors are rearranged for the right side of the sternum and a similar technique is utilized to mobilize the right vessel. Bilateral internal thoracic artery harvesting should be used with caution in the elderly, and particularly in those who are diabetic.

RADIAL ARTERIES

The left radial artery can be dissected and removed at the same time as mobilization of the left internal thoracic artery. The arm is abducted and the forearm pronated. The radial artery is dissected, together with the accompanying veins and soft tissues, dividing branches with scissors between clips. The mobilized radial artery is divided at one end and back-bleeding from the hand is confirmed before removal of the radial artery conduit. The conduit is stored in heparinized blood until required, and prior to use is gently flushed with heparinized blood. Subcutaneous tissues of the forearm are approximated with an absorbable suture prior to skin closure.

SAPHENOUS VEINS

All segments of the greater saphenous vein are commonly used for bypass conduit, but the vein below the knee is generally of more appropriate caliber and wall thickness. Vein from the lower leg is also preferable to vein from the thigh because of its greater distance from the perineum (a potential source of infection). The vein is easy to locate midway between the medial maleolus and tibialis anterior tendon. Exposure of the vein in the traditional fashion through a single long incision with minimal skin handling gives safe and easy access, though sometimes with cosmetically unattractive results. Important points in technique include keeping the skin incision directly over the vein, minimizing dissection, avoiding electrocautery, and ensuring hemostasis, thus reducing the opportunity for wound hematoma and infection. Side branches of the vein should be left long and securely ligated flush with the vein. The vein should not be directly grasped with instruments, stretched or overdistended, and is left in place until near to the time of use. It is flushed gently with heparinized blood prior to use. The saphenous nerve is closely applied to the vein in the lower leg, and should be gently separated without injuring the nerve.

Minimally invasive harvesting using endoscopic techniques,[91,92] often with only one or two short skin incisions, is feasible, effective and cosmetically acceptable, but may be slower and more expensive than the traditional method.[93,94] A number of reports indicate a lower risk of wound complications.[95–99] No deleterious effects on vein morphology[95,100] or endothelial and smooth muscle function have been reported with minimally invasive, compared to traditional open, harvesting.[101]

Cannulation for cardiopulmonary bypass

Arterial cannulation is usually at the most distal available portion of the ascending aorta. Division of the pericardial reflection enables the cannula to be placed well distally, leaving maximum space for proximal graft anastomoses. The tip of the cannula is directed into the aortic arch to minimize the risk of preferential perfusion of arch vessels. In view of the risk of atheroembolism, it is important not to place the cannula through calcified or atheromatous aortic wall. Palpation is unfortunately not an entirely reliable guide. Epi-aortic ultrasound scanning of the entire ascending aorta may reduce the risk of cannulating, cross-clamping or locating proximal anastomoses on hazardous atheromatous plaque. Though clinical proof of efficacy is still awaited, the use of an arterial cannula with integral filter, designed to trap liberated atheromatous material before it is circulated systemically (Embol-X), seems a valuable advance.[102]

Venous cannulation for systemic venous return is usually by a right atriocaval cannula, which drains blood from the inferior vena cava and the right atrium. Bi-caval cannulation, with snaring of the cavae around the cannulae, is useful if a long cross-clamp time is envisaged, and a cold cardioplegic technique supplemented with topical myocardial cooling is being used. This allows the cold cardioplegia effluent from the coronary sinus to cool the right atrium and right ventricle before being retrieved from a pulmonary artery vent.

Venting of the left heart is achieved by placing a purpose-made cannula in the ascending aorta, which is used for infusion of cardioplegia and for keeping the left ventricle decompressed by having gentle suction from a cardiotomy return sucker.

Conduct of cardiopulmonary bypass

Following the administration of heparin, and achievement of a satisfactory activated clotting time (ACT) of more than 480 seconds, cardiopulmonary bypass is commenced, ventilation is ceased and either the endotracheal tube is disconnected from the ventilator or the ventilator circuit is opened to the atmosphere. Blood temperature is reduced to the desired level in keeping with the practice of the center. During this time, the decompressed heart may be retracted to allow identification of distal target sites.

Flow rate is calculated as $2.4\,L\,m^{-1}\,min^{-1}$ at normothermia, and is reduced appropriately with hypothermia. There is a move towards using normothermic perfusion, or mild hypothermia, in some centers. Temperatures in the range of 28–34 °C are commonly used.[103–106]

Myocardial protective strategy and avoidance of injury

Blood cardioplegia and crystalloid cardioplegia are among the most popular of the many techniques for myocardial protection, though adherents of the intermittent cross-clamp fibrillation technique have shown excellent outcomes. The special problems with myocardial protection posed by coronary disease arise because of the risk of poor antegrade distribution of cardioplegic solution beyond severe or total coronary arterial obstructions. Retrograde administration of cardioplegia via the coronary sinus is a valuable technique when there is doubt about the adequacy of distribution of antegrade cardioplegia. Administration of cardioplegic solution via conduits inserted into the most severely obstructed coronary arteries is a further aid to achieving effective distribution of cardioplegia. With cold cardioplegic arrest, topical cooling of the heart is often used as an adjunct to cardioplegic protection. This is achieved by immersing the heart in cold saline within the pericardial well. Ice slush should probably be avoided, as excessive cooling risks damage to the phrenic nerves. Radial and internal thoracic artery conduits should not be exposed to excessive cooling as it may induce spasm.

Distension of the left ventricle is dangerous to the heart. Such distension can be induced by excessive bradycardia in the initial stages of surgery, or by leakage of cardioplegic solution through the aortic valve during infusion into the aortic root. Constant awareness of the state of the left ventricle is required to detect distension at an early stage. A functioning aortic root vent should prevent distension, but if it occurs, gentle compression of the left ventricle is needed.

Undue traction or twisting of the heart is a further source of injury to the myocardium. An important lesson from beating-heart surgery is that the heart can be very considerably displaced from its natural position without impeding its function, provided it is moved gently and gradually. These same precautions should be applied when exposing the coronary arteries, even when the heart is arrested.

Air in the coronary tree will impair myocardial perfusion. Grafts should be emptied of air by allowing backbleeding before completion of conduit anastomosis to the aorta. If there are obvious and excessive air bubbles in the conduits at the time of reperfusion, a small needle inserted into the graft will allow the air to escape. Otherwise, suspected air in the coronary arteries can be dissipated by allowing the heart to beat for several minutes while supported on cardiopulmonary bypass.

Akinetic or aneurysmal areas of the left ventricle may be lined with thrombus on the endocardial side. It is important not to handle these areas to avoid the risk of dislodging thrombus. Once the aorta has been cross-clamped and cardioplegia has been administered, any significant akinetic or aneurysmal area is opened and the interior aspect is inspected. If thrombus is present, it is removed and the scarred area is closed with strong, Teflon-buttressed sutures.

Loose atheromatous material can sometimes be identified in the effluent from the opened coronary artery during infusion of cardioplegia into the aortic root. This emphasizes the ease with which coronary atheroembolism can occur. Atheroembolism is particularly likely if previously placed, patent, diseased saphenous vein bypass grafts are handled or disturbed in any way.[27,28] Ligation of such grafts at an early stage of the re-operation, or early opening at their distal end, and retrograde rather than prograde administration of cardioplegia have all been advocated for reducing this risk.

Exposure and identification of target sites

The need for gentleness in retraction of the heart must be emphasized. The heart should be decompressed before it is retracted. A further useful lesson from beating-heart surgery is the value of placing sutures in the posterior pericardium on the left side and using them to pull the heart forward into view for exposure of the circumflex vessels. Before the heart is arrested, target vessels are marked with a scalpel to avoid identification error when the heart is empty and displaced. Precise location of the arteriotomy on the vessel involves judgment; a relatively straight, disease-free segment beyond angiographically demonstrated significant stenosis should be selected whenever possible. Angiographically demonstrable *significant stenosis* is not synonymous with *visibly diseased areas* apparent at surgery; it is often not practical to bypass all diseased segments.

Difficulty in finding the distal target is not uncommon with the anterior descending artery, which may be intramuscular or may be obscured by fat. Careful dissection over the anticipated course of the artery will often be successful. If not, a small incision into the artery near the apex (where it is nearly always visible) allows introduction of a small coronary probe that can be carefully advanced and palpated to facilitate more proximal exposure of the artery. This should not be done if the vessel is tortuous. However, the intramyocardial anterior descending artery is often relatively straight and a probe can usually be passed with care. The distal arteriotomy is subsequently closed by direct suture. Alternatively, dissection in a proximal direction over a diagonal vessel will lead to the anterior descending artery. Location of target areas should be undertaken before cross-clamping of the aorta, as dissection to find arteries may be time consuming.

The intermediate artery and the obtuse marginal branches of the circumflex artery often run below the epicardial surface in an intramyocardial location. They can usually be identified by the characteristic lighter color of the myocardium along the course of the vessel. Alternatively, as the proximal portions of these vessels are usually visible near their origins, they can be traced by dissection over the vessel, beginning at the place where the vessel disappears below the surface. The artery is frequently free from disease when it is intramyocardial, and conduit anastomosis can be undertaken in such a location.

The distal anastomosis

In general, the least accessible anastomoses (usually to lateral circumflex vessels) are constructed first to minimize the risk of exposure of the vessel inflicting inadvertent damage to grafts that have already been inserted. It may also be advisable to bypass the most critical stenoses early in the procedure to allow cardioplegia infusion via the conduits to the jeopardized myocardium that may be suboptimally perfused by antegrade administration via the aortic root.

The distal target artery is opened in its midline with a sharp scalpel. There are excellent purpose-designed scalpels available that are suitable for small thin-walled arteries. The midline of the vessel is usually identifiable by a pink or bluish color (Figure 11.13). Care is required to avoid damage to the posterior vessel wall. If the artery is opened while still filled with cardioplegic solution, there is less risk of posterior wall injury. Aortic root vent suction will usually clear the anastomotic site once the artery has been opened. Potts scissors are then used to extend the arteriotomy to approximately 3–5 mm in length, commensurate with the diameter of the artery (Figure 11.14).

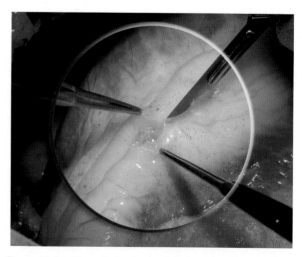

Figure 11.13 *The anterior descending artery has been exposed by incising the epicardium over it. The pink color of the lumen indicates the line of arteriotomy.*

Inadvertent injury to the posterior wall of the artery during opening should be handled by extending the arteriotomy slightly proximal and distal to the injury site. A fine (7/0) suture is placed from outside the artery into the lumen adjacent to the injury and the suture is used to approximate the edges of the injury region, before being passed outside again for tying. This achieves repair, prevents dissection or hematoma and minimizes the amount of suture material exposed to the blood (Figure 11.15).

Limited coronary endarterectomy may be required when localized plaque is apparent at the anastomotic site once the artery has been opened if it is at risk of delaminating during suturing, even if the lumen is of adequate size.

The choice of appropriate conduit is important, matching lumen size and wall thickness as far as possible. The end of the conduit is bevelled at about 45° and the 'heel' of the conduit may be cut back in line with the vessel if it is necessary to enlarge the conduit end to match the arteriotomy.

Interrupted sutures are recommended by some groups if the coronary artery is of small caliber and particularly if the wall is thin and delicate. The interrupted suture technique requires care and coordination by the surgical team, but avoids the risk, inherent in the continuous technique, of constricting the anastomotic area (Figure 11.16).

Precision in constructing the anastomosis is of over-riding importance. Magnification, good lighting, a clear surgical field and attention to detail are all essential. A continuous suture technique is used by most surgeons. It is quicker and simpler than the interrupted technique and

gives precision if care is taken to avoid undue tension on the suture. The most vulnerable parts of the anastomosis are at the 'heel' and at the 'toe'. Unduly wide spacing of sutures in these areas can result in constriction of the coronary artery at that site.

The author's preference is to keep the end of the conduit close to the arteriotomy during suturing (Figure 11.17). Sutures are placed at the heel first, with the conduit and coronary artery apart (Figure 11.18). After pulling the conduit and artery together, suturing is

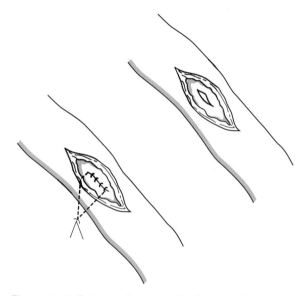

Figure 11.15 *Technique for repair of inadvertent injury to the posterior wall of the coronary artery.*

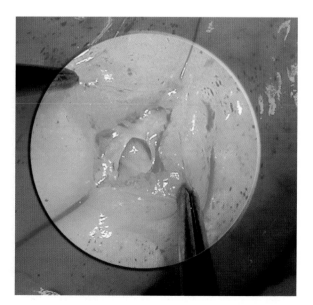

Figure 11.14 *The anterior descending artery has been opened for about 4 mm.*

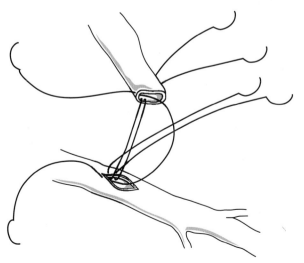

Figure 11.16 *Multiple double-armed sutures are placed through corresponding points in the conduit and the coronary artery in the interrupted technique of anastomosis.*

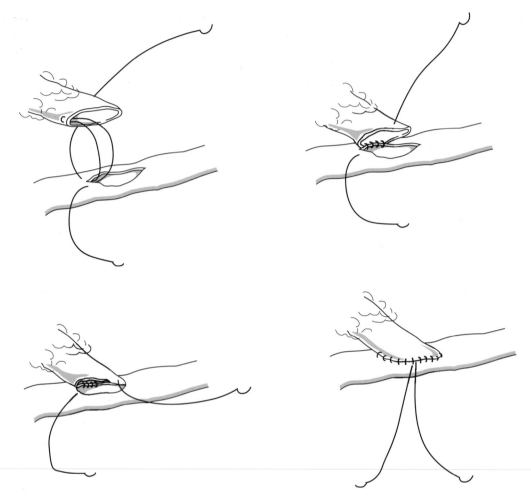

Figure 11.17 *The continuous suture technique for conduit–coronary anastomosis starting at the 'heel'.*

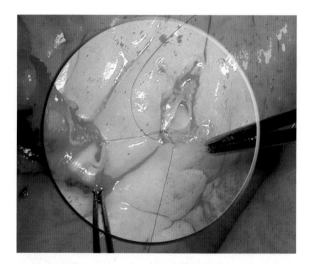

Figure 11.18 *A double-armed 7/0 polypropylene suture has been placed through the internal mammary artery at the heel end of the bevelled artery from outside. The sutures emerge inside the artery and are passed through the proximal end of the coronary arteriotomy in an anterior descending artery from inside to out.*

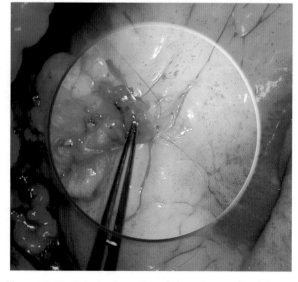

Figure 11.19 *Suturing is continued along the margin of the arteriotomy furthest from the surgeon.*

continued to the toe along the edge furthest away (Figures 11.19 and 11.20) and a little around the toe (Figure 11.21) before changing needles and completing the edge nearest to the surgeon (Figures 11.22 and 11.23). This is particularly applicable to the anterior descending artery. If the artery is running across the surgical field, as in the case of an obtuse marginal circumflex vessel, the suture may be conveniently commenced in the middle of the arteriotomy on the wall furthest from the surgeon (Figures 11.24–11.31). For a right coronary

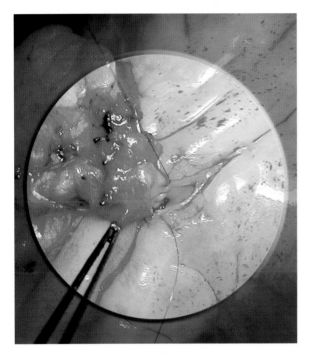

Figure 11.20 *The first quarter of the anastomosis is complete.*

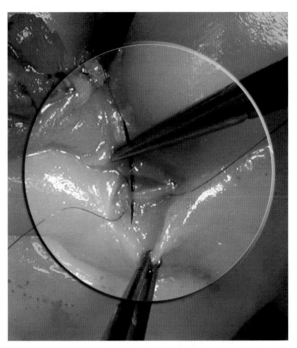

Figure 11.22 *Using the other needle, the anastomosis is continued from the 'heel' along the margin nearest the surgeon.*

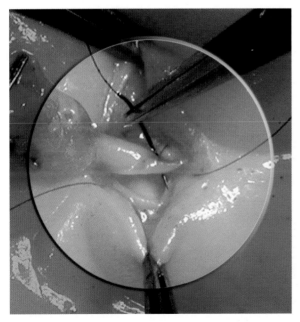

Figure 11.21 *The suture has been continued to the 'toe' and will be continued a short way along the margin nearest the surgeon.*

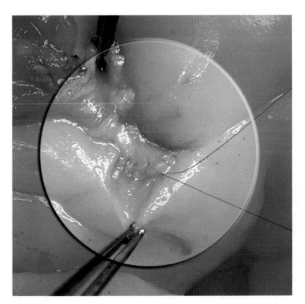

Figure 11.23 *The suture line is completed and the sutures are gently tensioned prior to ligation.*

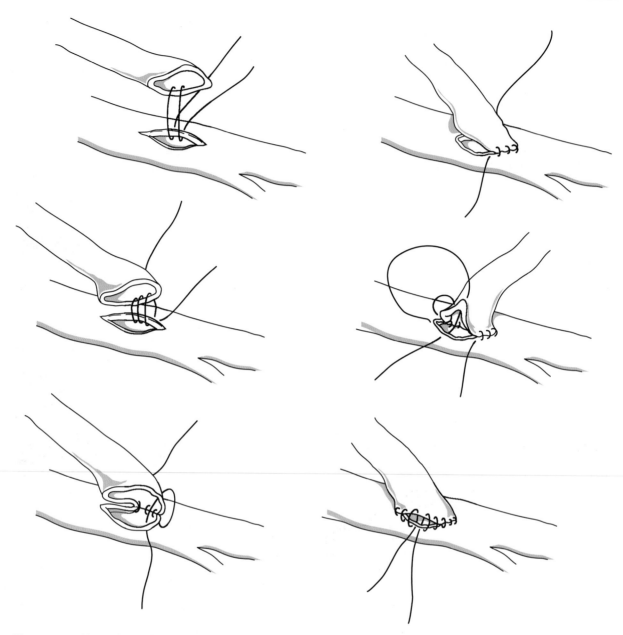

Figure 11.24 *Alternative continuous suture technique appropriate when the vessel runs from side to side across operating field.*

artery, which is running away from the surgeon, the suture is usually most conveniently commenced near the toe of the anastomosis (Figures 11.32–11.37, pages 179 and 180).

If the coronary lumen is narrow and the walls are thin, or if residual coronary blood is troublesome, it is often helpful to insert an appropriately sized coronary occluder into the coronary artery. This ensures that sutures are not encroaching into the lumen and helps to display the edges of the arteriotomy. The occluder is gently extracted before the anastomosing suture is tied.

Twisting and tension of the pedicled internal thoracic artery are prevented by suturing the peri-arterial thoracic fascia to the epicardium close to the anastomosis site.

The proximal anastomosis

Proximal anastomoses between the ascending aorta and free grafts are made with the patient still on cardiopulmonary bypass, using the time for rewarming, recovery from cardioplegic arrest, and allowing the non-working heart to beat without stimulation of pacing or inotropes. If necessary, a defibrillating shock is applied for conversion of ventricular fibrillation to regular rhythm, but a heart that has been well protected by cardioplegia will often beat spontaneously when reperfused. A side-biting clamp is applied, with the blood pressure temporarily lowered by slowing arterial input

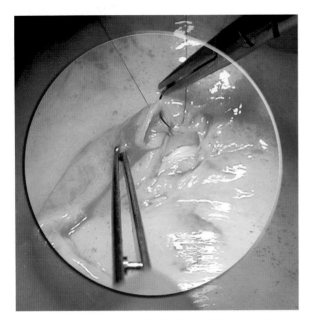

Figure 11.25 *A double-armed 7/0 polypropylene suture has been used to commence anastomosis of a saphenous vein conduit in the middle of the arteriotomy in the obtuse marginal branch of a circumflex artery.*

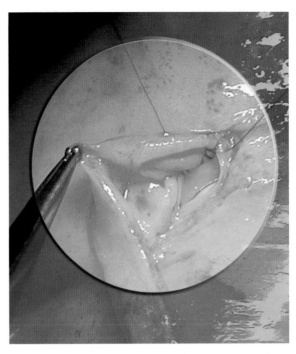

Figure 11.27 *Sutures have been placed around the 'toe' of the anastomosis.*

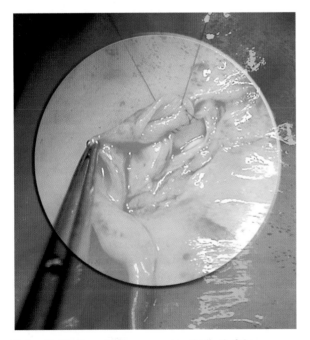

Figure 11.26 *The suturing approaches the 'toe' of the anastomosis.*

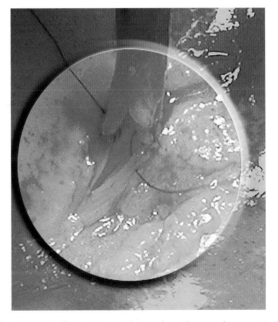

Figure 11.28 *The suture continues along the margin nearest the surgeon.*

from the pump. If at all possible, all proximal anastomoses are constructed with a single application of a side-biting clamp in order to minimize the risk of damage to a potentially diseased aorta and atheroembolism. Purpose-designed punches are available for removing a disc of aorta of appropriate size commensurate with the conduit. Proximal anastomoses may be made before commencing cardiopulmonary bypass, but the author's preference is to complete the distal anastomoses first.

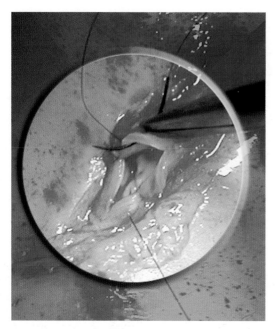

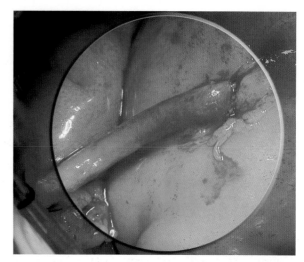

Figure 11.31 *The venous conduit is flushed with blood to confirm hemostasis and easy flow into the distal coronary bed.*

Figure 11.29 *Using the other needle, the remainder of the anastomosis is commenced towards the heel end.*

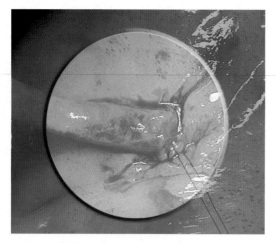

Figure 11.30 *The suture is tensioned prior to ligation.*

The heart should be distended to working dimensions (by temporarily restricting venous drainage to the extracorporeal circuit) before the conduit is cut to appropriate length prior to proximal anastomosis. The conduit is gently distended with a syringe to exclude the possibility of twisting. If back-bleeding is excessive, a soft vascular clamp is applied to the conduit.

The anastomosis is commenced at the heel of the beveled and slightly cut back conduit. With the sutures placed first through the conduit and then through the aorta, the endothelium of the conduit is pulled into the aorta, minimizing the area of cut aortic wall exposed to the blood (Figures 11.38 and 11.39). The suture is then continued around the edge of the aortic opening (Figure 11.40, page 181) and the two ends meet at the toe of the anastomosis and are tied after allowing back-bleeding to flush out air from the conduit (Figure 11.41, page 181).

Strategies to deal with the diseased or crowded aorta include avoidance of the aorta altogether, by siting the proximal ends of grafts onto the pedicled left or right internal thoracic artery, or onto the proximal end of a previously placed saphenous vein graft in repeat surgery.

Sequential grafting

There are circumstances in which it may be advantageous to anastomose a conduit to more than one distal coronary target – the procedure of sequential grafting. The advantages are:

- More efficient use can be made of scarce conduit. This may be particularly helpful in repeat coronary surgery, where previous surgery has left fewer options for conduit harvesting, or where potential conduits are diseased or missing (e.g. varicose veins or previous vein stripping).
- Scope for arterial grafting can be widened. Sequential grafting of a large, jeopardized diagonal artery together with the anterior descending artery using the left internal thoracic artery, or sequential grafting of two lateral circumflex branches using a radial artery, may make it possible to achieve predominant or even total arterial revascularization.
- A relatively small vessel that would be a questionable target may be revascularized by side-to-side anastomosis from a conduit that supplies a larger, predictable target, thus making complete revascularization more likely.

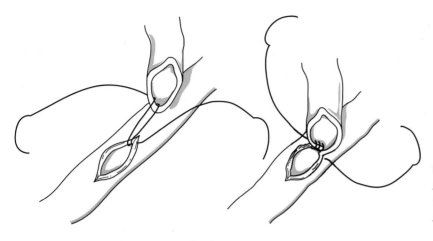

Figure 11.32 *Alternative continuous suture technique starting at the toe end for an artery running away from the surgeon.*

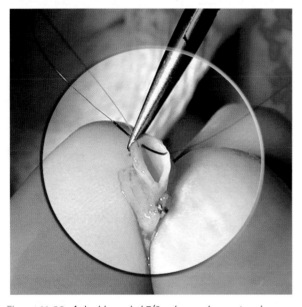

Figure 11.33 *A double-ended 7/0 polypropylene suture is placed at the toe end of a bevelled radial artery conduit from outside to inside.*

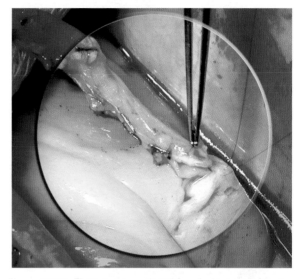

Figure 11.34 *The sutures are placed from inside to outside at the toe end of an arteriotomy in the distal right artery.*

- When a venous or radial conduit is used for sequential grafting, only one aortic anastomosis is required. This saves operative time and is helpful when suitable aortic sites are limited by disease or prior surgery.

Care is needed in the planning of sequential grafting, and judgment is necessary in selecting anastomotic sites on the conduit and the target coronary artery. The graft should end as an end-to-side anastomosis with a large coronary target (to ensure good flow down the length of the conduit). Undue angulation, or twisting, at the site of side-to-side anastomoses must be avoided, as must kinking or tension between anastomoses.

The most distal end-to-side anastomosis is constructed first. This makes it possible to confirm leak-free flow into the distal target vessel and also allows the conduit to be distended gently to ensure that it is not twisted. The proposed anastomotic site for the next coronary artery target is then selected. Ideally, the conduit should lie approximately in line with the target coronary artery, as this makes it possible to have a longer anastomosis and reduces the risks of conduit constriction and distortion.

It is possible to anastomose a conduit to an artery that crosses at right angles to the conduit. The coronary arteriotomy should then be relatively short (3–4 mm) and the opening in the conduit should be made in the same direction as the corresponding coronary artery. If this requires a transverse opening in the conduit, it is important to ensure that the diameter of the conduit is at least twice that of the planned opening in order to avoid constriction of the conduit.

Several side-to-side anastomoses between conduit and coronary artery targets are possible. In general, coronary

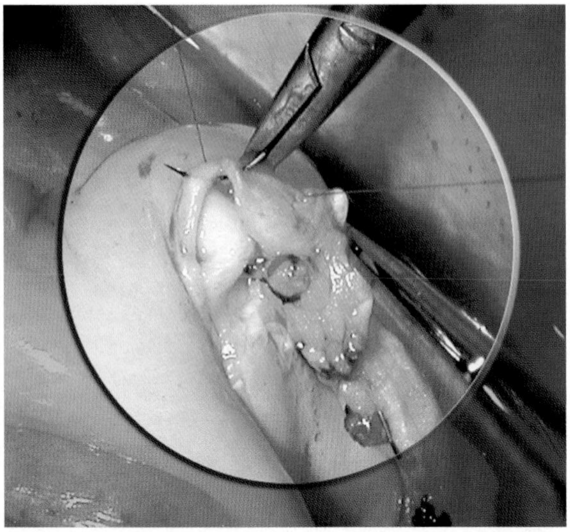

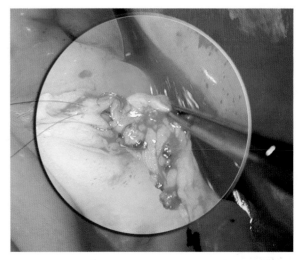

Figure 11.35 *Suturing commences along the first quadrant of the anastomosis.*

Figure 11.37 *Suturing is completed prior to tensioning of the suture and ligation.*

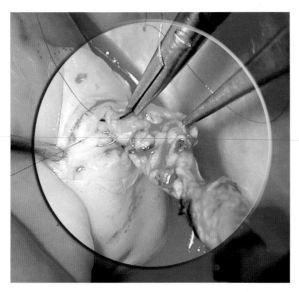

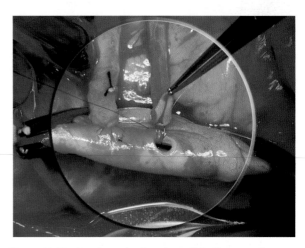

Figure 11.36 *The final quadrant is being completed towards the heel end.*

Figure 11.38 *Anastomosis of a vein graft to the ascending aorta. The suture commences at the 'heel' of the anastomosis, passing a double-ended 6/0 polypropylene suture through the vein conduit from outside to inside and from inside the aorta to outside. One vein graft anastomosis has been completed.*

targets lying deep in fat or muscle are unsatisfactory for side-to-side anastomosis with conduit. A technical problem arising at a proximally located anastomosis can jeopardize all distally located anastomoses. Thus, whenever there is doubt about the technical feasibility of undertaking sequential grafting, the distal targets should be individually bypassed with separate conduits.

In theory, the greater flow to be anticipated in a graft when it supplies more than one target coronary artery should reduce the risk of early thrombotic occlusion, which may affect individual conduits supplying the same distal targets. In practice, the use of sequential grafting has been shown to be associated with good graft patency.[107]

Routing of conduits

When planning the route of a conduit, it is important to avoid the conduit being too short or too long. A conduit that looks satisfactory with the heart empty may be stretched as the heart distends. This may twist, distort, occlude or tear the distal anastomosis.

An aid to correct judgment of conduit length is the placement of a suture or tape along the proposed conduit route to the anticipated coronary target over the beating heart prior to commencing cardiopulmonary bypass. The suture or tape is cut to the desired length and acts as a guide to the length of conduit required.

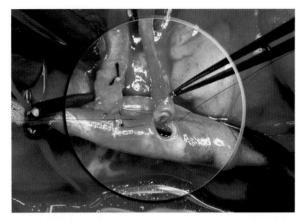

Figure 11.39 *When the sutures are tensioned, the vein graft is pulled into the aortic opening, bringing together intima of vein and aorta.*

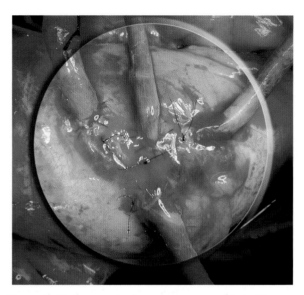

Figure 11.41 *Four proximal anastomoses completed with a single application of a side-biting clamp.*

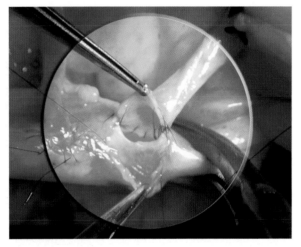

Figure 11.40 *The sutures are continued around the margins, to be tied at the toe end.*

In general, conduits running between the ascending aorta and a distal coronary artery should take a similar route to the grafted coronary artery, though with gentle curving to allow for cardiac distension. Typical conduit routes are illustrated in Figure 11.42.

Conduits anastomosed to descending limbs of the left ventricular branch of a dominant right artery often lie better, and with less chance of kinking, if routed behind the inferior vena cava. The conduit is then brought alongside the right atrium up to the right side of the ascending aorta.

The transverse sinus sometimes provides a preferable route for conduits to the circumflex branches (rather than around the left side of the heart and over the pulmonary artery), particularly when the heart is enlarged. If this route is used, the proximal anastomosis to the aorta should be located as far posteriorly as is feasible to

avoid kinking of the graft. The increased distortion of the ascending aorta necessary for applying a side-biting clamp in this position makes it advisable to lower arterial pressure during the proximal anastomosis. This route should be avoided if the aorta is diseased.

Endarterectomy

Coronary endarterectomy can often be successful in restoring a suitable lumen for anastomosing a graft, even if the proposed target vessel is totally occluded. The vessel (not necessarily its lumen) must be large (ideally 2 or 3 mm in diameter) for endarterectomy to be practical (Figure 11.43). If there is a suitable, adequately sized, patent, more distal segment of the artery, it is usually preferable to place a bypass graft to this segment rather than undertake endarterectomy. As endarterectomy is not a predictably successful procedure, surgery should be undertaken with caution if its success depends solely on the outcome of endarterectomy. Generally, there should be at least one other suitable major bypass target in another territory, which can be confidently bypassed, to avoid the risk of not being able to achieve any worthwhile bypass.

The artery is incised longitudinally until a lumen is encountered or until it is apparent that extensive atheroma is present without a lumen (Figure 11.44). A plane of dissection is developed between the atheromatous core and the remnants of the arterial wall, which is invariably extremely thin and often translucent. A blunt dissector is carefully inserted into this cleavage plane and the atheromatous core is freed from the wall of the artery (Figure 11.45). As soon as is possible, the core is grasped with

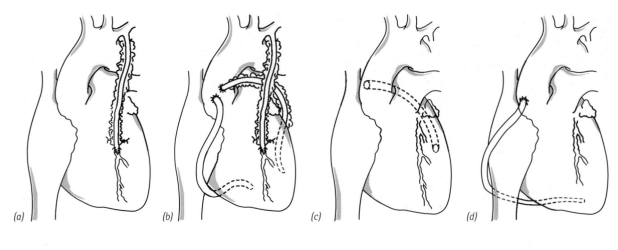

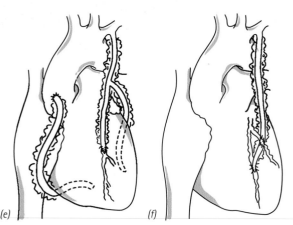

Figure 11.42 *Typical routes for coronary conduits. (a) Pedicled left internal thoracic artery to anterior descending artery. (b) Pedicled left internal thoracic artery to anterior descending artery, radial artery graft to obtuse marginal branch of circumflex and saphenous vein graft to distal right/posterior descending. (c) Conduit from posterior aspect of aorta via transverse sinus to obtuse marginal branch of circumflex. (d) Conduit to postero-lateral branch routed posterior to inferior vena cava. (e) Pedicled left internal thoracic artery to anterior descending artery, free right internal thoracic artery anastomosed to left internal thoracic artery, and radial artery graft to distal right artery. (f) Pedicled left internal thoracic artery anastomosed sequentially to diagonal and anterior descending arteries.*

blunt forceps (fine forceps will cut through the core: Figure 11.46). Gentle traction in the line of the vessel, aided by stroking of the vessel with a small swab (Figure 11.47), is usually rewarded by extraction of a tapering core of atheroma (Figure 11.48). If the core breaks off, it can sometimes be retrieved by a fine forceps within the lumen, but usually it is necessary to extend the arteriotomy to reach the residual core, or to make a second arteriotomy over the remaining atheromatous core.

It is possible to disobliterate occluded coronary arteries by endarterectomy anywhere in the coronary tree in this fashion (Figures 11.49–11.54). The proximal vessel should be disobliterated if possible, sufficiently to clear the anastomotic site. A bypass conduit should be anastomosed to the arteriotomy site. (Although it is sometimes possible to open the artery proximally, this is not generally advisable, as it is theoretically likely to increase the risk of bypass conduit occlusion.)

An alternative way of dealing with extensive coronary disease is opening the artery for as much as 5 or 6 cm and removing the atheromatous core by direct dissection. A patch is used to close the long arteriotomy. This patch is formed by the opened end of a bypass conduit (venous

or arterial), and the conduit perfuses the disobliterated artery. This technique is appropriate when a suitable core of atheroma cannot be extracted through a short arteriotomy.[108–111]

Weaning from cardiopulmonary bypass; heparin reversal

Once the heart is beating regularly at adequate rate and the systemic temperature is normal, cardiopulmonary bypass is gradually withdrawn. Excessive bradycardia should be avoided by the use of atropine, inotropic support or temporary pacing. Once all suture lines have been confirmed to be blood-tight, and the aortic and venous cannulas have been removed, heparin is reversed with protamine.

Chest closure and drainage

The pericardium is left open to avoid possible compression of grafts. On the left side, an incision is made laterally from the cut edge in the pericardium and its

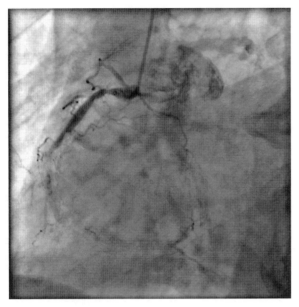

Figure 11.43 *Left anterior oblique view of right coronary artery shows occlusion at junction of proximal and mid-thirds, with very faint filling of the distal vessel which is calcified in places. The large proximal lumen suggests the possibility of endarterectomy, for the distal artery.*

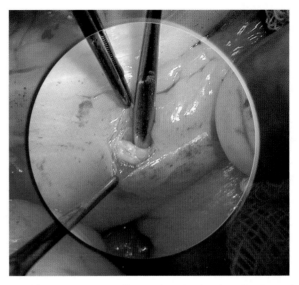

Figure 11.45 *A Watson–Cheyne dissector develops the plane of dissection.*

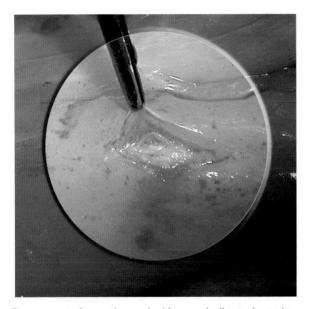

Figure 11.44 *An arteriotomy in this severely diseased anterior descending artery showing separation of atheromatous core from adventitia.*

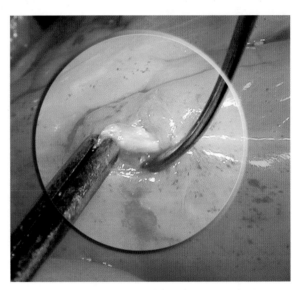

Figure 11.46 *The atheromatous core is grasped with a blunt Lahey forceps.*

overlying fat (taking care to avoid phrenic nerve injury) to allow a direct course for the left internal thoracic artery to the anterior descending artery. The pericardium is re-approximated at its free edge to keep the internal thoracic artery close to the heart and out of harm's way in the event of future surgery. The pleural space is widely opened to allow the left lung to expand anterior to the left internal thoracic artery pedicle, further reducing the risk of tension on the pedicle and keeping the pedicle away from the chest wall.

Chest drains are placed via stab incisions in the epigastric region – usually one into each opened pleural space and one into the anterior mediastinum.

Secure re-apposition of the two halves of the sternum is essential in ensuring prompt healing. This is not always easy to achieve in the obese, particularly when the upper part of the sternum has been elevated for internal thoracic artery mobilization. A number of techniques for

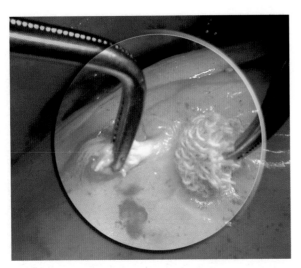

Figure 11.47 *Traction on the core is supplemented with counter-traction over the artery using a small swab.*

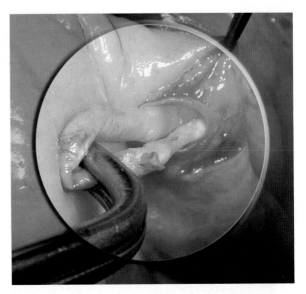

Figure 11.49 *This heavily diseased distal right artery has been opened and removal of the atheromatous core is in progress.*

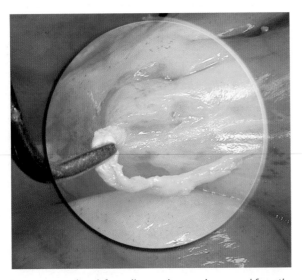

Figure 11.48 *A satisfactorily tapering core is removed from the distal artery.*

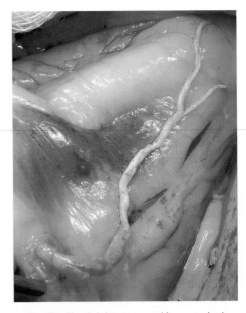

Figure 11.50 *The distal right artery and its posterior branch have been extensively disobliterated.*

sternal closure have been advocated and assessed in controlled laboratory conditions.[112–114] In the author's practice, heavy gauge (No. 7) stainless steel wires give secure closure. Two sutures are placed in the manubrium, passing through the bone well away from the cut edge. A further six sutures are placed around the body of the sternum and are twisted to approximate the sternum accurately and securely.

Postoperative management

Early postoperative management is directed at the observation of hemodynamic function, ventilatory adequacy, blood loss, urine output and fluid balance. The aim is to identify deviations from normal anticipated recovery patterns in order to intervene with appropriate therapy at an early stage. Inotropic support should not be delayed if there is any reason to expect poor cardiac output, or if the blood pressure, heart rate or cardiac output shows signs of falling to abnormal levels. Excessive blood loss is best managed by early re-opening of the sternotomy wound to identify localized bleeding sources, unless a correctable coagulation defect can be identified. Relief of pain and anxiety and early return to normal activity are important aspects of postoperative management.

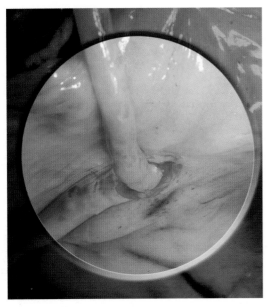

Figure 11.51 *The arteriotomy in the right artery has been anastomosed to a vein graft in this case.*

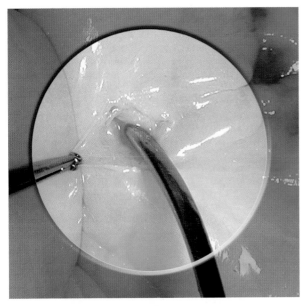

Figure 11.52 *Disobliteration of an occluded obtuse marginal branch of circumflex is started.*

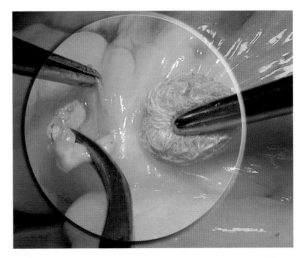

Figure 11.53 *Extraction of the core from the distal vessel is proceeding.*

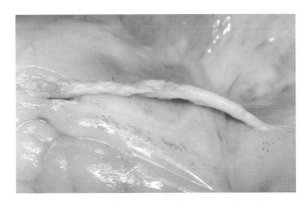

Figure 11.54 *The distal segment has been opened, with extraction of a satisfactorily tapering atheromatous plug.*

Strategies to enhance the outcome of coronary surgery

Although the adequacy of revascularization, choice of bypass conduits and conduct of surgical maneuvers are major influences on outcome, there are other important aspects of care that will enhance results. Ensuring good understanding by the patient of the disease and the operative procedure, optimizing co-morbid state and controlling unstable coronary syndromes will all improve the immediate outcome.

The early introduction of antiplatelet therapy has been shown to reduce early graft thrombosis. Preventative measures to combat disease progression in conduits and coronary arteries, as well as to retard myocardial deterioration, have an important influence on long-term outcome.

KEY REFERENCES

Barner HB, Sundt TM III, Bailey M, Zang Y. Midterm results of complete arterial revascularization in more than 1,000 patients using an internal thoracic artery/radial artery T graft. *Ann Surg* 2001; **234**:447–52.
One of the longer term outcome studies of the use of arterial revascularization, including the radial artery; provides powerful evidence for the safety and efficacy of the radial artery conduit.

Cameron A, Davis KB, Green G, Schaff HV. Coronary bypass surgery with internal-thoracic-artery grafts – effects on survival over a 15-year period. *N Engl J Med* 1996; **334**:216–19.

The Coronary Artery Surgery Study provides one of the best repositories of information on coronary disease and its management and outcomes. This paper highlights the value of this study and provides confirmation of the landmark paper from Loop's group a decade earlier firmly establishing the benefits of the internal thoracic artery conduit.

Eagle KA, Guyton RA, Davidoff R, Ewy GA, Fonger J, Gardner TJ, *et al.* ACC/AHA Guidelines for Coronary Artery Bypass Graft Surgery. A Report of the American College of Cardiology/American Heart Association Task Force on Practice Guidelines (Committee to Revise the 1991 Guidelines for Coronary Artery Bypass Graft Surgery). American College of Cardiology/ American Heart Association [Review – 753 refs]. *J Am Coll Cardiol* 1999; **34**:1262–347.

Essential reading and source of references for all coronary surgeons – a summary of 'state of the art' at the end of the twentieth century.

Leavitt BJ, O'Connor GT, Olmstead EM, Morton JR, Maloney CT, Dacey LJ, *et al.* Use of the internal mammary artery graft and in-hospital mortality and other adverse outcomes associated with coronary artery bypass surgery. *Circulation* 2001; **103**:507–12.

The Northern New England Cardiovascular Disease Study Group has used its extensive database and collaboration among six medical centers to report important lessons from coronary surgery practice. This example has the novelty of reinforcing the value of the internal thoracic artery conduit in enhancing perioperative outcome, in addition to its well-known long-term benefit.

Motwani JG, Topol EJ. Aortocoronary saphenous vein graft disease: pathogenesis, predisposition, and prevention. [Review – 133 refs.] *Circulation* 1998; **97**:916–31.

A comprehensive, well-referenced review of the problems and potential solutions associated with the conduits for coronary surgery.

REFERENCES

1. Eagle KA, Guyton RA, Davidoff R, Ewy GA, Fonger J, Gardner TJ, *et al.* ACC/AHA Guidelines for Coronary Artery Bypass Graft Surgery: A Report of the American College of Cardiology/American Heart Association Task Force on Practice Guidelines (Committee to Revise the 1991 Guidelines for Coronary Artery Bypass Graft Surgery). American College of Cardiology/American Heart Association. [Review – 753 refs.] *J Am Coll Cardiol* 1999; 34:1262–347.
2. Fihn SD, Williams SV, Daley J, Gibbons RJ, American College of Cardiology, American Heart Association, *et al.* Guidelines for the management of patients with chronic stable angina: treatment. *Ann Intern Med* 2001; 135(8 Pt 1):616–32.
3. Gibbons RJ, Chatterjee K, Daley J, Douglas JS, Fihn SD, Gardin JM, *et al.* ACC/AHA/ACP-ASIM guidelines for the management of patients with chronic stable angina: a report of the American College of Cardiology/American Heart Association Task Force on Practice Guidelines (Committee on Management of Patients With Chronic Stable Angina). *J Am Coll Cardiol* 1999; 33: 2092–197.
4. Pretre R, Turina MI. Choice of revascularization strategy for patients with coronary artery disease. *JAMA* 2001; 285:992–4.
5. Altman JD, Bache RJ. The coronary collateral circulation. *ACC Curr J Rev* 1997; 6:17–21.
6. Kersten JR, Pagel PS, Chilian WM, Warltier DC. Multifactorial basis for coronary collateralization: a complex adaptive response to ischemia. [Review – 149 refs.] *Cardiovasc Res* 1999; 43:44–57.
7. Favaloro RG. Saphenous vein graft in the surgical treatment of coronary artery disease. Operative technique. *J Thorac Cardiovasc Surg* 1969; 58:178–85.
8. Johnson WD, Lepley D Jr. An aggressive surgical approach to coronary disease. *J Thorac Cardiovasc Surg* 1970; 59:128–38.
9. Aldridge HE, Trimble AS. Progression of proximal coronary artery lesions to total occlusion after aorta-coronary saphenous vein bypass grafting. *J Thorac Cardiovasc Surg* 1971; 62:7–11.
10. Griffith LS, Achuff SC, Conti CR, Humphries JO, Brawley RK, Gott VL, *et al.* Changes in intrinsic coronary circulation and segmental ventricular motion after saphenous-vein coronary bypass graft surgery. *N Engl J Med* 1973; 288:589–95.
11. Maurer BJ, Oberman A, Holt JH Jr, Kouchoukos NT, Jones WB, Russell RO Jr, *et al.* Changes in grafted and nongrafted coronary arteries following saphenous vein bypass grafting. *Circulation* 1974; 50:293–300.
12. Glassman E, Spencer FC, Krauss KR, Weisinger B, Isom OW. Changes in the underlying coronary circulation secondary to bypass grafting. *Circulation* 1974; 50(2 Suppl.):II80–3.
13. Kakos GS, Oldham HN Jr, Dixon SH Jr, Davis RW, Hagen PO, Sabiston DC Jr. Coronary artery hemodynamics after aortocoronary artery vein bypass. An experimental evaluation. *J Thorac Cardiovasc Surg* 1972; 63:849–53.
14. Furuse A, Klopp EH, Brawley RK, Gott VL. Hemodynamics of aorta-to-coronary artery bypass. Experimental and analytical studies. *Ann Thorac Surg* 1972; 14:282–93.
15. Bourassa MG, Lesperance J, Corbara F, Saltiel J, Campeau L. Progression of obstructive coronary artery disease 5 to 7 years after aortocoronary bypass surgery. *Circulation* 1978; 58(Suppl. I):I100–6.
16. Bourassa MG, Enjalbert M, Campeau L, Lesperance J. Progression of atherosclerosis in coronary arteries and bypass grafts: ten years later. *Am J Cardiol* 1984; 53:102–7C.
17. Palac RT, Hwang MH, Meadows WR, Croke RP, Pifarre R, Loeb HS, *et al.* Progression of coronary artery disease in medically and surgically treated patients 5 years after randomization. *Circulation* 1981; 64(2 Pt 2):II17–21.
18. Frick MH, Valle M, Harjola PT. Progression of coronary artery disease in randomized medical and surgical patients over a 5-year angiographic follow-up. *Am J Cardiol* 1983; 52:681–5.
19. Alderman EL, Corley SD, Fisher LD, Chaitman BR, Faxon DP, Foster ED, *et al.* Five-year angiographic follow-up of factors associated with progression of coronary artery disease in the Coronary Artery Surgery Study (CASS). CASS Participating Investigators and Staff. *J Am Coll Cardiol* 1993; 22:1141–54.
20. Cosgrove DM, Loop FD, Saunders CL, Lytle BW, Kramer JR. Should coronary arteries with less than fifty percent stenosis be bypassed? *J Thorac Cardiovasc Surg* 1981; 82:520–30.

21. Hamada Y, Kawachi K, Yamamoto T, Nakata T, Kashu Y, Watanabe Y, et al. Effect of coronary artery bypass grafting on native coronary artery stenosis. Comparison of internal thoracic artery and saphenous vein grafts. J Cardiovasc Surg 2001; 42:159–64.

22. Singh RN, Beg RA, Kay EB. Physiological adaptability: the secret of success of the internal mammary artery grafts. Ann Thorac Surg 1986; 41:247–50.

23. Nwasokwa ON. Coronary artery bypass graft disease. [Review – 148 refs.] Ann Intern Med 1995; 123:528–45.

24. Motwani JG, Topol EJ. Aortocoronary saphenous vein graft disease: pathogenesis, predisposition, and prevention. [Review – 133 refs.] Circulation 1998; 97:916–31.

25. Grondin CM, Campeau L, Thornton JC, Engle JC, Cross FS, Schreiber H. Coronary artery bypass grafting with saphenous vein. [Review – 62 refs.] Circulation 1989; 79(6 Pt 2):I24–9.

26. Chen L, Theroux P, Lesperance J, Shabani F, Thibault B, De Guise P. Angiographic features of vein grafts versus ungrafted coronary arteries in patients with unstable angina and previous bypass surgery. J Am Coll Cardiol 1996; 28:1493–9.

27. Loop FD, Lytle BW, Cosgrove DM, Woods EL, Stewart RW, Golding LA, et al. Re-operation for coronary atherosclerosis. Changing practice in 2509 consecutive patients. Ann Surg 1990; 212:378–85.

28. Fitzgibbon GM, Kafka HP, Leach AJ, Keon WJ, Hooper GD, Burton JR. Coronary bypass graft fate and patient outcome: angiographic follow-up of 5,065 grafts related to survival and re-operation in 1,388 patients during 25 years. J Am Coll Cardiol 1996; 28:616–26.

29. Souza DS, Bomfim V, Skoglund H, Dashwood MR, Borowiec JW, Bodin, L et al. High early patency of saphenous vein graft for coronary artery bypass harvested with surrounding tissue. Ann Thorac Surg 2001; 71:797–800.

30. Loop FD, Lytle BW, Cosgrove DM, Stewart RW, Goormastic M, Williams GW, et al. Influence of the internal-mammary-artery graft on 10-year survival and other cardiac events. N Engl J Med 1986; 314:1–6.

31. Cameron A, Davis KB, Green G, Schaff HV. Coronary bypass surgery with internal-thoracic-artery grafts – effects on survival over a 15-year period. N Engl J Med 1996; 334:216–19.

32. Lytle BW, Loop FD. Superiority of bilateral internal thoracic artery grafting: it's been a long time comin'. Circulation 2001; 104:2152–4.

33. Danzer D, Christenson JT, Kalangos A, Khatchatourian G, Bednarkiewicz M, Faidutti B. Impact of double internal thoracic artery grafts on long-term outcomes in coronary artery bypass grafting. Tex Heart Inst J 2001; 28:89–95.

34. Endo M, Nishida H, Tomizawa Y, Kasanuki H. Benefit of bilateral over single internal mammary artery grafts for multiple coronary artery bypass grafting. Circulation 2001; 104:2164–70.

35. Barner HB, Sundt TM III, Bailey M, Zang Y. Midterm results of complete arterial revascularization in more than 1,000 patients using an internal thoracic artery/radial artery T graft. Ann Surg 2001; 234:447–52.

36. Tector AJ, McDonald ML, Kress DC, Downey FX, Schmahl TM. Purely internal thoracic artery grafts: outcomes. Ann Thorac Surg 2001; 72:450–5.

37. Wilson RF. Assessing the severity of coronary-artery stenoses. N Engl J Med 1996; 334:1735–7.

38. Botas J, Stadius ML, Bourassa MG, Rosen AD, Schaff HV, Sopko G, et al. Angiographic correlates of lesion relevance and suitability for percutaneous transluminal coronary angioplasty and coronary artery bypass grafting in the Bypass Angioplasty Revascularization Investigation study (BARI). Am J Cardiol 1996; 77:805–14.

39. Kern MJ. Definition of a critical coronary stenosis: implications for revascularization. Cor Europaeum – Eur J Card Intervent 1997; 6:47–51.

40. Marques KM, Spruijt HJ, Boer C, Westerhof N, Visser CA, Visser FC. The diastolic flow–pressure gradient relation in coronary stenoses in humans. J Am Coll Cardiol 2002; 39:1630–6.

41. Brosh D, Higano ST, Slepian MJ, Miller HI, Kern MJ, Lennon RJ, et al. Pulse transmission coefficient: a novel nonhyperemic parameter for assessing the physiological significance of coronary artery stenoses. J Am Coll Cardiol 2002; 39:1012–19.

42. Van Brussel BL, Plokker HW, Voors AA, Ernst SM, Kelder HC. Progression of atherosclerosis after venous coronary artery bypass graft surgery: a 15-year follow-up study. Cathet Cardiovasc Diagn 1997; 41:141–50.

43. Cashin WL, Sanmarco ME, Nessim SA, Blankenhorn DH. Accelerated progression of atherosclerosis in coronary vessels with minimal lesions that are bypassed. N Engl J Med 1984; 311:824–8.

44. Roth JA, Cukingnan RA, Brown BG, Gocka E, Carey JS. Factors influencing patency of saphenous vein grafts. Ann Thorac Surg 1979; 28:176–83.

45. Maniar HS, Sundt TM, Barner HB, Prasad SM, Peterson L, Absi T, et al. Effect of target stenosis and location on radial artery graft patency. J Thorac Cardiovasc Surg 2002; 123:45–52.

46. Jones EL, Weintraub WS. The importance of completeness of revascularization during long-term follow-up after coronary artery operations. J Thorac Cardiovasc Surg 1996; 112:227–37.

47. Whitlow PL, Dimas AP, Bashore TM, Califf RM, Bourassa MG, Chaitman BR, et al. Relationship of extent of revascularization with angina at one year in the Bypass Angioplasty Revascularization Investigation (BARI). J Am Coll Cardiol 1999; 34:1750–9.

48. Bertelsen CA, Kjoller M, Hoier-Madsen K, Folke K, Fritz-Hansen P. Influence of complete revascularization on long-term survival after coronary artery bypass surgery. Scand Cardiovasc J 1997; 31:271–4.

49. Lavee J, Rath S, Tran QH, Ra'anani P, Ruder A, Modan M, et al. Does complete revascularization by the conventional method truly provide the best possible results? Analysis of results and comparison with revascularization of infarct-prone segments (systematic segmental myocardial revascularization): the Sheba Study. J Thorac Cardiovasc Surg 1986; 92:279–90.

50. Bell MR, Gersh BJ, Schaff HV, Holmes DR Jr, Fisher LD, Alderman EL, et al. Effect of completeness of revascularization on long-term outcome of patients with three-vessel disease undergoing coronary artery bypass surgery. A report from the Coronary Artery Surgery Study (CASS) Registry. Circulation 1992; 86:446–57.

51. Osswald BR, Tochtermann U, Schweiger P, Thomas G, Vahl CF, Hagl S. Does the completeness of revascularization contribute to an improved early survival in patients up to 70 years of age? Thorac Cardiovasc Surg 2001; 49:373–7.

52. Scott R, Blackstone EH, McCarthy PM, Lytle BW, Loop FD, White JA, et al. Isolated bypass grafting of the left internal thoracic artery to the left anterior descending coronary artery: late consequences of incomplete revascularization. J Thorac Cardiovasc Surg 2000; 120:173–84.

53. Vander Salm TJ, Kip KE, Jones RH, Schaff HV, Shemin RJ, Aldea GS, et al. What constitutes optimal surgical revascularization? Answers from the Bypass Angioplasty Revascularization Investigation (BARI). J Am Coll Cardiol 2002; 39:565–72.

54. Moon MR, Sundt TM III, Pasque MK, Barner HB, Gay WA Jr, Damiano RJ Jr. Influence of internal mammary artery grafting and completeness of revascularization on long-term outcome in octogenarians. Ann Thorac Surg 2001; 72:2003–7.

55. Leavitt BJ, O'Connor GT, Olmstead EM, Morton JR, Maloney CT, Dacey LJ, et al. Use of the internal mammary artery graft and in-hospital mortality and other adverse outcomes associated with coronary artery bypass surgery. Circulation 2001; 103:507–12.

56. Cohn L. Use of the internal mammary artery graft and in-hospital mortality and other adverse outcomes associated with coronary artery bypass surgery. *Circulation* 2001; **103**:483–4.

57. Loop FD. Internal-thoracic-artery grafts. Biologically better coronary arteries. *N Engl J Med* 1996; **334**:263–5.

58. Hirose H, Amano A, Takanashi S, Takahashi A. Coronary artery bypass grafting using the gastroepiploic artery in 1,000 patients. *Ann Thorac Surg* 2002; **73**:1371–9.

59. Farrar DJ. Development of a prosthetic coronary artery bypass graft. [Review – 16 refs.] *Heart Surg Forum* 2000; **3**:36–40.

60. Royse AG, Royse CF, Tatoulis J. Total arterial coronary revascularization and factors influencing in-hospital mortality. *Eur J Cardiothorac Surg* 1999; **16**:499–505.

61. Wendler O, Hennen B, Demertzis S, Markwirth T, Tscholl D, Lausberg H, *et al*. Complete arterial revascularization in multivessel coronary artery disease with 2 conduits (skeletonized grafts and T grafts). *Circulation* 2000; **102**(19 Suppl. 3):III79–83.

62. Myers WO, Berg R, Ray JF, Douglas-Jones JW, Maki HS, Ulmer RH, *et al*. All-artery multigraft coronary artery bypass grafting with only internal thoracic arteries possible and safe: a randomized trial. *Surgery* 2000; **128**:650–9.

63. Dion R, Elias B, El Khoury G, Noirhomme P, Verhelst R, Hanet C. Surgical angioplasty of the left main coronary artery. *Eur J Cardiothorac Surg* 1997; **11**:857–64.

64. Hitchcock JF, Robles de Medina EO, Jambroes G. Angioplasty of the left main coronary artery for isolated left main coronary artery disease. *J Thorac Cardiovasc Surg* 1983; **85**:880–4.

65. Meseguer J, Hurle A, Fernandez-Latorre F, Alonso S, Llamas P, Casillas JA. Left main coronary artery patch angioplasty: midterm experience and follow-up with spiral computed tomography. *Ann Thorac Surg* 1998; **65**:1594–7.

66. Liska J, Jonsson A, Lockowandt U, Herzfeld I, Gelinder S, Franco-Cereceda A. Arterial patch angioplasty for reconstruction of proximal coronary artery stenosis. *Ann Thorac Surg* 1999; **68**:2185–9.

67. Loop FD, Lytle BW, Cosgrove DM, Mahfood S, McHenry MC, Goormastic M, *et al*. J. Maxwell Chamberlain memorial paper. Sternal wound complications after isolated coronary artery bypass grafting: early and late mortality, morbidity, and cost of care. *Ann Thorac Surg* 1990; **49**:179–86.

68. Ridderstolpe L, Gill H, Granfeldt H, Ahlfeldt H, Rutberg H. Superficial and deep sternal wound complications: incidence, risk factors and mortality. *Eur J Cardiothorac Surg* 2001; **20**:1168–75.

69. Kirklin JK, Westaby S, Blackstone EH, Kirklin JW, Chenoweth DE, Pacifico AD. Complement and the damaging effects of cardiopulmonary bypass. *J Thorac Cardiovasc Surg* 1983; **86**:845–57.

70. Bartels CG. Cardiopulmonary bypass: evidence or experience based? *J Thorac Cardiovasc Surg* 2002; **124**:20–7.

71. Cohen G, Borger MA, Weisel RD, Rao V. Intraoperative myocardial protection: current trends and future perspectives. [Review – 37 refs.] *Ann Thorac Surg* 1999; **68**:1995–2001.

72. Penttila HJ, Lepojarvi MV, Kiviluoma KT, Kaukoranta PK, Hassinen IE, Peuhkurinen KJ. Myocardial preservation during coronary surgery with and without cardiopulmonary bypass. *Ann Thorac Surg* 2001; **71**:565–71.

73. Filsoufi F, Aklog L, Adams DH. Minimally invasive CABG. [Review – 13 refs.] *Curr Opin Cardiol* 2001; **16**:306–9.

74. Oliveira SA, Lisboa LA, Dallan LA, Rojas SO, Poli de Figueiredo LF. Minimally invasive single-vessel coronary artery bypass with the internal thoracic artery and early postoperative angiography: midterm results of a prospective study in 120 consecutive patients. *Ann Thorac Surg* 2002; **73**:505–10.

75. Stamou SC, Corso PJ. Coronary revascularization without cardiopulmonary bypass in high-risk patients: a route to the future. [Review – 76 refs.] *Ann Thorac Surg* 2001; **71**:1056–61.

76. Hernandez F, Cohn WE, Baribeau YR, Tryzelaar JF, Charlesworth DC, Clough RA, *et al*. In-hospital outcomes of off-pump versus on-pump coronary artery bypass procedures: a multicenter experience. *Ann Thorac Surg* 2001; **72**:1528–33.

77. Cartier R, Brann S, Dagenais F, Martineau R, Couturier A. Systematic off-pump coronary artery revascularization in multivessel disease: experience of three hundred cases. *J Thorac Cardiovasc Surg* 2000; **119**:221–9.

78. Van Dijk D, Jansen EWL, Hijman R, Nierich AP, Diephuis JC, Moons KGM, *et al*. Cognitive outcome after off-pump and on-pump coronary artery bypass graft surgery: a randomized trial. *J Am Med Assoc* 2002; **287**:1405–12.

79. Al Ruzzeh S, George S, Bustami M, Nakamura K, Khan S, Yacoub M, *et al*. The early clinical and angiographic outcome of sequential coronary artery bypass grafting with the off-pump technique. *J Thorac Cardiovasc Surg* 2002; **123**:525–30.

80. Czerny M, Baumer H, Kilo J, Zuckermann A, Grubhofer G, Chevtchik O, *et al*. Complete revascularization in coronary artery bypass grafting with and without cardiopulmonary bypass. *Ann Thorac Surg* 2001; **71**:165–9.

81. Hart JC, Puskas JD, Sabik JF, III. Off-pump coronary revascularization: current state of the art. [Review – 50 refs.] *Semin Thorac Cardiovasc Surg* 2002; **14**:70–81.

82. Arom KV, Flavin TF, Emery RW, Kshettry VR, Janey PA, Petersen RJ. Safety and efficacy of off-pump coronary artery bypass grafting. *Ann Thorac Surg* 2000; **69**:704–10.

83. Cable DG, Mullany CJ, Schaff HV. The Allen test. *Ann Thorac Surg* 1999; **67**:876–7.

84. Ruengsakulrach P, Brooks M, Hare DL, Gordon I, Buxton BF. Preoperative assessment of hand circulation by means of Doppler ultrasonography and the modified Allen test. *J Thorac Cardiovasc Surg* 2001; **121**:526–31.

85. Culliford AT, Spencer FC. Guidelines for safely opening a previous sternotomy incision. *J Thorac Cardiovasc Surg* 1979; **78**:633–8.

86. Akl BF, Pett SB, Jr., Wernly JA. Use of a sagittal oscillating saw for repeat sternotomy: a safer and simpler technique. *Ann Thorac Surg* 1984; **38**:646–7.

87. Temeck BK, Katz NM, Wallace RB. An approach to re-operative median sternotomy. *J Card Surg* 1990; **5**:14–25.

88. Kulshrestha P, Garb JL, Rousou JA, Engelman RM, Wait RB. Re-operative median sternotomy using a cast spreader. *J Card Surg* 1999; **14**:185–6.

89. Follis FM, Pett SB Jr, Miller KB, Wong RS, Temes RT, Wernly JA. Catastrophic hemorrhage on sternal re-entry: still a dreaded complication? *Ann Thorac Surg* 1999; **68**:2215–19.

90. Gazzaniga AB, Palafox BA. Substernal thoracoscopic guidance during sternal re-entry. *Ann Thorac Surg* 2001; **72**:289–90.

91. Iafrati MM. Less-invasive saphenous harvest. [Review – 62 refs.] *Surg Clin North Am* 1999; **79**:623–44.

92. Jordan WD Jr, Goldberg SP. Video-assisted endoscopic saphenous vein harvest: an evolving technique. *Semin Vasc Surg* 2000; **13**:32–9.

93. Puskas JD, Wright CE, Miller PK, Anderson TE, Gott JP, Brown WM III, *et al*. A randomized trial of endoscopic versus open saphenous vein harvest in coronary bypass surgery. *Ann Thorac Surg* 1999; **68**:1509–12.

94. Hayward TZ III, Hey LA, Newman LL, Duhaylongsod FG, Hayward KA, Lowe JE, *et al*. Endoscopic versus open saphenous vein harvest: the effect on postoperative outcomes. *Ann Thorac Surg* 1999; **68**:2107–10.

95. Fabricius AM, Diegeler A, Doll N, Weidenbach H, Mohr FW. Minimally invasive saphenous vein harvesting techniques: morphology and postoperative outcome. *Ann Thorac Surg* 2000; **70**:473–8.

96. Bitondo JM, Daggett WM, Torchiana DF, Akins CW, Hilgenberg AD, Vlahakes GJ, *et al*. Endoscopic versus open saphenous vein

harvest: a comparison of postoperative wound complications. *Ann Thorac Surg* 2002; **73**:523–8.

97. Kan CD, Luo CY, Yang YJ. Endoscopic saphenous vein harvest decreases leg wound complication in coronary artery bypass grafting patients. *J Card Surg* 1999; **14**:157–62.

98. Schurr UP, Lachat ML, Reuthebuch O. Endoscopic saphenous vein harvesting for CABG – a randomized, prospective trial. *Thorac Cardiovasc Surg* 2002; **50**:160–3.

99. Felisky CD, Paull DL, Hill ME, Hall RA, Ditkoff M, Campbell WG, *et al.* Endoscopic greater saphenous vein harvesting reduces the morbidity of coronary artery bypass surgery. *Am J Surg* 2002; **183**:576–9.

100. Griffith GL, Allen KB, Waller BF, Heimansohn DA, Robison RJ, Schier JJ, *et al.* Endoscopic and traditional saphenous vein harvest: a histologic comparison. *Ann Thorac Surg* 2000; **69**:520–3.

101. Black EA, Guzik TJ, West NE, Campbell K, Pillai R, Ratnatunga C, *et al.* Minimally invasive saphenous vein harvesting: effects on endothelial and smooth muscle function. *Ann Thorac Surg* 2001; **71**:1503–7.

102. Reichenspurner H, Navia JA, Berry G, Robbins RC, Barbut D, Gold JP, *et al.* Particulate emboli capture by an intra-aortic filter device during cardiac surgery. *J Thorac Cardiovasc Surg* 2000; **119**:233–41.

103. Stensrud PE, Nuttall GA, de Castro MA, Abel MD, Ereth MH, Oliver WC Jr, *et al.* A prospective, randomized study of cardiopulmonary bypass temperature and blood transfusion. *Ann Thorac Surg* 1999; **67**:711–15.

104. Grimm M, Czerny M, Baumer H, Kilo J, Madl C, Kramer L, *et al.* Normothermic cardiopulmonary bypass is beneficial for cognitive brain function after coronary artery bypass grafting – a prospective randomized trial. *Eur J Cardiothorac Surg* 2000; **18**:270–5.

105. Gaudino M, Zamparelli R, Andreotti F, Burzotta F, Iacoviello L, Glieca F, *et al.* Normothermia does not improve postoperative hemostasis nor does it reduce inflammatory activation in patients undergoing primary isolated coronary artery bypass. *J Thorac Cardiovasc Surg* 2002; **123**:1092–100.

106. Birdi I, Caputo M, Underwood M, Angelini GD, Bryan AJ. Influence of normothermic systemic perfusion temperature on cold myocardial protection during coronary artery bypass surgery. *Cardiovasc Surg* 1999; **7**:369–74.

107. Christenson JT, Simonet F, Schmuziger M. Sequential vein bypass grafting: tactics and long-term results. *Cardiovasc Surg* 1998; **6**:389–97.

108. Mills NL. Coronary endarterectomy: surgical techniques for patients with extensive distal atherosclerotic coronary disease. [Review – 5 refs.] *Adv Card Surg* 1998; **10**:197–227.

109. Goldman BS, Christakis GT. Endarterectomy of the left anterior descending coronary artery. [Review – 4 refs.] *J Card Surg* 1994; **9**:89–96.

110. Sundt TM III, Camillo CJ, Mendeloff EN, Barner HB, Gay WA Jr. Reappraisal of coronary endarterectomy for the treatment of diffuse coronary artery disease. *Ann Thorac Surg* 1999; **68**:1272–7.

111. Shapira OM, Akopian G, Hussain A, Adelstein M, Lazar HL, Aldea GS, *et al.* Improved clinical outcomes in patients undergoing coronary artery bypass grafting with coronary endarterectomy. *Ann Thorac Surg* 1999; **68**:2273–8.

112. Casha AR, Gauci M, Yang L, Saleh M, Kay PH, Cooper GJ. Fatigue testing median sternotomy closures. *Eur J Cardiothorac Surg* 2001; **19**:249–53.

113. McGregor WE, Trumble DR, Magovern JA. Mechanical analysis of midline sternotomy wound closure. *J Thorac Cardiovasc Surg* 1999; **117**:1144–50.

114. Soroff HS, Hartman AR, Pak E, Sasvary DH, Pollak SB. Improved sternal closure using steel bands: early experience with three-year follow-up. *Ann Thorac Surg* 1996; **61**:1172–6.

12

Coronary surgery without cardiopulmonary bypass

MICHAEL J MACK

INTRODUCTION

Initial surgical revascularization of coronary arteries on the epicardial surface of the heart in the 1960s was performed while the heart was still beating. The introduction of cardiopulmonary bypass, with the ability to create a motionless, bloodless operative field, diverted attention from further efforts to develop techniques of beating-heart surgery. Over the ensuing 30 years, more than 10 million coronary revascularization procedures were performed, mostly with ischemic, cardioplegic arrest and cardiopulmonary bypass support.

With the success of catheter-based revascularization and the recognition in other surgical fields that operative procedures could be accomplished by less invasive means, a renewed interest in these early beating-heart techniques was generated. Initial attempts at making coronary revascularization less invasive, and therefore more patient friendly, were focused on limited access approaches, either on an arrested heart with peripheral cannulation (Port Access, HeartPort) or on a beating heart (minimally invasive direct coronary bypass grafting, MIDCAB). Suffice it to say that neither of these early efforts in minimally invasive cardiac surgery is commonly used today. The MIDCAB procedure, in which the left internal mammary artery is used to revascularize the left anterior descending (LAD) coronary artery through a limited anterior thoracotomy, now constitutes less than

2% of all surgical coronary revascularization.[1] The success of catheter-based revascularization of the LAD, the technical challenges of this approach, and the questionable benefit of an anterior thoracotomy compared with a median sternotomy have all served to limit its use. A variation of this procedure (in which a limited lateral thoracotomy is used to access the posterior surface of the heart, and branches of the circumflex coronary system are bypassed from a conduit placed from the descending thoracic aorta) does have a niche role.[2–6] The port-access approach, or variations thereof, have been largely relegated to mitral valve procedures only, having no significant place in coronary revascularization.[7]

It became recognized during the evolution of these techniques that the elimination of cardiopulmonary bypass may result in less procedural trauma to the patient than limiting the access incision.[8–12] Efforts therefore evolved to develop wide access beating-heart techniques (off-pump coronary artery bypass, OPCAB) as a treatment for multivessel disease. By the end of 2001, an estimated 23% of all surgical revascularization in the USA was performed without cardiopulmonary bypass on a beating heart, mostly though a median sternotomy approach.[13–16] Although the techniques are still being refined, a relatively standard operative choreography can be developed by an individual surgeon that will allow most, if not all, of coronary artery bypass to be performed safely and effectively by a beating-heart approach.

RATIONALE

Although the use of cardiopulmonary bypass creates optimal surgical conditions for coronary revascularization by creating a motionless, bloodless operative field, a significant systemic insult is incurred in creating these optimal surgical conditions. The surgical literature is replete with documentation of the incitement of the systemic inflammatory response induced by cardiopulmonary bypass, with the attendant systemic and pulmonary capillary leak, pulmonary, renal and neurological dysfunction as well as activation of the clotting cascade causing coagulation abnormalities.[17–19] As well as the side effects of cardiopulmonary bypass, the use of ischemic cardioplegic arrest creates global myocardial ischemia, which results in myocardial injury and dysfunction.[20,21] Although this can generally be tolerated for prolonged periods of time in patients with normal ventricular function, its use in patients with depressed ventricular function and/or acute myocardial ischemia can be a significant cause of perioperative mortality and morbidity.[22,23] Additionally, atherosclerotic disease of the ascending aorta is being increasingly recognized as a source of macroemboli leading to postoperative stroke and neurocognitive dysfunction.[24,25] Manipulation of the ascending aorta for cannulation, complete and partial cross-clamping and the 'jet' effects on intimal plaque by cannula flow have all been documented to lead to adverse neurological outcomes.

The following describes the techniques that have been developed to create conditions by which coronary artery surgical revascularization can be routinely performed on a beating heart without the attendant side effects of cardiopulmonary bypass, ischemic arrest and manipulation of the ascending aorta. There are, however, new complications of coronary surgery associated with beating-heart techniques, but careful attention to patient selection, the details of the operative technique and perioperative management can minimize or eliminate most of these consequences.

INDICATIONS

There are no absolute, only relative contraindications to off-pump coronary surgery. Institutional and individual surgeon experience and expertise dictate operative indication (Table 12.1). Without an extensive beating-heart surgical experience, optimal candidates for beating-heart approaches include patients who need a limited number of bypasses (one to three) on the anterior surface of the heart with large, relatively non-diseased target vessels and good left ventricular function. As surgeons become conversant with beating-heart surgery and greater experience

Table 12.1 *Patient selection for OPCAB*

With little experience:
- 1–3 bypasses
- Anterior cardiac surface
- Large target vessels
- Minimal distal disease
- Elective
- Hemodynamically stable

When experienced:
- Elderly
- Re-operative
- Poor left ventricular function
- Cerebral vascular disease
- Peripheral vascular disease
- Chronic lung disease
- Chronic renal insufficiency
- Significant co-morbidities

is gained, the techniques can be more widely applied to those patients who would most benefit from the elimination of cardiopulmonary bypass. These patients include the elderly ($\geq$75 years old),[26–28] re-operative patients,[29,30] patients with cerebral vascular disease,[31] peripheral vascular disease,[32] renal dysfunction,[33] pulmonary dysfunction[34] or other significant co-morbidities,[35] and patients with severe left ventricular dysfunction or presenting as an emergency after acute myocardial infarction.[36,37] Thus, the surgeon should develop a comfort level with beating-heart surgery in the more straightforward patients, until sufficient confidence has been acquired to apply the techniques to the patients who are most likely to benefit.

OPERATIVE TECHNIQUE

Successful coronary bypass without cardiopulmonary bypass is best accomplished by assembly of a dedicated surgical team. This team is led by a committed surgeon, a limited number of anesthesiologists who are also dedicated to developing the beating-heart approach, consistent first and second assistants and an experienced surgical nurse, who are all conversant with beating-heart techniques. The addition of a clinical care pathway nurse who is familiar with the innuendoes of postoperative care of the beating-heart surgery patient can optimize and catalyze the institutional experience.

Anesthetic management

Anesthetic techniques are focused on the maintenance of hemodynamic stability during the procedure, the consequences of local myocardial ischemia, the systemic nervous system activation, and the plans for early or immediate extubation. We have developed a pathway over the past 3 years in which immediate extubation without need for re-intubation is the goal in all beating-heart surgery patients who were not intubated or in cardiogenic shock preoperatively. This technique has been successful, with re-intubation being necessary in only 0.6% of 150 consecutive cases. Anesthetic management with short-acting agents, including sufentanyl, remifentinil or propofol-based techniques, as well as the use of shorter acting muscle relaxants facilitate early extubation. The use of thoracic epidural anesthesia for the early management of postoperative pain as well as liberal use of other methods of analgesia, including local techniques and intravenous anti-inflammatory agents, assist this technique.

Intraoperative efforts are focused on hemodynamic stability by maintaining cardiac output and normothermia (Table 12.2). In order to accomplish these goals, aggressive use of intraoperative hemodynamic monitoring is preferred. Our standard technique involves the use of pulmonary artery catheters capable of monitoring continuous cardiac output and the use of transesophageal echocardiography (TEE) to evaluate local wall motion abnormalities and distortion of ventricular geometry during various intraoperative maneuvers. Hemodynamic instability during surgical manipulation to access the posterior circulation is largely a consequence of right ventricular dysfunction due to inflow occlusion and/or distortion and compression of the right ventricle.[38–45] Early recognition of these causes and institution of appropriate remedies can minimize hemodynamic instability. Monitoring of the central venous pressure, pulmonary artery systolic pressure and mixed venous oxygen saturation and assessment of right ventricular compression by TEE can be helpful in modifying surgical technique. Optimization of right ventricular preload by the liberal use of intravenous fluids (3–4 L crystalloid) and reinfusion of shed blood to maintain the central venous pressure at 8–10 cmH$_2$O can optimize

right ventricular function. The use of intravenous nitroglycerin also aids right-sided preload. It is important for normothermia to be maintained because of the consequences of hypothermia and the absence of a heat exchanger to correct for heat loss. Maintenance of ambient operating room temperature warmer than is customary, the use of warming blankets and devices around the patient out of the immediate operative field and the use of heated intravenous fluids and heated inhalation gases are important to help maintain normothermia during the operative procedure.

Surgical technique

The standard OPCAB procedure is performed through a median sternotomy. Since the necessity for access to the ascending aorta is minimized, a shorter than standard skin incision can be performed (Figure 12.1). We typically perform an 8–10 cm skin incision beginning cephalad at the sterno-manubrial junction. Division of the sternum through this smaller access skin incision is made easier by the use of an oscillating saw. We have found no advantage in terms of improving postoperative pain or

Table 12.2 *Intraoperative measures to maintain hemodynamic stability*

Pulmonary artery catheter monitoring
Transesophageal echocardiography
Maintenance of normothermia
Volume loading to a CVP 8–10
Intravenous nitroglycerin
Trendelenburg table positioning
Avoidance of right ventricular compression distortion
Suction positioning devices
Slight re-adjustments
Avoidance of over-reacting

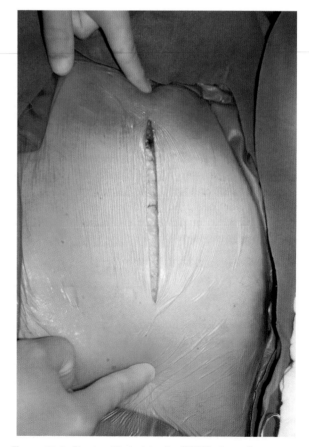

Figure 12.1 *Shorter skin incision for OPCAB via median sternotomy.*

morbidity in employing a partial sternotomy compared with a full sternotomy. Internal mammary artery grafts are harvested in the standard manner and a sternal retractor is placed in the lower portion of the sternal incision. Placement of the sternal retractor as low as possible causes less brachial plexus compression and allows easier subluxation of the apex of the heart for access to the posterior circulation. Specific retractors for off-pump surgery are helpful to allow the attachment of assorted beating-heart surgery hardware, including stabilizers and suction exposure devices, as well as providing suture holders that allow easy pericardial stay suture adjustment during the various maneuvers (Figure 12.2).

The pericardium is opened centrally in an inverted T manner. The lateral extensions of the pericardial incision are wider than usual. Opening to the left along the diaphragmatic surface towards the apex of the pericardium allows the apex of the heart to be distracted into the operative field more easily (Figure 12.3). Opening of the pericardium to the right along the diaphragmatic reflection creates more space for the right ventricle during access to the posterior circulation so that there is less compression (Figure 12.4). Three pericardial retraction sutures are placed on each side of the pericardium and

left untied. Frequent adjustments of these pericardial stays either to retract or slacken the pericardium are essential to optimize hemodynamics during the various maneuvers. As a general rule, all preliminary preparations are completed prior to distraction of the heart from its natural position. Graft preparation and positioning are performed before the heart is distracted so that the minimum amount of time is spent in the distracted stabilized position while performing the anastomosis.

The sequence by which the various anastomoses are performed is important. (Table 12.3).[46] Although individual surgeons may find their own choreography that increases their comfort level, we have found the following sequence to work quite well. We usually bypass the LAD coronary artery with the left internal mammary artery first. This target vessel is the easiest to expose and access and allows revascularization of the anterior wall and septum before any further maneuvers that may cause myocardial ischemia are performed. Care must be taken to avoid traction/torsion of the internal mammary artery pedicle during subsequent maneuvers. The exception to bypass of the LAD first is if the right coronary artery is totally occluded and the LAD serves as the sole blood supply to the anterior wall, septum and inferior walls.

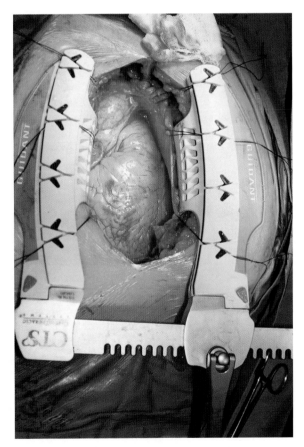

Figure 12.2 *OPCAB sternal retractor with 'stays' for pericardial suture adjustment and tracks for stabilizer and positioner.*

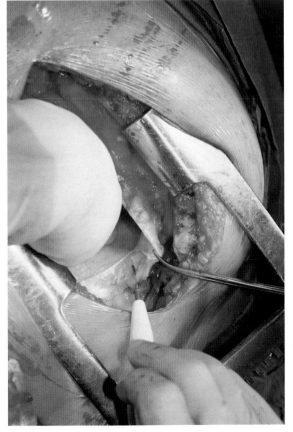

Figure 12.3 *Opening of pericardium laterally towards the apex to facilitate subluxation of the heart.*

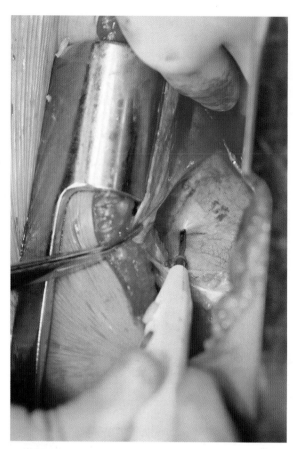

Figure 12.4 *Pericardium is divided on the right side posteriorly to the level of the phrenic nerve to allow more room for the right ventricle when the apex is elevated.*

Table 12.3 *Sequence of vessels to be bypassed*

LAD (if RCA not totally occluded)
RCA if totally occluded
Proximals
Diagonals
Posterior ventricular RCA branch
Obtuse marginals (2nd, 3rd)
Posterior descending branch RCA
High obtuse marginal branches
Ramus branches
RCA if not totally occluded (with shunt)

LAD, left anterior descending; RCA, right coronary artery.

In this instance, it is preferable to bypass the right coronary artery first, as occlusion of the already totally occluded right coronary artery is unlikely to cause adverse hemodynamic consequences; this zone of myocardium is then already perfused when the LAD coronary artery is subsequently occluded.

Before proceeding with the distal anastomoses, the patient is heparinized with $1–1.5\,mg\,kg^{-1}$ of heparin.

The LAD is brought earliest into the operative field by placement of a single, wet laparotomy sponge behind the heart (Figure 12.5). The right pericardial stays are slackened so that minimal compression of the right ventricle occurs (Figure 12.6). The operating table is then placed in the Trendelenburg position to maximize right ventricular preload. The left internal mammary artery has already been positioned, so the suturing of the distal anastomosis commences as soon as the arteriotomy is performed. A Silastic tape mounted on a blunt needle is then placed around the proximal LAD, which is carefully occluded. We have not found preconditioning to be necessary or advantageous. A mechanical stabilization foot is placed around the target landing zone on the LAD coronary artery and dissection of the vessel begins. An intramyocardial location of the LAD can be somewhat problematic. However, this vessel can be routinely located and bypassed on the beating heart if careful attention is paid to the details of exposure. An intramyocardial location can be reliably anticipated by careful examination of the preoperative angiogram. The presence of a straight mid-portion of the LAD without branch vessels containing an 'S' curve on each end is a signature of an intramyocardial location.

We never start dissection before stabilization is in place. The use of a misted carbon dioxide blower to keep a relatively bloodless field is also essential. We commence exposure by finding the LAD distally where it emerges on the epicardial surface near the apex of the heart. We then continue dissection more proximally, moving the stabilization device as we proceed, until an optimal sized vessel is found. There is usually a minimally diseased segment of vessel present in the intramyocardial location.

Once an optimal landing site is located and the proximal vessel is occluded, an arteriotomy is performed. We do not use distal occlusion because of concern about injuring the intima of the coronary artery.[47] Because distal coronary flow is present during the anastomosis, a misted carbon dioxide blower is used to keep the arteriotomy clear (Figure 12.7). A fair amount of shed blood usually accumulates during the anastomosis and we therefore use a cellsaver to salvage it. Alternatively, a shunt or 'seal' can be placed to minimize blood in the field and blood loss.[48] The anastomosis is performed using a continuous 7-0 suture, with three sutures placed in the heel of the internal mammary artery and three in the recipient coronary artery before approximation. The suture is then continued down the near side of the vessel towards the surgeon around the toe of the anastomosis, finishing on the far side. This technique and the use of the carbon dioxide blower allow a 'sail' effect to occur that keeps the vessels billowed open and retracted without the necessity for instrument traction on either vessel. With this 'no-touch' technique, care must be taken to use misted air so that desiccation of the intima does not

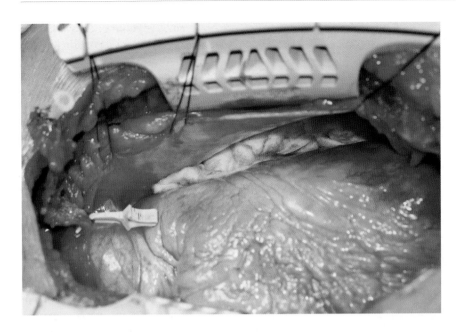

Figure 12.5 *A laparotomy sponge behind the heart and relaxation of the right pericardial stay sutures give excellent exposure of the LAD without hemodynamic compromise.*

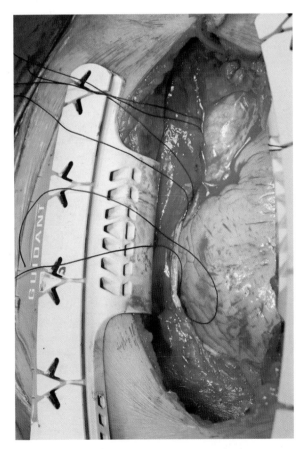

Figure 12.6 *Right pericardial stays are released prior to displacing the heart.*

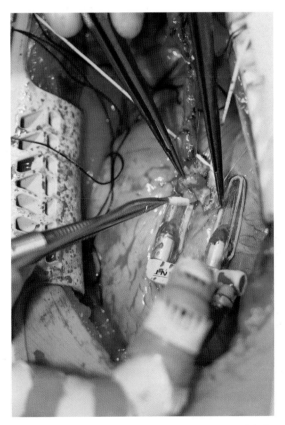

Figure 12.7 *Anastomosis of the LAD coronary artery with the LIMA. Note the stabilizer in place, proximal silastic snare, and CO_2 blower to allow visualization without blood.*

occur and so that the minimal amount of carbon dioxide flow is used to reduce the chance of vessel dissection.[49] Once the anastomosis is completed and the suture tied, a tacking suture is placed adjacent to the anastomosis so that torsion and excessive traction are minimized. The heart is then replaced in the natural position and allowed to fully recover hemodynamically before further maneuvers are performed.

We usually perform the proximal anastomoses next. Performance of proximal prior to distal anastomoses allows immediate reperfusion of ischemic myocardium at the completion of a distal anastomosis. Although judgment of graft length can be somewhat problematic initially, this assessment can be quickly mastered. It is essential to determine the exact distal anastomotic site before the graft is fashioned to its final length.

Frequently, a rebound hypertension occurs after the heart is placed back into the natural location after the LAD anastomosis. Care should be taken to ensure that systolic blood pressure is kept under 100 mmHg before a partial occlusion clamp is placed on the aorta. Prior to placement of a clamp, placement of a stabilizer on the right ventricular outflow tract may be helpful, both to expose the aorta and to minimize the motion during performance of the proximal anastomoses. The recent introduction of proximal anastomotic connectors has facilitated the performance of the anastomosis, obviating the necessity for a partial occlusion clamp and eliminating the hazard of aortic dissection, which has recently been described with placement of the partial occlusion clamp in beating-heart surgery (Figures 12.8 and 12.9). If a clamp is used, careful control of blood pressure to avoid hypertension is mandatory.

We then continue our distal anastomoses from easiest to hardest. Anastomoses to diagonal vessels on the anterior surface of the heart are relatively easy to perform. Next easiest are those vessels along the obtuse margin of the heart, including the distal circumflex, second or third obtuse marginal branches of the circumflex, and posterior ventricular branches of the right coronary artery. Posterior descending and first obtuse marginals follow next in degree of difficulty. Intermediate or ramus branches are somewhat more difficult due to some compression of the pulmonary artery and right ventricular outflow tract that may occur with exposure. Lastly, the right main coronary artery is bypassed.

During exposure and stabilization of the lateral and posterior surfaces, the same principles apply as for all anastomoses. Before positioning the heart, the graft length is assessed, sized and put in place so that the anastomosis can be performed immediately after the arteriotomy is made. The right pericardial stay sutures are

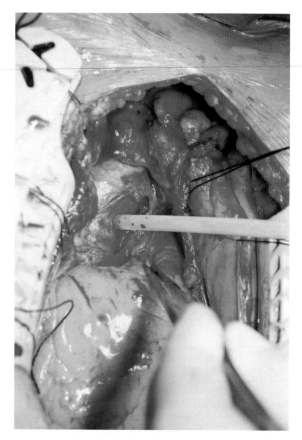

Figure 12.8 *Saphenous vein graft loaded in carrier being delivered into aortotomy for 'clampless' proximal anastomosis.*

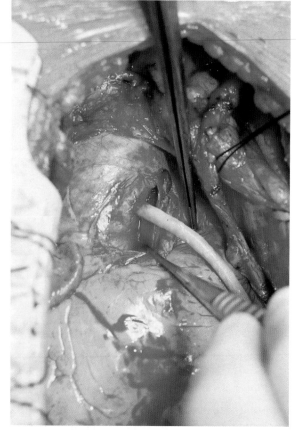

Figure 12.9 *Completed aorto-saphenous anastomosis with nitinol connector.*

slackened and the right pleura may even be opened to create more room for the right ventricle. The operating table is placed in the Trendelenburg position and rotated towards the surgeon so that exposure is optimized with the minimal amount of traction necessary. Opening the sternal retractor a little wider at this point may also help. One or two posterior pericardial sutures placed between the left inferior pulmonary vein and the inferior vena cava can serve as traction on the base of the heart to expose the posterior and lateral aspects with minimal compression of the ventricular chambers.[50–53] Alternatively, a suction exposure device placed on the apex of the heart can offer exposure to the posterior surface with maintenance of hemodynamics. The suction exposure devices elongate rather than compress the ventricular cavities and facilitate exposure without compression. Once optimal exposure of the target vessel has been obtained, the Silastic stay suture is placed proximally around the vessel to be bypassed, the mechanical stabilization foot is placed adjacent to the target area and the anastomosis is commenced in the usual manner (Figure 12.10). We usually replace the heart in its natural position after each

anastomosis and wait a few minutes to allow full hemodynamic recovery. We have not found the use of shunts to be necessary for most anastomoses and reserve them for heavily calcified vessels in which a proximal snare is unable to occlude the vessel, and for the right coronary artery (as discussed below).

Ischemia and hemodynamic collapse are most likely to occur during bypass of the distal right coronary artery. A few extra maneuvers are helpful to minimize the chance of this occurrence. Problems are most likely to occur when a large dominant, non-totally occluded right coronary artery is to be bypassed proximal to the crux. Proximal occlusion causes ischemia to the atrioventricular node, leading to heart block, loss of sinus rhythm, bradycardia, ventricular distention and eventual hemodynamic collapse. This can all be minimized by placement of temporary atrial and ventricular pacemaker wires before occlusion. The use of a shunt to maintain perfusion of the distal vessel during the arteriotomy is also helpful in this instance. For this anastomosis, we slacken the *left* pericardial stays, maintaining traction on the right stays. A suction exposure device placed on the acute margin of the heart allows adequate exposure without right ventricular compression. Alternatively, a felt-bolstered large suture placed through the acute margin of the heart for retraction can allow exposure of the distal right coronary artery.[54] Once proximal occlusion, optimal exposure and stabilization have occurred, the arteriotomy is performed and a shunt immediately placed. The distal anastomosis is then completed in the usual manner.

Upon completion of all anastomoses, assessment of hemodynamic stability, echocardiogram and wall motion abnormality is undertaken. Although some centers feel that transit-time flow measurements are helpful,[55] we do not routinely measure intraoperative graft flows, but rely on echocardiogram changes or wall motion abnormalities detected by TEE. We ascertain proper graft length and position and reverse the heparinization with protamine. Because immediate extubation is our rule, we place small drainage tubes in the pericardium (19 French Blake or Jackson–Pratt drains, Figure 12.11). Pacemaker wires are not placed unless they were previously used for bypass of the right coronary artery. The sternum is closed in the usual manner and any cellsaved blood is returned to the patient. Extubation is usually immediate unless the patient was intubated or hemodynamically unstable preoperatively.

ON-PUMP BEATING-HEART SURGERY

In patients who are hemodynamically unstable, due to cardiogenic shock, acute myocardial infarction or acute graft occlusion in a cardiac catheterization laboratory, the technique of on-pump beating-heart surgery can be

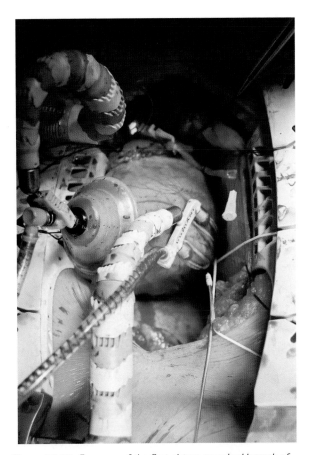

Figure 12.10 *Exposure of the first obtuse marginal branch of the circumflex. Note the suction positioner on the apex, suction stabilizer adjacent to the artery, silastic snare proximally, and SVG positioned to begin anastomosis.*

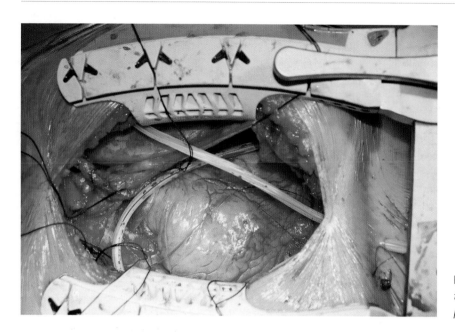

Figure 12.11 *Small silastic drainage tubes in the pericardium and left pleural cavity.*

helpful. In these situations, the risk is due to global myocardial ischemic arrest rather than to the use of cardiopulmonary bypass. Cannulation and commencement of cardiopulmonary bypass in the usual manner and then performance of coronary bypass using the standard stabilization techniques allow hemodynamic stability that minimizes myocardial ischemia. There is limited experience in some centers with the use of right heart support in unstable patients to improve hemodynamic stability during the performance of beating-heart coronary surgery, in the hope of minimizing some of the effects of standard cardiopulmonary bypass.[41,42,44]

LATERAL THORACOTOMY FOR BEATING-HEART REVASCULARIZATION OF THE CIRCUMFLEX SYSTEM

The clinical situation can arise in which isolated revascularization of the circumflex system is necessary and not amenable to catheter-based techniques. The usual situation is in the re-operative patient who has a previously placed, patent left internal mammary artery to the LAD and recurrent in-stent restenosis of the circumflex or a chronic total occlusion of the circumflex system and lateral wall ischemia. The use of beating-heart techniques via a limited lateral thoracotomy through the intercostal space is a nice solution to this clinical problem.[2,4–6] In this instance, a short, 7–8 cm, segment of saphenous vein graft or radial artery is placed from the descending aorta just above the diaphragm to an obtuse marginal branch of the circumflex. The procedure is performed through the 7th intercostal space, with exposure of the lateral surface of the heart posterior to the phrenic nerve. Frequently, a previously placed saphenous vein graft serves

as a marker to locate the target vessel, and this area of the heart is usually remarkably free of pericardial adhesions. The inferior pulmonary ligament is divided to allow straight access from the descending aorta to the lateral surface of the heart. This operation has been facilitated by the introduction of anastomotic connectors to allow placement of the graft off the descending aorta without the necessity for placement of a partial occlusion clamp (Figure 12.12). Using a stabilization device for the distal coronary artery, the anastomosis is performed in the usual manner. Because of the distance of the operative site from the chest wall, some technical challenges can be present. However, this operation can be routinely performed with ease in most circumstances.

POSTOPERATIVE CARE

With the avoidance of cardiopulmonary bypass and the attendant systemic inflammatory response, pulmonary and systemic capillary leak, and pulmonary white blood cell sequestration, as well as the diminution in blood loss, early or immediate extubation becomes a more viable option. Beginning in late 1999, we moved from a fast-track protocol, in which all patients were extubated early, to one in which immediate extubation in the operating room is performed. We currently have experience, with a single anesthesiologist, of 150 consecutive patients managed in this way, who were not intubated preoperatively or in cardiogenic shock. One patient who developed a postoperative pneumothorax required intubation. Mortality in this series is 0.67%.

When patients reach the intensive care unit, a 3-day clinical care pathway is initiated. Close attention to the

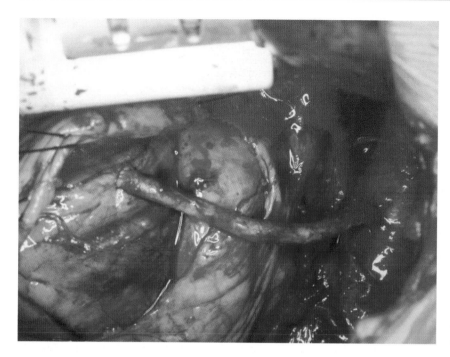

Figure 12.12 *Saphenous vein graft from descending aorta to an obtuse marginal branch of the circumflex coronary artery using an anastomotic connector for the proximal anastomosis.*

management of early postoperative pain is mandatory. The use of epidural analgesia and local analgesia and the liberal use of intravenous anti-inflammatory agents are essential for successful pain management. Early mobilization, within 3–6 hours of surgery, is encouraged. It is unusual to have significant postoperative bleeding, and all monitoring lines can usually be removed within 4 hours of surgery to facilitate mobilization. If there is significant bleeding after off-pump surgery, a mechanical source of bleeding is likely because coagulopathy is unusual and a prompt return to the operating room should be considered.

There appears to be an increase in thromboembolic complications after beating-heart surgery.[56,57] The loss of the 'post-pump coagulopathy' results in a postoperative hypercoagulable state after beating-heart coronary artery bypass similar to that which occurs after any other major surgical procedure. The consequences of this include deep vein thrombosis, pulmonary embolism and embolic stroke – related to either atrial fibrillation or rupture of the ascending aortic plaque during partial occlusion clamping.[58] As a prophylactic measure, we maintain all patients on aspirin preoperatively and continue it postoperatively. In the immediate postoperative period, patients are given a loading dose of clopidogrel and maintained on this antiplatelet agent for 30 days postoperatively. Although it appears that the incidence of atrial fibrillation is lower than with arrested heart surgery,[59,60] we do employ low-dose beta-blockers as prophylaxis. Approximately 50% of our patients are able successfully to complete this 3-day postoperative care pathway.

COMPLICATIONS

The goal of beating-heart surgery is to eliminate complications associated with the use of cardiopulmonary bypass. The outcomes are discussed more fully under 'Results' below, but suffice it to say that there is a preponderance of evidence that at least some complications associated with coronary bypass surgery decrease with the elimination of cardiopulmonary bypass, whereas other complications appear to be unchanged or have a minimal decrease.[13,15] In addition, there is an increase in some complications and new complications are being described that appear to be associated with off-pump techniques.[58]

There are published series in the literature clearly demonstrating a decrease in blood loss and transfusion rate,[61–70] inotrope use and intra-aortic balloon support,[13,15] new-onset renal failure[13] and mortality in specific subgroups, including the elderly,[26,28] patients with renal dysfunction[71] and re-do surgery patients.[29,30] In addition, it appears that there is approximately a 1-day hospital length of stay benefit and cost savings.[64] Complications that appear to be increased or new with beating-heart surgery include an incidence of aortic dissection related to placement of a partial occlusion clamp on the distended, pulsatile aorta leading to intimal injury.[58] As well as dissection, placement of this clamp may lead to rupture of plaque, with subsequent embolic neurological consequences. There are reports of intestinal ischemia, probably related to low flow states with beating-heart surgery. Avoidance of hypotension and low cardiac output, especially in elderly patients with potentially diseased mesenteric vessels, should avert this complication. A postoperative hypercoagulable state may result in an increased incidence of deep vein thrombosis and pulmonary embolus, stroke and graft occlusion.[56,57] Overall, complications appear to be less than with on-pump surgery,[72] and appropriate recognition of new complications and prophylactic measures to prevent their occurrence can lead to an overall benefit.

RESULTS

Evaluation of the effects of any treatment occurs by outcome analysis. In the hierarchy of research designs, the results of randomized, controlled trials are considered to be evidence of the highest grade, whereas observational studies are viewed as having less validity because they reportedly overestimate treatment effects.[73–75] The grades of evidence rank from the highest (grade 1), which is evidence obtained from properly randomized, controlled trials, followed by evidence from well-designed controlled trials without randomization, through evidence from well-designed cohort or case-controlled analytic studies, to the evidence gained from the results of observational studies. Based upon this descending hierarchy of therapy evaluation, we will review the current published results of off-pump surgery. The group in Bristol, England, led by Angelini has published seven articles regarding controlled, randomized trials of beating-heart surgery versus conventional coronary bypass. The numbers of patients in these trials range from 40 to 200, with varying findings. One study of 60 patients has shown a decreased inflammatory response in beating-heart patients as evidenced by lower interleukin-8, white blood cell and monocyte counts, and decreased wound infections in beating-heart patients.[78] A randomized trial of 200 patients showed that blood loss was 1.6 times higher in the on-pump group, with 52% of the on-pump patients and 23% of the off-pump patients ($P < 0.01$) requiring transfusion.[62] A study of 60 randomized patients showed superior renal protection in off-pump patients, as evidenced by creatinine clearance and urinary microalbumin:creatinine ratio.[73] Randomized studies of 80 patients and 200 patients have shown improved myocardial function and lower cost with beating-heart surgery compared with conventional coronary artery bypass grafting (CABG) respectively.[76,77] Two additional randomized trials have shown no difference in pulmonary gas exchange in 52 patients or in neurological and neuropsychological outcomes in 60 patients.[78,79] Diegeler randomized 80 patients to off-pump versus on-pump surgery and found that there was a decreased incidence of cerebral emboli, as measured by transcranial Doppler, in beating-heart surgery (compared with conventional CABG), which correlated with improved neurocognitive

outcomes.[80] Casati has shown in a randomized group of 40 beating-heart patients that tranexamic acid use results in less blood loss compared with control.[81]

There are a number of observational series of larger experiences in off-pump surgery. A recent review of 12 cohort studies and 11 intervention studies yielded a pooled analysis showing 22.5% of patients with significant cognitive deficit 2 months after conventional CABG.[82] The authors concluded that the relationship of cardiopulmonary bypass to this complication was unclear, and called for a randomized study that directly compared off-pump and on-pump surgery.

Magee, from our group, published our results of off-pump surgery in 1983 patients operated on in our center and at the Washington Hospital Center from 1998 through July 2000.[13] In an effort to identify and address selection bias, preoperative risk factors found by logistic regression to be associated with OPCAB selection were weighted by odds ratio and a propensity score calculated for each patient. Off-pump and on-pump patients were then computer matched by propensity score, institution and number of bypasses in a 1–2 ratio. Use of cardiopulmonary bypass was found to be independently associated with a 1.9 (95% CI 1.2–3.1) times increased risk of death. In another computer-matched cohort, Puskas compared 200 consecutive off-pump bypass patients and computer matched those to a contemporary group of 1000 patients.[64] Mortality rate for off-pump patients was 1.0% (vs 2.2% in on-pump), postoperative stroke 1.5% (vs 2.3%), and myocardial infarction 1.0% (vs 0.8%). There was a statistically significant reduction in the rate of blood transfusion (33% cf. 70%), and no deep sternal wound infection in the off-pump group (0% cf. 2.2%). Four hundred and twenty-one grafted arteries were also analyzed by angiography in 167 of the OPCAB patients prior to discharge, with a patency rate of 98.8% and perfect patency in 93.3%. All 163 internal mammary artery grafts were patent. In addition, there was a reduced postoperative hospital stay, from 5.7 days in the on-pump group to 3.9 days in the off-pump group, with a decrease in hospital cost of 15%.

We recently reviewed our own total off-pump experience from inception in 1995 through to the end of 2000.[15] One thousand nine hundred and fifteen of 12 540 (15%) patients underwent coronary bypass grafting during that period without cardiopulmonary bypass. By the year 2000, we were performing 34% of all isolated coronary bypass grafting off-pump. We found a significant decrease in observed and risk-adjusted mortality off-pump (1.9 vs 3.5, $P < 0.001$) as well as a decreased need for blood transfusion, blood products, prolonged ventilation and re-operation for bleeding, and shorter hospital stay.

Other groups have reviewed their general experience with beating-heart surgery with series ranging between

100 and 300 patients, all of which show a decreased mortality and complication rate, albeit in selected groups.[83–86]

The effect of beating-heart surgery in various subgroups has been analyzed. Two series of OPCAB in left main disease have shown improved outcomes. Retrospective reviews of 387 patients by Yeatman[87] and of 100 patients by Dewey[88] have shown a trend towards lower mortality and identical lower requirements for postoperative inotropes, less blood product usage and wound infection, and shorter hospital stay.

Magee found that in the 346 of 2891 (12%) diabetic patients having isolated CABG using the beating-heart technique, there was no difference in mortality compared with the on-pump group, but there was reduced blood product use and a decrease in complication rates, including prolonged ventilation, atrial fibrillation and postoperative renal failure.[89]

Other series have retrospectively analyzed large databases for beating-heart outcomes. A recent series by Plomondon reviewed 680 off-pump CABG procedures from 43 experienced centers. Off-pump mortality rate (2.7% vs 4.0%) and complication rates (8.8% vs 14%) were lower compared with those for on-pump patients.[90] Risk-adjusted mortality and morbidity were also improved, with multivariable odds ratios of 0.52 and 0.56 for off-pump versus on-pump respectively ($P < 0.05$). Review of nearly 17 000 isolated coronary artery bypass operations performed in 72 hospitals of the HCA Hospital System in the USA in 1999 reported that 16.4% were performed off-pump. There was a lower mortality (2.33% vs 2.97%) in the off-pump group ($P = 0.058$). In addition, there was a statistically significant decrease in stroke, new-onset renal failure and re-operation for bleeding, shorter length of stay and lower cost in the off-pump group. These outcomes hold true for both high-volume and low-volume centers.[91]

Neurological and neurocognitive outcomes have been an area of intense interest over the years with conventional CABG and, in more recent years, with the increasing use of off-pump techniques. Roach in 1996 demonstrated a 6.4% incidence of adverse neurological outcomes equally divided between focal deficits (stroke) and diffuse neurocognitive dysfunction following conventional CABG.[92] These adverse neurological outcomes were age related, so that in patients >80 years old the incidence of neurological complications was 16% after routine elective coronary bypass surgery. Adverse outcomes after on-pump CABG were further substantiated by Newman.[93] He longitudinally assessed neurocognitive function after coronary bypass surgery, finding that the adverse effects on cognitive function persisted for up to 5 years. In Diegeler's randomized series comparing off versus on pump, adverse neurocognitive changes were present in 90% of the on-pump patients, compared with none of the off-pump patients, and this correlated with cerebral emboli as measured by transcranial Doppler. Other retrospective series have demonstrated fewer cerebral microemboli,[24] less evidence of brain injury,[94,95] less neurocognitive dysfunction,[24] and improved clinical neurological outcomes.[96] The effect of eliminating cardiopulmonary bypass is to reduce the number of gaseous and platelet emboli to the brain as well as of atherosclerotic microemboli from cannulation or clamping of the aorta. However, additional measures can be taken to improve neurological outcomes, including the avoidance of grafts placed on the ascending aorta, the use of protective filters, anastomotic connectors and pharmacological agents that minimize the inflammatory response.

The incidence of atrial fibrillation in off-pump surgery has been shown in some series to be approximately half that in on-pump surgery.[13,15] However, this is not a universal finding in published series, with some centers finding that there is no decrease in the incidence of atrial fibrillation with off-pump surgery.[97]

A number of centers have looked at methods of safely integrating beating-heart surgery into established on-pump programs.[98,99] As well as examining methods of integration, they have tackled the tough issue of resident training.[100,101] It appears that with gradual integration of beating-heart techniques in a planned, careful approach, any 'learning curve' can be safely surmounted, first by the staff surgeons and subsequently by the resident trainees.

FUTURE CONSIDERATIONS

It is anticipated that the percentage of coronary artery bypass surgery performed without cardiopulmonary bypass will continue to increase in the foreseeable future. Although the adoption rate will not be as great as that of the last 3 or 4 years, numerous factors will tend to cause a shift towards the performance of more off-pump surgery. Drivers of this adoption include the introduction of new technology and refinements in technique that facilitate the user friendliness of the procedure. In the past few years, there have been refinements in stabilizers, the addition of apical suction exposure and positioning devices, the use of carbon dioxide blowers and shunts, and refinement of anesthetic techniques, all of which facilitate execution of the procedure. The addition of other technology, including anastomotic connectors, may further help facilitate off-pump techniques by minimizing the time necessary to perform anastomoses and mitigate the need for exacting operating field conditions.[102,103] As more surgeons become educated in beating-heart techniques, adoption rates are anticipated to increase. Surgeons currently entering the field who have already become conversant with minimally invasive techniques in their general surgical backgrounds are more likely to adopt these techniques than surgeons with no previous exposure. This shift will be further accelerated by the impending retirement of a generation of surgeons whose predominant mode of revascularization was by on-pump techniques. Numerous thrusts in postgraduate education regarding the effective education of surgeons in these new techniques are underway.

Another factor affecting adoption is clinical validation of outcomes. As cited in this chapter, only a few small, randomized series exist demonstrating clinical validity. One large, single-center, randomized study is now closed and the results should be available in early 2003. Large series observational outcomes analyses tend to show benefit, but a large, multicenter, randomized study has not yet been initiated. Such a study may never be forthcoming due to surgeons being firmly entrenched in either technique and therefore unwilling to randomize patients. Other effective procedures have been introduced and subsequently widely adopted in cardiac surgery without randomized studies, including the use of the left internal thoracic artery and mitral valve repair. It may be that continuing adoption of beating-heart surgery will occur without the assistance of evidence-based medicine.

KEY REFERENCES

Ascione R, Lloyd CT, Underwood MJ, Lotto AA, Pitsis AA, Angelini GD. Inflammatory response after coronary revascularization with or without cardiopulmonary bypass. *Ann Thorac Surg* 2000; **69**:1198–204.
This is one of the series of articles from the group at Bristol that randomized patients to beating-heart versus on-pump surgery. This and the accompanying five articles by these authors are the first to randomize patients between off-pump and on-pump.

Diegeler A, Hirsch R, Schneider F, Schilling LO, Falk V, Rauch T, *et al.* Neuromonitoring and neurocognitive outcome in off pump versus conventional coronary bypass operation. *Ann Thorac Surg* 2000; **69**:1162–6.
This is a randomized study looking at neurocognitive outcomes in on-pump versus off-pump surgery that shows potential benefit of the beating-heart approach.

Grundeman PF, Borst C, Verlaan CWJ, Meijburg H, Moues CM, Jansen EWL. Exposure of circumflex branches in the tilted, beating porcine heart: echocardiographic evidence of right ventricular deformation and the effect of right or left heart bypass. *J Thorac Cardiovasc Surg* 1999; **118**:316–23.
This is the original work establishing the reason for hemodynamic instability associated with beating-heart surgery. It was the first work to turn the focus on the right ventricle as

a cause of hemodynamic instability and the corrective measures for this.

Murkin JM, Boyd WD, Ganapathy S, Adams SJ, Peterson RC. Beating heart surgery: why expect less central nervous system morbidity? *Ann Thorac Surg* 1999; **68**:1498–501.
This is a good summary article that addresses all the issues of the central nervous system in coronary bypass surgery and why beating-heart surgery can be expected to improve some aspects of the adverse neurological consequences.

Puskas JD, Thourani VH, Marshall JJ, Dempsey SJ, Steiner MA, Sammons BH, *et al.* Clinical outcomes, angiographic patency, and resource utilization in 200 consecutive off pump coronary bypass patients. *Ann Thorac Surg* 2001; **71**:1477–84.
This is a relatively large consecutive study with computer matching that includes angiographic follow-up that documents angiographic patency as well as some benefits of beating-heart surgery.

REFERENCES

1. Diegeler A, Spyrantis N, Matin M, Falk V, Hambrecht R, Autschbach R, *et al.* The revival of surgical treatment for isolated proximal high grade LAD lesions by minimally invasive coronary artery bypass grafting. *Eur J Cardiothorac Surg* 2000; **17**:501–4.
2. Baumgartner FJ, Gheissari A, Panagiotides GP, Capouya ER, Declusion RJ, Yokoyama T. Off pump obtuse marginal grafting with local stabilization: thoracotomy approach in re-operations. *Ann Thorac Surg* 1999; **68**:946–8.
3. Pitsis AA, Angelini GD. Off pump coronary bypass grafting of the circumflex artery. *Eur J Cardiothorac Surg* 1999; **16**:478–9.
4. Byrne JG, Aklog L, Adams DH, Cohn LH, Aranki SF. Re-operative CABG using left thoracotomy: a tailored strategy. *Ann Thorac Surg* 2001; **71**:196–200.
5. Cartier R, Blain R. Off pump revascularization of the circumflex artery: technical aspect and short-term results. *Ann Thorac Surg* 1999; **68**:94–9.
6. Dewey TM, Magee MJ, Edgerton JR, Vela R, Prince SL, Acuff TE, *et al.* Left mini-thoracotomy for beating heart bypass grafting: a safe alternative to high-risk intervention for selected grafting of the circumflex artery distribution. *Circulation* 2001; **104**(12 Suppl. I):I99–101.
7. Reichenspurner H, Boehm DH, Welz A, Schmitz C, Wildhirt S, Schulze C, *et al.* Minimally invasive coronary artery bypass grafting: port-access approach versus off pump techniques. *Ann Thorac Surg* 1999; **66**:1036–40.
8. Ascione R, Lloyd CT, Underwood MJ, Lotto AA, Pitsis AA, Angelini GD. Inflammatory response after coronary revascularization with or without cardiopulmonary bypass. *Ann Thorac Surg* 2000; **69**:1198–204.
9. Lockowandt U, Owall A, Franco-Cereceda A. Myocardial outflow of prostacyclin in relation to metabolic stress during off pump coronary artery bypass grafting. *Ann Thorac Surg* 2000; **70**:206–11.
10. Czerny M, Baumer H, Kilo J, Lassnig A, Hamwi A, Vukovich T, *et al.* Inflammatory response and myocardial injury following coronary artery bypass grafting with or without cardiopulmonary bypass. *Eur J Cardiothorac Surg* 2000; **17**:737–42.

11. Matata BM, Sosnowski AW, Galinanes M. Off pump bypass graft operation significantly reduces oxidative stress and inflammation. *Ann Thorac Surg* 2000; **69**:785–91.

12. Wan S, Izzat MB, Lee TW, Wan IYP, Tang NLS, Yim APC. Avoiding cardiopulmonary bypass in multivessel CABG reduces cytokine response and myocardial injury. *Ann Thorac Surg* 1999; **68**:52–6.

13. Magee MJ, Jablonski KA, Stamou SC, Pfister AJ, Dewey TM, Dullum MKC, *et al.* Elimination of cardiopulmonary bypass improves early survival for multivessel coronary artery bypass patients. *Ann Thorac Surg* 2002; **73**:1196–202.

14. Sabik JF, Gillinov AM, Blackstone EH, Vacha C, Houghtalling P, Navia J, *et al.* Does off-pump coronary surgery reduce morbidity and mortality. *J Thorac Cardiovasc Surg* 2002; **124**:698–707.

15. Mack MJ, Bachand D, Acuff TE, Edgerton JR, Prince SL, Dewey TM. Improved outcomes in coronary artery bypass grafting with beating heart techniques. *J Thorac Cardiovasc Surg* 2002; **124**:598–607.

16. Tasdemir O, Vural KM, Karagoz H, Bayazit K. Coronary artery bypass grafting on the beating heart without the use of extracorporeal circulation: review of 2052 cases. *J Thorac Cardiovasc Surg* 1998; **116**:68–73.

17. Kirklin JK. Prospects for understanding and eliminating the deleterious effects of cardiopulmonary bypass. *Ann Thorac Surg* 1999; **51**:529–31.

18. Chenoweth DE, Cooper SW, Hughi TE, Stewart RW, Blackstone EH, Kirklin JW. Complement activation during cardiopulmonary bypass; evidence for generation of C3a and C5a anaphylatoxins. *N Engl J Med* 1981; **304**:497–503.

19. Ohri SK. The effects of cardiopulmonary bypass on the immune system. *Perfusion* 1999; **8**:121–37.

20. Delva E, Maille JG, Solymoss BC, Chabot M, Grondin CM, Bourassa MG. Evaluation of myocardial damage during coronary artery grafting with serial determinations of serum CPK MB isoenzymes. *J Thorac Cardiovasc Surg* 1978; **75**:467–75.

21. Daily PO, Pfeffer TA, Wisniewski JB, Steinke TA, Kinney TB, Moores WY, *et al.* Clinical comparisons of methods of myocardial protection. *J Thorac Cardiovasc Surg* 1987; **93**:324–36.

22. Gundry SR, Kirsh MM. A comparison of retrograde cardioplegia versus antegrade cardioplegia in the presence of coronary artery obstruction. *Ann Thorac Surg* 1984; **38**:124–7.

23. Rosenkranz ER, Okamoto F, Buckberg GD, Robertson JM, Vinten-Johansen J, Bughi HI. Safety of prolonged aortic clamping with blood cardioplegia. III. Aspartate enrichment of glutamate-blood cardioplegia in energy-depleted hearts after ischemic and reperfusion injury. *J Thorac Cardiovasc Surg* 1986; **91**:428–35.

24. Murkin JM, Boyd WD, Ganapathy S, Adams SJ, Peterson RC. Beating heart surgery: why expect less central nervous system morbidity? *Ann Thorac Surg* 1999; **68**:1498–501.

25. Trehan N, Mishra M, Kasliwal RR, Mishra A. Reduced neurological injury during CABG in patients with mobile aortic atheromas: a five-year follow-up study. *Ann Thorac Surg* 2000; **70**:1558–64.

26. Ricci M, Karamanoukian HL, Abraham R, Fricken KV, D'Ancona G, Choi S, *et al.* Stroke in octogenarians undergoing coronary artery surgery with and without cardiopulmonary bypass. *Ann Thorac Surg* 2000; **69**:1471–5.

27. Stamou SC, Dangas G, Dullum MKC, Pfister AJ, Boyce SW, Bafi AS, *et al.* Beating heart surgery in octogenarians: perioperative outcome and comparison with younger age groups. *Ann Thorac Surg* 2000; **69**:1140–5.

28. Koutlas TC, Elbeery JR, Williams JM, Moran JF, Francalancia NA, Chitwood WR. Myocardial revascularization in the elderly using beating heart coronary artery bypass surgery. *Ann Thorac Surg* 2000; **69**:1042–7.

29. Mack MJ, Dewey TM, Magee MJ. Facilitated anastomosis for re-operative circumflex coronary revascularisation on the beating heart through a left thoracotomy. *J Thorac Cardiovasc Surg* 2002; **123**:816–17.

30. Stamou SC, Pfister AJ, Dangas G, Dullum MKC, Boyce SW, Bafi AS, *et al.* Beating heart versus conventional single-vessel re-operative coronary artery bypass. *Ann Thorac Surg* 2000; **69**:1383–7.

31. Trehan N, Mishra M, Kasliwal RR, Mishra A. Surgical strategies in patients at high risk for stroke undergoing coronary artery bypass grafting. *Ann Thorac Surg* 2000; **70**:1037–45.

32. Stamou SC, Corso PJ. Coronary revascularization without cardiopulmonary bypass in high-risk patients: a route to the future. *Ann Thorac Surg* 2001; **71**:1056–61.

33. Ascione R, Lloyd CT, Underwood MJ, Gomes WJ, Angelini GD. On pump versus off pump coronary revascularization: evaluation of renal function. *Ann Thorac Surg* 1999; **68**:493–8.

34. Guler M, Kirali K, Toker ME, Bozbuga N, Omeroglue, Akinci E, *et al.* Different CABG methods in patients with chronic obstructive pulmonary disease. *Ann Thorac Surg* 2001; **71**:152–7.

35. Yokoyama T, Baumgartner FJ, Gheissari A, Capouya ER, Panagiotides GP, Declusin RJ. Off pump versus on pump coronary bypass in high-risk subgroups. *Ann Thorac Surg* 2000; **70**:1546–50.

36. Locker C, Shapira I, Paz Y, Kramer A, Gurevitch J, Matsa M, *et al.* Emergency myocardial revascularization for acute myocardial infarction: survival benefit of avoiding cardiopulmonary bypass. *Eur J Cardiothorac Surg* 2000; **17**:234–8.

37. Mohr R, Moshkovitch Y, Shapira I, Amir G, Hod H, Gurevitch J. Coronary artery bypass without cardiopulmonary bypass for patients with acute myocardial infarction. *J Thorac Cardiovasc Surg* 1999; **118**:50–6.

38. Watters MPR, Ascione R, Ryder IG, Ciulli F, Pitsis AA, Angelini GD. Hemodynamic changes during beating heart coronary surgery with the 'Bristol Technique'. *Eur J Cardiothorac Surg* 2001; **19**:34–40.

39. Mathison M, Edgerton JR, Horswell JL, Akin JJ, Mack MJ. Analysis of hemodynamic changes during beating heart surgical procedures. *Ann Thorac Surg* 2000; **70**:1355–60.

40. Grundeman PF, Borst C, Verlaan CWJ, Meijburg H, Moues CM, Jansen EWL. Exposure of circumflex branches in the tilted, beating porcine heart: echocardiographic evidence of right ventricular deformation and the effect of right or left heart bypass. *J Thorac Cardiovasc Surg* 1999; **118**:316–23.

41. Porat E, Sharony R, Ivry S, Ozaki S, Meyns BP, Flameng WJ, *et al.* Hemodynamic changes and right heart support during vertical displacement of the beating heart. *Ann Thorac Surg* 2000; **69**:1188–91.

42. Seumatsu Y, Ohtsuka T, Miyaji K, Murakami A, Miyairi T, Eyileten Z, *et al.* Right heart mini-pump bypass for coronary artery bypass grafting: experimental study. *Eur J Cardiothorac Surg* 2000; **18**:276–81.

43. Grundeman PF, Borst C, van Herwaarden JA, Verlaan CW, Jansen EW. Vertical displacement of the beating heart by the Octopus tissue stabilizer: influence on coronary flow. *Ann Thorac Surg* 1998; **65**:1348–52.

44. Mathison M, Buffolo E, Jatene AD, Jatene FB, Reichenspurner H, Matheny RG, *et al.* Right heart circulatory support facilitates coronary artery bypass without cardiopulmonary bypass. *Ann Thorac Surg* 2000; **70**:1083–5.

45. Nierich AP, Diephuis J, Jansen EW, Borst C, Knape JT. Heart displacement during off pump CABG: how well is it tolerated? *Ann Thorac Surg* 2000; **70**:466–72.

46. Baumgartner FJ, Gheissari A, Capouya ER, Panagiotides GP, Katouzian A, Yokoyama T. Technical aspects of total revascularization in off pump coronary bypass via sternotomy approach. *Ann Thorac Surg* 1999; **67**:1653–8.

47. Hangler HB, Pfaller K, Antretter H, Dapunt OE, Bonatti JO. Coronary endothelial injury after local occlusion on the human beating heart. *Ann Thorac Surg* 2001; **71**:122–7.

48. Heijmen RH, Borst C, van Dalen R, Verlaan CW, Moues CM, van der Helm YJ, *et al.* Temporary luminal arteriotomy seal: II. Coronary artery bypass grafting on the beating heart. *Ann Thorac Surg* 1998; **66**:471–6.

49. Okazaki Y, Takarabe K, Murayama, Suenaga E, Furukawa K, Rikitake K, *et al.* Coronary endothelial damage during off pump CABG related to coronary-clamping and gas insufflation. *Eur J Cardiothorac Surg* 2001; **19**:834–9.

50. Shennib H, Bastawisy A. Coronary artery bypass grafting on the beating heart: simple technique for subluxating the heart. *Ann Thorac Surg* 1999; **67**:870–1.

51. Bergsland J, Karamanoukian HL, Soltoski PR, Salerno TA. Single suture for circumflex exposure in off pump coronary artery bypass grafting. *Ann Thorac Surg* 1999; **68**:1428–30.

52. Ricci M, Karamanoukian HL, D'Ancona G, Bergsland J, Salerno TA. Exposure and mechanical stabilization in off pump coronary artery bypass grafting via sternotomy. *Ann Thorac Surg* 2000; **70**:1736–40.

53. Rama A, Mohammadi S, Leprince P, Gandjbakhch I. A simple method for heart stabilization during off pump multi-vessel coronary artery bypass grafting: surgical technique and short-term results. *Eur J Cardiothorac Surg* 2001; **19**:105–7.

54. Rousou JA, Engelman RM, Flack JE, Deaton DW. Fenestrated felt facilitates anastomotic stability and safety in off pump coronary bypass. *Ann Thorac Surg* 1999; **68**:272–3.

55. D'Ancona G, Karamanoukian HL, Ricci M, Schmid S, Bergsland J, Salerno TA. Graft revision after transit time flow measurement in off pump coronary artery bypass grafting. *Eur J Cardiothorac Surg* 2000; **17**:287–93.

56. Mariani MA, Gu YJ, Boonstra PW, Grandjean JG, van Oeveren W, Ebels T. Procoagulant activity after off pump coronary operation: is the current anticoagulation adequate? *Ann Thorac Surg* 1999; **67**:1370–5.

57. Cartier R, Robitaille D. Thrombotic complications in beating heart operations. *J Thorac Cardiovasc Surg* 2001; **121**:920–2.

58. Chavanon O, Carrier M, Cartier R, Hebert Y, Pellerin M, Page P, *et al.* Increased incidence of acute ascending aortic dissection with off pump aortocoronary bypass surgery? *Ann Thorac Surg* 2001; **71**:117–21.

59. Jedeus L, Blomstrom P, Niilsson L, Stridsberg M, Hansell P, Blomstrom-Lundqvist C. Tachyarrhythmias and triggering factors for atrial fibrillation after coronary artery bypass operations. *Ann Thorac Surg* 2000; **69**:1064–9.

60. Siebert J, Rogowski J, Jagielak D, Anisimowicz L, Lango R, Narkiewicz M. Atrial fibrillation after coronary artery bypass grafting without cardiopulmonary bypass. *Eur J Cardiothorac Surg* 2000; **17**:520–3.

61. Cartier R, Brann S, Dagenais F, Martineau R, Couturier A. Systematic off pump coronary artery revascularization in multivessel disease: experience of three hundred cases. *J Thorac Cardiovasc Surg* 2000; **119**:221–9.

62. Ascione R, Williams S, Lloyd CT, Sundaramoorthi T, Pitsis AA, Angelini GD. Reduced postoperative blood loss and transfusion requirement after beating heart coronary operations: a prospective randomized study. *J Thorac Cardiovasc Surg* 2001; **121**:689–96.

63. Hernandez F, Clough RA, Klemperer JD, Blum JM. Off pump coronary artery bypass grafting: initial experience at one community hospital. *Ann Thorac Surg* 2000; **70**:1070–2.

64. Puskas JD, Thourani VH, Marshall JJ, Dempsey SJ, Steiner MA, Sammons BH, *et al.* Clinical outcomes, angiographic patency, and resource utilization in 200 consecutive off pump coronary bypass patients. *Ann Thorac Surg* 2001; **71**:1477–84.

65. Turner WF. Off pump coronary artery bypass grafting: the first one hundred cases of the Rose City experience. *Ann Thorac Surg* 1999; **68**:1482–5.

66. Puskas JD, Wright CE, Ronson RS, Brown WM, Gott JP, Guyton RA. Off pump multivessel coronary bypass via sternotomy is safe and effective. *Ann Thorac Surg* 1998; **66**:1068–72.

67. Spooner TH, Hart JC, Pym J. A two-year, three institution experience with the Medtronic Octopus: systematic off pump surgery. *Ann Thorac Surg* 1999; **68**:1478–81.

68. Cartier R. Systematic off pump coronary artery revascularization: experience of 275 cases. *Ann Thorac Surg* 1999; **68**:1494–7.

69. Hart JC, Spooner TH, Pym J, Flavin TF, Edgerton JR, Mack MJ, *et al.* A review of 1,582 consecutive Octopus off pump coronary bypass patients. *Ann Thorac Surg* 2000; **70**:1017–20.

70. Nader ND, Khadra WZ, Reich NT, Bacon DR, Salerno TA, Panos AL. Blood product use in cardiac revascularization: comparison of on and off pump techniques. *Ann Thorac Surg* 1999; **68**:1640–3.

71. Mack MJ. Unpublished data.

72. Mack MJ. Pro: beating heart surgery for coronary revascularization: is it the most important development since the introduction of the heart–lung machine? *Ann Thorac Surg* 2000; **70**:1774–8.

73. Benson K, Hartz AJ. A comparison of observational studies and randomized, controlled trials. *N Engl J Med* 2000; **342**:1878–86.

74. Concato J, Shah N, Horwitz RI. Randomized, controlled trials, observational studies, and the hierarchy of research designs. *N Engl J Med* 2000; **342**:1887–92.

75. Pocock SJ, Elbourne DR. Randomized trials or observational tribulations? *N Engl J Med* 2000; **342**:1907–9.

76. Ascione R, Lloyd CT, Gomes WJ, Caputo M, Bryan AJ, Angelini GD. Beating versus arrested heart revascularization: evaluation of myocardial function in a prospective randomized study. *Eur J Cardiothorac Surg* 1999; **15**:685–90.

77. Ascione R, Lloyd CT, Underwood MJ, Lotto AA, Pitsis AA, Angelini DG. Economic outcome of off pump coronary artery bypass surgery: a prospective randomized study. *Ann Thorac Surg* 1999; **68**:2237–42.

78. Cox CM, Ascione R, Cohen AM, Davies IM, Ryder IG, Angelini GD. Effect of cardiopulmonary bypass on pulmonary gas exchange: a prospective randomized study. *Ann Thorac Surg* 2000; **69**:140–5.

79. Lloyd CT, Ascione R, Underwood MJ, Gardner F, Black A, Angelini GD. Serum S100 protein release and neuropsychologic outcome during coronary revascularization on the beating heart: a prospective randomized study. *J Thorac Cardiovasc Surg* 2000; **119**:148–54.

80. Diegeler A, Hirsch R, Schneider F, Schilling LO, Falk V, Rauch T, *et al.* Neuromonitoring and neurocognitive outcome in off pump versus conventional coronary bypass operation. *Ann Thorac Surg* 2000; **69**:1162–6.

81. Casati V, Gerli C, Franco A *et al.* Tranexamic acid in off pump coronary surgery: a preliminary randomized, double-blind, placebo-controlled study. *Ann Thorac Surg* 2000; **72**:470–5.

82. Van Dijk D, Keizer AMA, Diephuis JC, Durand C, Vos LJ, Hijman R. Neurocognitive dysfunction after coronary artery bypass surgery: a systematic review. *J Thorac Cardiovasc Surg* 2000; **120**:632–9.

83. Cremer JT, Wittwer T, Boning A, Anssar MB, Kofidis T, Mugge A, *et al.* Minimally invasive coronary artery revascularization on the beating heart. *Ann Thorac Surg* 2000; **69**:1787–91.

84. Detter C, Reichenspurner H, Boehm DH, Thalhammer M, Schutz A, Reichart B. Single vessel revascularization with beating heart techniques – minithoracotomy or sternotomy? *Eur J Cardiothorac Surg* 2001; **19**:464–70.

85. Jansen EWL, Borst C, Lahpor JR, Grundeman PF, Eeftling FD, Nierich A. Coronary artery bypass grafting without cardiopulmonary bypass using the Octopus method: results in the first one hundred patients. *J Thorac Cardiovasc Surg* 1998; **116**:60–7.

86. Caputo M, Chamberlain MH, Ozalp F, Underwood MJ, Ciulli F, Angelini G. Off pump coronary operations can be safely taught to cardiothoracic trainees. *Ann Thorac Surg* 2001; **71**:1215–19.

87. Yeatman M, Caputo M, Ascione R, Ciulli F, Angelini GD. Off pump coronary artery bypass surgery for critical left main stem disease: safety, efficacy and outcome. *Eur J Cardiothorac Surg* 2001; **19**:239–44.

88. Dewey TM, Magee MJ, Edgerton JR, Mathison M, Tennison D, Mack MJ. Off pump bypass grafting is safe in patients with left main coronary disease. *Ann Thorac Surg* 2001; **72**:788–92.

89. Magee MJ, Dewey TM, Acuff TE, Edgerton JR, Hebeler JF, Prince SL, *et al.* Influence of diabetes on mortality and morbidity: off pump coronary artery bypass grafting versus coronary artery bypass grafting with cardiopulmonary bypass. *Ann Thorac Surg* 2001; **72**:776–81.

90. Plomondon ME, Cleveland JC, Ludwig ST, Grunwald GK, Kiefe CI, Grover FL, *et al.* Off pump coronary artery bypass is associated with improved risk-adjusted outcomes. *Ann Thorac Surg* 2001; **72**:114–19.

91. Brown PP, Mack MJ, Simon AW, Battaglia SL, Tarkington LG, Culler SD, *et al.* Comparing clinical outcomes in high-volume and low-volume off pump coronary bypass programs. *Ann Thorac Surg* 2001; **72**:S1009–15.

92. Roach GW, Kanchuger M, Mangano CM, Newman, M, Nussmeier N, Wolman R, *et al.* Adverse cerebral outcomes after coronary bypass surgery. *N Engl J Med* 1996; **335**:1857–64.

93. Newman MF, Kirchner JL, Phillips-Bute B, Gaver V, Grocott H, Jones RH, *et al.* Longitudinal assessment of neurocognitive function after coronary artery bypass surgery. *N Engl J Med* 2001; **344**:395–402.

94. Wandschneider W, Thalmann M, Trampitsch E, Zievogel G, Kobinia G. Off pump coronary bypass operations significantly reduces S100 release: an indicator for less cerebral damage? *Ann Thorac Surg* 2000; **70**:1577–9.

95. Anderson RE, Hanson LO, Vaage J. Release of S100B during coronary artery bypass grafting is reduced by off pump surgery. *Ann Thorac Surg* 1999; **67**:1721–5.

96. Trehan N, Mishra M, Sharma OP, Mishra A, Kasliwal RR. Further reduction in stroke after off pump coronary artery bypass grafting: a 10-year experience. *Ann Thorac Surg* 2001; **72**:S1026–32.

97. Siebert J, Anisimowicz L, Lango R, Rogowski J, Pawlaczyk R, Brzezinski M, *et al.* Atrial fibrillation after coronary artery bypass grafting: does the type of procedure influence the early postoperative incidence? *Eur J Cardiothorac Surg* 2001; **19**:455–9.

98. Novick RJ, Fox SA, Stitt LW, Swinamer SA, Lehnhardt KR, Rayman R, *et al.* Cumulative sum failure analysis of a policy change from on pump to off pump coronary artery bypass grafting. *Ann Thorac Surg* 2001; **72**:S1016–21.

99. Sergeant P, de Worm E, Meyns B, Wouters P. The challenge of departmental quality control in the reengineering towards off pump coronary artery bypass grafting. *Eur J Cardiothorac Surg* 2001; **20**:538–43.

100. Izzat MB, El-Zufari MH, Yim AP. Training model for beating heart coronary artery anastomoses. *Ann Thorac Surg* 1998; **66**:580–1.

101. Ricci M, Karamanoukian HL, D'Ancona G, DeLaRosa J, Karamanoukian RL, Choi S, *et al.* Survey of resident training in beating heart operations. *Ann Thorac Surg* 2000; **70**:479–82.

102. Solem JO, Boumzebra D, Al-Buraiki J, Nakeeb S, Rafeh W, Al-Halees Z. Evaluation of a new device for quick sutureless coronary artery anastomosis in surviving sheep. *Eur J Cardiothorac Surg* 2000; **17**:312–18.

103. Eckstein FS, Bonilla LF, Englerger L, Stauffer E, Berg TA, Schmidli J, *et al.* Minimizing aortic manipulation during OPCAB using the symmetry aortic connector system for proximal vein graft anastomoses. *Ann Thorac Surg* 2001; **72**:S995–8.

13

Minimally invasive techniques for coronary surgery

VICTOR F CHU, L WILEY NIFONG AND W RANDOLPH CHITWOOD JR

INTRODUCTION

Heightened interest in minimally invasive coronary operations began in the 1990s in response to emerging patient challenges and new technological opportunities. Early successes of minimally invasive and endoscopic techniques have fostered an expanding trend towards less invasive and patient-friendlier[1] operations in many surgical specialties. Contemporaneously, catheter-based technologies were rapidly expanding[2] and redefining the indications for surgical and percutaneous revascularization. Minimally invasive cardiac surgery (MICS) can be categorized according to the use (or not) of cardiopulmonary bypass or, alternatively, by the size and location of incision. The authors consider that MICS is the culmination of minimal to no perfusion, small incisions, minimal to no musculo-skeletal retraction, and careful hemostasis with blood conservation. When combined with altered anesthetic and critical care pathways, a 'new philosophy' of surgery has evolved. Innovations in retraction, exposure, cardiac motion stabilization, cardiopulmonary perfusion, assisted visualization, creation of anastomoses, hemostasis, tissue adhesives, cardiac support and instrumentation have placed this new cardiac surgery era within the reach of most surgeons. This chapter provides an overview of both the technical and clinical aspects of MICS, including the latest experimental studies and clinical trials.

MINIMALLY INVASIVE APPROACHES IN CORONARY SURGERY

Conventional approaches for coronary surgery have consisted of a complete median sternotomy, central cardiopulmonary bypass and cardioplegic arrest. Surgical trauma from a median sternotomy can be associated with significant postoperative morbidity and patient discomfort. This can be problematic, especially in diabetics, with osteoporotic sternums, following irradiation, and with sternal abnormalities. Discomfort is related to both the length of the musculo-skeletal incision and the extent of sternal spreading. Ribs hinge at the thoracic vertebrae, therefore wide sternal spreading increases paraspinal and posterior thoracic pain. Cardiopulmonary bypass has been the mainstay of coronary surgery but is considered to be the predominant cause of postoperative systemic inflammatory responses and bleeding. Moreover, cannulation and manipulation of the aorta can cause intraoperative embolic debris and strokes. Cardioplegia provides a quiescent heart during coronary anastomoses but, even with the best protective strategies, may not prevent postoperative myocardial depression. Moreover, hypothermic perfusion can cause coagulopathies leading to postoperative bleeding. To minimize these detrimental effects of conventional coronary surgery, innovative minimally invasive techniques have been developed to enable revascularization through smaller incisions with or without cardiopulmonary bypass.

MINIMALLY INVASIVE DIRECT CORONARY ARTERY BYPASS (MIDCAB) AND VARIATIONS

In 1967, the Russian surgeon Vasili Kolessov[3] performed the first internal thoracic artery to coronary artery anastomosis on a beating heart via a left anterior thoracotomy. The surgical community did not appreciate his ingenuity for nearly 30 years, when his technique was revisited. His operation is now known as the minimally invasive direct coronary artery bypass, or MIDCAB. Various terms and acronyms have been used to describe this procedure and the many subsequent variations (Table 13.1).

The most common indication for a MIDCAB is isolated coronary artery disease (CAD), occurring in the left anterior descending (LAD) artery distribution, where a single left internal thoracic artery (LITA) bypass alone is needed. Sequential anastomosis or composite Y-grafts to both the LAD and diagonal branches can be performed as well. In selected patients, isolated proximal right coronary artery disease is also an indication for a right-sided MIDCAB, using the right internal thoracic artery (RITA).

A typical MIDCAB is performed through a small (3.5–12 cm) left anterior thoracotomy made in the 4th or 5th intercostal space (Figure 13.1).[4–6] Either resection or division of the 4th costal cartilage has been used to improve exposure. More recently, surgeons have preferred to avoid cartilage resection and division. Dissection of the LITA is done either under direct vision[7,8] or using thoracoscopic assistance.[4,9] Specially designed 'lift' retractors may improve exposure of the proximal LITA by elevating the 3rd and 4th ribs and simultaneously depressing the 1st

and 2nd ribs. Early in the development of the MIDCAB procedure, local coronary snares were used to control bleeding. Currently, however, clip devices (Myoclip™) have been designed to compress the myocardium around the vessel, thus avoiding intimal damage (Medtronic Corp., Minneapolis, MN). Also, specialized intracoronary shunts have been designed to provide continuous distal myocardial perfusion. In the MIDCAB procedure, the coronary anastomosis is completed through the incision, using conventional instruments and magnified direct vision with or without mechanical stabilization.

Mechanical heart stabilization has become the most important enabling technology for beating-heart coronary surgery. With mechanical stabilization, it is much easier to achieve a locally motionless operative field without affecting global contractility. Numerous types of stabilizers are available commercially for beating-heart surgery (Figure 13.2).

Even early clinical outcomes of MIDCAB operations *without* stabilization were encouraging. Both Benetti[4] and Buffolo[6] reported a 2.3% mortality with no neurological complications. Despite this early work, Gundry found patency was limited severely in his first attempts at off-pump coronary surgery.[10] More recently, Gill reported that at 9.6 months a 95.4% angiographic patency could be achieved without using a stabilizer during beating-heart LITA to LAD anastomoses.[11] Despite these successes, mechanical stabilization facilitates coronary anastomoses and significantly improves both early graft patency rate and overall clinical outcomes. Calafiore and co-workers[12] reported 92.4% graft patency and 87% perfect anastomosis

Table 13.1 *Minimally invasive direct coronary artery bypass procedures*

Acronym	Procedure
MIDCAB	Minimally invasive direct coronary artery bypass
LAST operation	Left anterior small thoracotomy (same as MIDCAB)
H-Graft, T-Graft	Interposition graft, ITA–LAD
SAXCAB	Subclavian–axillary coronary artery bypass

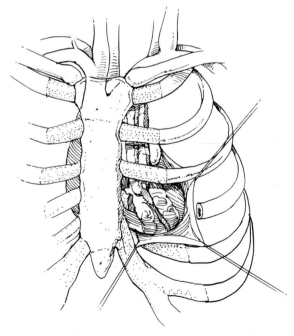

Figure 13.1 *Minimally invasive direct coronary artery bypass, surgical exposure.*

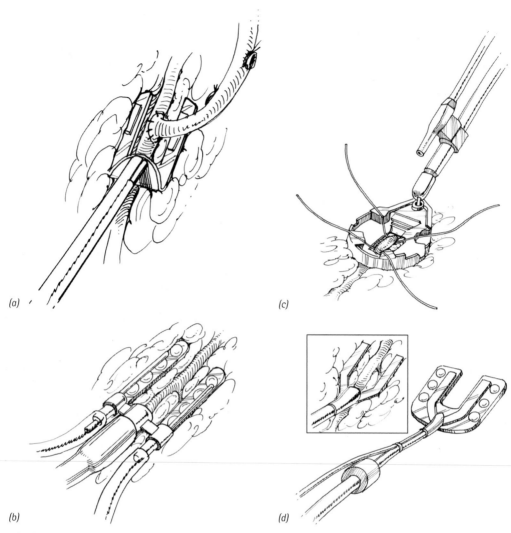

Figure 13.2 *Different types of mechanical heart stabilizers: (a) pusher type; (b) sucker type; (c) pusher–puller type; (d) pusher–sucker type.*

before LAD stabilization, compared to 98.2% patency and 95.4% perfect anastomosis after the employment of stabilizers. Others also reported similar improved early patency rates using mechanical stabilization.[13,14] In these patients, the early mortality has been reported to be approximately 1.0%.[12–15]

Intermediate-term clinical results and graft patency rates have compared favorably to those of conventional coronary artery bypass grafting (CABG). Mehran and co-workers[14] reported 7.8% adverse cardiac events and a 2.5% mortality at 1 year. Similarly, Vassiliades and co-workers[16] reported a 6-month angiographic patency of 98.3%.

When compared to perfusion-based CABG operations, the clinical benefits of the MIDCAB operation have included better postoperative pulmonary function,[17] shorter lengths of hospital stay and fewer blood transfusions.[18] A lower rate of postoperative atrial fibrillation was reported by some authors,[19] but was refuted by others.[20] Many reports have shown comparatively lower incidences

of neurological complications.[4–6] However, when compared to conventional single-vessel operations on cardiopulmonary bypass, neurological differences were not observed.[21] Most assuredly, age differences in these populations may contribute to the discrepancy. Potential pitfalls of MIDCAB include greater incisional pain when compared to sternotomy,[17] longer operating and myocardial ischemic times,[18] subclinical myocardial damage[22] and target vessel misidentification, leading to incorrect vessel grafting.[23]

It is generally agreed that the MIDCAB technique reduces overall hospital cost.[24] Most of the cost saving comes from eliminating cardiopulmonary bypass and providing a shorter hospital length of stay. King et al.[25] compared MIDCAB and conventional CABG operations and found a significant decrease in hospitalization (2.7 vs 4.8 days, respectively) and a commensurate large cost reduction ($10 129 vs $17 816, respectively). Similarly, del Rizzo et al. reported a cost saving of almost 50% in

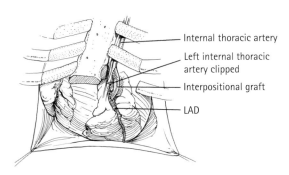

Internal thoracic artery

Left internal thoracic artery clipped

Interpositional graft

LAD

Figure 13.3 *Variations of MIDCAB. Interposition graft from LITA to LAD. T-graft has occluding clip on the LITA distal to the graft.*

high-risk patients undergoing a MIDCAB when compared to conventional CABG.[26]

MIDCAB *multivessel* bypass operations have been reported using either complex composite grafts[27] or multiple incisions.[28] The latter approach is particularly valuable in re-operative situations.[29] The 'hybrid' approach, combining MIDCAB and percutaneous transluminal balloon angioplasty (PTCA), is an alternative strategy for multivessel revascularization in high-risk patients.[30]

In certain high-risk situations, complete dissection and mobilization of the ITA can be avoided by placing an interposition graft between the chest wall-based *in situ* ITA and the target vessel via a MIDCAB approach (H-graft, T-MIDCAB, TRUCAB; Figure 13.3).[31,32] Another interesting MIDCAB variation is the subclavian-axillary artery to coronary artery bypass (SAXCAB) with a saphenous vein.[33] This is particularly attractive when the ITA is unavailable or of poor quality.

The MIDCAB approach combines small surgical incisions with beating-heart coronary surgery. Compared to conventional coronary surgery, the MIDCAB has been shown to have either equivalent or superior early and intermediate clinical results. In properly selected patients, the MIDCAB is an ideal choice for the treatment of single-vessel coronary disease, especially in the LAD distribution.

OFF-PUMP CORONARY ARTERY BYPASS (OPCAB)

Off-pump coronary artery bypass, commonly known as OPCAB, refers to coronary operations done without cardiopulmonary bypass or cardioplegia. By convention, OPCAB implies a median sternotomy approach, whereas MIDCAB connotes a small anterior thoracotomy approach. OPCAB procedures were performed in the early 1960s and before cardiopulmonary perfusion was used. However, after the heart–lung machine was developed and improved, only a few surgeons in the world continued to perform coronary operations without the

pump. Benetti[4] in Argentina and Buffolo[6] in Brazil were among the first to use off-pump coronary surgical techniques routinely. Their results demonstrated that beating-heart coronary bypass operations were feasible technically, and could be performed with satisfactory clinical outcomes.

The success of MIDCAB and the availability of improved mechanical stabilization have popularized beating-heart, multivessel coronary bypass operations. A full median sternotomy remains the preferred route for OPCAB surgery, allowing access to all regions of the coronary system. In these operations, grafts to the circumflex region offer the greatest challenges, and hemodynamic positioning can be achieved with generous cardiac access. Choices of conduits in OPCAB are not different from those of conventional coronary operations. However, pedicled arterial grafts are preferable in OPCABs as these grafts obviate the need for proximal anastomoses and provide immediate myocardial perfusion following completion of each distal anastomosis. Thus, regions at most jeopardy can be reperfused first before beginning to graft less vulnerable myocardium. Complete arterial revascularization using combinations of the RITA and LITA, as well as gastro-epiploic arteries,[34] is possible in selected patients. Most recently, radial arteries have been used in conjunction with pedicle arterial grafts to provide all arterial grafting.

Proper patient selection is crucial for OPCAB operations to ensure success. Although there is no consensus, some surgeons would exclude patients with severely depressed left ventricular function (ejection fraction <25%) and small (<1 mm) or diffusely diseased target vessels. Moreover, intramyocardial coronary vessels or the need for an endarterectomy increase the difficulty of the procedure significantly. Centers with considerable beating-heart coronary experience have reported OPCAB success in more than 95% of cases.[35,36]

Target vessel exposure on a contracting heart remains one of the most difficult technical skills during OPCAB procedures. Nevertheless, proper coronary exposure is particularly important for quality grafting. Several maneuvers have been shown to achieve optimal exposure while maintaining hemodynamic stability. The heart will often tolerate twisting and elevation of ventricular chambers during retroflexion, whereas significant compression more often causes hemodynamic instability. This ability to distort the heart radially probably relates to the countercurrent 'belted-spiral' motion of ventricular muscle layers.[37] Retraction using deep pericardial sutures placed in the oblique sinus and left inferior surfaces, combined with tilting the operating table 'head down', will deflect the heart into a vertical position with the apex pointing ventrad (Figure 13.4).[38] This 'verticalization' of the heart allows satisfactory exposure of both the circumflex and right coronary artery systems. Again, cardiac twisting is

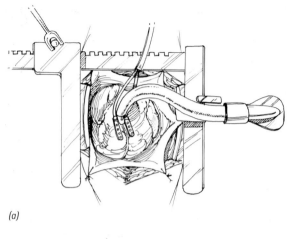

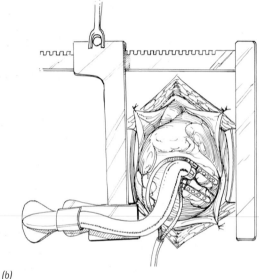

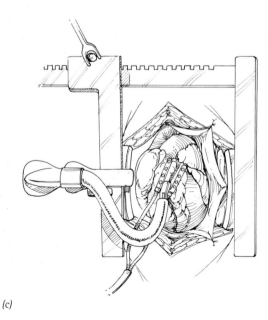

(a)

(b)

(c)

Figure 13.4 *Exposures for OPCAB: (a) anterior vessels; (b) lateral vessels; (c) inferior vessels.*

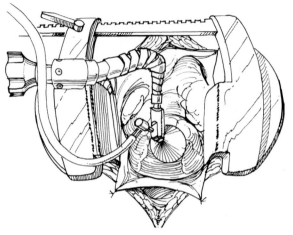

Figure 13.5 *Cardiac traction device, Xpose™ (Guidant Inc., Indianapolis, IN).*

preferable to compression. Not uncommonly, lifting the heart causes compression of the right chambers. During these maneuvers, incising the right basal pericardium widely, opening the right pleura, and volume loading the ventricle will generally stabilize the patient hemodynamically. Soft atraumatic slings placed through both the transverse and oblique sinuses have been used to improve circumflex vessel exposure. Specially designed cardiac positioning devices, employing apical or cardiac margin suction traction, have been developed to further improve exposure (Figure 13.5). With proper manipulation, it is possible to expose all coronary artery territories, including the circumflex and proximal obtuse marginals, which are particularly difficult.[39,40] Today, nearly all OPCAB procedures are performed using mechanical stabilizers, which have improved significantly in the last few years.

Clinical results of OPCAB operations in the *post-stabilizer era* compare favorably to those of conventional coronary artery surgery. In 1582 consecutive OPCAB cases, Hart *et al.*[41] showed 1% operative mortality, 0.6% permanent strokes, 1.2% myocardial infarctions and 2.6% conversions to conventional perfusion methods. In 2800 OPCAB operations carried out over a 10-year period, Trehan *et al.*[42] reported an overall hospital mortality of 2.14%, with only 0.14% neurological complications. These excellent results are similar to those reported by other OPCAB surgeons.[36,43]

The OPCAB technique has been hypothesized to reduce neurological complications markedly because of fewer cerebrovascular embolic events. However, clinical evidence supporting this theory remains inconsistent. Ricci *et al.*[44] reported no strokes in 97 OPCAB cases, compared with 9.3% strokes in 172 matched patients undergoing conventional CABG surgery in the same institution. Trehan *et al.* reported no strokes in 88 high-risk patients with preoperatively identified mobile aortic atheroma.[45] These authors suggested that, by eliminating cardiopulmonary bypass, OPCAB markedly decreases both the chance and occurrence of atheroemboli. In contradistinction, Arom et al.[46] showed no such difference in a retrospective review of 3521 consecutive coronary cases (including 350 OPCABs). These discrepancies could result from different patient populations.

Reported benefits of the OPCAB include fewer overall complications[47] and blood transfusions,[36] as well as shorter intensive care unit and hospital lengths of stay.[48] Clearly, the OPCAB appears to reduce the overall cost associated with the treatment of CAD.[24] The potential disadvantages of eliminating the pump during coronary artery surgery include a significant learning curve, longer operative times, a greater incidence of incomplete revascularization, and greater risks of ascending aortic dissection,[49] possibly related to partial aortic clamp occlusion during proximal anastomoses.

The OPCAB has the advantage of avoiding cardiopulmonary bypass and associated complications. Using modern operative techniques and instrumentation, multivessel complete coronary revascularization can be achieved with superior clinical results in properly selected patients. Currently, the OPCAB is the most frequent minimally invasive coronary procedure performed, now comprising 15–20% of all coronary cases. This percentage has constantly increased since the late 1990s, and some predict that most surgeons will perform well over 70% of their coronary operations using these new methods.

PORT-ACCESS™ CORONARY SURGERY

The Port-Access™ (Cardiovations, Johnson and Johnson Inc., Sommerville, NJ) system is comprised of peripheral cardiopulmonary perfusion cannulas, balloon aortic occlusive devices and specialized instruments, all of which permit cardiac operations to be done through small 'port' incisions on an arrested heart. The initial intent of the Port-Access™ system was to provide a totally endoscopic platform for cardiac surgery. Unlike mitral valve surgery, this approach became impractical for coronary surgery because of long-instrument tremor amplification and two-dimensional endoscopic visualization. Thus, most Port-Access™ coronary operations have been performed through small incisions, under direct vision, by displacing the arrested target vessel nearer to the incision. This allows the use of short instruments and direct vision, which provide the anastomotic accuracy and speed of conventional surgery. Following the initial Stanford University experience, several institutions used the Port-Access™ system for multivessel coronary operations,[50] most commonly through a small left thoracotomy.[51–57]

The Port-Access™ system uses peripheral cannulation for cardiopulmonary bypass and a catheter-based balloon

EndoClamp™ for aortic occlusion and cardioplegia delivery.[58] Arterial cannulas are placed either via the femoral artery or transthoracically into the ascending aorta. The balloon occlusion catheter is guided from the femoral artery to the proximal aorta, either under fluoroscopy or transesophageal echocardiography (TEE). Constant intraoperative TEE monitoring is necessary to avoid balloon migration and either dislodgement or innominate artery occlusion. Venous return is established via a single femoral vein cannula, passed into the right atrium using the Seldinger method. A small (6–7 cm) left anterior thoracotomy is generally used to access the heart and proximal aorta.

Galloway[50] reported one of the largest Port-Access™ coronary experiences. This multicenter international registry described 555 isolated Port-Access™ coronary bypass patients. The operative mortality, stroke rate and incidence of myocardial infarctions were 1.0%, 2.2% and 1.0%, respectively. These results are in agreement with others reported in the literature and compared favorably to that of the predicted outcomes of conventional CABG.[51–55,59]

Early in the history of this technique, endoaortic balloon occlusion became a common source of technical difficulties, not only because it required fluoroscopic or TEE guidance for placement, but also because the balloon can migrate into the ventricle, occlude the innominate artery, or even rupture during critical parts of the operation. These risks were resolved partially by design improvements, including the introduction of the Endodirect™ cannula.[60] This device consists of a knife-tipped cannula with an adjunctive occluding balloon, which is inserted through the chest wall and directly into the ascending thoracic aorta (Figure 13.6a). Other surgeons have modified the Port-Access™ technique by deploying a transthoracic aortic clamp,[57] eliminating completely the need for balloon occlusion. Modified aorta occluding balloon catheters, which also provide antegrade perfusion through multiple side orifices, are promising (Remote Access Perfusion(R), ESTECH Inc. Danville, CA; Figure 13.6b)

The advantage of the Port-Access™ method is that precise coronary anastomosis can be performed on an arrested decompressed heart without a median sternotomy. However, cardiopulmonary bypass is still required and remains the major morbidity and mortality factor during both conventional and Port-Access™ surgery. Thus far, Port-Access™ CABG clinical reports have not shown sufficient superior results to conventional operations to justify the added technical complexities and significant costs. Consequently, many centers have abandoned Port-Access™ coronary operations in favor of MIDCAB and OPCAB procedures, which are less costly than any on-pump operation.

Despite these data, Port-Access™ or alternative balloon-perfusion methods for coronary surgery could

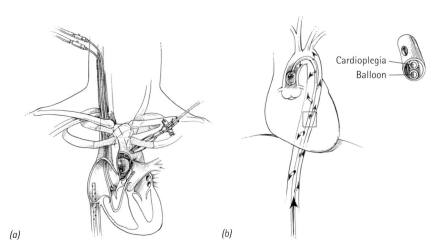

(a)   (b)

Figure 13.6 *Port-Access™ system: (a) Endodirect™ arterial cannula; (b) modified peripheral arterial cannula (Remote Access Perfusion®, ESTECH Inc., Danville, CA).*

enjoy a renaissance in the near future. Robotic methods are being shown to be efficacious for endoscopic coronary surgery, albeit at a slow pace. As balloon occlusive methods do not require direct access to the aorta, they seem particularly advantageous in closed chest coronary surgery and especially in totally endoscopic coronary artery bypass (TECAB) operations using computer-assisted surgical robotics. Early reports combining this tele-manipulative technology with closed chest aortic balloon occlusion and perfusion seem promising for future surgeons.

TOTALLY ENDOSCOPIC CORONARY ARTERY BYPASS (TECAB) AND ROBOTICS

Early in the course of totally endoscopic coronary surgery, efforts using conventional instruments were discouraging and were hampered by anastomotic imprecision because of two-dimensional visualization. Conventional endoscopic instruments and videoscopes were limited by several factors:

1 the 'fulcrum' effect of long instruments makes a microscopic anastomosis difficult,
2 two-dimensional endoscopic imaging is inadequate, and
3 the bony thorax limits exact placement and instrument movements.

The development of computer-assisted tele-manipulation devices and three-dimensional visualization has helped to overcome these technical limitations.

The *da Vinci*™ (Intuitive Surgical Inc., Mountain View, CA) and *Zeus*™ robotic systems (Computer Motion Inc., Goleta, CA) are in the early stages of clinical application for coronary surgery. Despite very different designs, both systems employ three-dimensional high-definition video visualization and computer-assisted remotely controlled microsurgical instruments with either 7° (*da Vinci*™) or 6° (*Zeus*™) of freedom motion. Both *da Vinci*™ and *Zeus*™ are master-slave remote tele-manipulators. The master control units are coupled to slave robotic arms via a computerized interface, which receives motion input from the surgeon. This input is processed digitally before transmitting complex fine-motion commands to the instrument tips at the surgical site. Through this human-to-digital interface, the system emulates the surgeon's motion either in real time or at a reduced ratio (motion scaling). Moreover, high-frequency unintentional movements are filtered (tremor filtration), allowing the operator the benefits of electronic ambidexterity. The net result is tremor-free, high-precision, well-controlled and wide-ranging movements at instrument tips. As instrument articulation and movements are within the bony thorax, the fulcrum effect is eliminated completely. Visual feedback is transmitted to the master console as magnified high-resolution three-dimensional videoscopic images. Robotically controlled endoscopic vision provides virtual 'tele-presence' for the surgeon. The surgeon now appears to become part of the operative topography. Superior visualization and precise instrument control are the key advantages of these robotic surgical systems.

Several authors have shown that excellent coronary anastomoses can be constructed using robotic tele-manipulation. Damiano[61] and Falk[62] have shown clinically that high-quality grafts can be constructed without endothelial injury. These studies encouraged the further development of totally endoscopic robotic coronary operations (Figure 13.7). To date, TECAB operations have been performed either on arrested hearts, using the Port-Access™ system,[62,63] or on beating hearts, using specially designed endoscopic stabilizers.[64,65] Initial clinical studies, conducted in Europe and Canada, have demonstrated both feasibility and safety of TECAB procedures. Similarly, clinical trials of both beating and arrested heart robotically assisted TECABs are currently

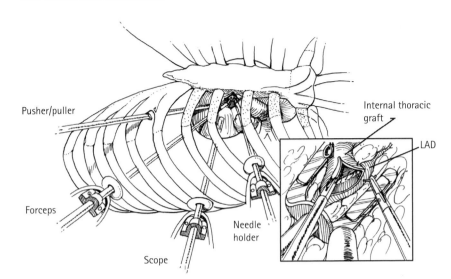

Figure 13.7 *Totally endoscopic coronary artery bypass.*

underway in Europe and North America. We are planning to begin Food and Drug Administration (FDA)-based coronary bypass trials soon, and consider that complete revascularization must be the goal for the benefits of robotic surgery to be realized fully.

MINIMALLY INVASIVE CONDUIT HARVESTING

The pedicled internal thoracic artery is the conduit of choice for coronary operations. Since the early reports of Okies and Lytle, a >98% patency rate at 10 years has been reported in conventional coronary surgery.[66,67] Harvesting of the ITA has commonly required forceful chest wall retraction, especially in MIDCAB procedures, and video-assisted visualization[9] can facilitate the ITA dissection in these operations. Endoscopic ITA dissection is a logical step towards the development of TECAB surgery. Recently, several authors have shown that the harvest can be facilitated by computer-assisted surgical robotic systems.[68–70] Both the *da Vinci*™ and *Zeus*™ systems have been used in Europe and have received FDA approval in the USA for ITA harvest and preparation. Clinical experience from robotically assisted ITA takedown procedures has shown that it is safe and reduces patient discomfort.[71]

Traditional methods of greater saphenous vein harvesting, using long incisions, are frequent causes of wound complications, patient discomfort and hospital readmissions.[72,73] Many patients complain of their long leg incisions more than of their sternotomy. With minimum conventional technique modifications and instrument development, it is possible to harvest the entire saphenous vein using sequential small incisions (Figure 13.8a). In a prospective randomized study, Tevaearai *et al.* reported shorter additive incision length, less incisional hematoma

and less pain using small, interrupted incisions.[74] Specially developed endoscopic vein harvesting instruments can further reduce the size of leg skin incisions and the rate of complications (Figure 13.8b).[73,75] Initial concerns regarding damage to saphenous vein grafts during minimally invasive vein harvesting have been alleviated somewhat by reports revealing intact endothelial and smooth muscle function following minimally invasive vein harvests.[76,77] The success of endoscopic vein harvesting has encouraged the development of minimally invasive techniques for radial and gastro-epiploic artery harvesting.[78,79] As cosmesis is important for radial harvest patients, these devices seem particularly exciting.

ANESTHESIA AND POSTOPERATIVE CARE IN MINIMALLY INVASIVE CARDIAC SURGERY

With the arrival of minimally invasive techniques, it has been necessary to modify anesthetic techniques to provide safety and maximize the benefits. In many beating-heart operations, especially in MIDCAB procedures, it is possible to extubate most patients in the operating room. However, early extubation requires digression from traditional narcotic-based deep cardiac anesthesia, in which early extubation was not possible, and depends on a strategy based upon shorter acting agents, such as propofol.[80] Lighter anesthesia and earlier extubation also change the practice of intensive care unit postoperative care.[81] Supplemental perioperative metabolic support using insulin, magnesium, milrinone and norepinephrine has also been proposed to optimize off-pump surgeries.[82] Moreover, the nursing staff must be aware that this is a different type of postoperative cardiac patient and must use a different pain management protocol than previously employed in the management of heavily

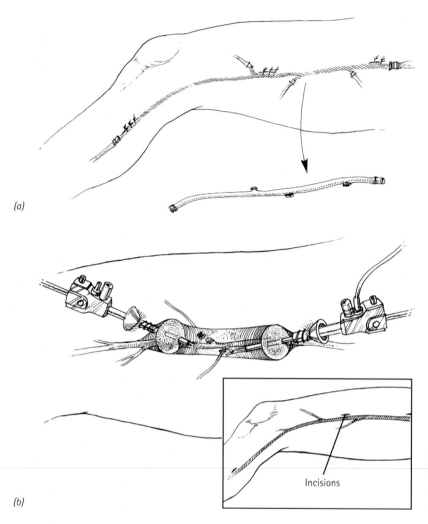

(a)

(b)

Incisions

Figure 13.8 *Minimally invasive saphenous vein harvesting: (a) sequential small incisions; (b) endoscopic vein harvesting instrument.*

sedated patients. Minimally invasive cardiac surgery is not a technique but a global patient care philosophy and strategy.

During off-pump surgery, anesthesiologists must be aware of the altered physiology patterns induced by the manipulation of cardiac chambers. Generally, volume loading and/or mild inotropic support can correct these hemodynamic changes. Also, regional ischemia is created during serial grafting, and thus observant arrhythmia management and heart rate control are a must. The posture that many anesthesiologists assumed during cardiopulmonary bypass can no longer exist and constant vigilance is paramount during cardiac manipulation.

Limited surgical incisions also limit direct visual assess to the heart. Intraoperative TEE[83,84] offers real-time, objective measurements of cardiac contractility, ventricular volume and valvular function. During Port-Access™ procedures and other method of percutaneous intracardiac catheter insertions, TEE is necessary for safe guidance.[85] Lastly, in open cardiac procedures, during which limited manipulation of the heart impedes air evacuation, intraoperative echocardiography is essential.

ENABLING TECHNOLOGIES IN MINIMALLY INVASIVE CORONARY SURGERY

Technological innovations have been the 'springboard' for the development of MICS. Enabling devices have been designed to facilitate performance and/or expedite these procedures. We are at the developmental beginning of exciting new devices, methods and techniques dedicated to performing coronary surgery more quickly, less invasively, more accurately and with fewer complications.

Mechanical stabilizers and exposure devices

In order to achieve high-quality, reproducible, optimal results, coronary anastomoses must be constructed in a near-motionless operative field. During the early development of beating-heart surgery, ingenious methods were developed to alter heart rate and contractility, thus minimizing coronary movement. Beta-blockers, calcium-channel blockers, adenosine[86] and vagal stimulation[87] were used to either reduce or temporarily arrest global contraction. Local coronary snares and retraction sutures were also used to achieve local stabilization, but met with limited success. Moreover, surgeons became concerned about the potential of coronary endothelial injuries. Reports of the use of mechanical stabilization appeared in the literature in 1997.[88–90] The mechanical stabilization concept is simple: to immobilize the local target area at the anastomotic site without affecting global contractility. Subsequent clinical experiences confirmed the effectiveness of this concept, which revolutionized the practice of beating-heart coronary surgery.[36,41,91,92]

There are three basic types of mechanical stabilizers. The 'pusher' type reduces wall motion locally by compressing the ventricle on both sides of the target vessel. Many 'pusher'-type stabilizers are available commercially. This stabilizer is composed of a U-shaped pusher plate connected to the chest retractor via a rigid rod with universal joints. Tightening of these joints provides optimal coronary positioning and stability. Although the basic concept remains unchanged, the newer generation of devices has a lower profile, is more versatile and is easier to operate. The 'pusher–puller' type additionally has a 'coronary cage' at the pusher end. Here, the frame or 'cage' device pushes down around the artery, while Silastic snares pull the artery into the frame to further immobilize it and create hemostasis. 'Sucker'-type stabilizers immobilize the target area using epicardial vacuum suction. These tend to evert the epicardium away from the vessel, whereas the 'pusher' compression plates tend to invert surface epicardium over the artery. All three types are capable of creating a motionless local operative field. The 'pusher' type is simple and straightforward in its application. However, positioning of this device on lateral and posterior walls is often more difficult than either 'suction' or 'pusher–puller' methods. Moreover, the 'sucker' type seems to have the advantage of obtaining better hemodynamic stability in certain positions, as it avoids pushing the ventricular wall. Newer stabilizers could combine 'pusher' and 'sucker' mechanisms. We have found when doing circumflex coronary anastomoses that during relaxation the heart tolerates twisting better than firm compression. Jansen determined both the reasons for and corrections of abnormal hemodynamics affected by alterations in cardiac position.[93,94]

The Medtronic Octopus™ stabilizer typifies the 'sucker'-type device. As its name implies, the Octopus™ is made of suction cups attached to a flexible coaxial arm, which becomes rigid when locked. The first-generation Octopus™ stabilizers were attached to the operating table and were both bulky and encumbering. The current generation, the Octopus IV™ device, is much smaller, attaches directly to the chest retractor and is as easy to apply. It seems that suction stabilization enables cardiac retraction better than other devices and often does not require pericardial retraction or myocardial sutures. To

assist further in cardiac positioning during beating-heart operations, suction-type heart positioning devices have been developed. The Xpose™ (see Figure 13.5; Guidant Inc., Indianapolis, IN) and Starfish™ (Medtronic Inc., Minneapolis, MN) devices help manipulate target sites in all myocardial regions without unwanted myocardial compression. These positioning devices are then *combined* with stabilizer systems to provide optimal coronary target position and stabilization. Advanced heart positioning techniques are particularly helpful during circumflex coronary grafting.

Intracoronary and aortocoronary shunts

During beating-heart coronary operations, snares and vessel clips are often used to temporarily occlude vessels in order to achieve a bloodless field. However, resulting myocardial ischemia may be poorly tolerated, especially when incomplete atherosclerotic occlusions of the proximal LAD and/or right coronary arteries exist.[95] To establish distal perfusion while maintaining a bloodless operative field, intracoronary shunts (Figure 13.9) have been devised.[96] Studies have shown that intracoronary shunting does not cause more endothelial injury when compared to external compression hemostatic methods.[97]

To improve hemodynamic stability further by maintaining distal myocardial perfusion during beating-heart operations, aortocoronary perfusion devices have also been developed. Van Aarnhem *et al.* proposed using simple, passive aortocoronary shunts[95] placed in the distal coronary artery to alleviate ischemia during off-pump coronary grafting. Active perfusion of both anastomosed vein grafts[98] and distal coronary vessels has been proposed as well. These perfusion devices may enable more

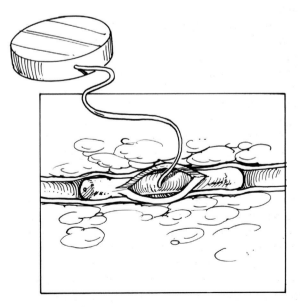

Figure 13.9 *Intracoronary shunt.*

complete revascularization during complex multivessel OPCAB operations, especially in the presence of poor ventricular function.

Anastomotic devices

Currently, most OPCAB operations still require the use of partial occlusion clamps to construct proximal vein graft anastomosis. This method is a potential source of embolic debris, and may also pose an increased risk of aortic dissection in pressurized aortas.[49] Sutureless mechanical anastomotic devices,[99] such as the Symmetry™ Bypass System (St Jude Medical Inc., St Paul, MN), allow attachment of proximal vein grafts to the aorta without clamping. This device is deployed in two steps and requires no aortic manipulation, except of the direct aortotomy site. These devices significantly reduce aortic manipulation, enhance vein conservation, and may potentially become a significant factor in the expansion of off-pump coronary surgery.

Experiences from TECAB operations have shown that robotic suture handling and endoscopic knot tying remain cumbersome and time consuming. Active research and clinical trials are underway currently to develop alternative sutureless anastomotic techniques. Coalescent™ clips (Coalescent Inc., Sunnyvale, CA) are Nitinol™-based alloy clips, which replace traditional running coronary anastomotic sutures with interrupted self-closing clips. Totally sutureless, distal anastomotic connectors are also in the late phase of animal studies. Some of these deploy stent-like connections, while others use magnetic connectors to fuse graft to coronary artery. Recent unpublished experimental studies by Adams and clinical applications by Mohr have been encouraging using the magnetic anastomotic couplers (Ventrica Inc., Fremont, CA). These new technologies are bringing us closer to a future of totally sutureless and potentially robotic endoscopic coronary surgery.

Cardiac support devices

Hemodynamic deterioration during OPCAB operations can occur as a result of either poor ventricular function[100] or compression of right-sided heart chambers during exposure of posterior vessels.[94] Left and right heart mechanical support has been shown to improve hemodynamic stability during some OPCAB operations. Lonn et al.[100] reported the use of the Hemopump™ (Texas Heart Institute, Houston, TX) for left ventricular support in patients with depressed left ventricular function. The Hemopump™ is a percutaneously inserted axial-flow pump, capable of generating up to 3.5 L min^{-1} of support. Currently, this device is not available for clinical use in the USA.

Right heart dysfunction may be encountered during OPCAB procedures. The A-Med Coaxial™ cannula is a cable-driven, centrifugal pump used for right heart support during OPCAB procedures (A-Med Inc., Sacramento, CA). Recently, Lima et al.[101] reported their initial multicenter clinical experience of beating-heart coronary surgery with the A-Med pump. They reported that the system improved hemodynamics and reduced inotropic support requirements, especially during circumflex anastomoses. Further clinical studies are needed to elucidate the clinical indications and benefits of these ventricular support systems in beating-heart coronary surgeries.

GRAFT VERIFICATION

Conventional CABG operations have achieved excellent short-term and long-term graft patency and clinical outcomes. It is imperative that any reduction of surgical invasiveness must not come at the expense of graft quality. Intraoperative and postoperative verification of graft patency is an indispensable safeguard for anyone performing MICS.

Selective coronary angiography is considered to be the 'gold standard' for the assessment of graft patency. Intraoperative angiography can be performed, without significant added cost, by the surgeon[102] or the cardiologist.[103] Using radial artery-based angiography, Elbeery[102] showed a number of angiographic ITA–coronary imperfections that were not obvious from Doppler studies and required acute graft revisions. However, some causes of early angiographic stenosis, such as vessel spasm, edema, mural hematoma or luminal clot, are potentially reversible without re-intervention. Thus, routine intraoperative angiography may result in unnecessary revisions. Comparison of early angiographic patency and long-term graft patency is difficult due to the heterogeneity of published studies. Nevertheless, intraoperative angiography provides surgeons with direct visual assessment of entire graft quality before leaving the operating room.

Intraoperative Doppler has been used widely for the verification of graft flow. Lin et al.[104] have shown a 100% correlation of hand-held Doppler patency and intraoperative angiography in a series of 35 patients. However, Elbeery[102] showed that qualitative Doppler ultrasound failed to identify some anastomotic stenoses definitively. Doppler ultrasound is less invasive and much easier to perform intraoperatively than coronary angiography.

Transit time flow measurement (TTFM) is an ultrasound-based technology, which determines graft flow independently of vessel size, shape and Doppler angle.[105] By carefully analyzing the flow curves, the pulsatile index and mean flow values obtained intraoperatively, it is possible to identify a significant number of unsatisfactory grafts before leaving the operating room. D'Ancona et al.[106] reported a 3.2% revision rate in 1145 grafts based on TTFM studies. In 35 of the 37 revisions, technical or anatomical problems were identified and corrected. TTFM is a simple and reproducible method of intraoperative flow measurement, which is capable of influencing surgical decision-making in a significant number of patients.

In MICS, graft verification is an important quality-control mechanism. With currently available technologies, it is possible to attain near the goal of 100% early graft patency.

SUMMARY

Considerable progress has been made over the past decade in reducing the surgical invasiveness of coronary operations. Cardiac surgeons today have an armamentarium of multiple less invasive approaches, which can be tailored to individual patient needs. The continued developments of new devices and enabling technologies will further facilitate minimally invasive coronary operations. The addition of computer-assisted remote manipulation will bring us even closer to the 'ideal' coronary operation, which may be a totally endoscopic beating-heart multivessel bypass method. Continued technical innovations, unrelenting pursuit of leading-edge technologies and meticulous attention to clinical outcomes will secure the success and competitiveness of coronary operations in the twenty-first century. In order to remain competitive in the treatment of coronary disease, cardiothoracic surgeons must continue to develop less invasive methods that have superior long-term results to catheter-based techniques.

KEY REFERENCES

Detter C, Reichenspurner H, Boehm DH, Thalhammer M, Raptis P, Schutz A, *et al.* Minimally invasive direct coronary artery bypass grafting (MIDCAB) and off-pump coronary artery bypass grafting (OPCAB): two techniques for beating heart surgery. *Heart Surg Forum* 2002; **5**:157–62.

An evaluation of two approaches – MIDCAB and OPCAB. The need for the careful selection of patients for MIDCAB is emphasized and it is shown that OPCAB gives better exposure to all vessels.

Diegeler A, Thiele H, Falk V, Hambrecht R, Spyrantis N, Sick P, *et al.* Comparison of stenting with minimally invasive bypass surgery for stenosis of the left anterior descending artery. *N Engl J Med* 2002; **347**:561–6.

A randomized trial in 220 patients evaluated stenting or bypass surgery with a minimally invasive approach. One-year outcome indicated a higher need for repeat intervention with stenting, though this treatment had fewer peri-procedural adverse events.

Iakovou I, Dangas G, Mehran R, Lansky AJ, Stamou SC, Pfister AJ, *et al.* Minimally invasive direct coronary artery bypass (MIDCAB) versus coronary artery stenting for elective revascularization of the left anterior descending artery. *Am J Cardiol* 2002; **90**:885–7.

A non-randomized study of 542 patients comparing MIDCAB and stenting for the anterior descending artery confirms a greater need for revascularization with current stents.

Stamou SC, Jablonski KA, Pfister AJ, Hill PC, Dullum MK, Bafi AS, *et al.* Stroke after conventional versus minimally invasive coronary artery bypass. *Ann Thorac Surg* 2002; **74**:394–9.

A large experience of 2320 OPCAB patients is compared with 8069 on-pump patients using propensity score matching. Off-pump CABG was associated with a substantially lower stroke rate.

REFERENCES

1. Hornberger J, Bloch DA, Hlatky MA, Baumgartner W. Patient preferences in coronary revascularization. *Am Heart J* 1999; **137**:1153–62.
2. Holubkov R, Detre KM, Sopko G, Sutton-Tyrrell K, Kelsey SF, Frye RL. Trends in coronary revascularization 1989 to 1997: the Bypass Angioplasty Revascularization Investigation (BARI) survey of procedures. *Am J Cardiol* 1999; **84**:157–61.
3. Kolessov VI. Mammary artery–coronary artery anastomosis as method of treatment for angina pectoris. *J Thorac Cardiovasc Surg* 1967; **54**:535–44.
4. Benetti F, Mariani MA, Sani G, Boonstra PW, Grandjean JG, Giomarelli P, *et al.* Video-assisted minimally invasive coronary operations without cardiopulmonary bypass: a multicenter study. *J Thorac Cardiovasc Surg* 1996; **112**:1478–84.
5. Calafiore AM, Teodori G, Di Giammarco G, Vitolla G, Iaco' A, Iovino T, *et al.* Minimally invasive coronary artery bypass grafting on a beating heart. *Ann Thorac Surg* 1997; **63**(6 Suppl.):S72–5.
6. Buffolo E, Gerola LR. Coronary artery bypass grafting without cardiopulmonary bypass through sternotomy and minimally invasive procedure. *Int J Cardiol* 1997; **62**(Suppl 1.):S89–93.
7. Garrett HE Jr, Gilmore JC, Lowdermilk GA, McCoy D. Complete direct mammary harvest for minimally invasive coronary artery bypass. *Ann Thorac Surg* 1997; **64**:864–6.
8. Qaqish NK, Pagni S, Spence PA. Instrumentation for minimally invasive internal thoracic artery harvest. *Ann Thorac Surg* 1997; **63**(6 Suppl.):S97–9.
9. Nataf P, Lima L, Regan M, Benarim S, Ramadan R, Pavie A, *et al.* Thoracoscopic internal mammary artery harvesting: technical considerations. *Ann Thorac Surg* 1997; **63**(6 Suppl.):S104–6.
10. Gundry SR, Romano MA, Shattuck OH, Razzouk AJ, Bailey LL. Seven-year follow-up of coronary artery bypasses performed with and without cardiopulmonary bypass. *J Thorac Cardiovasc Surg* 1998; **115**:1273–8.

11. Gill IS, Higginson LA, Maharajh GS, Keon WJ. Early and follow-up angiography in minimally invasive coronary bypass without mechanical stabilization. *Ann Thorac Surg* 2000; **69**:56–60.

12. Calafiore AM, Teodori G, Di Giammarco G, Vitolla G, Contini M. Minimally invasive coronary artery surgery: the last operation. *Semin Thorac Cardiovasc Surg* 1997; **9**:305–11.

13. Cremer JT, Wittwer T, Boning A, Anssar MB, Kofidis T, Mugge A, *et al.* Minimally invasive coronary artery revascularization on the beating heart. *Ann Thorac Surg* 2000; **69**:1787–91.

14. Mehran R, Dangas G, Stamou SC, Pfister AJ, Dullum MK, Leon MB, *et al.* One-year clinical outcome after minimally invasive direct coronary artery bypass. *Circulation* 2000; **102**:2799–802.

15. Chitwood WR Jr, Wixon CL, Elbeery JR, Franalancia NA, Lust RM. Minimally invasive cardiac operation: adapting cardioprotective strategies. *Ann Thorac Surg* 1999; **68**:1974–7.

16. Vassiliades TA Jr, Nielsen JL. Alternative approaches in off-pump redo coronary artery bypass grafting. *Heart Surg Forum* 2000; **3**:203–6.

17. Lichtenberg A, Hagl C, Harringer W, Klima U, Haverich A. Effects of minimal invasive coronary artery bypass on pulmonary function and postoperative pain. *Ann Thorac Surg* 2000; **70**:461–5.

18. Bonatti J, Ladurner R, Antretter H, Hormann C, Friedrich G, Moes N, *et al.* Single coronary artery bypass grafting – a comparison between minimally invasive 'off pump' techniques and conventional procedures. *Eur J Cardiothorac Surg* 1998; **14**(Suppl. 1):S7–12.

19. d'Amato TA, Savage EB, Wiechmann RJ, Sakert T, Benckart DH, Magovern JA. Reduced incidence of atrial fibrillation with minimally invasive direct coronary artery bypass. *Ann Thorac Surg* 2000; **70**:2013–16.

20. Tamis-Holland JE, Homel P, Durani M, Iqbal M, Sutandar A, Mindich BP, *et al.* Atrial fibrillation after minimally invasive direct coronary artery bypass surgery. *J Am Coll Cardiol* 2000; **36**:1884–8.

21. Andrew MJ, Baker RA, Kneebone AC, Knight JL. Neuropsychological dysfunction after minimally invasive direct coronary artery bypass grafting. *Ann Thorac Surg* 1998; **66**:1611–17.

22. Bonatti J, Hangler H, Hormann C, Mair J, Falkensammer J, Mair P. Myocardial damage after minimally invasive coronary artery bypass grafting on the beating heart. *Ann Thorac Surg* 1998; **66**:1093–6.

23. Schmid C, Tjan TD, Henrichs KJ, Boppert D, Scheld HH. Anastomosis to the wrong vessel during off-pump bypass surgery via mini-thoracotomy. *Ann Thorac Surg* 1999; **67**:831–2.

24. Reichenspurner H, Boehm D, Detter C, Schiller W, Reichart B. Economic evaluation of different minimally invasive procedures for the treatment of coronary artery disease. *Eur J Cardiothorac Surg* 1999; **16**(Suppl. 2):S76–9.

25. King RC, Reece TB, Hurst JL, Shockey KS, Tribble CG, Spotnitz WD, *et al.* Minimally invasive coronary artery bypass grafting decreases hospital stay and cost. *Ann Surg* 1997; **225**:805–11.

26. Del Rizzo DF, Boyd WD, Novick RJ, McKenzie FN, Desai ND, Menkis AH. Safety and cost-effectiveness of MIDCABG in high-risk CABG patients. *Ann Thorac Surg* 1998; **66**:1002–7.

27. Watanabe G, Misaki T, Kotoh K, Kawakami K, Yamashita A, Ueyama K. Multiple minimally invasive direct coronary artery bypass grafting for the complete revascularization of the left ventricle. *Ann Thorac Surg* 1999; **68**:131–6.

28. Subramanian VA, Patel NU. Transabdominal minimally invasive direct coronary artery bypass grafting (MIDCAB). *Eur J Cardiothorac Surg* 2000; **17**:485–7.

29. Subramanian VA. Clinical experience with minimally invasive reoperative coronary bypass surgery. *Eur J Cardiothorac Surg* 1996; **10**:1058–63.

30. Wittwer T, Cremer J, Boonstra P, Grandjean J, Mariani M, Mugge A, *et al.* Myocardial 'hybrid' revascularisation with minimally invasive direct coronary artery bypass grafting combined with coronary angioplasty: preliminary results of a multicentre study. *Heart* 2000; **83**:58–63.

31. Coulson AS, Bakhshay SA. The 'T-MIDCAB' procedure. Use of extension grafts from the undisturbed internal mammary artery in high-risk patients. *Heart Surg Forum* 1998; **1**:54–9.

32. Cohn WE, Suen HC, Weintraub RM, Johnson RG. The 'H' graft: an alternative approach for performing minimally invasive direct coronary artery bypass. *J Thorac Cardiovasc Surg* 1998; **115**: 148–51.

33. Coulson AS, Glasgow EF, Bonatti J. Minimally invasive subclavian/axillary artery to coronary artery bypass (saxcab): review and classification. *Heart Surg Forum* 2001; **4**:13–25.

34. Akhter M, Lajos TZ, Grosner G, Bergsland J, Visco J. Minimally invasive coronary artery bypass grafting using the right gastroepiploic artery without pump. *Eur J Cardiothorac Surg* 1998; **14**(Suppl. 1):S58–61.

35. Puskas JD, Wright CE, Ronson RS, Brown WM 3rd, Gott JP, Guyton RA. Off-pump multivessel coronary bypass via sternotomy is safe and effective. *Ann Thorac Surg* 1998; **66**:1068–72.

36. Cartier R, Brann S, Dagenais F, Martineau R, Couturier A. Systematic off-pump coronary artery revascularization in multivessel disease: experience of three hundred cases. *J Thorac Cardiovasc Surg* 2000; **119**:221–9.

37. Torrent-Guasp F, Ballester M, Buckberg GD, Carreras F, Flotats A, Carrio I, *et al.* Spatial orientation of the ventricular muscle band: physiologic contribution and surgical implications. *J Thorac Cardiovasc Surg* 2001; **122**:389–92.

38. Cartier R, Blain R. Off-pump revascularization of the circumflex artery: technical aspect and short-term results. *Ann Thorac Surg* 1999; **68**:94–9.

39. Ricci M, Karamanoukian HL, D'Ancona G, Bergsland J, Salerno TA. Exposure and mechanical stabilization in off-pump coronary artery bypass grafting via sternotomy. *Ann Thorac Surg* 2000; **70**:1736–40.

40. Watters MP, Ascione R, Ryder IG, Ciulli F, Pitsis AA, Angelini GD. Haemodynamic changes during beating heart coronary surgery with the 'Bristol Technique'. *Eur J Cardiothorac Surg* 2001; **19**:34–40.

41. Hart JC, Spooner T, Edgerton J, Milsteen SA. Off-pump multivessel coronary artery bypass utilizing the Octopus tissue stabilization system: initial experience in 374 patients from three separate centers. *Heart Surg Forum* 1999; **2**:15–28.

42. Trehan N, Mishra M, Sharma OP, Mishra A, Kasliwal RR. Further reduction in stroke after off-pump coronary artery bypass grafting: a 10-year experience. *Ann Thorac Surg* 2001; **72**: S1026–32.

43. Stanbridge RD, Hadjinikolaou LK. Technical adjuncts in beating heart surgery comparison of MIDCAB to off-pump sternotomy: a meta-analysis. *Eur J Cardiothorac Surg* 1999; **16**(Suppl. 2):S24–33.

44. Ricci M, Karamanoukian HL, Abrham R, von Fricken K, D'Ancona G, Choi S, *et al.* Stroke in octogenarians undergoing coronary artery surgery with and without cardiopulmonary bypass. *Ann Thorac Surg* 2000; **69**:1471–5.

45. Trehan N, Mishra M, Kasliwal RR, Mishra A. Reduced neurological injury during CABG in patients with mobile aortic atheromas: a five-year follow-up study. *Ann Thorac Surg* 2000; **70**: 1558–64.

46. Arom KV, Flavin TF, Emery RW, Kshettry VR, Janey PA, Petersen RJ. Safety and efficacy of off-pump coronary artery bypass grafting. *Ann Thorac Surg* 2000; **69**:704–10.

47. Plomondon ME, Cleveland JC Jr, Ludwig ST, Grunwald GK, Kiefe CI, Grover FL, *et al.* Off-pump coronary artery bypass is associated with improved risk-adjusted outcomes. *Ann Thorac Surg* 2001; **72**:114–19.

48. Kilger E, Weis FC, Goetz AE, Frey L, Kesel K, Schutz A, *et al.* Intensive care after minimally invasive and conventional coronary

surgery: a prospective comparison. *Intensive Care Med* 2001; 27:534–9.

49. Chavanon O, Carrier M, Cartier R, Hebert Y, Pellerin M, Page P, *et al.* Increased incidence of acute ascending aortic dissection with off-pump aortocoronary bypass surgery? *Ann Thorac Surg* 2001; **71**:117–21.

50. Galloway AC, Shemin RJ, Glower DD, Boyer JH Jr, Groh MA, Kuntz RE, *et al.* First report of the Port Access International Registry. *Ann Thorac Surg* 1999; **67**:51–8.

51. Diegeler A, Falk V, Krahling K, Matin M, Walther T, Autschbach R, *et al.* Less-invasive coronary artery bypass grafting: different techniques and approaches. *Eur J Cardiothorac Surg* 1998; **14**(Suppl. 1):S13–19.

52. Grossi EA, Zakow PK, Ribakove G, Kallenbach K, Ursomanno P, Gradek CE, *et al.* Comparison of post-operative pain, stress response, and quality of life in port access vs. standard sternotomy coronary bypass patients. *Eur J Cardiothorac Surg* 1999; **16**(Suppl. 2):S39–42.

53. Gulielmos V, Wagner FM, Waetzig B, Solowjowa N, Tugtekin SM, Schroeder C, *et al.* Clinical experience with minimally invasive coronary artery and mitral valve surgery with the advantage of cardiopulmonary bypass and cardioplegic arrest using the Port Access technique. *World J Surg* 1999; **23**:480–5.

54. Reichenspurner H, Gulielmos V, Wunderlich J, Dangel M, Wagner FM, Pompili MF, *et al.* Port-Access coronary artery bypass grafting with the use of cardiopulmonary bypass and cardioplegic arrest. *Ann Thorac Surg* 1998; **65**:413–19.

55. Ribakove GH, Miller JS, Anderson RV, Grossi EA, Applebaum RM, Cutler WM, *et al.* Minimally invasive port-access coronary artery bypass grafting with early angiographic follow-up: initial clinical experience. *J Thorac Cardiovasc Surg* 1998; **115**:1101–10.

56. Schwartz DS, Ribakove GH, Grossi EA, Schwartz JD, Buttenheim PM, Baumann FG, *et al.* Single and multivessel port-access coronary artery bypass grafting with cardioplegic arrest: technique and reproducibility. *J Thorac Cardiovasc Surg* 1997; **114**:46–52.

57. Zapolanski A, Korver K, Pliam MB, Mengarelli L, Shaw R. Multiple coronary artery bypass via mini left thoracotomy with conventional aortic occlusion. *Heart Surg Forum* 2001; **4**:109–12.

58. Ribakove GH, Galloway AC, Grossi EA, Cutler W, Miller JS, Baumann FG, *et al.* Port-Access coronary artery bypass grafting. *Semin Thorac Cardiovasc Surg* 1997; **9**:312–19.

59. Groh MA, Sutherland SE, Burton HG 3rd, Johnson AM, Ely SW. Port-access coronary artery bypass grafting: technique and comparative results. *Ann Thorac Surg* 1999; **68**:1506–8.

60. Glower DD, Komtebedde J, Clements FM, Debruijn NP, Stafford-Smith M, Newman MF. Direct aortic cannulation for port access mitral or coronary artery bypass grafting. *Ann Thorac Surg* 1999; **68**:1878–80.

61. Prasad SM, Ducko CT, Stephenson ER, Chambers CE, Damiano RJ Jr. Prospective clinical trial of robotically assisted endoscopic coronary grafting with 1-year follow-up. *Ann Surg* 2001; **233**: 725–32.

62. Falk V, Diegeler A, Walther T, Banusch J, Brucerius J, Raumans J, *et al.* Total endoscopic computer enhanced coronary artery bypass grafting. *Eur J Cardiothorac Surg* 2000; **17**:38–45.

63. Loulmet D, Carpentier A, d'Attellis N, Berrebi A, Cardon C, Ponzio O, *et al.* Endoscopic coronary artery bypass grafting with the aid of robotic assisted instruments. *J Thorac Cardiovasc Surg* 1999; **118**:4–10.

64. Kappert U, Cichon R, Tugtekin SM, Schueler S. Closed chest coronary artery bypass on the beating heart. *Heart Surg Forum* 2001; **4**:89–90.

65. Boyd WD, Rayman R, Desai ND, Menkis AH, Dobkowski W, Ganapathy S, *et al.* Closed-chest coronary artery bypass grafting on the beating heart with the use of a computer-enhanced

surgical robotic system. *J Thorac Cardiovasc Surg* 2000; **120**:807–9.

66. Okies JE, Page US, Bigelow JC, Krause AH, Salomon NW. The left internal mammary artery: the graft of choice. *Circulation* 1984; **70**:I213–21.

67. Lytle BW, Blackstone EH, Loop FD, Houghtaling PL, Arnold JH, Akhrass R, *et al.* Two internal thoracic artery grafts are better than one. *J Thorac Cardiovasc Surg* 1999; **117**:855–72.

68. Dogan S, Aybek T, Westphal K, Mierol S, Moritz A, Wimmer-Greinecker G. Computer-enhanced totally endoscopic sequential arterial coronary artery bypass. *Ann Thorac Surg* 2001; **72**:610–11.

69. Falk V, Fann JI, Grunenfelder J, Daunt D, Burdon TA. Endoscopic computer-enhanced beating heart coronary artery bypass grafting. *Ann Thorac Surg* 2000; **70**:2029–33.

70. Cichon R, Kappert U, Schneider J, Schramm I, Gulielmos V, Tugtekin SM, *et al.* Robotically enhanced 'Dresden technique' with bilateral internal mammary artery grafting. *Thorac Cardiovasc Surg* 2000; **4**:189–92.

71. Cichon R, Kappert U, Schneider J, Schramm I, Gulielmos V, Tugtekin SM, *et al.* Robotic-enhanced arterial revascularization for multivessel coronary artery disease. *Ann Thorac Surg* 2000; **70**:1060–2.

72. Paletta CE, Huang DB, Fiore AC, Swartz MT, Rilloraza FL, Gardner JE. Major leg wound complications after saphenous vein harvest for coronary revascularization. *Ann Thorac Surg* 2000; **70**:492–7.

73. Allen KB, Heimansohn DA, Robinson RJ, Schierr JJ, Griffith GL, Fitzgerald EB, *et al.* Risk factors for leg wound complications following endoscopic versus traditional saphenous vein harvesting. *Heart Surg Forum* 2000; **3**:325–30.

74. Tevaearai HT, Mueller XM, von Segesser LK. Minimally invasive harvest of the saphenous vein for coronary artery bypass grafting. *Ann Thorac Surg* 1997; **63**(6 Suppl.): S119–21.

75. Isgro F, Weisse U, Voss B, Kiessling AH, Saggau W. Minimally invasive saphenous vein harvesting: is there an improvement of the results with the endoscopic approach? *Eur J Cardiothorac Surg* 1999; **16**(Suppl. 2): S58–60.

76. Black EA, Guzik TJ, West NE, Campbell K, Pillai R, Ratnatunga C, *et al.* Minimally invasive saphenous vein harvesting: effects on endothelial and smooth muscle function. *Ann Thorac Surg* 2001; **71**:1503–7.

77. Fabricius AM, Diegeler A, Gerber W, Mohr FW. Functional and morphologic assessment of saphenous veins harvested with minimally invasive techniques using a modified laryngoscope. *Heart Surg Forum* 2000; **3**:32–5.

78. Galajda Z, Peterffy A. Minimally invasive harvesting of the radial artery as a coronary artery bypass graft. *Ann Thorac Surg* 2001; **72**:91–3.

79. Gomes WJ, Goldenberg A, Buffolo E, Losso LC, Marcondes W, Rolla F, *et al.* Video-endoscopic dissection of multiple pedicled arterial grafts for use in minimally invasive coronary artery bypass surgery. *J Cardiovasc Surg (Torino)* 2000; **41**:7–9.

80. Pawlowski J, Haering JM, Comunale ME, Mashikian J, Reynolds D, Johnson R, *et al.* Minimally invasive anesthesia should accompany minimally invasive surgery. *J Cardiothorac Vasc Anesth* 1997; **11**:536–7.

81. Jara FM, Klush J, Kilaru V. Intrathecal morphine for off-pump coronary artery bypass patients. *Heart Surg Forum* 2001; **4**:57–60.

82. Perkowski DJ, Marcus AO, Wagner SL, Gorman LM. Optimizing off-pump coronary artery bypass graft: technical and metabolic aspects. *Heart Surg Forum* 2001; **4**:80–8.

83. Gillam LD. Intraoperative transesophageal echocardiography. *Cardiol Rev* 2000; **8**:269–78.

84. Siegel LC, St Goar FG, Stevens JH, Pompili MF, Burdon TA, Reitz BA, *et al.* Monitoring considerations for port-access cardiac surgery. *Circulation* 1997; **96**:562–8.

85. Schulze CJ, Wildhirt SM, Boehm DH, Weigand C, Kornberg A, Reichenspurner H, *et al.* Continuous transesophageal echocardiographic (TEE) monitoring during port-access cardiac surgery. *Heart Surg Forum* 1999; 2:54–9.

86. Robinson MC, Thielmeier KA, Hill BB. Transient ventricular asystole using adenosine during minimally invasive and open sternotomy coronary artery bypass grafting. *Ann Thorac Surg* 1997; **63**(6 Suppl.):S30–4.

87. Bufkin BL, Puskas JD, Vinten-Johansen J, Shearer ST, Guyton RA. Controlled intermittent asystole: pharmacologic potentiation of vagal-induced asystole. *Ann Thorac Surg* 1998; **66**:1185–90.

88. Boonstra PW, Grandjean JG, Mariani MA. Local immobilization of the left anterior descending artery for minimally invasive coronary bypass grafting. *Ann Thorac Surg* 1997; **63**(6 Suppl.):S76–8.

89. Cremer J, Struber M, Wittwer T, Ruhparwar A, Harringer W, Zuk J, *et al.* Off-bypass coronary bypass grafting via minithoracotomy using mechanical epicardial stabilization. *Ann Thorac Surg* 1997; **63**(6 Suppl.):S79–83.

90. Jansen EW, Grundeman PF, Borst C, Eefting F, Diephuis J, Nierich A, *et al.* Less invasive off-pump CABG using a suction device for immobilization: the 'Octopus' method. *Eur J Cardiothorac Surg* 1997; **12**:406–12.

91. Bedi HS, Suri A, Kalkat MS, Sengar BS, Mahajan V, Chawla R, *et al.* Global myocardial revascularization without cardiopulmonary bypass using innovative techniques for myocardial stabilization and perfusion. *Ann Thorac Surg* 2000; **69**:156–64.

92. Whitman GJ, Hart JC, Crestanello JA, Spooner TH. Uniform safety of beating heart surgery using the Octopus tissue stabilization system. *J Card Surg* 1999; **14**:323–9.

93. Nierich AP, Diephuis J, Jansen EW, Borst C, Knape JT. Heart displacement during off-pump CABG: how well is it tolerated? *Ann Thorac Surg* 2000; **70**:466–72.

94. Grundeman PF, Borst C, van Herwaarden JA, Mansvelt Beck HJ, Jansen EW. Hemodynamic changes during displacement of the beating heart by the Utrecht Octopus method. *Ann Thorac Surg* 1997; **63**(6 Suppl.):S88–92.

95. van Aarnhem EE, Nierich AP, Jansen EW. When and how to shunt the coronary circulation in off-pump coronary artery bypass grafting. *Eur J Cardiothorac Surg* 1999; **16**(Suppl. 2): S2–6.

96. Rivetti LA, Gandra SM. Initial experience using an intraluminal shunt during revascularization of the beating heart. *Ann Thorac Surg* 1997; **63**:1742–7.

97. Perrault LP, Desjardins N, Nickner C, Geoffroy P, Tanguay J, Carrier M. Effects of occlusion devices for minimally invasive coronary artery bypass surgery on coronary endothelial function of atherosclerotic arteries. *Heart Surg Forum* 2000; **3**:287–92.

98. Puskas JD, Thourani VH, Vinten-Johansen J, Guyton RA. Active perfusion of coronary grafts facilitates complex off-pump coronary artery bypass surgery. *Heart Surg Forum* 2001; **4**:65–8.

99. Bonilla LF, Sullivan DJ. New approaches for vascular anastomoses. *Curr Interv Cardiol Rep* 2001; **3**:44–9.

100. Lonn U, Peterzen B, Carnstam B, Casimir-Ahn H. Beating heart coronary surgery supported by an axial blood flow pump. *Ann Thorac Surg* 1999; **67**:99–104.

101. Lima LE, Jatene F, Buffolo E, Vanky F, Casimir-Ahn E, Lohn U, *et al.* A multicenter initial clinical experience with right heart support and beating heart coronary surgery. *Heart Surg Forum* 2001; **4**:60–4.

102. Elbeery JR, Brown PM, Chitwood WR Jr. Intraoperative MIDCABG arteriography via the left radial artery: a comparison with Doppler ultrasound for assessment of graft patency. *Ann Thorac Surg* 1998; **66**:51–5.

103. Mack MJ, Magovern JA, Acuff TA, Landreneau RJ, Tennison DM, Tinnerman EJ, *et al.* Results of graft patency by immediate angiography in minimally invasive coronary artery surgery. *Ann Thorac Surg* 1999; **68**:383–90.

104. Lin JC, Fisher DL, Szwerc MF, Magovern JA. Evaluation of graft patency during minimally invasive coronary artery bypass grafting with Doppler flow analysis. *Ann Thorac Surg* 2000; **70**:1350–4.

105. Walpoth BH, Bosshard A, Genyk I, Kipfer B, Berdat PA, Hess OM, *et al.* Transit-time flow measurement for detection of early graft failure during myocardial revascularization. *Ann Thorac Surg* 1998; **66**:1097–100.

106. D'Ancona G, Karamanoukian HL, Ricci M, Schmid S, Bergsland J, Salerno TA. Graft revision after transit time flow measurement in off-pump coronary artery bypass grafting. *Eur J Cardiothorac Surg* 2000; **17**:287–93.

14

Avoidance of visceral injury in coronary surgery

FRIEDHELM BEYERSDORF AND GERALD D BUCKBERG

INTRODUCTION

Coronary artery surgery is one of the most frequently performed operations worldwide and has benefited many thousands of patients by reducing symptoms and prolonging life. Prerequisites for a successful operation include:

- perfect surgical construction of bypass grafts,
- avoidance of myocardial injury during the construction of grafts, and
- avoidance of visceral injury.

Over many years, surgical techniques to construct bypass grafts have improved substantially and today even patients of advanced age with diffuse coronary artery disease can be successfully operated upon, if attention is given to the details summarized in this chapter.

TYPES OF POTENTIAL INJURY DURING CORONARY SURGERY

Myocardial injury

HEMODYNAMIC UPSETS IN THE PERIOPERATIVE PERIOD

Adequate cardiac output is the central issue in avoiding myocardial and visceral injury before, during or after cardiac surgery. Low cardiac output is diagnosed best by a thermodilution catheter (Swan–Ganz), but indirect measures such as mixed venous oxygen levels, urine flow, skin temperature, metabolic acidosis and lactic acidemia should also be considered perioperatively.

Low cardiac output may be defined as a cardiac index below $2.0\,L\,min^{-1}\,m^{-2}$. The cardiac stroke volume is determined by the ventricular preload, afterload and myocardial contractility.

- *Ventricular preload.* In patients with normal atrioventricular valves, right or left atrial pressures are a reliable measure of right and left ventricular preload. Furthermore, in the absence of pulmonary vascular disease and pulmonary edema, diastolic pulmonary artery pressure or pulmonary capillary wedge pressure (Swan–Ganz catheter) is a reasonable approximation of left atrial pressure.
- *Ventricular afterload.* Increased afterload results in decreased stroke volume. Therefore afterload measurements should be performed and treatment instituted in any individual in a compromised hemodynamic state.
- *Myocardial contractility.* If a reference value exists, contractility of the right and left ventricle can be assessed by echocardiography. Impaired contractility is treated mostly by the administration of inotropic drugs.

Low cardiac output before, during or after surgery is a significant risk factor for both morbidity and mortality and should therefore be treated aggressively. Treatment options include pharmaceutical manipulations of preload, afterload and contractility as well as adequate treatment of rhythm disturbances. Mechanical circulatory support using the intra-aortic balloon pump (IABP) is the next step in treating low output and should be used liberally. Preoperative use of the IABP will often improve cardiac performance and avoid periods of cardiogenic shock prior to surgery. In this patient group, the use of warm blood cardioplegic induction with substrate enhancement has been shown to be of benefit. Additionally, intravenous solutions such as glucose–insulin–potassium (GIK) and substrate enhancement will improve the energy state of the myocardium significantly. If all these maneuvers fail, ventricular assist devices (left, right or biventricular) may allow survival of the patient.

PERIODS OF LOW CARDIAC OUTPUT IN BEATING–HEART SURGERY

During off-pump coronary revascularization, periods of low output may occur during grafting of circumflex branches, as well as of branches of the right coronary artery. Although appropriate anesthetic techniques will reduce these periods (temporary inotropic support, increased central venous pressure by volume loading), awareness of this potentially dangerous low cardiac output state may prompt the use of circulatory support devices or a change to an on-pump technique.

MYOCARDIAL ISCHEMIA AND REPERFUSION INJURY WITH CARDIOPLEGIC TECHNIQUE

Inadequate myocardial protection can lead to myocyte and endothelial injury, and the two are interrelated.[1] This, in turn, may lead to delayed recovery of contractility (stunning), resulting in problems coming off bypass, postoperative low cardiac output, the need for pharmacological or even mechanical circulatory support and, in some instances, a higher mortality. Inadequate protection of the heart during surgery will lead to ischemic damage that is further aggravated during reperfusion after removal of the aortic clamp. Strict adherence to modern techniques of myocardial protection (see below) is mandatory for the patient to benefit from complex cardiac procedures.

In damaged hearts, conventional cardioplegic solutions can completely prevent myocyte injury, yet fail to prevent endothelial damage, with resultant white blood cell adherence. A principal underlying mechanism is endothelial loss of nitric oxide production. This allows neutrophil and platelet adherence, and changing vasoactivity, to impair subsequent vasodilatation. White blood cell adhesion is only one step in this injury.

Neutrophil filters interfere with the process once it has been initiated; strategies that focus on maintaining the intrinsic endothelium-dependent protective component, nitric oxide generation, may be useful.[1] Some studies have shown that delivery of the natural nitric oxide precursor,

L-arginine, limits endothelial and myocyte injury, even without leukocyte depletion. Ideally, future developments should prevent endothelial injury rather than treating the damage.

EXCESSIVE TRACTION OR HANDLING OF THE HEART

Some surgeons like to touch the heart and 'feel' the aorta, the coronaries or other parts of the heart during the cardioplegia induction or reinfusion. Some even try to save time by starting the revascularization procedure during cardioplegic delivery. This, in fact, may lead to overdistension of the ventricles (by causing mild aortic insufficiency), impaired view of the coronary anastomosis and inadequate delivery of cardioplegia to jeopardized myocardial regions. Difficulties in coming off bypass and a prolonged reperfusion period may be the result of such maneuvers.

Neurological injury

CEREBRAL INJURY

Central nervous system injury after cardiac surgery may involve clinically apparent events – type I (stroke, seizures, stupor or coma), or more subtle but also more common (type II) injuries such as intellectual deterioration, memory deficit or seizures.[2] In several studies the incidence of cerebral injury after coronary artery bypass grafting (CABG) has been reported to be 3.1% for type I injuries and 3%–42% for type II injuries.[3,4] Patients with adverse cerebral outcomes are reported to have a higher mortality, longer hospitalization and a higher rate of discharge to facilities for intermediate or long-term care.[3] The cause of both types of cerebral injuries after CABG is most likely to be multifactorial in origin and includes cerebral embolization, hypoperfusion and both localized and systemic inflammatory processes.

Atherosclerotic embolization
Coronary artery bypass graft patients are among those with a very high probability of having the typical risk factors for atheroemboli, such as type II diabetes, advanced age and vascular disease. Preoperative detection of aortic atheroma is of great importance in planning the conduct of the operation. Manual palpation, even though the most frequently applied method for the detection of aortic calcification, is the least reliable. Intraoperative epi-aortic ultrasound scanning provides accurate images of the aortic wall, but requires special equipment and trained personnel. Preoperative computerized tomographic scanning of the thoracic aorta in high-risk patients is another reliable method for the detection of aortic atherosclerotic lesions.

Surgical strategies to reduce the incidence of cerebral embolization include:

- proper selection of the cannulation site,
- decision between on-pump and off-pump surgery,
- single-clamp technique,
- avoidance of manual manipulations of the aorta,
- specialized clamp for thick-walled aorta (e.g. Fogarty-type clamp), and
- new aortic cannulas.

In the opinion of the authors, the new type of aortic cannulas, which avoid the 'water-hose effect' and reduce the velocity of aortic inflow, are of great importance in reducing the incidence of macroembolic events. Whether other new cannulas, such as those with intra-aortic filters or with flexible shields, are able to significantly reduce type I neurological injuries is currently being assessed in several clinical studies.

Microemboli

Current evidence would seem to favor diffuse microembolization as a significant contributor to type II cognitive dysfunction after cardiac surgery.[2] Arterial filters have been shown to be effective in decreasing the microembolic load.

PERIPHERAL NEURAL INJURY

Phrenic nerve injury

Cardiac hypothermia (by systemic cooling) has unequivocal value during ischemia because it reduces damage by slowing cardiac metabolic rate. However, several studies have shown that *topical* hypothermia, especially with ice slush, can injure the phrenic nerve.[5] In addition, it has been shown that topical hypothermia does not add to the quality of myocardial protection at all, but increases the prevalence of pulmonary complications (i.e. atelectasis, pleural effusion and diaphragmatic paralysis).

Phrenic nerve damage is known to be due to demyelinization when the temperature is lowered below 4 °C, and recovery of damaged axons may be delayed for up to 1 year. Therefore, routine surface cooling of the heart should be abandoned, especially in critically ill patients.

Saphenous nerve injury

The saphenous nerve runs alongside the greater saphenous vein. To avoid postoperative paresthesia, special care should be taken not to divide it. There is some evidence that endoscopic minimally invasive harvesting of the greater saphenous vein will reduce the incidence of nerve injury.

Respiratory injury

After CABG, changes in the respiratory system are almost inevitable. Even though these changes are mild and transient and of no clinical relevance in the majority of patients who are at no special risk for respiratory dysfunction, the lungs are the organs most likely to have dysfunction postoperatively. This risk seems to be higher in on-pump compared with off-pump cases. Respiratory dysfunction is the result of damage to various components of the respiratory system, including the chest wall and intercostal muscles, diaphragm, airways and lungs (Table 14.1).

The multiple causes of respiratory dysfunction can be divided into surgery-specific and patient-specific causes.

SURGERY-SPECIFIC CAUSES

Our group[6] as well as others have described a significant decrease in *bronchial blood flow* during extracorporeal circulation, as well as a decrease in *pulmonary blood flow* during total and partial cardiopulmonary bypass.

- *Atelectasis*, either segmental or lobar, may occur and, in particular, the left lower lobe has a tendency to atelectasis.
- *Direct trauma to the lung* (rupture of bullae, iatrogenic injury during internal thoracic artery takedown) will also result in various degrees of dysfunction.
- *Left* (rarely right) *phrenic nerve injury* and/or *diaphragmatic dysfunction* are almost always the result of topical cold solutions used for myocardial protection. However, there are several reports showing that cold topical solutions

Table 14.1 *Various components of the respiratory system potentially damaged during coronary artery bypass grafting*

Respiratory system component	Cause of injury
Chest wall and intercostal muscles	Sternotomy, thoracotomy, postoperative pain
Phrenic nerve damage and/or diaphragmatic dysfunction	Cold topical solution
Airways	Absence of pulmonary artery blood flow
	Reduction of bronchial artery blood flow
	Secretions
Lungs	Absence of pulmonary artery blood flow
	Reduction of bronchial artery blood flow
	Atelectasis
	Direct trauma (rupture of bullae, iatrogenic injury)
	Secretions
	Cardiogenic pulmonary edema

are of no additional value when modern techniques of myocardial protection (e.g. blood cardioplegia) are used.[5] Topical cooling should therefore be abandoned in order to reduce pulmonary injury.

- *Secretions* are a well-known cause of acute pulmonary dysfunction in the immediate postoperative period and need vigorous tracheal suctioning.
- *Pulmonary edema* will be the result of elevated left atrial pressures associated with low output states postoperatively.
- *Procedural risk factors* include the use of oxygenators other than the membrane type, absence of filters in the arterial line and longer duration of cardiopulmonary bypass.

PATIENT-SPECIFIC CAUSES

- *Older age*, particularly age over 60 years, has been associated with an increased prevalence of pulmonary dysfunction after cardiac surgery.
- *Chronic obstructive lung disease* is an important risk factor for postoperative pulmonary dysfunction as well as for sternal instability with subsequent pulmonary dysfunction.
- Some *drugs* (e.g. amiodarone) have caused rapidly fatal pulmonary dysfunction after cardiac surgery in some patients.

Renal injury

During a well-conducted cardiac operation, there should be no procedure-specific cause of renal dysfunction. However, several patient-specific, intraoperative and postoperative circumstances may lead to acute renal failure (Table 14.2).

The treatment of renal injury consists mainly of appropriate fluid intake, dopamine, diuretics and, importantly, maintenance of good cardiac function.

Table 14.2 *Risk factors for acute renal failure*[20]

I Patient specific	Preoperative impairment of renal function
	Chronic heart failure
	Cyanotic heart disease
	Young age
	Older age
II Intraoperative	Long period of cardiopulmonary bypass
	Priming with whole blood
	High plasma hemoglobin levels
III Postoperative	Acute reduction in cardiac output
	Some antibiotics

Gastrointestinal injury

Gastrointestinal (GI) complications after bypass surgery are uncommon and occur in approximately 1%.[7] However, the mortality associated with GI complications is very high, reaching 50%.

In the majority of patients, no clinically apparent changes in GI function are detected after coronary procedures with cardiopulmonary bypass, and most patients are eating 12–24 hours postoperatively. However, even in asymptomatic patients, studies have shown transient elevations in liver function tests,[8] and hyperamylasemia without overt pancreatitis.[9] In addition, decrease in gastric pH,[10] decreased GI organ blood flow and the appearance of endotoxins in the circulation[11] do occur, but are of little importance in 99% of coronary patients.

Evidence of abdominal distension, absence of peristalsis, and hyperperistalsis are signs of GI malfunction, and immediate discontinuation of alimentation, institution of investigations and intravenously administered hyperalimentation should be considered.

The spectrum of GI complications includes:

- GI bleeding,
- acute cholecystitis,
- acute pancreatitis,
- hepatic necrosis,
- intestitinal necrosis,
- esophagitis,
- watery diarrhea,
- abdominal distension.

All of these dysfunctions are the result of hypoperfusion of the GI tract, the liver, or both.

The single most important predictor of such adverse outcome is the duration of hypotension, i.e. the development of a low-output state. In addition, advanced age, long duration of cardiopulmonary bypass and the need for prolonged inotropic support increase the risk of these complications.

Skeletal muscle injury

Skeletal muscle injury of the lower limb most often occurs as a consequence of IABP insertion in a patient with peripheral vascular disease. In rare cases it may also be apparent after the application of a tight bandage in a limb from which a vein was removed, or after thromboembolism.

Besides symptomatic treatment, therapy has more recently addressed the cause, dealing with both the ischemic and reperfusion injuries (controlled limb reperfusion).[12] With this treatment modality, revascularization is achieved, first with embolectomy, thromboendarterectomy or any bypass procedure necessary, followed by a reperfusion strategy over a 30-minute period in order to reduce (or even avoid) the consequences of post-ischemic syndrome.

CURRENT TECHNIQUES FOR MYOCARDIAL MANAGEMENT DURING CORONARY SURGERY

Inadequate myocardial protection resulting in perioperative cardiac damage and dysfunction has always been a major cause of morbidity and mortality after technically successful correction of acquired heart disease. In the past, many techniques have been described dealing with pharmaceutical and mechanical ways to improve cardiac output and methods to manage postoperative renal, hepatic and respiratory failure resulting from impaired postoperative cardiac performance.[13] Considerable progress has been made since then, and currently multi-organ failure, even in critically ill coronary patients, is rather rare. In the following sections of this chapter, current techniques for myocardial management during coronary surgery are described.

With cardiopulmonary bypass

The tremendous change in the spectrum of patients requiring cardiac surgery today has led to an evolution of advanced cardioprotective techniques, including pharmacological additives, oxygenated cardioplegia, antegrade and retrograde delivery, and the use of warm blood cardioplegia to resuscitate the heart and limit reperfusion damage. These techniques have reduced, but not avoided completely, the low output syndrome, which remains the leading cause of perioperative death.

Advanced cardiac management during operations with cardiopulmonary bypass includes the following cornerstones.

TYPE OF CARDIOPLEGIC SOLUTION

There are innumerable cardioplegic solutions in clinical use today. However, only those solutions that have been tested extensively both in the experimental and clinical setting can be used safely in clinical practice. No other mixtures or solutions should be used.

Blood cardioplegia has many advantages and is therefore used in most modern centers worldwide today. Oxygen delivery is only one attribute of blood cardioplegia, and many more are enumerated, including minimal hemodilution, natural oncotic pressure due to the protein content of blood, buffering capacity of blood (especially histidine/imidazole groups), and endogenous free oxygen radical scavengers (e.g. superoxide dismutase, catalase and glutathione).

TEMPERATURE OF THE CARDIOPLEGIC SOLUTION

The two axioms concerning myocardial protection that have often prevailed among cardiac surgeons are that 'all is well if the heart is made as cold as possible' and that there 'is a battle against the clock' during aortic cross-clamping.[13] However, the development of more advanced techniques of myocardial protection has resulted in a different approach. This is evident experimentally from the complete functional recovery after 4 hours of aortic clamping when cold blood cardioplegia is used, whereas severe functional depression follows 45 minutes of normothermic ischemia (which has also been documented clinically).

The myocardial protective effect of cardiac hypothermia is a result of:

- reduction of the rate of myocardial metabolism and oxygen consumption,
- reduction of the rate and force of the process leading to myocardial cell death, and
- promotion of electromechanical quiescence.

Cardiac hypothermia has no favorable effects on coronary endothelium or vascular resistance, or on the rate of recovery of ischemically injured myocardial cells.

The most potentially harmful belief is the myth that profound hypothermia confers a blanket of protection with such intrinsic value that other aspects of myocardial protection can be disregarded without incurring the risk of avoidable ischemic/reperfusion damage.

The versatility of blood as the cardioplegic vehicle allows normothermic delivery (37 °C) to provide 'active cardiac resuscitation', either to better prepare the heart for the cold ischemic periods needed for the technical procedure, or to 'limit reperfusion damage' in jeopardized myocardium.[13] The purpose of normothermia during blood cardioplegic induction and reperfusion is to optimize the metabolic rate of repair and thereby provide an appropriate environment for the constituents of the cardioplegic solutions to exert their desired effects.

Blood cardioplegic solutions can be given cold, warm or tepid, according to the metabolic state of the heart and the surgical requirements.

THE ISSUE OF TOPICAL COOLING

Topical cooling does not improve the quality of myocardial protection, nor does it decrease transmural myocardial temperature for a prolonged period of time. Only the epicardial layers may be reduced in temperature. However, pulmonary complications may follow topical cooling techniques (especially with ice slush), such as phrenic nerve injury, atelectasis, pleural effusions, etc. We have therefore, like others, abandoned topical hypothermia as an adjunct to myocardial protection.

ROUTE OF DELIVERY

Cardioplegic myocardial protection in patients with coronary artery disease is only effective if there is adequate delivery of the cardioplegic solution beyond coronary stenoses or occlusions. The limitations of antegrade delivery of cardioplegia can be overcome by:

- delivery of cardioplegia by direct graft perfusion,
- performing proximal grafting before aortic clamping and administering cardioplegic solutions via the aorta after each distal graft, or
- performing sequential distal and proximal anastomoses during aortic clamping and giving cardioplegia via the aorta after each proximal and distal connection is complete.

However, these strategies do not ensure adequate distribution of antegrade cardioplegia if there is diffuse coronary artery disease or if arterial grafts are the desired conduits.

Retrograde cardioplegia has been used routinely for over 10 years and is probably the best solution for ensuring the adequate distribution of cardioplegic solutions in various settingss, including redo-surgery, diffuse coronary artery disease, and complete arterial revascularization. The advantages of retrograde cardioplegia over antegrade cardioplegia in coronary surgery include:

- distribution of cardioplegia to jeopardized myocardium,
- facility to perform distal anastomoses without interruption by the delivery of antegrade cardioplegia (and the necessity to stop retracting the heart in order to avoid aortic valve insufficiency), and
- retrograde flushing of atheroma and air emboli, especially in redo cases.

The combined techniques of antegrade and retrograde cardioplegia, administered alternatively or simultaneously, allow benefits to be derived from both routes of delivery, and clinical application of this combined strategy has provided satisfying clinical results.

INTERVENTIONS DURING THE INITIAL REPERFUSION PERIOD

Reperfusion injury is defined as the functional, metabolic and structural alteration caused by reperfusion after a period of ischemia; it can occur whenever the aorta is clamped to produce a motionless, bloodless field. Reperfusion damage is characterized by:

- intracellular calcium accumulation,
- cell swelling with low coronary reflow and reduced ventricular compliance,
- inability to use delivered oxygen, even when coronary flow and oxygen content are ample, and

- oxygen-mediated damage, including neutrophil adherence and activation.

Studies in globally and regionally ischemic hearts show that the fate of jeopardized myocardium is determined more by careful control of the conditions and the composition of the reperfusate than by the duration of ischemia itself.

Interventions during the initial reperfusion period can be performed as warm terminal reperfusions ('hot shot') in elective patients or as controlled reperfusion in patients with acute coronary occlusions in order to avoid transmural myocardial infarction.

SINGLE CROSS-CLAMP PERIOD

In the authors' practice, all coronary operations are performed entirely with a single-clamp technique. The advantages are threefold.

1 Improved myocardial protection despite prolonged cross-clamp period: this underscores again that the duration of aortic cross-clamp is not as important as the technique used for protection during that interval. However, this does not imply that cross-clamp time is of no interest at all. Surgical steps that do not necessarily require cross-clamping or cardiopulmonary bypass (e.g. complete preparation of all bypass conduits) should be completed before cross-clamping.
2 Cessation of cardiopulmonary bypass shortly (i.e. 3–5 minutes) after removal of the cross-clamp.
3 Improved neurological outcome, probably due to reduced emboli from the ascending aorta.

SYSTEMIC TEMPERATURE

In the past, systemic hypothermia was an indispensable adjunct in cardiac surgery, but current advances in myocardial protection have rendered it redundant. In routine cardiac procedures, systemic normothermia (34–35 °C) is standard in all cases.

During beating-heart surgery

Beating-heart surgery uses local coronary occlusion without cardiopulmonary bypass by:

- minimally invasive direct coronary artery bypass (MIDCAB) grafting with strategically placed minimal access incisions, i.e. mini left and right thoracotomy (left internal thoracic to anterior descending and right internal thoracic to right coronary artery grafts), mini-sternotomy, subxiphoid incision and mini left lateral thoracotomy; or

- coronary artery bypass surgery via midline sternotomy without cardiopulmonary bypass (off-pump CABG, OPCAB).[14]

Despite its advantages, the beating-heart technique creates three surgical problems:

1 the motion of the coronary target site hampers accurate anastomosis suturing,
2 collateral blood flow from the side branches of the isolated coronary artery segment carries blood into the arteriotomy and obscures the view, and
3 for surgical access to posterior anastomosis sites, the beating heart needs to be lifted, which causes a precipitous drop in arterial pressure.[14]

Currently, temporary intracoronary shunts are in use for myocardial protection and creation of a bloodless field. During the period of local coronary occlusion, the depth of anesthesia is increased to reduce left ventricular contractility, blood pressure and heart rate. This is accomplished with the use of intravenous beta-blockers or calcium-channel blockers.[14] (In our early beating-heart surgery practice, we used adenosine for short-term cardiac arrest but no longer use it.) Volume loading as well as routine hemodynamic monitoring, including trans-esophageal echocardiography and mapping of ST segments, are maintained throughout the entire operation.

Ischemic preconditioning (5 minutes of local coronary occlusion followed by 5 minutes of reperfusion before occlusion of the coronary artery for coronary anastomosis) has been advocated by some groups before coronary occlusion. However, we have not used this technique during the past 2 years, and have not been able to demonstrate any clinically relevant difference.

With port-access surgery

Port-access bypass surgery with minithoracotomy uses peripheral cannulation, cardiopulmonary bypass, endoluminal ascending aortic occlusion and cardioplegic arrest. This technique is most often used in coronary revascularization and mitral valve surgery. The endoaortic device is a triple-lumen catheter with a distal inflatable balloon for aortic occlusion. Antegrade cardioplegia is delivered through the central lumen, which also serves as an aortic vent. A percutaneous coronary sinus catheter can be placed if retrograde cardioplegia is desired.

In general, the myocardial protective techniques used in port-access surgery are similiar to those used for cardiac operations with cardiopulmonary bypass via full sternotomy. However, as the average cross-clamp, cardiopulmonary bypass and total operating room times are typically longer as compared to conventional cardiac surgery, the quality of myocardial protection must be at least as good as for the conventional procedures.

Several limitations are still present with port-access surgery:

- percutaneous placement of the pulmonary artery vent and the retrograde coronary sinus catheter requires fluoroscopic and transesophageal echocardiographic guidance and clinical expertise,
- proper positioning of the endovascular aortic occlusion catheter is important because misplacement can potentially result in aortic valve incompetence and left ventricular distension, inability to deliver cardioplegia, or compromised perfusion of the arch vessels.[15]

OPTIMAL USE OF MYOCARDIAL PROTECTION AND CARDIOPULMONARY BYPASS FOR CORONARY SURGERY

Myocardial protection techniques are designed to:

- provide a bloodless and motionless field for optimal anatomical repair,
- avoid injury to the myocardium and other organs during aortic cross-clamping, and
- be used for different surgical presentations (elective, urgent, emergency cases).

Blood cardioplegic techniques are those most frequently used worldwide and these strategies are described below.

In the past, many different cardioplegic solutions were in clinical use, even though they had not been thoroughly tested experimentally and clinically for intracoronary use during cardiac surgery. During recent years, proven solutions have been produced by different companies worldwide, ensuring a solution with consistent composition, pyrogen-free and stable. Only these tested solutions should be used clinically.

Routine coronary artery surgery

In elective coronary patients, immediately after commencement of cardiopulmonary bypass, the aorta is clamped and the myocardial protection sequence, consisting of cold induction, multiple reinfusions and warm terminal reperfusion, is started.

COLD BLOOD CARDIOPLEGIC INDUCTION

For cold induction, 8–12 °C blood cardioplegic solution is used and delivered 2 minutes antegrade (200–300 mL min^{-1}, 60–80 mmHg) and 2 minutes retrograde (200 mL min^{-1}, 30–50 mmHg). Immediately after achieving asystole, the perfusionist changes from a high-K^+ to a low-K^+ solution.

COLD BLOOD CARDIOPLEGIC REINFUSIONS

Approximately every 20 minutes cardioplegia is given for 2 minutes (200 mL min^{-1}, 50 mmHg), preferably 1 minute antegrade and 1 minute retrograde. The mode of delivery depends upon the type of grafts used, for example in arterial revascularization, retrograde delivery is preferred, whereas in combined venous and arterial revascularization, the authors use retrograde delivery combined with antegrade delivery via vein grafts (combined delivery).

WARM TERMINAL REPERFUSION

Warm terminal reperfusion is used in all operations before opening the aortic clamp to counteract possible reperfusion damage. In coronary operations the proximal anastomoses are performed with the single-clamp technique and warm terminal reperfusion is started immediately prior to completion of the last proximal anastomosis. The warm terminal reperfusate is given for 3 minutes (1.5 minutes antegrade and 1.5 minutes retrograde) at a temperature of 37 °C and a flow rate of 150 mL min^{-1}.

Thereafter the aortic clamp is removed and sinus rhythm resumes, in most cases spontaneously. After checking all anastomotic sites for bleeding, cardiopulmonary bypass is stopped.

Patients with acute coronary syndromes

The cardioplegic strategy depends upon the type of acute coronary syndrome – unstable angina or acute coronary occlusion.

UNSTABLE ANGINA

In patients with unstable angina, warm blood cardioplegic induction is used before the protection sequence is continued with cold induction (see above). The rationale for warm induction is to provide the myocardium with a phase of 'active resuscitation' before an ischemic period is added for graft construction for complete coronary revascularization.

For warm induction, a substrate-enriched blood cardioplegic solution at a temperature of 37 °C is used at an initial flow of 300–350 mL min^{-1} until asystole has occurred. After asystole, the flow is reduced to 150 mL min^{-1} for a total of 5 minutes (2.5 minutes antegrade and 2.5 minutes retrograde), followed by 3 minutes of cold induction.

ACUTE CORONARY OCCLUSION

Complete coronary revascularization of the acutely ischemic area as well as the remote myocardium is of great importance. Failure to completely revascularize the myocardium (e.g. coronary arteries less than 1 mm and unsuitable for grafting, left anterior descending dissections

after percutaneous transluminal balloon angioplasty failure with occlusion of larger septal branches, peripheral occlusions) may result in persistent hypokinesia or akinesia and will cause inadequate reversal of cardiogenic shock.

The surgical strategy for acute coronary occlusion can be separated into the phases of:

- total vented bypass,
- aortic cross-clamping,
- regional controlled reperfusion, and
- prolonged beating empty state.[16]

Total vented bypass

Cardiopulmonary bypass is established as quickly as possible and the left ventricle is vented routinely via the right superior pulmonary vein. To ensure optimal cardioplegic distribution, a retrograde coronary sinus cannula is always inserted. For bypass conduits we only use vein grafts into the segment undergoing infarction, because the controlled reperfusate has to be administered through these conduits. Internal thoracic artery grafts are feasible only for a small remote segment, because (unlike vein grafts) they cannot immediately accommodate the high flows that might be needed to supply remote segments with a large muscle mass.

Aortic cross-clamping

The phase of aortic cross-clamping is divided into induction, maintenance and global reperfusion.

- *Induction.* For induction, either cold or warm blood cardioplegic induction is used, depending upon the condition of the patient. Patients in cardiogenic shock due to acute coronary occlusion always receive warm induction, whereas in hemodynamically stable patients asystole is induced with cold induction.
- *Maintenance.* After each distal anastomosis, or after 20 minutes, cold blood cardioplegic reinfusion is delivered as described above.
- *Global reperfusion.* After the last distal anastomosis has been performed, warm (37 °C) substrate-enriched blood cardioplegia is given into the aorta and all grafts for 2 minutes at 150 mL min^{-1}. Thereafter, the aortic clamp is removed.

Regional controlled reperfusate

After removal of the aortic clamp, controlled regional blood cardioplegic solution is given at a flow rate of 50 mL min^{-1}, only into the graft supplying the region revascularized for acute coronary occlusion, for an additional 18 minutes. In patients with acute coronary occlusion of the left main coronary artery, or with acute occlusions of two coronary arteries, flow is increased to 100 mL min^{-1} and given into both vein grafts. Normal blood is delivered into the remainder of the heart via the aortic segment not included in the tangential clamp.

Cannulation of a side branch of the vein graft allows delivery of the controlled blood cardioplegic reperfusate while the proximal anastomosis is performed so that no additional ischemic time is imposed upon the previously ischemic area. The proximal anastomosis of the vein graft supplying the ischemic region is always constructed first.

Prolonged beating empty state

The heart is kept in the beating empty state for 30 more minutes after completion of the controlled regional reperfusion. Recovery of jeopardized myocardium is best achieved by lowering the oxygen demands and increasing oxygen delivery.

A two-stage venous cannula, or separate cannulation of the superior and inferior venae cavae, will not ensure complete left heart decompression, because coronary sinus return and/or bronchial flow will enter the left ventricle, distend it, allow wall tension to develop, and result in occasional ejection despite apparent right heart decompression. Therefore, effective left heart decompression is required by directly venting the left ventricle.

Extracorporeal circulation is discontinued after 30 minutes of beating empty state. If cardiac output is not satisfactory, cardiopulmonary bypass is resumed and appropriate methods to support the failing ventricle are instituted (pharmacological or mechanical support).

Patients with severely impaired left ventricular function

For patients with severely impaired left ventricular function, consideration should be given to warm cardioplegic induction, preoperative IABP and surgical anterior ventricular reconstruction to reduce left ventricular end-diastolic diameter. In general, protection techniques are similar to those described above.

Managing patients for repeat coronary surgery

Re-operations are accompanied by difficult problems deriving from substernal and pericardial adhesions, severely compromised heart function with advanced, diffuse coronary artery disease, and non-coronary atherosclerosis. In addition, these patients are older and sicker, with other organ dysfunction.[17] Severe aortic atherosclerosis can create the risk of intraoperative atherosclerotic embolization and multi-organ failure. These patients often require prolonged cardiopulmonary bypass and aortic cross-clamping. In such circumstances, preservation of cardiac function with advanced techniques of myocardial protection is of utmost importance.[18]

It is important to be aware that the single most important cause of morbidity and mortality during coronary

Table 14.3 *Frequent causes of myocardial infarction during coronary reoperations*

- Graft injury
- Incomplete revascularization
- Embolization:
  - from atherosclerotic vein grafts
  - from an atherosclerotic aorta
- Inadequate delivery of cardioplegia
- Devascularization by graft removal
- Early graft failure
- Technical error

re-operations is perioperative myocardial infarction (Table 14.3). Re-operative patients differ from primary coronary patients in many ways, which makes the intraoperative myocardial protection strategy more demanding.

For the conduct of a successful repeat coronary artery operation, special consideration should be given to the following operative steps.

STERNAL RE-ENTRY

In order to reduce the possibility of injuring the free wall of the right ventricle, the aorta, patent vein grafts or arterial grafts, it is helpful to assess the substernal anatomy by lateral chest x-rays (look for hemoclips on the grafts) and CT scans. In addition, the preoperative coronary angiograms, including all grafts, show their anatomical location in relation to the substernal space.

Sternal re-entry is performed with an oscillating saw and it is helpful to leave the sternal wires intact posteriorly while cutting the sternum, to avoid damage to the underlying structures.

In cases where there is a high probability of injury to these structures during re-entry, it is important to prepare the groin (or use the axillary approach) for possible emergency femoro-femoral bypass in the event of excessive bleeding. The establishment of cardiopulmonary bypass before sternal re-entry decompresses the heart, thereby keeping cardiac structures, including patent graft conduits, away from the sternum. In addition, hemodynamic stability can be maintained by cardiopulmonary bypass, even if serious injury to substernal structures occurs.[18] In the event of severe injury to substernal cardiac structures, the chest should not be opened forcefully with the retractor, because this only lacerates the right ventricle or aorta even more. Instead, sharp dissection should be continued until a retractor can be safely inserted and opened.

ATHEROSCLEROTIC EMBOLIZATION

Atherosclerotic embolization from patent or stenosed grafts represents one of the main challenges during re-operation. Compression trauma or direct injury during dissection may cause intraoperative myocardial infarction by interruption of the blood supply or embolization of easily detachable atheromatous debris.[17] Therefore, extensive intrapericardial dissection, especially around bypass conduits, should be delayed until cardiopulmonary bypass is established, or even until cardioplegic arrest occurs.[19]

The delivery of retrograde blood cardioplegia has been shown to significantly reduce mortality in coronary re-operations[19] due to a reduction in embolization from grafts, and should be used in all cases of cardiac surgery re-operation. The delivery of antegrade cardioplegia into the aortic root may not fully protect the heart in re-operative patients and, in the presence of atherosclerotic vein grafts, may also create the risk of embolization.

If embolization is to be expected, functioning grafts should be divided even before the administration of antegrade cardioplegia and myocardial protection is achieved through retrograde delivery of blood cardioplegia.

FUNCTIONING ARTERIAL GRAFTS

Patent arterial grafts tend to reduce the quality of myocardial protection and hamper the operative procedure by continuously supplying non-cardioplegic blood to the myocardium. This, in turn, delays cardioplegic arrest and leads to an early return of electromechanical activity.

If technically possible without injuring the grafts, careful dissection and temporary occlusion by a vascular clamp may overcome these problems. However, if dissection is difficult and may damage the integrity of the arterial graft, systemic hypothermia and frequent reinfusions of retrograde cold blood cardioplegia is the preferred alternative method.

MYOCARDIAL PROTECTION STRATEGY

The authors use intermittent cold antegrade and retrograde blood cardioplegia combined with terminal warm reperfusion for all coronary re-operations. All anastomoses are performed with the single cross-clamp technique. Antegrade cardioplegic delivery through the aortic root and down atherosclerotic grafts may have the following disadvantages:

- it may cause embolization from atherosclerotic vein grafts into the coronary circulation, and
- in the presence of patent arterial grafts to occluded coronary arteries, distribution of cardioplegic solution may be inhomogeneous.

Therefore, retrograde administration of cardioplegia has been of benefit to ensure a more homogeneous distribution of the cardioplegic solution. However, there are experimental data showing incomplete protection of the

right ventricle if only retrograde cardioplegia has been used. Even though we have not experienced this potential disadvantage of retrograde administration clinically, the combination of antegrade with retrograde delivery seems to offer the optimal protection.

KEY REFERENCES

Buckberg GD (Guest Editor). Myocardial preservation. *Semin Thorac Cardiovasc Surg* 2001; **13**:29–88.
A series of papers describing myocardial preservation techniques in different surgical settings, including re-operation, poor left ventricular function, and off-pump coronary surgery.

Buckberg GD. Development of blood cardioplegia and retrograde techniques: the experimenter/observer complex. *J Card Surg* 1998; **13**:163–70.
Review article.

Murkin JM. Attenuation of neurologic injury during cardiac surgery. *Ann Thorac Surg* 2001;**72**:S1838–44.
An up-to-date review of the current understanding of surgically relevant risk factors for cerebral complications after coronary surgery, with recommendations for the management of those at particularly high risk.

Schlensak C, Doenst T, Beyersdorf F. Clinical experience with blood cardioplegia. *Thorac Cardiovasc Surg* 1998; **46**(Suppl. 2):282–5.
Further description of the authors' technique, with indications for use of the different protocols.

REFERENCES

1. Buckberg GD. Editorial: Endothelial and myocardial stunning. *J Thorac Cardiovasc Surg* 2000; **120**:640–1.
2. Murkin JM. Attenuation of neurologic injury during cardiac surgery. *Ann Thorac Surg* 2001; **72**:S1838–44.
3. Roach GW, Kanchuger M, Mangano CM, Newman M, Nussmeier N, Wolman R, *et al.* Adverse cerebral outcomes after coronary bypass surgery. *N Engl J Med* 1996; **335**:1857–63.
4. Newman MF, Kirchner JL, Phillips-Bute B, Gaver V, Grocott H, Jones RH, *et al.* Longitudinal assessment of neurocognitive function after coronary artery bypass surgery. *N Engl J Med* 2001; **344**:395–402.
5. Allen BS, Buckberg GD, Rosenkranz ER, Plested W, Skow J, Mazzei E, et al. Topical cardiac hypothermia in patients with coronary disease. *J Thorac Cardiovasc Surg* 1992; **104**:626–31.
6. Schlensak C, Doenst T, Preußer S, Wunderlich M, Kleinschmidt M, Beyersdorf F. Bronchial artery perfusion during cardiopulmonary bypass does not prevent ischemia of the lungs in piglets. Assessment of bronchial artery blood flow with fluorescent microspheres. *Eur J Cardiothorac Surg* 2001; **19**:326–32.
7. Mora CT. *Cardiopulmonary Bypass. Principles and Techniques of Extracorporeal Circulation.* New York: Springer-Verlag, 1995.
8. Collins JD, Bassendine MF, Ferner R, Blesovsky A, Murray A, Pearson DT, *et al.* Incidence and prognostic importance of jaundice

after cardiopulmonary bypass surgery. *Lancet* 1983;
1(8334):1119–23.

9. Rattner DW, Gu Z-Y, Vlahakes GJ, Warshaw AL. Hyperamylasemia after cardiac surgery. *Ann Surg* 1989; 209:279–83.

10. Fiddian-Green RG, Baker S. The predictive value of measurements of pH in the wall of the stomach for complications after cardiac surgery: a comparison with other forms of monitoring. *Critical Care Med* 1987; 15:153–6.

11. Karlstad MD, Patteson SK, Guszczan JA, Langdon R, Chesney JT. Methylprednisolone does not influence endotoxin translocation during cardiopulmonary bypass. *J Cardiothorac Vasc Anesth* 1993; 7:23–7.

12. Beyersdorf F, Mitrev Z, Eckel L, Sarai K, Satter P. Controlled limb reperfusion as a new surgical technique to reduce postischemic syndrome. *J Thorac Cardiovasc Surg* 1993; 106:378–80.

13. Buckberg GD. Introduction. *Semin Thorac Cardiovasc Surg* 1993; 5:97.

14. Subramanian VA. Minimally invasive coronary artery bypass grafting. In: *Advanced Therapy in Cardiac Surgery*, KL Franco, ED Verrier (eds). St Louis, MI: B.C. Decker, 1999, 118–28.

15. Fann JI, Pompili MF, Burdon TA, Reitz BA. Minimally invasive cardiac surgery: Port-Access method. In: *Advanced Therapy in Cardiac Surgery*, KL Franco, ED Verrier (eds). St Louis, MI: B.C. Decker, 1999, 135–44.

16. Beyersdorf F, Buckberg GD. Myocardial protection in patients with acute myocardial infarction and cardiogenic shock. *Semin Thorac Cardiovasc Surg* 1993; 5:151–61.

17. Loop FD. The value and conduct of reoperations for coronary atherosclerosis. *Semin Thorac Cardiovasc Surg* 1994; 6:116–19.

18. Okamoto F, Sakai K. Protection strategies in reoperations. In: *Ischemia-Reperfusion Injury in Cardiac Surgery*, F. Beyersdorf (ed.). Georgetown, TX: Landes Bioscience, 2001, 203–9.

19. Savage EB, Cohn LH. 'No touch' dissection, antegrade–retrograde blood cardioplegia, and single aortic cross-clamp significantly reduce operative mortality of reoperative CABG. *Circulation* 1994; 90:II-140–3.

20. Kirklin J, Barrett-Boyes BG. *Cardiac Surgery*, 2nd edn. New York: Churchill Livingstone, 1993.

15

The complications of coronary surgery

DAVID J WHEATLEY

Although most patients go through coronary surgery without apparent difficulty, evidence of a number of adverse effects of the surgical procedure can frequently be shown with detailed sensitive testing. The spectrum of these effects ranges from mild biochemical abnormalities or subtle functional changes, through more obvious though transitory functional deficit, to frank complications that may leave lasting disability or cause death. Coronary surgery in the aged, or those with serious co-morbidity or advanced ischemic heart disease, carries increased risk of major complications. Besides the obvious distress, anxiety and lost time, there is the added demand on hospital resources and hence costs – estimated at about 10% of the total expenditure on surgical treatment of coronary disease in the USA.[1]

INTRODUCTION

It is important for the surgeon to be aware of the incidence and nature of complications associated with coronary surgery in order to be able to obtain truly informed patient consent and to advise patients and their families about the likely course of the complications should they arise. Awareness of causes and predisposing factors may make it possible to adopt techniques that will reduce complications. If they do occur, early detection and intervention will often reduce their impact.

The goal must be to avoid complications, primarily by careful patient selection, meticulous anesthetic and perioperative care, as well as accurate, appropriate and expeditious surgery. Where age, infirmity, co-morbidity or coronary pathology makes a good surgical outcome

unlikely, other management strategies should be examined. Operative techniques themselves influence outcome, as is illustrated by the now well-recognized beneficial effect of the internal thoracic artery conduit, not only on long-term event-free survival,[2] but also on perioperative mortality.[3] Some groups advocate beating-heart surgery to avoid the risks associated with cardiopulmonary bypass in the hope of reducing mortality and at least some complications,[4,5] though further experience is needed to determine the best policy for individual patients.

Even in the best of practices, complications do arise.[6] Many of the components of coronary surgery impose a challenge to the body, which may or may not be well tolerated, depending on the physiological reserves and co-morbidity of the individual patient. The atherosclerotic process for which coronary surgery is undertaken is usually not confined to the coronary arteries but is more widespread in the body. Cerebrovascular, ischemic visceral and peripheral vascular complications are therefore more likely in coronary surgery patients than in those undergoing other, comparable major surgery.

RISK FACTORS

The prevalence of coronary disease increases with age, and elderly patients comprise a substantial proportion of surgical practice. There is a natural loss of physiological reserves in the organs of the body with aging. Measures of cardiac performance and pulmonary, renal and cerebral function show deterioration in the elderly.[7] Co-morbidity, if only at a minor, subclinical level, is common in the elderly. Thus, *advanced age* features prominently as a risk factor for most complications following coronary surgery.

Another powerful risk factor is the *urgency of surgery*. It may be possible to reduce surgical risk by measures that lessen the urgency of operation. One of the most effective strategies in coronary surgery is improving the supply/demand balance for myocardial perfusion in unstable angina. Reduction of myocardial work with systemic vasodilators, beta-blocking drugs and sedation, together with antiplatelet therapy and coronary vasodilators, may avoid the need for urgent surgery and allow elective surgery at lower risk. Intra-aortic balloon pump support may similarly convert an emergency presentation of unstable angina, evolving infarction, or complication of infarction, into a less urgent one, with improved myocardial supply/demand balance and lower operative hazard.[8]

Some *co-morbid conditions* may be amenable to treatment that would lessen or abolish their impact. Infection of any nature (e.g. colds, flu-like illnesses, skin infection) should be treated or allowed to subside before elective surgery. Infection and bronchospasm associated with *chronic obstructive airways disease* can be treated with appropriate antibiotics, physiotherapy and bronchodilators, with benefit in the postoperative course. Optimal control of *diabetes* can lower the risk of wound infection, including deep sternal infection.[9,10] There is usually not sufficient time to implement cessation of smoking or weight loss, but when feasible, such intervention is advisable.

Ongoing audit of outcomes is of great value in detecting unfavorable trends in complication rates and prompting measures to identify causes and remedial action. A good example of a multicenter collaborative audit initiative resulting in clinical improvement comes from a Northern New England Cardiovascular Disease Study Group report on bleeding following coronary surgery.[11]

ADVERSE EVENTS FOLLOWING CORONARY SURGERY

Death

Death in the perioperative period (within 30 days or within the hospitalization period, however long) is the most serious and indisputable adverse outcome of coronary surgery. It can usually be ascribed to a definite cause. Low cardiac output and its consequences, stroke, pulmonary insufficiency and renal failure are the common causes of death following coronary surgery. The likelihood of hospital mortality can be predicted with some accuracy from knowledge of preoperative factors. The most powerful predictive factors include age, urgency of operation, previous cardiac surgery, degree of left ventricular dysfunction, female gender, left main coronary stenosis, and extent of coronary disease.[12] A number of preoperative scoring systems have been developed that allow prediction of hospital mortality and provide the basis for improvement of preoperative decision making.[12–14] In many countries, hospital mortality has been used as a quality marker for surgery, adding further impetus to the development of accurate measures for predicting mortality.[15]

The risk of hospital death for elective coronary surgery in men under 60 years of age and without co-morbidity is less than 0.5% in the Northern New England Cardiovascular Disease Study Group risk prediction, based on more than 7000 patients having coronary surgery between 1996 and 1998.[16] In North American experience, compared to risk for those under 65, risk doubles for the 65–74-year group, and quadruples for the over-75-year group. Women have about 1.5 times the risk of men, and previous heart surgery triples the risk.[16] Data for coronary surgery in the UK for 1996–1999[17] show crude mortality of 1.5% for the 56–60-year group; 2.7% for the 66–70 group, and 6.8% for those over 75 years of age. Men had a crude mortality of 2.4% and women 3.6%. For first-time coronary surgery, mortality was 2.5%; following previous cardiac surgery it was 7.4%.

Low cardiac output syndrome

CLINICAL FEATURES

The clinical syndrome of low cardiac output is a result of the heart ejecting insufficient blood to maintain normal metabolism of the tissues of the body and normal visceral function. Normal cardiac index at rest is about $2.4\,L\,m^{-2}\,min^{-1}$. This sustains aerobic metabolism and visceral function at normothermia, with normal vascular resistance and blood pressure. Cardiac output can be measured with reasonable accuracy from an indwelling pulmonary artery catheter (either intermittently or continuously), and the measurement is often combined with mixed venous saturation, a useful confirmatory assessment of tissue perfusion. Such measurements are often part of monitoring of cardiac surgical patients. However, cardiac output measurement must be interpreted in the context of the clinical and physiological status, taking account of the relationship between cardiac output, vascular resistance and blood pressure for rational assessment and management.

The recognition of low cardiac output syndrome in the operating room requires a high index of suspicion. Low blood pressure, bradycardia or tachycardia, visible evidence of either an underfilled, hyperactive heart or a dilated, sluggish heart, and low mixed venous saturation, while weaning from cardiopulmonary bypass should alert the surgeon and anesthesiologist to the possibility of low output. Unduly low (or high) left heart filling pressure can be suspected from palpation of the pulmonary artery. Measurement of left atrial pressure (directly or indirectly), cardiac output and mixed venous saturation adds greater precision to the clinical estimate. Early attention to heart rate, intravascular filling and contractile state is more important than awaiting conclusive evidence of low cardiac output.

In the recovery period, clinical recognition of low cardiac output is easier, though residual effects of anesthesia and hypothermia may confound assessment. Evidence of skin perfusion (color, temperature, visible capillary and venous filling), renal perfusion (urine output) and acid–base status, combined with observation of trends in blood pressure, heart rate and venous filling pressure, should allow reasonable assessment of adequacy of cardiac output.

INCIDENCE

Low cardiac output syndrome is the commonest cause of hospital mortality in most reported surgical experience. Mild degrees are relatively common, are present for a few hours only, and respond to simple management such as fluid administration or inotrope support. The need for inotrope or mechanical support of the circulation is a reasonable surrogate marker for low cardiac output and may be a reflection of the adequacy of myocardial protective strategies. Preoperative left ventricular dysfunction is one of the most powerful predictors of postoperative low output syndrome. Yau and colleagues[18] have reported a prevalence of low output syndrome of about 5% following coronary surgery in patients with left ventricular ejection fraction greater than 40% for the period 1992–1997; for those with ejection fraction of 20–40%, low output syndrome occurred in about 12%; and in those with ejection fraction below 20%, about 22% had low output syndrome after surgery.

NATURAL HISTORY

Most instances resolve or respond to treatment, recovering within hours or days. Inability of the heart to sustain an adequate cardiac output in the early period following cardiac surgery results in poor perfusion of tissues throughout the body. The most vulnerable are those of the heart itself, the brain, the kidneys and the abdominal viscera. Impaired perfusion of each of these may result in organ-specific complications. Under-perfusion of skeletal muscle and other tissues results in metabolic acidosis, which in turn can adversely affect vital organs, including the heart. Low cardiac output leads to increasing venous desaturation, as tissue oxygen extraction exceeds delivery. Severe mixed venous desaturation may initiate arterial desaturation as a result of intrapulmonary right-to-left shunting as well as of the inability of alveolar ventilation to replenish fully the oxygen capacity of the alveolar capillary blood, particularly if pulmonary edema develops. Hypoxic cardiac arrest, cerebral damage, renal failure and abdominal ischemic complications are possible consequences, and each can lead to death.

CAUSES AND PREDISPOSING FACTORS

The causes of low cardiac output following coronary surgery include the following.

1 Inadequate filling of the vascular compartment (hypovolemia), due to incomplete restoration of blood volume following cardiopulmonary bypass, blood loss or drug-induced vasodilatation.
2 Cardiac dysfunction. Following coronary surgery, frequent causes are:
   * abnormal heart rhythm – bradycardia, tachycardia or dysrhythmia;
   * primary myocardial dysfunction (temporary stunning, perioperative infarction):
     – *global injury* due to ischemia, inadequate cardioplegic protection, distension or excessive retraction,
     – *regional injury* due to flawed coronary anastomosis, atheroembolism, or thrombotic coronary occlusion on atheromatous plaque;
   * secondary myocardial depression due to electrolyte imbalance, acidosis or myocardial depressive drugs;
   * cardiac tamponade from blood clot around the heart.

AVOIDANCE

Measures to maintain normal myocardial oxygen supply/demand balance prior to surgery have great benefit. Careful attention to all aspects of myocardial protection, care in handling the heart and ascending aorta, and avoidance of ventricular distension during surgery are essential in minimizing postoperative low cardiac output. Avoidance of underfilling or overfilling of the circulation when weaning from cardiopulmonary bypass, and measures to maintain a normal heart rate and blood pressure (e.g. pacing, cardioversion, inotrope support) may forestall the initiation of the cycle of events leading to low cardiac output. In high-risk patients (those with acutely or chronically impaired left ventricular function), a period of controlled reperfusion of the non-working heart without inotrope stimulation may mitigate or avoid low output syndrome.

MANAGEMENT

Rational management requires identification of the cause. Inadequate left heart filling pressure is treated by appropriate fluid replacement (e.g. blood, plasma or plasma expander) or pharmacological vasoconstriction (e.g. with norepinephrine), depending on the cause.

Excessive left heart filling pressure implies poor left ventricular function. If due to severe bradycardia, tachycardia or dysrhythmias such as uncontrolled atrial fibrillation, drug therapy, pacing or cardioversion may be appropriate. If due to myocardial dysfunction, inotrope support, optimization of blood electrolytes, acid–base balance and oxygenation are necessary. Intra-aortic balloon pumping[8] will reduce the need for inotropic drive by favorably altering afterload and coronary filling pressure.

Rising central venous pressure with falling blood pressure may be due to cardiac tamponade. Echocardiography may distinguish a failing, dilated heart from a heart restricted by blood or thrombus. Clinical assessment can be difficult as the tachycardia commonly present with tamponade may be attenuated by beta-blockade. If there is any reason to suspect tamponade, the chest should be re-opened and blood or thrombus should be removed. An open pericardial and pleural cavity does not prevent cardiac compression from retained thrombus.

Alterations in systemic vascular resistance and blood pressure are frequently present in the perioperative period and must be borne in mind when assessing the adequacy of cardiac output and deciding management. For example, a low cardiac output in the presence of high systemic vascular resistance can be improved by vasodilatation and intravascular fluid infusion. However, a normal (or even increased) cardiac output in a patient with low systemic vascular resistance may be associated with hypotension and be inadequate for visceral perfusion.

If there is reason to suspect a perioperative infarct due to a faulty bypass graft or thrombotic occlusion on a plaque, urgent coronary angiography may be indicated, and re-intervention (thrombolysis, percutaneous catheter intervention or re-operation) may be necessary.[19]

OUTCOME

Outcome ranges from complete recovery in mild and appropriately treated cases, to death or lasting disability. More severe manifestations may be complicated by acute renal failure, cerebral injury, abdominal complications such as bowel ischemia, myocardial infarction or peripheral limb ischemic necrosis (especially if peripheral arterial disease or the presence of an intra-aortic balloon pump further compromises circulation). In the most severe cases, increasing hypoxia and acidosis may cause death by cardiac arrest or multi-organ failure with its attendant risk of septicemia.

Preoperatively impaired left ventricular function, the major predisposing factor for postoperative low cardiac output, has an important effect on outcome. In UK practice during 1996–1999, patients with an ejection fraction

of 50% or more had a crude mortality of 1.8%; for those with an ejection fraction of 30–49%, it was 3.4%; and for those with an ejection fraction below 30%, mortality was 9.8%.[17]

Perioperative myocardial infarction

Perioperative myocardial infarction is one of the causes of low cardiac output syndrome and ventricular dysrhythmias following coronary surgery. Localized, regional infarction can occur as a result of technical deficiencies in grafting (occluded recipient artery, kinked graft), or thrombotic occlusion in a graft or recipient artery, or in an ungrafted artery. Atheroembolism is another cause of localized infarction. Diffuse, global injury can affect the myocardium as a consequence of preoperative and postoperative ischemia due to imbalance of blood supply and myocardial demand. This can occur during induction of anesthesia, during surgery, particularly off-pump surgery, or due to inadequate cardioplegic protection. There is a spectrum of myocardial injury, from the clinically obvious transmural infarct causing low output syndrome, to more subtle degrees of global injury that are detectable only with sensitive test methods. The reported incidence varies between 5% and 12% and depends on the sensitivity of the methods used for detection.[20–22] A 7% incidence of definite or probable perioperative myocardial infarction following coronary surgery has been reported[23] in a study which showed the immediate effect on mortality (14% hospital death rate) and predisposing factors (recent myocardial infarction, emergency surgery). Diagnosis of perioperative myocardial infarction may be made on the basis of electrocardiography (evolving ST-segment changes, new Q waves), cardiac-specific enzyme changes (e.g. creatine phosphokinase) or troponins, or infarct-avid radionuclide imaging.[21]

Patients with ongoing myocardial ischemia prior to surgery (unstable angina, evolving infarction) are at greater risk of perioperative myocardial infarction. Poor left ventricular function and widespread coronary disease increase the risk of this complication. Coronary endarterectomy, prolonged aortic cross-clamping, incomplete revascularization, inadequate myocardial protection and ventricular distension have all been identified as risk factors.[21] During surgery, ST-segment trending devices, pulmonary artery catheters and transesophageal echocardiography have all been advocated for early detection of myocardial ischemia, elevation of left ventricular end-diastolic pressure, or development of regional wall abnormalities suggestive of ischemia.

Preoperative heparin and antiplatelet therapy for those with ongoing ischemic events undergoing surgery, avoidance of tachycardia, and beta-blockade have protective effects against perioperative infarction.[21]

Hemodynamic compromise from perioperative myocardial infarction may require inotropic support, control of dysrhythmias, intra-aortic balloon pump assistance or left heart assistance. Urgent re-angiography has been used to identify incomplete revascularization or graft-related problems leading to further emergency surgery.[19,20]

Perioperative myocardial infarction has a detrimental effect on event-free survival, which can be predicted on the basis of adequacy of revascularization and left ventricular ejection fraction.[22] In a study of outcome of nearly 5000 coronary surgical patients, in whom hospital mortality was 1.9%, there were new Q waves in 2.1% of the entire group. Elevated cardiac-specific enzymes on the first postoperative day increased the risk of both early death (odds ratio 6 or 9, depending on enzyme) and late death (odds ratio 1.4 or 1.5) during the 5-year mean follow-up period.[24]

Dysrhythmias

Changes in serum potassium level are common after coronary surgery, and low serum potassium may result in ventricular extrasystoles. Non-sustained ventricular tachyarrhythmias are often associated with previous infarction or perioperative ischemia, inotropes, low serum potassium or low serum magnesium. The administration of beta-blocking drugs and intravenous magnesium sulphate is a prophylactic measure. Specific anti-arrhythmic drugs may be required (e.g. lignocaine, amiodarone) and electrical defibrillation is needed promptly for ventricular fibrillation.[25]

Atrial fibrillation

Atrial fibrillation has been reported to occur in 23–33% of patients following coronary surgery.[26] It occurs most frequently on the second or third postoperative day, often resulting in breathlessness and feeling unwell. It is a rapidly self-terminating event within 24 hours in many patients. Poor myocardial preservation during surgery, postoperative hypoxia and old age are predisposing factors. There is an associated risk of thromboembolism. The consequences of increased hospital stay, complications, costs, prophylaxis and treatment are well reviewed.[26,27] Beating-heart techniques have been shown not to reduce the incidence of this complication in at least one study,[28] but to have lowered its frequency in another.[29]

Beta-blocking drugs, given preoperatively and restarted immediately after surgery, have been shown to reduce the incidence of atrial fibrillation following coronary surgery by more than 75%.[30] Magnesium replenishment has also been shown to reduce the incidence.[31] Amiodarone or electrical cardioversion are the most commonly effective treatment methods. If atrial fibrillation persists, anticoagulation is indicated.[26]

The inflammatory response to cardiopulmonary bypass

CLINICAL FEATURES

It has been recognized for many years that cardiopulmonary bypass induces an inflammatory response in the body, with activation of the complement system.[32] Many factors are now recognized as having a role, including kallikrein, neutrophil and monocyte activation, endotoxin, inflammatory mediators and oxygen-free radicals. There is plugging of capillary beds with activated neutrophils, generalized increased capillary permeability, edema of the heart, lungs, brain, kidneys and other viscera and tissues, bleeding and thromboembolism.[33,34] Clinically, impaired pulmonary gas exchange is probably the most frequent early indication of severe inflammatory response, and this may occasionally progress to acute respiratory distress syndrome.

INCIDENCE

An inflammatory response is probably initiated in all patients undergoing cardiopulmonary bypass, but in most there is little clinical impact. Increased capillary permeability, causing widespread edema, impairment of pulmonary gas exchange, and cerebral, renal and hepatic dysfunction, is commoner with prolonged cardiopulmonary bypass time.

NATURAL HISTORY

The changes are usually self-limiting, but when acute respiratory distress syndrome occurs, widespread pulmonary consolidation leads to life-threatening hypoxia. The cardiopulmonary bypass inflammatory response may exacerbate morbidity and mortality of other complications.

CAUSES AND PREDISPOSING RISK FACTORS

Exposure to the foreign surfaces of the extracorporeal circuit is the initiating cause.

AVOIDANCE

A number of pharmacological strategies have been tried in order to mitigate the problem. Steroids are probably protective, and the use of aprotinin is thought to have a beneficial effect. Heparin-coated extracorporeal circuits and leukodepletion have been shown to reduce the deleterious effect of cardiopulmonary bypass, though the clinical benefit is not dramatic.[33,34] Improved materials and designs over the years have lowered the injurious effects of cardiopulmonary bypass, including reduction of gaseous and particulate microembolic load and trauma to proteins and cellular elements in blood.

Hopes of avoiding the problem altogether by dispensing with cardiopulmonary bypass have been a major reason for the development of beating-heart techniques. Reduced activation of inflammatory markers and white cells[35,36] has been shown in beating-heart surgical patients compared with cardiopulmonary bypass patients. However, the relatively small clinical differences in outcome for coronary surgery with cardiopulmonary bypass or with beating-heart techniques in randomized trials indicate that the problem of the inflammatory response to cardiopulmonary bypass is not the only factor of clinical significance in most patients in modern practice.

MANAGEMENT

Severe impairment of pulmonary gas exchange may require prolonged ventilation with increased inspired oxygen concentration. Most of the changes elsewhere in the body are self-limiting.

OUTCOME

Transient visceral dysfunction becomes more important when combined with pre-existing co-morbidity. Fever, general malaise, confusion, hypoxia, oliguria and increased hospital stay are clinical manifestations of the inflammatory response to cardiopulmonary bypass. A fatal outcome can occur when acute respiratory distress syndrome is the predominant manifestation.

Bleeding

CLINICAL FEATURES

Blood loss during and immediately after coronary surgery is inevitable. Insertion of chest drains into the mediastinal space and pleural cavities (if opened) is routinely undertaken to prevent the compressive or restrictive effects of retained intrathoracic blood. The volume of blood loss that constitutes excessive bleeding is arbitrary; of more significance is the rate of loss and the physiological effect of the loss. In general, a total postoperative blood loss following elective coronary surgery of up to 1500 mL, and a rate of loss of up to 200 mL h^{-1} in the first 3 or 4 hours would not be considered excessive.

Strategies to minimize bleeding and the decision about when to intervene for unexpected blood loss are important aspects of management protocols. Although the risk of transmission of viral or prion disease via blood transfusion is low in most countries, public anxiety provides a powerful motivation for reducing or avoiding transfusion whenever possible. Cardiac surgery has been reported to account for 10% of all transfusion in the USA.[37] A similar proportion is used in cardiac surgical centers in England.[38] Costs for blood and blood products are an important component of overall coronary surgical costs – particularly if bleeding complications occur.

INCIDENCE

Allogeneic blood transfusion following cardiac surgery is common.[39] The proportion of patients receiving blood transfusion following elective coronary surgery has been reported to be 80% or more in some centers.[38] It may be argued that the need for transfusion *per se* indicates excessive blood loss. The need for re-exploration for bleeding is a widely accepted marker of excessive bleeding. Re-exploration rates after coronary surgery in over 12 500 patients in a Northern New England Cardiovascular Disease Study Group report were shown to have fallen from 3.6% to 2% over the study period of 1992–1997.[11] Another study of coronary surgical practice involving more than 8500 patients over a 25-year period showed 4.4% requiring re-operation for bleeding, with those over 80 years of age having a re-operation rate of 8.6%.[40]

NATURAL HISTORY

Excessive bleeding will often subside spontaneously without intervention. Severe bleeding may lead directly to a fatal outcome as a result of oligemic shock, or sometimes as a result of cardiac tamponade. If chest drainage is efficient and blood replacement adequate, the bleeding may continue for many hours. There is then an increasing risk of depletion of coagulation factors and platelets, and a vicious circle ensues with further bleeding. Disseminated intravascular hemolysis may occur, with the risk of multi-organ failure.

CAUSES AND PREDISPOSING RISK FACTORS

As coronary surgery involves multiple anastomoses at arterial sites and division of small arteries for mobilization of arterial conduits, the propensity for bleeding is far greater than for most other major surgical procedures. In addition, heparinization, cardiopulmonary bypass-induced changes in hemostatic and thrombotic mechanisms, hemodilution and hypothermia impair the natural ability of the body to achieve hemostasis.

Antiplatelet agents (aspirin, clopidogrel), which are nearly always used in patients with coronary disease, as well as the more potent anti-thrombotic and antiplatelet regimes used for acute coronary events and percutaneous catheter interventions, are predisposing factors for excessive bleeding, as are advanced age, prolonged cardiopulmonary bypass and re-operation.[16]

AVOIDANCE

Careful surgical technique, with confirmation of hemostasis prior to closing the chest, is an important aspect of keeping bleeding complications to a minimum. However, bleeding complications occur even with the most meticulous surgery. Cessation of aspirin or other antiplatelet drugs for a week before surgery is often advocated to reduce bleeding risk.[16]

A number of pharmacological methods, including antifibrinolytics (aprotinin, epsilon aminocaproic acid and tranexamic acid) and erythropoietin, have been advocated to attenuate the deficiencies in hemostasis that follow cardiopulmonary bypass.[41,42]

High-dose tranexamic acid and epsilon aminocaproic acid have both been shown to reduce blood loss and exposure to allogeneic blood products following coronary surgery.[43] A low dose of tranexamic acid has also been shown to have similar benefit to a high dose.[44]

Use of either epsilon aminocaproic acid or low-dose aprotinin in a randomized study involving patients having valve surgery with or without coronary surgery showed similar efficacy in reducing bleeding.[45] In another randomized study, a high dose and a low dose of aprotinin were equally effective in reducing bleeding in coronary surgery.[46]

Non-pharmacological methods for minimizing blood loss include pre-hospitalization autologous blood donation, pre-cardiopulmonary bypass blood removal (acute perioperative normovolemic hemodilution), intraoperative shed blood salvage, and salvage of postoperative mediastinal drainage.[47–49]

A randomized study of 252 patients undergoing elective coronary surgery with either intraoperative cell salvage or intraoperative cell salvage combined with removal of blood prior to cardiopulmonary bypass, and a control group, showed that intraoperative cell salvage resulted in halving of the number of patients requiring allogeneic blood transfusion. Adding acute perioperative normovolemic hemodilution showed no additional benefit.[38]

As cardiopulmonary bypass is implicated in the cause of excess bleeding following coronary surgery, it is not surprising that a number of reports have shown decreased blood loss for coronary surgery without cardiopulmonary bypass.[50–53]

MANAGEMENT

If cardiac tamponade is suspected, the chest should be promptly re-opened for evacuation of blood and thrombus. A bleeding site should be sought.

A sudden increase in chest drainage in a patient who was not previously bleeding unduly suggests a 'surgical' cause. The chest should be re-opened and the bleeding source identified and dealt with. In general, a consistent loss of more than 200 mL of blood per hour or the radiological finding of a substantial pleural accumulation requires re-opening of the chest for evacuation of blood

and a search for a bleeding source. It is not uncommon not to find any obvious site of bleeding.

Excessive bleeding may be due to a hemostatic defect. This is particularly likely if bleeding is a feature from the time of discontinuation of cardiopulmonary bypass, especially if there are predisposing factors such as long bypass time or preoperative antiplatelet therapy. Full reversal of heparin should be confirmed by measuring the activated clotting time, and corrected if necessary with protamine. Measurement of platelet count and a clotting screen (activated clotting time, prothrombin time and partial thromboplastin time) may identify specific deficiencies. Transfusion of fresh frozen plasma and platelets is usually helpful in restoring hemostatic function.

OUTCOME

Promptly controlled bleeding is often not associated with adverse outcome or delayed discharge, but severe postoperative bleeding is associated with longer hospital stay and increased morbidity (especially infective complications) and mortality.[54]

Cerebral complications

CLINICAL FEATURES

Two general types of cerebral complication are described following coronary surgery.[55] Major, focal cerebral dysfunction (type 1 deficit) is characterized by loss of regional function, most commonly stroke (hemiplegia, hemiparesis, monoparesis), delirium or coma. Type 1 deficits are usually all too apparent soon after surgery when the patient fails to awake as promptly as expected, or fails to move limbs. Less commonly, the onset is in the first few days following surgery. Diffuse cerebral dysfunction (type 2 deficit) is characterized by intellectual impairment (personality change, memory loss, inability to concentrate or perform mental tasks) or seizures, which may not be immediately apparent clinically. Type 2 deficits may only come to light days or weeks after surgery, sometimes at the instigation of family members. Careful and detailed neuropsychological tests are often needed to identify these deficits.[56]

INCIDENCE

Quoted incidences of 0.4–5.4% for stroke, and 25–90% for neuropsychological dysfunction can be found in the literature.[55,57] The Multicenter Study of Perioperative Ischemia report on 2108 patients revealed a 6.1% incidence of cerebral complications (half of which were type 1 and half type 2) during hospitalization for coronary surgery.[55] Hogue and colleagues,[58] reporting prospective findings from a study of more than 5000 patients, showed postoperative stroke rates of 2.5% for men and 3.2% for women. Stamou and colleagues,[59] in reviewing more than 16 500 patients having coronary surgery with cardiopulmonary bypass relevant to contemporary practice, showed a 2.0% stroke incidence. The Northern New England Cardiovascular Disease Study Group risk estimation for cerebrovascular accident varies from 0.3% (elective coronary operation in a man under 60 years of age without co-morbidity) to over 6.5%, with advanced age being the major predictor.[16]

The incidence of cognitive dysfunction is less easy to define, largely accounting for the wide range in reported incidence.[60] In a review of reports from the literature, it has been suggested that 22.5% of patients have a cognitive defect 2 months after surgery.[61] A more authoritative report, based on 261 patients having elective coronary surgery, has shown an incidence of neurocognitive defect of 53% at discharge.[56]

NATURAL HISTORY

The natural history of stroke and other type 1 deficits varies considerably depending on the severity of the original insult, from complete recovery to permanent disability or death. Though cognitive dysfunction (type 2 deficit) may not be immediately apparent, there is disturbing evidence that such dysfunction can persist or worsen after early improvement: although the 53% incidence at discharge reported by Newman and colleagues[56] had fallen to 24% at 6-month follow-up, at 5 years the incidence was found to be 42%.

CAUSES AND PREDISPOSING RISK FACTORS

Focal manifestations (type 1 deficits) are thought to be related to macroembolism (atheroma or thrombus), intracerebral hemorrhage, or thrombotic occlusion on atheromatous plaque in the intracranial or extracranial cerebral circulation. Predisposing factors recognized by Stamou and colleagues[59] included older age, chronic renal insufficiency, recent myocardial infarction, previous stroke, carotid disease, hypertension, diabetes, moderate or severe left ventricular dysfunction and, in the postoperative period, low cardiac output and new onset of atrial fibrillation. Others have shown the importance of aortic atherosclerosis and atheroembolism as a risk factor for stroke.[55,62]

Diffuse changes (type 2) are thought to be related to cardiopulmonary bypass,[57] though even this commonly held belief has been questioned on the basis of similar neuropsychological test changes in patients having coronary surgery with or without cardiopulmonary bypass in the same center.[63] Suspected mechanisms include changes in perfusion pressure and flow, gaseous or particulate microembolism, hypoxia and the inflammatory response to cardiopulmonary bypass. Fluoroscein

retinoscopy in the early postoperative period has shown widespread microvascular embolic occlusion.[64]

AVOIDANCE

The importance of aortic atherosclerosis as a particular risk factor has led to recommendations for minimal handling of the ascending aorta, the use of epi-aortic ultrasound scanning for the detection of lesions,[55,65] and the development of an aortic cannula incorporating a filter designed to trap liberated atheromatous material.[66]

Maintainance of physiological pressure and flow during cardiopulmonary bypass, use of an arterial filter, and avoidance of cardiotomy suction return (which adds a gaseous microembolic burden to the extracorporeal circuit) are probably important factors in the conduct of cardiopulmonary bypass.[67,68] The effect of perfusate temperature is unclear; two recent studies show conflicting results in comparing neurological outcome with hypothermia and normothermia.[69,70]

In view of the recognized potential of cardiopulmonary bypass for causing cerebral injury, off-pump techniques might be expected to reduce the risk of both types of cerebral complications. There are studies that address the impact of off-pump surgery on type 1 deficits. Patel and colleagues have shown an incidence of focal neurological deficit of 1.6% in 1210 coronary operations with cardiopulmonary bypass, and of 0.4% or 0.5% (depending on whether the ascending aorta was manipulated) for 520 beating-heart operations.[71] A study by Stamou and colleagues based on more than 10 000 patients undergoing coronary surgery, in which 'off-pump' and 'on-pump' patients were matched by propensity score, has produced evidence of a risk reduction for stroke when the beating-heart technique is used (odds ratio of 1.8).[72] Randomized trials of coronary surgery with and without cardiopulmonary bypass have not shown unequivocal differences in neuropsychological complications to date.[53,68,73] This may be related to the power of the studies or to the multifactorial nature of the etiology of cerebral injury related to coronary surgery. However, in a study of 40 patients randomly allocated to have coronary surgery with cardiopulmonary bypass or with an off-pump technique, 18 of the 20 in the cardiopulmonary bypass group were reported to have impaired cognitive performance, while those in the off-pump group had no impairment. There was also a striking reduction in high-intensity transient signals detected by ultrasonic imaging of the middle cerebral artery during surgery, and reduction in the S-100 protein, a marker of cerebral injury, in the off-pump group.[57]

MANAGEMENT

Management of type 1 deficits includes maintenance of physiological parameters of ventilation and cardiovascular status. Mechanical ventilation, care of the airway and good nursing practice to avoid pressure area, bladder and bowel complications are necessary. Specialist advice and CT or nuclear magnetic imaging of the brain may be necessary to plan further management and to distinguish embolic from hemorrhagic pathology, a distinction which may have a bearing on anticoagulant or antiplatelet therapy. Physiotherapy and rehabilitation are important in the longer term.

OUTCOME

Cerebral complications following coronary surgery are associated with increased hospital mortality, morbidity and hospital stay, poor long-term outcome and increased healthcare costs.[74] Puskas and colleagues report a prospective study of 10 860 patients having coronary surgery. Stroke occurred in 2.2%, and their hospital mortality was 22.5%. Their 1-year and 5-year survival were 64% and 44%. For those who did not have a stroke, hospital mortality was 2.0% and 1-year and 5-year survival were 94% and 81%. In the study reported by Roach and colleagues,[55] type 1 deficits had a 21% mortality; type 2 had a 10% hospital mortality. Prolonged hospitalization and continued disability are often further features of both types of deficit,[56] and the possibility that type 2 deficits may increase the late risk of dementia has been raised.[68]

Pulmonary complications and ventilatory insufficiency

CLINICAL FEATURES

A degree of pulmonary dysfunction, demonstrable by measuring alveolar-arterial oxygen gradient, shunt fraction or lung compliance, is present in most patients following coronary surgery with cardiopulmonary bypass, though this is usually not clinically obvious.[75] The most severe form, acute respiratory distress syndrome, is associated with severe dyspnea, hypoxia and widespread radiographic changes in the lungs.

Preferential ventilation of the right main bronchus due to the endotracheal tube moving downward, atelectasis, particularly of the lower lobes, retained secretions, tracheobronchitis, bronchopneumonia, phrenic nerve injury from exposure to cold topical fluid, retained blood in the pleural space and pneumothorax are commonly encountered abnormalities following coronary surgery. All impair ventilation and gas exchange and contribute to the clinical presentation of respiratory or ventilatory insufficiency. Chest x-ray will usually show the nature and extent of the pulmonary problems (pleural effusion, pulmonary atelectasis or consolidation).

Difficulty in weaning from mechanical ventilation, inability to maintain physiological blood gas indices on spontaneous ventilation, excessive work of breathing, dyspnea and arterial desaturation are the usual clinical manifestations of these abnormalities. Unheralded hypoxic cardiac arrest may be the first presentation if desaturation is not rectified.

INCIDENCE

Mild degrees of clinically inapparent pulmonary insufficiency are common.[75] Acute respiratory distress syndrome has been reported in up to 2% of patients following cardiopulmonary bypass.[76]

The respiratory and ventilatory consequences of a thoracic operation (endotracheal ventilation, open pleural spaces, postoperative pain) and the atelectatic and infective pulmonary changes that occur in many coronary patients (often overweight and recent smokers) are manifest to some degree in the majority of coronary surgical patients.

NATURAL HISTORY

Mild degrees of pulmonary insufficiency resolve spontaneously, but may take several weeks to disappear altogether.[75] More serious dysfunction may be complicated by prolonged dependence on mechanical ventilation, atrial and ventricular dysrhythmias, hypoxic cardiac arrest and death.

CAUSES AND PREDISPOSING RISK FACTORS

Changes induced by cardiopulmonary bypass, as part of a general systemic inflammatory response, have usually been implicated in the cause.[33] A comprehensive review of the causes and possible therapeutic interventions is available.[77] It is apparent from recent randomized trials of beating-heart surgery and surgery with cardiopulmonary bypass, that the extracorporeal circulation is not responsible for all the deleterious changes in the lungs following cardiac surgery. Although shorter postoperative ventilation times and lower pulmonary infection rates have been reported, no difference has been shown in alveolar-arterial oxygen gradients with beating-heart surgery.[36,78,79] Telectasis, retained secretions, bronchopneumonia, pleural effusion, phrenic nerve injury, obesity, chest wall or wound pain, and the depressant effect of analgesia may all have a causative role in ventilatory and pulmonary dysfunction. Chronic obstructive airways disease, chronic bronchitis and cigarette smoking are predisposing risk factors.

AVOIDANCE

Although the use of beating-heart techniques for coronary surgery, to avoid the use of cardiopulmonary bypass, has been suggested as a strategy for reducing pulmonary complications, this has not shown dramatic effects in randomized trials.[36,78,79] Few interventions, including steroid administration, leukocyte depletion and heparin-coated circuits, have shown significant amelioration of cardiopulmonary bypass-related lung dysfunction in clinical practice, with the possible exception of aprotinin priming of the extracorporeal circuit.[77]

Avoidance of pleural accumulations by properly located chest drains, humidification of inspired gas, adequate pain relief, physiotherapy, incentive spirometry and preoperative antibiotic therapy for chronic infection are the main methods of mitigating these complications.

Continuous pulse oximetry is a wise precaution in those at risk of pulmonary or ventilatory insufficiency, as it allows early detection of deterioration in arterial saturation.

MANAGEMENT

Mechanical ventilatory support may need to be prolonged. Mini-tracheostomy is often helpful in weaning from prolonged ventilation, as it allows ready aspiration of secretions. Antibiotic therapy, based on culture and sensitivity testing of organisms from secretions, and physiotherapy are the mainstays of therapy.

OUTCOME

The majority of patients recover fully from mild or moderate degrees of ventilatory insufficiency with correct management. However, ventilatory insufficiency is an important cause of hospital mortality. An increase in mortality and prolonged hospital stay, with the need for re-intubation and reventilation as a result of pulmonary insufficiency following coronary surgery, are predictable in patients with chronic obstructive airways disease. Acute respiratory distress syndrome carries an extremely high mortality (50–90%)[76] and the risk of prolonged disability.[80]

Renal dysfunction

CLINICAL FEATURES

Oliguria (failure to pass more than 0.5 mL of urine $kg^{-1}h^{-1}$ for more than an hour or two in the average adult soon after coronary surgery, in the presence of satisfactory postoperative hemodynamic status), rising serum creatinine and urea, and impaired ability to handle potassium and acid–base homeostasis are the immediate features. High serum potassium levels may precipitate cardiac arrest. Fluid retention results in pulmonary, cerebral, visceral and peripheral edema, each with its own consequences.

INCIDENCE

Acute renal failure needing dialysis has been reported to occur in 1–5% of cardiac surgical patients.[81] A report from Bent and colleagues showed acute renal failure needing renal replacement therapy to have occurred in 2.1% of more than 3000 patients undergoing cardiac surgery in a 5-year period (the majority having coronary surgery).[82] A recent multicenter prospective study of 2222 patients, who did not have preoperative renal failure or dysfunction, undergoing coronary surgery (with or without valve surgery) provides good data relevant to contemporary practice. This study showed that 7.7% of patients developed postoperative renal dysfunction – defined as serum creatinine of 177 μmol L^{-1} (2.0 mg dL^{-1}) or more, or an increase of 62 μmol L^{-1} (0.7 mg dL^{-1}) or more over preoperative levels. Eighteen percent of these patients (1.4% of all patients) needed dialysis.[83]

NATURAL HISTORY

Although the majority of patients improve spontaneously, given satisfactory hemodynamic status and attention to fluid, electrolyte and acid–base balance, postoperative renal dysfunction is a dangerous complication of coronary surgery. Sepsis is an ever-present threat, and hemodynamic instability may further complicate dialysis in those requiring renal replacement therapy.

CAUSES AND PREDISPOSING RISK FACTORS

Decreased renal blood flow and reduced glomerular filtration have been demonstrated in patients following cardiopulmonary bypass.[84] Proposed mechanisms include non-physiological renal perfusion, presence of cardiopulmonary bypass-induced inflammatory mediators, microemboli, free haemoglobin, and changes in catecholamine levels. Increasing age, insulin-dependent diabetes, hyperglycemia, serum creatinine levels above normal, congestive cardiac failure and prior coronary surgery were risk factors in the multicenter study of Mangano and colleagues.[83] In this study, the deleterious effects of cardiopulmonary bypass on renal dysfunction were evident. Omission of arterial filtration, hemodynamic instability in the operative and early postoperative period, and prolonged cardiopulmonary bypass time all increased the risk of renal impairment.

AVOIDANCE

Minimizing exposure to cardiopulmonary bypass and avoidance of intraoperative and postoperative hemodynamic instability are currently the only effective measures. Drugs with known nephrotoxicity should be avoided in the perioperative period in those with recognized risk factors. Contrary to widespread belief, the use of dopamine has no proven renal protective effect.[85] Using sensitive biochemical markers, leukodepletion has been shown to have a renal protective effect during non-pulsatile cardiopulmonary bypass.[86] Avoidance of bypass by the use of beating-heart techniques has been shown to give improved creatinine clearance, better micro-albumin:creatinine ratio and improved renal tubular function in a randomized evaluation of coronary surgery with or without cardiopulmonary bypass.[87]

MANAGEMENT

Every effort should be made to optimize fluid balance and hemodynamic state at the first suspicion of renal dysfunction. Assessment of indirect left atrial pressure, cardiac output and systemic vascular resistance makes rational intervention possible. Potassium administration should be avoided, and dangerous elevations of serum potassium level should be treated with intravenous glucose–insulin infusion. Failure of more conservative methods requires renal replacement therapy until recovery of renal function occurs. Intermittent hemodialysis in the cardiac surgical patient is often plagued by hemodynamic instability; methods for continuous renal replacement therapy have been developed, and continuous veno-venous hemofiltration currently appears to be the best technique.[82]

OUTCOME

The multicenter study reported by Mangano *et al.*[83] showed a 0.9% mortality for those not developing renal dysfunction, 19% mortality for those who did develop renal dysfunction, but not needing dialysis, and 63% mortality for those who were dialysed. Increased hospital stay and increased costs are inevitable when renal dysfunction requiring dialysis occurs.

Pre-existing renal dysfunction increases the risk of coronary surgery. The Northern New England Cardiovascular Disease Study Group reported 279 dialysis-dependent renal failure patients having coronary surgery. They were more than four times more likely to die (hospital mortality 12.2% vs 3.0% for other coronary patients) and had increased risk of mediastinitis and stroke.[88] In the UK, crude mortality for 1996–1999 for coronary surgery in those with no pre-existing renal disease was 2.3%; for those with elevated creatinine, 7.6%; and for those on renal dialysis, 10.8%.[17]

Abdominal complications

CLINICAL FEATURES

Abdominal complications include gastroduodenal inflammation, ulceration, bleeding or perforation, cholecystitis, pancreatitis, liver dysfunction, paralytic ileus and intestinal ischemia or infarction. These complications may be manifest as hematemesis, abdominal distension and tenderness, frequently occurring in the setting of a generally complicated recovery with hemodynamic instability or signs of multi-organ failure. Recognition of such complications is often delayed for many days into the postoperative course. Elevated serum amylase suggests pancreatitis; high lactate levels occur with necrotic bowel. Plain abdominal x-ray may show intraperitoneal gas if bowel perforation has occurred.

INCIDENCE

An incidence of 0.3–3.0% has been reported.[89] A report of outcome of more than 4000 cardiac surgical patients,[90] in which the overall incidence of abdominal complications was 1.4%, showed an incidence of 1.06% for coronary surgery, and is typical of a number of reports over the past decade. More than a third of the complications were paralytic ileus.

NATURAL HISTORY

The general status of the patient has a strong influence on the clinical course. Paralytic ileus usually resolves spontaneously. Upper gastrointestinal bleeding may be mild and self-terminating, but may be lethal if blood loss continues unabated. If abdominal complications occur in the setting of multi-organ failure, a fatal outcome is common. Ischemic bowel is often complicated by perforation, peritonitis and death.

CAUSES AND PREDISPOSING RISK FACTORS

Advanced age, heart failure and prolonged cardiopulmonary bypass time are among the commoner risk factors.[91–93] Poor perfusion of the abdominal viscera during cardiopulmonary bypass and loss of pulsatile flow are usually implicated. Atheroembolism (from the proximal aorta) and thromboembolism (resulting from atrial fibrillation) are other causative factors. Pre-existing atheroma in the celiac and mesenteric arteries may accentuate the hypoperfusion of cardiopulmonary bypass.

AVOIDANCE

Antacid and H2 receptor blockers are advised if there is a recent history of peptic ulcer or reflux esophagitis, but routine use is not recommended.[94] If severe abdominal aortic disease is suspected, the use of cardiopulmonary bypass should be avoided, if possible, by using a beating-heart technique.

MANAGEMENT

Paralytic ileus is managed with nasogastric suction and intravenous fluid maintenance. If bowel ischemia or perforation is suspected, laparotomy should not be delayed. Resection of infarcted or perforated bowel carries a high mortality in this setting, but is the only hope of survival. Upper gastrointestinal bleeding can usually be managed by local control at endoscopy. Acute cholecystitis may settle with conservative management, but cholecystectomy may be required if resolution is not prompt.

OUTCOME

Outcome depends on the cause and its severity. Milder manifestations such as gastritis or paralytic ileus have a good outlook. The most dangerous complication is intestinal ischemia, for which high mortality is reported.[89,95]

Peripheral nerve complications

BRACHIAL PLEXUS INJURY

Clinical features and recognition
The most vulnerable peripheral nerves during coronary surgery are those of the brachial plexus. A spectrum of symptoms occurs, from minor changes in sensation to loss of movement due to paralysis of muscle groups. There may be predominant upper or lower plexus injury, and even Horner's syndrome.[96] Lower trunk injuries are commonest, with a C8-T1 distribution.[97,98]

Incidence
Brachial plexus injuries following median sternotomy have been variously reported as occurring in 1.4% to as many as 38% of patients.[96,99,100] Using intraoperative somatosensory monitoring in a study of coronary surgery patients, electrophysiological changes were found to be common during surgery (70%), though most resolved by the end of operation.[101]

Natural history
Some degree of injury to the brachial plexus is common, but usually not clinically evident. Spontaneous resolution is the usual outcome. The extent and degree of injury are likely to dictate the speed and completeness of recovery.

Causes and predisposing risk factors
A number of mechanisms have been proposed, including traction and compression of the brachial plexus, positioning of the arms and head, fracture of first rib, and central venous cannulation.[96,101] Spreading of the sternal retractor is the major common factor, though the literature is inconsistent about the influence of the extent of spreading or the positioning of the retractor.[96] Previous neuropathies, wide sternal spreading and long operation times have been considered to be predisposing factors.[102] Asymmetrical opening of the chest, particularly as

required for internal thoracic artery mobilization, has been implicated as an important risk factor.[100]

Avoidance
Despite some inconsistencies in the literature, there is considerable agreement that the degree of sternal opening should be kept to a minimum, that time of retraction should be as short as possible, that placement of the retractor towards the caudal (epigastric) end of the incision (rather than towards the cranial or head end) is preferable, and that asymmetrical retraction (necessary for internal thoracic artery harvesting) should be as brief and limited as possible.[100] Somatosensory evoked potential monitoring during surgery has been used to assess the propensity of different types of asymmetric sternal retractors to cause impairment of brachial plexus function.[103] This study has suggested that a retractor design that simultaneously pushes down on the non-operative side whilst pushing the operative side up causes less brachial plexus functional impairment than designs that only lift the operative side of the sternotomy incision.

Management
Most patients require little specific management. Physiotherapy may have a role. Specialized advice should be sought when it is apparent that spontaneous recovery is not occurring.

Outcome
Rapid recovery is usual, and most patients show spontaneous recovery within 4 months.[96] However, persistent symptoms may be a problem.[100]

ULNAR NERVE INJURY

Postoperative ulnar nerve injury has long been described following different types of surgery, and has been shown to be common after cardiac surgery.[104] It has been thought to be due to nerve compression at the elbow, though the role of padding at the elbow and the most advisable position for the forearm during surgery are unclear.

Ulnar neuropathy after coronary surgery may be difficult to distinguish clinically from brachial plexus injury. Nerve conduction studies may be required to locate the site of injury. Pre-existing neuropathy of a minor degree may well be a predisposing factor, and minor ulnar nerve injury may be exacerbated by minor injury to the brachial plexus.[105] Injury may not be apparent for several days postoperatively. Sensory loss on the ulnar side of the hand and forearm and weakness of the small muscles of the hand are the clinical manifestations. Spontaneous recovery is usual.[106–108]

OTHER PERIPHERAL NERVES

The saphenous nerve is vulnerable to injury when harvesting the saphenous vein, and the superficial branch of the radial nerve is similarly vulnerable during radial artery harvesting. Loss of sensation in the territory of the nerve results from injury, and may not recover if the nerve has been divided.

Wound infection

Wound infections are not specific to coronary surgery, although cardiopulmonary bypass, with its immunode-pressant effect, together with the prolonged time needed for most operations and the extensive exposure of tissues during operation make the coronary surgical patient a vulnerable target for infection. Diabetes, particularly if poorly controlled, and peripheral vascular disease are important risk factors. Preoperative skin preparation, careful aseptic surgical technique and avoidance of tissue devitalization from electrocautery, hematoma, under-mining of skin edges and crushing of skin with inappropriate instruments are all important in reducing the risk of wound infection.

The donor sites for saphenous vein conduit are the most common to suffer infective complications. Minimally invasive techniques of vein harvesting have been shown to reduce the risk of infection.[109] Management of the infected saphenous vein donor sites may require local dressings, antibiotics or even skin grafts and tissue flaps. The sternotomy wound is less at risk. Radial artery donor sites are relatively free from infective complications.

Deep sternal wound infection

CLINICAL FEATURES

Systemic signs of infection (fever, leukocytosis, raised C-reactive protein level), together with local symptoms and signs of infection or sternal instability, and pericardial or pleural effusion are the main features suggesting the diagnosis. Presentation is usually within the first 2–4 weeks following surgery, often after hospital discharge, and for as long as 2–3 months postoperatively.[110] The Center for Disease Control and Prevention has published diagnostic criteria for deep sternal wound infection.[111] Chest x-ray and CT scanning are helpful in identifying sternal changes and fluid collections.[112]

INCIDENCE

Though a range from 0.15% to 5% has been reported, an incidence of 0.75–2.5% of cardiac operations seems representative of most recently reported practice.[113–118] The Northern New England Cardiovascular Disease Study Group has provided a risk estimation for mediastinitis from 0.4% to more than 6.5%, dependent on patient characteristics and urgency of surgery.[16]

NATURAL HISTORY

Early and milder mediastinal infection may respond to appropriate antibiotic treatment alone. By the time the diagnosis becomes apparent, there is often spreading mediastinal and sternal infection, with recurrent sinuses and purulent discharge, which, if inadequately managed, may last for years. Sternal separation is common, with ventilatory compromise. Often there is total breakdown of the wound with exposure of the heart. Secondary bleeding from graft anastomoses may be fatal. Septicemia and death from overwhelming sepsis is a possible outcome, particularly if drainage of infection is delayed.

CAUSES AND PREDISPOSING RISK FACTORS

Devascularization of the sternum as a result of internal thoracic artery mobilization (particularly if bilateral), excessive use of electrocautery or bone wax, insecure sternal closure and poor aseptic technique are likely predisposing factors in surgical technique. Diabetes, obesity, advanced age, chronic obstructive airways disease, heart failure, renal failure, peripheral vascular disease, prolonged surgery, excessive blood transfusion and re-operation or re-opening of the chest for bleeding have all been identified as possible risk factors.

AVOIDANCE

Correct surgical technique should minimize factors likely to risk sternal devascularization or bacterial contamination. Preoperative skin preparation, careful aseptic technique in the operating room,[114] use of prophylactic antibiotics (usually a cephalosporin) for the first 48–72 hours, commencing at the start of operation before skin incision, and secure sternal closure are important measures for the avoidance of this complication.[16,112,114] Careful control of hyperglycemia in diabetic patients has been shown to lower their risk of mediastinitis.[10] Prompt management of the complication may reduce the risk of a fatal or protracted course.

MANAGEMENT

Appropriate antibiotic administration, based on culture and sensitivity of the identified organism – commonly a *Staphylococcus aureus* or *epidermidis* – (from culture of wound exudate, CT-guided needle aspiration, sinus discharge or blood culture), is implemented immediately the diagnosis is suspected. Re-opening of the wound for debridement of infected material and sternal rewiring with prolonged local irrigation via mediastinal drainage tubes is successful in milder cases. For more extensive infection, the sternum is left open to allow better irrigation.[116] Gradual healing and stabilization of the sternum by fibrous union will occur in most cases, and transfer of omentum, rectus abdominis or pectoral flaps when infection is under control will hasten healing.[112,119–121] A single-stage debridement and closure with either pectoralis musculo-cutaneous flaps[122] or a latissimus dorsi musculo-cutaneous flap, leaving the sternum to unite secondarily, has also been described as having good results.[123]

OUTCOME

Mortality rates of 7% to 70% have been reported, though recent series with current management strategies have shown rates below 10%.[110,116,117] The Northern New England Cardiovascular Disease Study Group has shown a 1-year mortality of 22% for patients with mediastinitis, compared to a 5% mortality for coronary surgery patients not developing this complication.[116] The long-term cosmetic result is not ideal, particularly if a muscle flap procedure is required. Healing is a prolonged process, even with the best of management in a reasonably fit patient. Sepsis may be overwhelming and fatal, particularly in the elderly, obese and diabetic patient.

Sternal dehiscence

Separation of the sternum, in the absence of infection, is most commonly seen in overweight patients, particularly when poor respiratory function increases the work of breathing and the stresses on the sternum. Patients with advanced osteoporosis are also at increased risk of sternal dehiscence. Unequal division of the sternum is a potent risk factor, and inadequate technique of sternal closure is a further risk factor. Pain, particularly when lying on the side, and awareness of instability or clicking of the anterior chest wall are features.

Keeping sternal separation to a minimum and avoiding extension into the epigastrium will reduce the likelihood and the consequences of sternal dehiscence. Such measures are consistent with safe coronary surgery[124] and have benefits in terms of cosmetic results and postoperative pain.

Thick (7 gauge) stainless steel wires passed around the sternum or sternal bands which encircle the sternum provide secure closure by spreading pressure over a wider area and by including sternal cortical bone within the closure. Fine wire has a 'cheese-wire' effect, and anchorage through the sternum is more likely to be insecure than closure methods that encircle the sternum.[125–127]

Sternal dehiscence of a minor nature will usually fuse by fibrous union. More severe forms that cause pain and distress should be re-closed under careful aseptic conditions.

General complications of surgery

Cardiac surgical patients are not immune to the complications that may follow most major procedures. The effects of alcohol withdrawal, psychiatric disturbance, musculo-skeletal injury, pressure point ulceration, venous thrombosis,[128] urinary tract infection and drug sensitivity are some of the unwanted accompaniments that may delay a satisfactory outcome of coronary surgery.

Iatrogenic injury

The surgical treatment of coronary disease is complex and involves many individuals of differing disciplines. It requires correct interpretation of clinical information and cardiological investigations, as well as competent technical interventions for monitoring, anesthesia and drug administration, and the surgical procedure itself gives considerable scope for life-threatening injury. Errors or accidental injuries are therefore not surprising. Examples are injury during cannulation for invasive monitoring, endotracheal intubation and urethral catheterization, injury to intrathoracic structures (heart and major vessels, previously placed grafts), cardiopulmonary bypass accidents (inadequate perfusion, selective perfusion of aortic arch vessels, air embolism, thromboembolism, atheroembolism, aortic wall injury), retained foreign material, failure to give necessary drugs (e.g. heparin), inappropriate drug administration, and anaphylactic reactions. Keeping such mishaps to a minimum requires training and the development of skills, adherence to protocols, audit of outcomes, and regular review of practice.[129]

KEY REFERENCES

Carthey J, De Leval MR, Reason JT. The human factor in cardiac surgery: errors and near misses in a high technology medical domain. *Ann Thorac Surg* 2001; **72**:300–5.

This report offers a helpful and new insight into a systematic approach to the human factors that may impact on the safe conduct of cardiac surgery, drawing on lessons from similar high-risk fields of human endeavor such as the airline industry. Patient safety and the avoidance of complications play a major part in the delivery of coronary surgical care.

Jones RH, Hannan EL, Hammermeister KE, Delong ER, O'Connor GT, Luepker RV, *et al.* Identification of preoperative variables needed for risk adjustment of short-term mortality after coronary artery bypass graft surgery. The Working Group Panel on the Cooperative CABG Database Project. [Review – 35 refs.] *J Am Coll Cardiol* 1996; **28**:1478–87.

This report shows the predictive value of seven core clinical variables and describes the relative contribution of these and other variables in predicting death after coronary surgery, using data from seven different databases.

Losanoff JE, Richman BW, Jones JW. Disruption and infection of median sternotomy: a comprehensive review. *Eur J Cardiothorac Surg* 2002; **21**:831–9.

Problems with the sternotomy wound are indisputably the responsibility of the surgeon and may affect any patient. This review of a persistent problem describes current methods for the prevention and treatment of disrupted and infected sternal wounds.

Maisel WH, Rawn JD, Stevenson WG. Atrial fibrillation after cardiac surgery. [Review – 104 refs.] *Ann Intern Med* 2001; **135**:1061–73.

A comprehensive review of mechanisms and methods for the prevention and treatment of one of the commonest problems following coronary surgery.

Newman MF, Kirchner JL, Phillips-Bute B, Gaver V, Grocott H, Jones RH, *et al*. Longitudinal assessment of neurocognitive function after coronary artery bypass surgery. *N Engl J Med* 2001; **344**:395–402.

This report, from an authoritative group, draws attention to the magnitude of the problem of subtle injury to the brain, which may have effects many years after coronary surgery. The mechanisms of neurocognitive decline are still unclear; cardiopulmonary bypass is implicated and off-pump techniques may show improved outcomes. This will remain an area of research for many years to come.

REFERENCES

1. Mangano DT. Cardiovascular morbidity and CABG surgery – a perspective: epidemiology, costs, and potential therapeutic solutions. *J Card Surg* 1995; 10(Suppl.):366–8.
2. Cameron A, Davis KB, Green G, Schaff HV. Coronary bypass surgery with internal-thoracic-artery grafts – effects on survival over a 15-year period. *N Engl J Med* 1996; 334:216–19.
3. Leavitt BJ, O'Connor GT, Olmstead EM, Morton JR, Maloney CT, Dacey LJ, *et al*. Use of the internal mammary artery graft and in-hospital mortality and other adverse outcomes associated with coronary artery bypass surgery. *Circulation* 2001; 103:507–12.
4. Hart JC, Puskas JD, Sabik JF III. Off-pump coronary revascularization: current state of the art. [Review – 50 refs.] *Semin Thorac Cardiovasc Surg* 2002; 14:70–81.
5. Magee MJ, Jablonski KA, Stamou SC, Pfister AJ, Dewey TM, Dullum MK, *et al*. Elimination of cardiopulmonary bypass improves early survival for multivessel coronary artery bypass patients. *Ann Thorac Surg* 2002; 73:1196–202.
6. Pepper J. Severe morbidity after coronary artery surgery. [Review – 33 refs.] *Curr Opin Cardiol* 2000; 15:400–5.
7. Wheatley DJ, Taggart D. Surgery. In: *Geriatric Cardiology, Principles and Practice*, Martin A, Camm AJ (eds). London: John Wiley and Sons Ltd, 1994; 623–47.
8. Ferguson JJ III, Cohen M, Freedman RJ Jr, Stone GW, Miller MF, Joseph DL, *et al*. The current practice of intra-aortic balloon counterpulsation: results from the Benchmark Registry. *J Am Coll Cardiol* 2001; 38:1456–62.
9. Zerr KJ, Furnary AP, Grunkemeier GL, Bookin S, Kanhere V, Starr A. Glucose control lowers the risk of wound infection in diabetics after open heart operations. *Ann Thorac Surg* 1997; 63:356–61.
10. Furnary AP, Zerr KJ, Grunkemeier GL, Starr A. Continuous intravenous insulin infusion reduces the incidence of deep sternal wound infection in diabetic patients after cardiac surgical procedures. *Ann Thorac Surg* 1999; 67:352–60.
11. Munoz JJ, Birkmeyer NJ, Dacey LJ, Birkmeyer JD, Charlesworth DC, Johnson ER, *et al*. Trends in rates of reexploration for hemorrhage after coronary artery bypass surgery. Northern New England Cardiovascular Disease Study Group. *Ann Thorac Surg* 1999; 68:1321–5.
12. Jones RH, Hannan EL, Hammermeister KE, Delong ER, O'Connor GT, Luepker RV, *et al*. Identification of preoperative variables needed for risk adjustment of short-term mortality after coronary artery bypass graft surgery. The Working Group Panel on the Cooperative CABG Database Project. [Review – 35 refs.] *J Am Coll Cardiol* 1996; 28:1478–87.
13. Nashef SA, Roques F, Michel P, Gauducheau E, Lemeshow S, Salamon R. European system for cardiac operative risk evaluation (EuroSCORE). *Eur J Cardiothorac Surg* 1999; 16:9–13.
14. Baretti RP. Risk stratification scores for predicting mortality in coronary artery bypass surgery. *Thorac Cardiovasc Surg* 2002; 50:237–46.
15. Chassin MR, Hannan EL, DeBuono BA. Benefits and hazards of reporting medical outcomes publicly. *N Engl J Med* 1996; 334:394–8.
16. Eagle KA, Guyton RA, Davidoff R, Ewy GA, Fonger J, Gardner TJ, *et al*. ACC/AHA Guidelines for Coronary Artery Bypass Graft Surgery: A Report of the American College of Cardiology/American Heart Association Task Force on Practice Guidelines (Committee to Revise the 1991 Guidelines for Coronary Artery Bypass Graft Surgery). American College of Cardiology/American Heart Association. [Review – 753 refs.] *J Am Coll Cardiol* 1999; 34:1262–347.
17. Keogh BE, Kinsman R. National Adult Cardiac Surgical Database Report 1999–2000. Reading: Dendrite Clinical Systems Ltd, 2001.
18. Yau TM, Fedak PW, Weisel RD, Teng C, Ivanov J. Predictors of operative risk for coronary bypass operations in patients with left ventricular dysfunction. *J Thorac Cardiovasc Surg* 1999; 118:1006–13.
19. Bonchek LI. How should we manage suspected perioperative infarction after coronary bypass surgery? *Am J Cardiol* 2001; 87:761–2.
20. Rasmussen C, Thiis JJ, Clemmensen P, Efsen F, Arendrup HC, Saunamaki K, *et al*. Significance and management of early graft failure after coronary artery bypass grafting: feasibility and results of acute angiography and re-re-vascularization. *Eur J Cardiothorac Surg* 1997; 12:847–52.
21. Tuman KJ. Perioperative myocardial infarction. *Semin Thorac Cardiovasc Surg* 1991; 3:47–52.
22. Force T, Hibberd P, Weeks G, Kemper AJ, Bloomfield P, Tow D, *et al*. Perioperative myocardial infarction after coronary artery bypass surgery. Clinical significance and approach to risk stratification. *Circulation* 1990; 82:903–12.
23. Greaves SC, Rutherford JD, Aranki SF, Cohn LH, Couper GS, Adams DH, *et al*. Current incidence and determinants of perioperative myocardial infarction in coronary artery surgery. *Am Heart J* 1996; 132:572–8.
24. Steuer J, Horte LG, Lindahl B, Stahle E. Impact of perioperative myocardial injury on early and long-term outcome after coronary artery bypass grafting. *Eur Heart J* 2002; 23:1219–27.
25. Willems S, Weiss C, Meinertz T. Tachyarrhythmias following coronary artery bypass graft surgery: epidemiology, mechanisms,

and current therapeutic strategies. [Review – 46 refs.] *Thorac Cardiovasc Surg* 1997; **45**:232–7.

26. Maisel WH, Rawn JD, Stevenson WG. Atrial fibrillation after cardiac surgery. [Review – 104 refs.] *Ann Intern Med* 2001; **135**:1061–73.

27. Hogue CW Jr, Hyder ML. Atrial fibrillation after cardiac operation: risks, mechanisms, and treatment. [Review – 94 refs.] *Ann Thorac Surg* 2000; **69**:300–6.

28. Mueller XM, Tevaearai HT, Ruchat P, Stumpe F, von Segesser LK. Did the introduction of a minimally invasive technique change the incidence of atrial fibrillation after single internal thoracic artery–left anterior descending artery grafting? *J Thorac Cardiovasc Surg* 2001; **121**:683–8.

29. Ascione R, Caputo M, Calori G, Lloyd CT, Underwood MJ, Angelini GD. Predictors of atrial fibrillation after conventional and beating heart coronary surgery: a prospective, randomized study. *Circulation* 2000; **102**:1530–5.

30. Andrews TC, Reimold SC, Berlin JA, Antman EM. Prevention of supraventricular arrhythmias after coronary artery bypass surgery. A meta-analysis of randomized control trials. *Circulation* 1991; **84**(Suppl.):III236–44.

31. Wistbacka JO, Koistinen J, Karlqvist KE, Lepojarvi MV, Hanhela R, Laurila J, *et al*. Magnesium substitution in elective coronary artery surgery: a double-blind clinical study. *J Cardiothorac Vasc Anesth* 1995; **9**:140–6.

32. Kirklin JK, Westaby S, Blackstone EH, Kirklin JW, Chenoweth DE, Pacifico AD. Complement and the damaging effects of cardiopulmonary bypass. *J Thorac Cardiovasc Surg* 1983; **86**:845–57.

33. Wan S, LeClerc JL, Vincent JL. Inflammatory response to cardiopulmonary bypass: mechanisms involved and possible therapeutic strategies. *Chest* 1997; **112**:676–92.

34. Edmunds LH Jr. Inflammatory response to cardiopulmonary bypass. *Ann Thorac Surg* 1998; **66**(Suppl.):S12–16.

35. Ascione R, Lloyd CT, Underwood MJ, Lotto AA, Pitsis AA, Angelini GD. Inflammatory response after coronary revascularization with or without cardiopulmonary bypass. *Ann Thorac Surg* 2000; **69**:1198–204.

36. Taggart DP. Respiratory dysfunction after cardiac surgery: effects of avoiding cardiopulmonary bypass and the use of bilateral internal mammary arteries. *Eur J Cardiothorac Surg* 2000; **18**:31–7.

37. Graves EJ. National hospital discharge survey: annual summary, 1991. *Vital Health Stat* 1993; **13**:1–62.

38. McGill N, O'Shaughnessy D, Pickering R, Herbertson M, Gill R. Mechanical methods of reducing blood transfusion in cardiac surgery: randomised controlled trial. *BMJ* 2002; **324**:1299.

39. Thurer RL. Blood transfusion in cardiac surgery. *Can J Anaesth* 2001; **48**(Suppl.):S6–12.

40. Sellman M, Intonti MA, Ivert T. Reoperations for bleeding after coronary artery bypass procedures during 25 years. *Eur J Cardiothorac Surg* 1997; **11**:521–7.

41. Despotis GJ, Avidan MS, Hogue CW Jr. Mechanisms and attenuation of hemostatic activation during extracorporeal circulation. *Ann Thorac Surg* 2001; **72**:S1821–31.

42. Hardy JF. Pharmacological strategies for blood conservation in cardiac surgery: erythropoietin and antifibrinolytics. *Can J Anaesth* 2001; **48**(Suppl.):S24–31.

43. Hardy JF, Belisle S, Dupont C, Harel F, Robitaille D, Roy M, *et al*. Prophylactic tranexamic acid and epsilon-aminocaproic acid for primary myocardial revascularization. *Ann Thorac Surg* 1998; **65**:371–6.

44. Lambert W, Brisebois FJ, Wharton TJ, Carrier RC, Boyle D, Rowe BH. The effectiveness of low dose tranexamic acid in primary cardiac surgery. *Can J Anaesth* 1998; **45**:571–4.

45. Ray MJ, O'Brien MF. Comparison of epsilon aminocaproic acid and low-dose aprotinin in cardiopulmonary bypass: efficiency, safety and cost. *Ann Thorac Surg* 2001; **71**:838–43.

46. Santamaria A, Mateo J, Oliver A, Litvan H, Murillo J, Souto JC, *et al*. The effect of two different doses of aprotinin on hemostasis in cardiopulmonary bypass surgery: similar transfusion requirements and blood loss. *Haematologica* 2000; **85**:1277–84.

47. Cross MH. Autotransfusion in cardiac surgery. *Perfusion* 2001; **16**:391–400.

48. Eichert I, Isgro F, Kiessling AH, Saggau W. Cell saver, ultrafiltration and direct transfusion: comparative study of three blood processing techniques. *Thorac Cardiovasc Surg* 2001; **49**:149–52.

49. Ruel MA, Rubens FD. Non-pharmacological strategies for blood conservation in cardiac surgery. *Can J Anaesth* 2001; **48**(Suppl.):S13–23.

50. Bonatti J, Ladurner R, Antretter H, Hormann C, Friedrich G, Moes N, *et al*. Single coronary artery bypass grafting – a comparison between minimally invasive 'off pump' techniques and conventional procedures. *Eur J Cardiothorac Surg* 1998; **14**(Suppl. 1):S7–12.

51. Puskas JD, Wright CE, Ronson RS, Brown WM III, Gott JP, Guyton RA. Off-pump multivessel coronary bypass via sternotomy is safe and effective. *Ann Thorac Surg* 1998; **66**:1068–72.

52. Nader ND, Khadra WZ, Reich NT, Bacon DR, Salerno TA, Panos AL. Blood product use in cardiac revascularization: comparison of on- and off-pump techniques. *Ann Thorac Surg* 1999; **68**:1640–3.

53. Abu-Omar Y, Taggart DP. Off-pump coronary artery bypass grafting. [Review – 31 refs.] *Lancet* 2002; **360**:327–30.

54. Hall TS, Brevetti GR, Skoultchi AJ, Sines JC, Gregory P, Spotnitz AJ. Re-exploration for hemorrhage following open heart surgery differentiation on the causes of bleeding and the impact on patient outcomes. *Ann Thorac Surg* 2001; **7**:352–7.

55. Roach GW, Kanchuger M, Mangano CM, Newman M, Nussmeier N, Wolman R, *et al*. Adverse cerebral outcomes after coronary bypass surgery. Multicenter Study of Perioperative Ischemia Research Group and the Ischemia Research and Education Foundation Investigators. *N Engl J Med* 1996; **335**:1857–63.

56. Newman MF, Kirchner JL, Phillips-Bute B, Gaver V, Grocott H, Jones RH, *et al*. Longitudinal assessment of neurocognitive function after coronary artery bypass surgery. *N Engl J Med* 2001; **344**:395–402.

57. Diegeler A, Hirsch R, Schneider F, Schilling LO, Falk V, Rauch T, *et al*. Neuromonitoring and neurocognitive outcome in off-pump versus conventional coronary bypass operation. *Ann Thorac Surg* 2000; **69**:1162–6.

58. Hogue CW Jr, Sundt T III, Barzilai B, Schechtman KB, Davila-Roman VG. Cardiac and neurologic complications identify risks for mortality for both men and women undergoing coronary artery bypass graft surgery. *Anesthesiology* 2001; **95**:1074–8.

59. Stamou SC, Hill PC, Dangas G, Pfister AJ, Boyce SW, Dullum MKC, *et al*. Stroke after coronary artery bypass: incidence, predictors, and clinical outcome. *Stroke* 2001; **32**:1508–12.

6_. _____ ognitive disorders after _____ *Cardiol* 2001; **16**:271–6.

6_ _____ | C, Vos LJ, _____ r coronary artery bypass _____ refs.]

6_. _____ NB, Boylan M, _____ the ascending aorta. _____ *Thorac Cardiovasc Surg*

6_. _____ e DT. Is cardiopulmonary bypass still the cause of cognitive dysfunction after cardiac operations? *J Thorac Cardiovasc Surg* 1999; **118**:414–20.

64. Blauth CI, Arnold JV, Schulenberg WE, McCartney AC, Taylor KM. Cerebral microembolism during cardiopulmonary bypass. Retinal microvascular studies in vivo with fluorescein angiography. *J Thorac Cardiovasc Surg* 1988; **95**:668–76.

65. Kouchoukos NT, Wareing TH, Daily BB, Murphy SF. Management of the severely atherosclerotic aorta during cardiac operations. *J Card Surg* 1994; **9**:490–4.

66. Reichenspurner H, Navia JA, Berry G, Robbins RC, Barbut D, Gold JP, *et al.* Particulate emboli capture by an intra-aortic filter device during cardiac surgery. *J Thorac Cardiovasc Surg* 2000; **119**: 233–41.

67. Nussmeier NA. A review of risk factors for adverse neurologic outcome after cardiac surgery. *J Extra Corpor Technol* 2002; **34**:4–10.

68. Mark DB, Newman MF. Protecting the brain in coronary artery bypass graft surgery. *JAMA* 2002; **287**:1448–50.

69. Gaudino M, Martinelli L, Di Lella G, Glieca F, Marano P, Schiavello R, *et al.* Superior extension of intraoperative brain damage in case of normothermic systemic perfusion during coronary artery bypass operations. *J Thorac Cardiovasc Surg* 1999; **118**:432–7.

70. Engelman RM, Pleet AB, Hicks R, Rousou JA, Flack JE III, Deaton DW, *et al.* Is there a relationship between systemic perfusion temperature during coronary artery bypass grafting and extent of intraoperative ischemic central nervous system injury? *J Thorac Cardiovasc Surg* 2000; **119**:230–2.

71. Patel NC, Deodhar AP, Grayson AD, Pullan DM, Keenan DJ, Hasan R, *et al.* Neurological outcomes in coronary surgery: independent effect of avoiding cardiopulmonary bypass. *Ann Thorac Surg* 2002; **74**:400–5.

72. Stamou SC, Jablonski KA, Pfister AJ, Hill PC, Dullum MK, Bafi AS, *et al.* Stroke after conventional versus minimally invasive coronary artery bypass. *Ann Thorac Surg* 2002; **74**:394–9.

73. Lloyd CT, Ascione R, Underwood MJ, Gardner F, Black A, Angelini GD. Serum S-100 protein release and neuropsychologic outcome during coronary revascularization on the beating heart: a prospective randomized study. *J Thorac Cardiovasc Surg* 2000; **119**:148–54.

74. Puskas JD, Winston AD, Wright CE, Gott JP, Brown WM III, Craver JM, *et al.* Stroke after coronary artery operation: incidence, correlates, outcome, and cost. *Ann Thorac Surg* 2000; **69**:1053–6.

75. Taggart DP, el Fiky M, Carter R, Bowman A, Wheatley DJ. Respiratory dysfunction after uncomplicated cardiopulmonary bypass. *Ann Thorac Surg* 1993; **56**:1123–8.

76. Asimakopoulos G, Smith PL, Ratnatunga CP, Taylor KM. Lung injury and acute respiratory distress syndrome after cardiopulmonary bypass. *Ann Thorac Surg* 1999; **68**:1107–15.

77. Ng CS, Wan S, Yim AP, Arifi AA. Pulmonary dysfunction after cardiac surgery. *Chest* 2002; **121**:1269–77.

78. Van Dijk D, Nierich AP, Jansen EW, Nathoe HM, Suyker WJ, Diephuis JC, *et al.* Early outcome after off-pump versus on-pump coronary bypass surgery: results from a randomized study. *Circulation* 2001; **104**:1761–6.

79. Angelini GD, Taylor FC, Reeves BC, Ascione R. Early and midterm outcome after off-pump and on-pump surgery in Beating Heart Against Cardioplegic Arrest Studies (BHACAS 1 and 2): a pooled analysis of two randomised controlled trials. *Lancet* 2002; **359**:1194–9.

80. Mortelliti MP, Manning HL. Acute respiratory distress syndrome. *Am Fam Physician* 2002; **65**:1823–30.

81. Fortescue EB, Bates DW, Chertow GM. Predicting acute renal failure after coronary bypass surgery: cross-validation of two risk-stratification algorithms. *Kidney Int* 2000; **57**:2594–602.

82. Bent P, Tan HK, Bellomo R, Buckmaster J, Doolan L, Hart G, *et al.* Early and intensive continuous hemofiltration for severe renal failure after cardiac surgery. *Ann Thorac Surg* 2001; **71**:832–7.

83. Mangano CM, Diamondstone LS, Ramsay JG, Aggarwal A, Herskowitz A, Mangano DT. Renal dysfunction after myocardial revascularization: risk factors, adverse outcomes, and hospital resource utilization. The Multicenter Study of Perioperative Ischemia Research Group. *Ann Intern Med* 1998; **128**:194–203.

84. Mazzarella V, Gallucci MT, Tozzo C, Elli M, Chiavarelli R, Marino B, *et al.* Renal function in patients undergoing cardiopulmonary bypass operations. *J Thorac Cardiovasc Surg* 1992; **104**:1625–7.

85. Tang AT, El Gamel A, Keevil B, Yonan N, Deiraniya AK. The effect of 'renal-dose' dopamine on renal tubular function following cardiac surgery: assessed by measuring retinol binding protein (RBP). *Eur J Cardiothorac Surg* 1999; **15**:717–21.

86. Tang AT, Alexiou C, Hsu J, Sheppard SV, Haw MP, Ohri SK. Leukodepletion reduces renal injury in coronary revascularization: a prospective randomized study. *Ann Thorac Surg* 2002; **74**:372–7.

87. Ascione R, Lloyd CT, Underwood MJ, Gomes WJ, Angelini GD. On-pump versus off-pump coronary revascularization: evaluation of renal function. *Ann Thorac Surg* 1999; **68**:493–8.

88. Liu JY, Birkmeyer NJ, Sanders JH, Morton JR, Henriques HF, Lahey SJ, *et al.* Risks of morbidity and mortality in dialysis patients undergoing coronary artery bypass surgery. Northern New England Cardiovascular Disease Study Group. *Circulation* 2000; **102**:2973–7.

89. Zacharias A, Schwann TA, Parenteau GL, Riordan CJ, Durham SJ, Engoren M, *et al.* Predictors of gastrointestinal complications in cardiac surgery. *Tex Heart Inst J* 2000; **27**:93–9.

90. Simic O, Strathausen S, Hess W, Ostermeyer J. Incidence and prognosis of abdominal complications after cardiopulmonary bypass. *Cardiovasc Surg* 1999; **7**:419–24.

91. Byhahn C, Strouhal U, Martens S, Mierdl S, Kessler P, Westphal K. Incidence of gastrointestinal complications in cardiopulmonary bypass patients. *World J Surg* 2001; **25**:1140–4.

92. Christenson JT, Schmuziger M, Maurice J, Simonet F, Velebit V. Gastrointestinal complications after coronary artery bypass grafting. *J Thorac Cardiovasc Surg* 1994; **108**:899–906.

93. Perugini RA, Orr RK, Porter D, Dumas EM, Maini BS. Gastrointestinal complications following cardiac surgery. An analysis of 1477 cardiac surgery patients. *Arch Surg* 1997; **132**:352–7.

94. van der Voort PH, Zandstra DF. Pathogenesis, risk factors, and incidence of upper gastrointestinal bleeding after cardiac surgery: is specific prophylaxis in routine bypass procedures needed? *J Cardiothorac Vasc Anesth* 2000; **14**:293–9.

95. Klempnauer J, Grothues F, Bektas H, Wahlers T. Acute mesenteric ischemia following cardiac surgery. *J Cardiovasc Surg (Torino)* 1997; **38**:639–43.

96. Stangl R, Altendorf-Hofmann A, von der EJ. Brachial plexus lesions following median sternotomy in cardiac surgery. *Thorac Cardiovasc Surg* 1991; **39**:360–4.

97. Tomlinson DL, Hirsch IA, Kodali SV, Slogoff S. Protecting the brachial plexus during median sternotomy. *J Thorac Cardiovasc Surg* 1987; **94**:297–301.

98. Levin KH, Wilbourn AJ, Maggiano HJ. Cervical rib and median sternotomy-related brachial plexopathies: a reassessment. *Neurology* 1998; **50**:1407–13.

99. Stoelting RK. Brachial plexus injury after median sternotomy: an unexpected liability for anesthesiologists. *J Cardiothorac Vasc Anesth* 1994; **8**:2–4.

100. Vahl CF, Carl I, Muller-Vahl H, Struck E. Brachial plexus injury after cardiac surgery. The role of internal mammary artery preparation: a prospective study on 1000 consecutive patients. *J Thorac Cardiovasc Surg* 1991; **102**:724–9.

101. Hickey C, Gugino LD, Aglio LS, Mark JB, Son SL, Maddi R. Intraoperative somatosensory evoked potential monitoring predicts peripheral nerve injury during cardiac surgery. *Anesthesiology* 1993; **78**:29–35.

102. Seyfer AE, Grammer NY, Bogumill GP, Provost JM, Chandry U. Upper extremity neuropathies after cardiac surgery. *J Hand Surg [Am]* 1985; **10**:16–19.

103. Jellish WS, Blakeman B, Warf P, Slogoff S. Somatosensory evoked potential monitoring used to compare the effect of three asymmetric sternal retractors on brachial plexus function. *Anesth Analg* 1999; **88**:292–7.

104. Wey JM, Guinn GA. Ulnar nerve injury with open-heart surgery. *Ann Thorac Surg* 1985; **39**:358–60.

105. Casscells CD, Lindsey RW, Ebersole J, Li B. Ulnar neuropathy after median sternotomy. *Clin Orthop* 1993; **291**:259–65.

106. Alvine FG, Schurrer ME. Postoperative ulnar-nerve palsy. Are there predisposing factors? *J Bone Joint Surg Am* 1987; **69**:255–9.

107. Warner MA, Warner DO, Matsumoto JY, Harper CM, Schroeder DR, Maxson PM. Ulnar neuropathy in surgical patients. *Anesthesiology* 1999; **90**:54–9.

108. Watson BV, Merchant RN, Brown WF. Early postoperative ulnar neuropathies following coronary artery bypass surgery. *Muscle Nerve* 1992; **15**:701–5.

109. Bitondo JM, Daggett WM, Torchiana DF, Akins CW, Hilgenberg AD, Vlahakes GJ, *et al.* Endoscopic versus open saphenous vein harvest: a comparison of postoperative wound complications. *Ann Thorac Surg* 2002; **73**:523–8.

110. Loop FD, Lytle BW, Cosgrove DM, Mahfood S, McHenry MC, Goormastic M, *et al.* J. Maxwell Chamberlain memorial paper. Sternal wound complications after isolated coronary artery bypass grafting: early and late mortality, morbidity, and cost of care. *Ann Thorac Surg* 1990; **49**:179–86.

111. Garner JS, Jarvis WR, Emori TG, Horan TC, Hughes JM. CDC definitions for nosocomial infections, 1988. *Am J Infect Control* 1988; **16**:128–40.

112. Losanoff JE, Richman BW, Jones JW. Disruption and infection of median sternotomy: a comprehensive review. *Eur J Cardiothorac Surg* 2002; **21**:831–9.

113. Risk factors for deep sternal wound infection after sternotomy: a prospective, multicenter study. *J Thorac Cardiovasc Surg* 1996; **111**:1200–7.

114. Baskett RJ, MacDougall CE, Ross DB. Is mediastinitis a preventable complication? A 10-year review. *Ann Thorac Surg* 1999; **67**:462–5.

115. Borger MA, Rao V, Weisel RD, Ivanov J, Cohen G, Scully HE, *et al.* Deep sternal wound infection: risk factors and outcomes. *Ann Thorac Surg* 1998; **65**:1050–6.

116. Braxton JH, Marrin CA, McGrath PD, Ross CS, Morton JR, Norotsky M, *et al.* Mediastinitis and long-term survival after coronary artery bypass graft surgery. *Ann Thorac Surg* 2000; **70**:2004–7.

117. Levi N, Olsen PS. Primary closure of deep sternal wound infection following open heart surgery: a safe operation? *J Cardiovasc Surg (Torino)* 2000; **41**:241–5.

118. De Feo M, Renzulli A, Ismeno G, Gregorio R, Della CA, Utili R, *et al.* Variables predicting adverse outcome in patients with deep sternal wound infection. *Ann Thorac Surg* 2001; **71**:324–31.

119. Francel TJ, Kouchoukos NT. A rational approach to wound difficulties after sternotomy: reconstruction and long-term results. *Ann Thorac Surg* 2001; **72**:1419–29.

120. Francel TJ, Kouchoukos NT. A rational approach to wound difficulties after sternotomy: the problem. *Ann Thorac Surg* 2001; **72**:1411–18.

121. Rand RP, Cochran RP, Aziz S, Hofer BO, Allen MD, Verrier ED, *et al.* Prospective trial of catheter irrigation and muscle flaps for sternal wound infection. *Ann Thorac Surg* 1998; **65**:1046–9.

122. Jeevanandam V, Smith CR, Rose EA, Malm JR, Hugo NE. Single-stage management of sternal wound infections. *J Thorac Cardiovasc Surg* 1990; **99**:256–62.

123. Dejesus RA, Paletta JD, Dabb RW. Reconstruction of the median sternotomy wound dehiscence using the latissimus dorsi myocutaneous flap. *J Cardiovasc Surg (Torino)* 2001; **42**:359–64.

124. Akins CW. Full sternotomy through a minimally invasive incision: a cardiac surgeon's true comfort zone. *Ann Thorac Surg* 1998; **66**:1429–30.

125. Casha AR, Gauci M, Yang L, Saleh M, Kay PH, Cooper GJ. Fatigue testing median sternotomy closures. *Eur J Cardiothorac Surg* 2001; **19**:249–53.

126. McGregor WE, Trumble DR, Magovern JA. Mechanical analysis of midline sternotomy wound closure. *J Thorac Cardiovasc Surg* 1999; **117**:1144–50.

127. Soroff HS, Hartman AR, Pak E, Sasvary DH, Pollak SB. Improved sternal closure using steel bands: early experience with three-year follow-up. *Ann Thorac Surg* 1996; **61**:1172–6.

128. Shammas NW. Pulmonary embolus after coronary artery bypass surgery: a review of the literature. *Clin Cardiol* 2000; **23**:637–44.

129. Carthey J, De Leval MR, Reason JT. The human factor in cardiac surgery: errors and near misses in a high technology medical domain. *Ann Thorac Surg* 2001; **72**:300–5.

16

Conduits for coronary surgery

BRIAN F BUXTON AND JAMES TATOULIS

INTRODUCTION

The choice of graft and surgical technique influence the late patency of a coronary artery bypass graft (CABG) and patient survival. The internal thoracic artery (ITA), radial artery and saphenous vein are the most commonly used conduits. These are employed as *in situ* or free grafts using standard aorta-coronary, Y-graft, sequential anastomotic and graft extension techniques. Early arteriosclerotic changes in vein grafts have encouraged surgeons to adopt extensive arterial or even complete arterial grafting techniques.

The move away from conventional coronary artery bypass to off-pump coronary artery surgery and pump-assisted techniques has reduced the risk of neurological complications. Further reduction of stroke may result from reconstructions that avoid attaching grafts to the aorta. When combined with sequential grafting, these techniques have reduced the need for extensive harvesting of precious conduits by using them more efficiently. At present there are few late postoperative graft patency results using arterial conduits other than the ITA, and there is little validation of the efficacy of complex arterial reconstructions.

Surgeons continue to explore and extend the application of complex reconstructive techniques on the assumption that arterial grafts are superior to saphenous veins. The description of arterial graft harvesting, coronary artery reconstructive techniques and the clinical results form the basis of this chapter.

INTERNAL THORACIC ARTERY

The ITA has been long recognized as a conduit to bypass lesions in the coronary arteries. In 1946, the cut end of the ITA was inserted directly into the myocardium by Vineberg in an attempt to promote a collateral circulation between the systemic and coronary circulations. Demikov described an anastomotic technique between the ITA and the left anterior descending (LAD) artery in the dog in 1952. Human ITA coronary artery bypass grafts were reported by Spencer, Goetz and Longmire,[1–3] and the first series was by George Green.[4] Kolessov, from the then USSR, reported an off-pump technique implanting the right internal thoracic artery (RITA) to the LAD coronary artery.[5]

The durability of the left internal thoracic artery (LITA) when used as a coronary artery bypass graft was recognized by Loop and others in 1986. This led to the widespread application of the LITA and subsequently the RITA as a bypass graft.

Anatomy

The ITA descends vertically from its origin from the subclavian artery about 1 cm lateral to the sternal border behind the first six costal cartilages and intervening intercostal spaces, and terminates behind the sixth costal cartilage as the superior epigastric and musculophrenic branches. The ITA is separated from the pleura by the endothoracic fascia and also by the transversus thoracis muscle and fascia between the third and sixth intercostal spaces. The other named branches are the pericardio-phrenic and anterior intercostal branches. There are also many unnamed branches that supply the upper mediastinum, thyroid muscle, manubrium and pleura. In addition to the classic, sternal, perforating and anterior intercostal branches, other vessels have been described in the anterior intercostal space: these are the sternal perforating, sternal intercostal and persisting posterior branches.[6]

Variations have been described at the lower end of the ITA. The ITA may terminate above the level of the sixth costal cartilage. A watershed exists between the distal ITA branches and the intercostal arteries laterally and the abdominal wall vessels inferiorly. Division of the terminal branches of the ITA may cause ischemia following mobilization of one or both ITAs in elderly and diabetic patients in whom the collateral supply is poor.

Harvesting

The current trend is to mobilize the ITA with a small pedicle to reduce the damage to the chest wall and collateral circulation and reduce the risk of sternal infection.[7,8] Predictors include age, lung disease, obesity, graft choice and re-operation.[9,10] Semi-skeletonization is a technique which mobilizes only the ITA and its collateral veins. The artery and associated veins are dissected from the chest wall after reflecting the transversus thoracis muscle and pleura posteriorly. Skeletonization mobilizes only the ITA and leaves the venous drainage on the chest wall.

Our preferred technique is to use both ITAs in younger patients because of the excellent outcome.[11] The ITA and veins are routed within the mediastinum (extrapleurally) in the line of the phrenic nerve. Semi-skeletonization preserves the chest wall structures and protects the lung. The semi-skeletonized extrapleural technique allows the maximum length of ITA and is the technique of choice in elderly or diabetic patients. Located within the mediastinum, the LITA and RITA are protected from damage during sternal re-entry.

The sternum is divided and the cut edge elevated. The pedicle is exposed by detaching the origin of the transversus thoracis muscle from the sternum and costal cartilages between clips. The ITA and venae comitantes are mobilized by division of the perforating, anterior intercostal and sternal branches and associated veins. Mobilization of the ITA and veins may be commenced proximally or distally. The musculophrenic and superior epigastric arteries and veins are divided at the inferior end of the pedicle. Dissection is continued superiorly to the inferior border of the subclavian vein. At this point, the phrenic nerve lies immediately posterior to the artery and must be avoided. The artery can be seen disappearing proximally beneath the inferior border of the subclavian vein. The internal thoracic vein terminates in the brachiocephalic vein on the left and near the junction of the brachiocephalic and superior vena cava on the right. A tunnel is created within the mediastinum between the lateral side of the thymus and the mediastinal parietal pleura (Figure 16.1). The pleura is separated from the structures of the mediastinum to display the phrenic nerve. A window is made in the pericardium through which the semi-skeletonized pedicle is threaded, avoiding rotation. The ITA is located on the aorta, posterior to the thymus (Figure 16.2), away from the sternum.

Grafting techniques

Graft patency data suggest that *in situ* grafts have an advantage over the use of free arterial grafts. It is therefore desirable to use both the RITA and LITA *in situ*.[12] The LITA can be used to graft the LAD, diagonal, intermediate or circumflex marginal branches. Commonly, the LITA graft is attached as a single graft using an end-to-side anastomotic technique. When the circumflex marginal artery is to be grafted, the LITA is routed extrapleurally, anterior to the phrenic nerve, or transpleurally, posterior to the phrenic nerve, before being sutured to the marginal branch.[13]

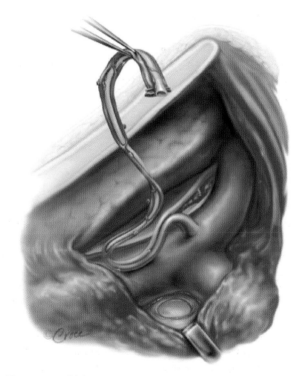

Figure 16.1 *Right upper anterior mediastinum with separation of the mediastinal pleura by retracting the thymus medially. The internal thoracic artery and vein and phrenic nerve are visible. The pleura remains intact.*

The LITA may be used as a sequential graft to a medially placed diagonal branch using a side-to-side technique, terminating in the distal LAD. Usually the side-to-side anastomosis is performed first, followed by the end-to-side anastomosis. This technique is suitable when the proposed anastomotic sites on the diagonal branch and the LAD are in a direct line. Excessive angulation at the site of the diagonal anastomosis may cause kinking and obstruction at the site of the side-to-side anastomosis. Under these circumstances the Y-graft technique is more suitable.

Use of the *in situ* RITA graft is more restricted because of the asymmetric shape of the heart; the graft length is often insufficient to reach either the posterior descending or the postero-lateral branch of the right coronary artery. The graft extension technique is particularly suitable under these circumstances. A segment of free arterial graft such as the radial, the inferior epigastric artery (IEA) or unused

distal LITA is sutured end-to-end to the RITA to provide an additional length. The extension graft can be anastomosed to the postero-lateral branch as a single graft or as a sequential graft to the posterior descending artery terminating in the postero-lateral branch. Alternatively, a Y-graft can be based on the *in situ* RITA, in a manner similar to that used on the LITA.[14]

The RITA may be used as a free graft to reach distal target arteries. The upper end of the RITA and vein are divided. The arterial inflow for the free RITA is from the aorta or from the LITA. When the ascending thoracic artery is disease free, the RITA is attached to the anterior aspect of the aorta using a running 6/0 Prolene suture. When it is desirable to avoid clamping or suturing the aorta, the RITA is sutured to the LITA on its anterior surface at about the level of its entry into the pericardium using a running 7/0 Prolene suture. This is angled at about 45° in a 'Y' fashion; the angle between the RITA and LITA is supported with a suture. The free RITA graft, sutured to the left-sided vessels, will usually reach the postero-lateral and posterior descending branches.

Graft patency

SINGLE ARTERIAL GRAFTS

In situ LITAs and RITAs, when grafted to the LAD with a stenosis of greater than 70%, have a 10-year patency of about 95%.[15] The target artery also influences ITA graft patency, with a higher failure rate when grafts are used to bypass lesions in the non-LAD arteries. The highest failure rate was associated with right coronary artery grafting, with a near fourfold increase in graft failure (Table 16.1, Figure 16.3a).

Competitive flow markedly reduces arterial graft patency. Free RITA grafts are affected adversely by grafting vessels with a low-grade stenosis. Grafts to vessels with non-critical lesions <60% are associated with a fourfold increase in graft failure (Figure 16.3b).[15] When used as

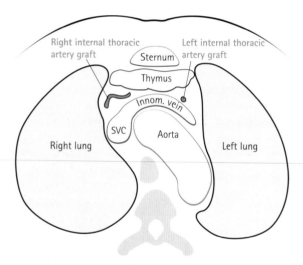

Figure 16.2 *Transverse section of the mediastinum at the level of the aortic arch showing the internal thoracic artery passing posterior to the thymus, anterior to the SVC, aorta and pulmonary artery to reach the left heart.*

Table 16.1 *Kaplan–Meier estimates: internal thoracic graft patency at 10 years*

Single graft	Target	Patency (%)	Reference
In situ[a]			
LITA (*n* = 530)	LAD ⩾80% stenosis	95	Buxton (2000)[15]
RITA (*n* = 70)	LAD ⩾80% stenosis	95	Buxton (2000)[15]
RITA (*n* = 321)	LAD, C[x], RCA	83	University of Melbourne Database, J Fuller 2003
Free[b]			
RITA (*n* = 284)	LAD, C[x], RCA	80	University of Melbourne Database, J Fuller 2003

[a]*In situ* graft: subclavian origin.
[b]Free graft: aortocoronary anastomosis.
University of Melbourne database.
LAD, left anterior descending; RCA, right coronary artery; LITA, left internal thoracic artery; RITA, right interior thoracic artery.

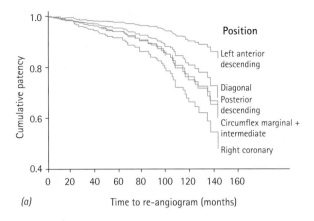

(a)

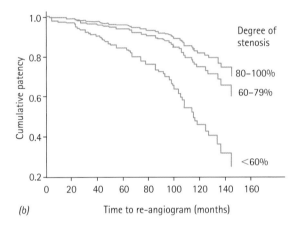

(b)

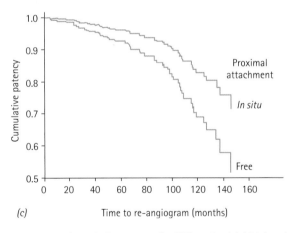

(c)

Figure 16.3 *Cumulative patency for RITA grafts. (a) A higher risk of graft failure was associated with non-LAD arteries; the highest rate was observed within the right coronary artery at its distal branches. (b) Effect of the native coronary artery stenosis on coronary artery bypass patency. A non-critical stenosis of 60% or less incurred a fourfold increase in risk. (c) Patency of free versus in situ RITA grafts was associated with a twofold increase in graft failure. Reprinted from Buxton B, et al. The right internal thoracic artery graft – benefits of grafting the left coronary system and native vessels with a high grade stenosis. Eur J Cardiothorac Surg 2000; 18:255–61, with permission from Elsevier Science.*

an aortocoronary bypass, RITA showed a twofold increase in graft failure compared with *in situ* grafts (Figure 16.3c).

Y-GRAFTING

The adequacy of flow reserve with LITA and RITA Y-grafts has been confirmed by Ochi, Maniar, Markwith and Prifti and challenged by others.[14,16–18] Calafiore reported excellent angiographic results when the RITA was attached to the LITA.[19]

EXTENSION GRAFTING

Extension grafting is a safe and effective technique.[19] Late patency was verified in 22 of 23 (96%) composite lengthened conduits.

SEQUENTIAL GRAFTING

Sequential ITA anastomoses have shown excellent patency except for the distal circumflex marginal and distal branches of the right coronary artery. In general, parallel sequential anastomoses were superior to diamond anastomoses.[20]

Clinical results

In-hospital mortality of less than 1% has been reported for bilateral and ITA grafting. Re-operation and percutaneous intervention were more frequent in patients with single compared with bilateral ITA grafting. Survival was improved with bilateral ITA grafts and this remained despite adjustment for patient selection sampling and follow-up. A major benefit was the reduction in re-operation for bilateral ITA grafting.[21] The differences between the benefits of bilateral over single ITA grafting was seen in the first 10 years in older patients with multiple risk factors, compared with younger patients for whom there is little difference in the first 10 years after surgery.[22] Cardiac events and angiographic patency are similar for bilateral ITAs when they are used either *in situ* or as 'Y'-grafts.[23]

RADIAL ARTERY

The radial artery (RA) was first used by Carpentier and reported in 1973.[24] Unfortunately, the early results were suboptimal, probably due to endothelial damage of the RA by mechanical dilatation, and also because strategies to deal with RA spasm were inadequate.[25] The RA was successfully revived as a conduit by Acar *et al.* with a landmark report in 1992.[26]

Since that time, the use of the RA in coronary surgery has increased, with high rates of total arterial coronary revascularization.[27–32] It has also been extensively used in beating-heart (or off-pump) coronary surgery. The main

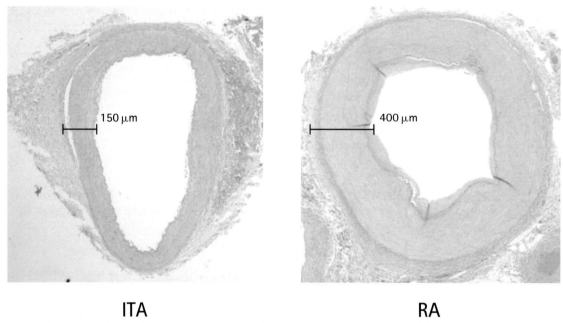

ITA   RA

Figure 16.4 *Comparison of the wall structure and thickness of a normal internal thoracic artery (ITA) and the radial artery (RA), at their distal ends.*

attractions of the RA include availability, appropriate size, excellent length and handling characteristics. The RA is robust, resistant to kinking and ideal for sequential anastomoses. Avoidance of leg incisions allows rapid ambulation.[29]

Anatomy

The RA originates from the brachial artery, at the elbow, just medial to the biceps tendon. It runs distally, deep to the brachioradialis muscle, in loose areolar tissue between the brachioradialis laterally and pronator teres and flexor carpi radialis medially. In the distal third, the RA is superficial, and at the wrist it lies 1 cm medial to the styloid process of the radius, placed between the tendons of brachioradialis laterally and flexor carpi radialis medially.

The branches are numerous but constant. From proximal to distal, there is a lateral recurrent branch. One or two deep branches run medially to the muscles and interosseous space. The central part of the radial has several small branches, which are readily identifiable in the loose areolar tissue. This area is where the RA can be most rapidly harvested. Near the wrist, the number of branches increases, and they are smaller and shorter. They are usually deep on either side but rarely on the superficial aspect. Beyond the wrist, the RA terminates in the superficial and deep palmar arches. Variations of the RA anatomy occur in up to 3% of people.[33,34] These include a high origin and aberrant branches, particularly to the hand.

It is important that the hand circulation is carefully evaluated before harvesting the RA.[29]

Histopathologically, the RA is a muscular artery. It has an endothelial layer, a thin intima and then an internal elastic lamina, which has numerous fenestrations. The media, with predominantly smooth muscle cells and few elastic fibers, is thick and constitutes the bulk of the wall thickness. Vasa vasorum are found in the adventitia. There is a pronounced, fenestrated external elastic lamina and finally an adventitia of modest thickness. The wall thickness of the RA is 400–500 μm (60–70% of which is media) – as compared to the ITA wall thickness of 150–200 μm (Figure 16.4).[29,35]

Calcification of a varying degree occurs in up to 5% of patients, ranging from microscopic calcification to a rigid calcific wall. Rarely, atheromatous plaques may also be present. These changes, when present, are more pronounced distally, and are more common in older diabetic males who also have peripheral vascular disease (Figure 16.5).[36,37] The internal diameter of the RA is usually 2.5 mm distally and 3.5–4 mm proximally. The average length from its origin to the wrist is 25 cm.

An absent or weak radial pulse may indicate a small size, aberrance or wall disease. The modified Allen's test (or a variation) is mandatory to ensure adequate ulnar collateral blood supply to the hand. Index finger pulse oximetry and plethysmography can also be used, noting the waveform, pressures and oxygen saturations during RA compression. These constitute a further refinement of the modified Allen's test.[38] Ultrasound and Doppler

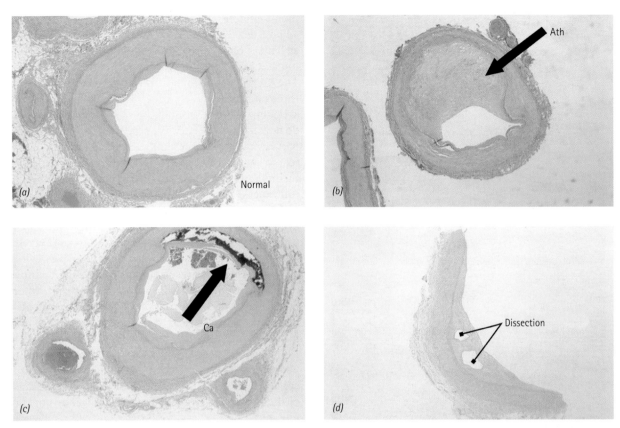

Figure 16.5 *Normal structure and pathological changes in radial arteries. (a) Normal radial artery (distal end). (b) Atheromatous and fibrotic plaque with a greater than 75% occlusion, at the distal end of the radial artery. (c) Medial calcification affecting a quarter of the circumference of the radial artery distally. (d) Dissection channels in the distal radial artery wall after prior (9 years) cannulation of the RA for arterial blood pressure monitoring. Ath, atheroma; Ca, calcium.*

evaluation of the RAs is particularly useful if calcification or other abnormalities are suspected preoperatively.

Inadequate ulnar collateral circulation to the hand, dense calcification, trauma (from prior RA cannulation) and the possibility that the patient may require a forearm fistula for chronic hemodialysis in the future are contraindications to RA harvesting. Raynaud's disease, scleroderma, poor peripheral circulation in a patient who lives in a particularly cold environment, prior trauma or surgery to the relevant upper limb, and known subclavian or axillary artery stenoses are relative contraindications.

Mobilization and harvest

The forearm is marked preoperatively for the RA harvest and the arm abducted 70–80°. Usually the left (non-dominant) RA is harvested simultaneously with the sternotomy and ITA harvest. If both RAs are used, harvesting and closure are completed prior to the sternotomy.

If the entire RA length is required, it is first exposed distally above the wrist, proximal to the skin crease, to ensure freedom from calcification. The incision is then extended proximally along the length of the RA, from a point 1 cm proximal and medial to the styloid process of the radius, in a curvilinear fashion to 1 cm distal to the biceps tendon at the elbow. The incision curves medially to avoid the lateral cutaneous nerve of the forearm. Mobilization commences near the wrist and proceeds retrogradely. We prefer to enter the fascia surrounding the RA and mobilize the vessel with precise dissection using scissors. Only the RA and its accompanying venae comitantes are taken. Smaller branches are secured with low-power cautery. Larger branches are divided between two metal vascular clips. Two small self-retaining retractors enhance exposure. The central portion of the RA can be harvested rapidly as it lies in an excellent plane with loose areolar tissue surrounding it, and has few, readily accessible branches. Proximally, mobilization is ceased 2 cm below the brachial bifurcation, to avoid damage to the ulnar artery and to ensure good control of the proximal RA stump. The venae comitantes that accompany the RA join together proximally over the anterior (superficial) surface of the RA. This plexus coincides with the proximal

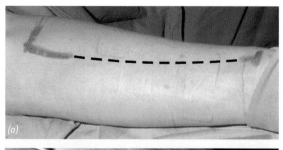

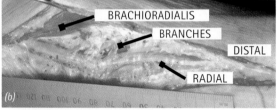

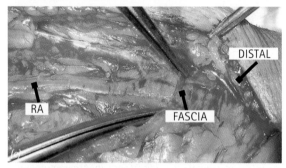

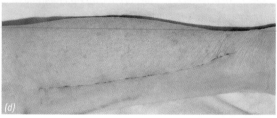

Figure 16.6 *Radial artery (RA) harvest. (a) Landmarks for the curvilinear incision. (b) The RA exposed and branches identified. The brachioradialis muscle lies laterally. Note tendency for spasm in the RA. (c) Subfascial harvest of the RA. (d) Healing forearm wound (5 days).*

mobilization of a wide pedicle with adjacent fascial and adipose tissue – using low-power cautery – the theoretical advantage of this being avoidance of spasm and damage to the RA, and provision of support to the vascular wall. The RA can also be mobilized with the Harmonic scalpel (Ethicon, Somerville, NJ, USA). Some workers completely skeletonize the RA without the venae comitantes. There do not appear to be any clear practical advantages for one harvest technique over another.[28,29,38,39] Recently, endoscopic harvesting of the RA has been undertaken, with incisions at the mid-forearm, wrist and elbow; however, this experience has been limited.

Before transection of the RA, a retrograde pulse is confirmed by temporarily occluding the artery proximally with a soft vascular clamp. Distally, the accompanying veins are isolated and divided between clips, followed by division of the RA after securing the distal stump with two medium-sized vascular clips or a 2/0 transfixion suture tie. Five milliliters of a papaverine solution, $2\,\mathrm{mmol\,L^{-1}}$ ($1\,\mathrm{mg\,mL^{-1}}$) in warm ($37\,^{\circ}\mathrm{C}$) heparinized arterial blood, is injected intraluminally into the RA with a blunt-tipped 1 mm vascular needle. The RA is clipped and then left to pulsate against the occluded end. A similar solution is applied topically. Papaverine in saline is avoided because of the very acidic pH. The distal stump will be noted to pulsate.

Residual proximal branches are divided while the RA is dilating, and the proximal end is secured by dividing first the veins and then the RA between clips. Again, two medium vascular clips or a transfixion suture of 2/0 polyglycolic acid (Vicryl, Ethicon) are used. The fascia and any other adventitial tissues over the RA are incised for several centimeters at either end in preparation for anastomosis (Figure 16.7). Additionally, fascial and adventitial tissues are incised for several centimeters at points for anticipated sequential anastomoses. The RA is then stored in an identical solution of heparinized arterial blood with papaverine $2\,\mathrm{mmol\,L^{-1}}$ ($1\,\mathrm{mg\,mL^{-1}}$) solution at room temperature until use.

ANTI-SPASM MEASURES

The RA has a pronounced muscular wall, and is prone to spasm. The maximal vasoconstrictor response of the RA *in vitro* is double that of the ITA.[40,41] Spasm is prevented or treated by using a 'no-touch' technique during harvest and by the use of vasodilator drugs perioperatively. We prefer to apply papaverine in blood intraluminally, topically, and for storage as detailed above, for its simplicity. Alternatively, nitroglycerine (GTN) and Verapamil can be used. Intraoperatively, GTN infusion $30–100\,\mathrm{\mu g\,min^{-1}}$ is used during surgery and for the first 24 hours. Alternatively, intravenous Diltiazem is used, but may not be as effective as GTN.[42] It is important to avoid topical ice-slush or cold saline in the pericardium, as this may cause arterial graft spasm.

limit of the mobilization. If a shorter length of RA is required, the central portion of the RA is removed to maximize collateral blood supply.

The superficial radial nerve runs parallel and approximately 10 mm lateral to the RA, deep to the brachioradialis. It should be looked for, and avoided. The lateral cutaneous nerve of the forearm runs in this subcutaneous tissue, and is lateral to the skin incision and thus avoided. However, the lateral cutaneous nerve of the forearm or its branches may cross anterior to the RA near the wrist. Traction or damage to these branches may result in numbness of the thumb (Figure 16.6).

The RA pedicle harvested in this way is thin, and without bulk and fat. Alternative methods of harvest include

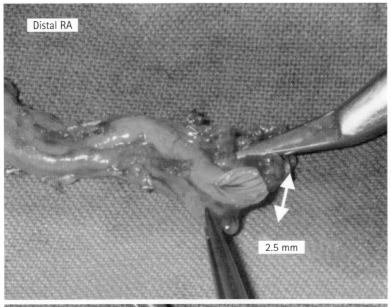

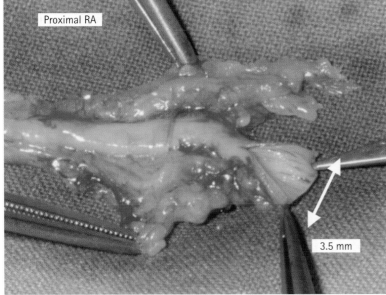

Figure 16.7 *The radial artery prepared for anastomosis distally (2.5 mm internal diameter) and proximally (3.5 mm internal diameter).*

We recommend a once-daily calcium-channel blocker, amlodipine 5–10 mg per day for 6 months. Although the use of long-term oral calcium-channel blockers is empirical, we and others have noted isolated instances of localized RA spasm in RA angiograms early postoperatively and at 1–4 months. Conversely, RA graft spasm has not been seen on RA angiograms performed more than 12 months postoperatively.[26,29]

Grafting

AORTOCORONARY GRAFTS

The RA is an ideal conduit to graft the circumflex marginal branches. If the lie is appropriate, a proximal marginal may be grafted sequentially (side-to-side) with an end-to-side anastomosis for a distal marginal.

The RA is also an ideal graft for the posterior descending branch of the right coronary artery as it will reach distally beyond any stenosis. Occasionally, the RA may reach the left ventricular branch of the right coronary artery. Bilateral RA grafts may also be used with a LITA to the LAD, one RA to the circumflex marginal system and the second RA to the posterior descending artery. This is useful where there is paucity of other conduit or in a re-operation (Figure 16.8).[43,44]

Y-GRAFTS

The commonest Y-graft or T-graft arrangement is an in-flow anastomosis from the LITA. The LITA supplies

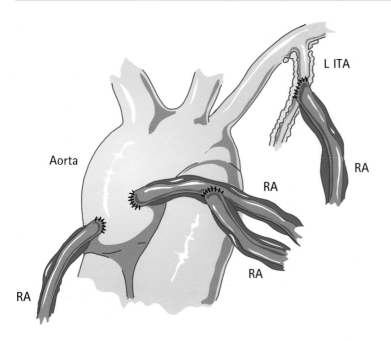

Figure 16.8 *Sites of proximal (inflow) radial artery anastomosis, directly to the aorta, left internal thoracic artery (LITA)–radial artery Y-graft, radial artery–radial artery (RA–RA) Y-graft.*

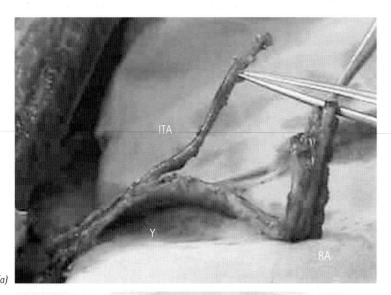

(a)

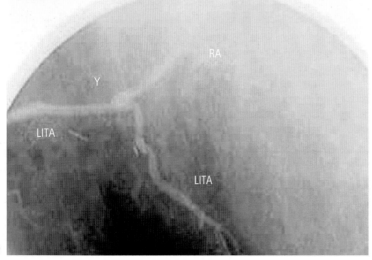

(b)

Figure 16.9 *(a) A left internal thoracic artery–radial artery (LITA–RA) Y-graft. Note the generous length of RA available. (b) Angiographic depiction of the LITA–RA composite Y-graft, the LITA to the anterior aspect of the heart (left anterior descending artery) and the RA passing posteriorly to the circumflex territory.*

the LAD/diagonal system, with the RA coursing laterally and posteriorly to revascularize the circumflex marginal vessels, and terminate on the posterior descending artery (Figure 16.9).[45]

Special technical issues

An RA-to-RA Y-graft can be used if the position of the occlusive lesions in the circumflex marginals is such that the lie of a sequential graft would be difficult.[29] An inverted LITA/RA U-graft can be used where a short LITA may provide the inflow to both ends of the RA.

ITA/RA END-TO-END EXTENSION GRAFT

This may be used on the right side allowing the RA to readily reach the posterior descending artery, the left ventricular branch of the right coronary artery, and even distal circumflex branches.[31] It is a particularly useful technique to provide inflow to right-sided and inferior wall grafts in beating-heart surgery, without the need for any proximal manipulation, clamps or anastomoses on the ascending thoracic aorta. Construction of Y pedicled or end-to-end extension grafts is performed after appropriate heparinization, and before the institution of cardiopulmonary bypass if conventional coronary surgery is employed.

The deployment of the RA as described above can be used in either conventional or beating-heart surgery. However, the Y and extension graft techniques avoid the aorta and also reduce the conduit requirements. The anterior (superficial) aspect of the RA is more suitable for the construction of sequential anastomoses as it is devoid of branches.

ADVANTAGES AND DISADVANTAGES

Additional advantages reported of the RA are that it is an arterial conduit and the forearm wound heals well, leg incisions are avoided and rapid ambulation is possible. Harvest can be efficiently accomplished at the same time as the sternotomy and ITA harvest.[28,29,37–39]

Disadvantages include additional forearm incisions and the tendency to spasm. There is also a theoretical risk of finger ischemia if the hand circulation has not been correctly evaluated.[29,38]

Clinical results

PERIOPERATIVE

The operative and 30-day mortality for primary coronary artery surgery in which the RA was a key conduit in our experience of almost 7000 surgeries was 0.9%.[46] Similar perioperative mortality has been reported by other workers.[47–49]

In coronary bypass re-operations, use of the RA is associated with a perioperative mortality of 3.3%.[43] The perioperative morbidity when the RA is used is also low, with a myocardial infarction rate of 1% and a stroke rate of 1.4%.

Myocardial hypoperfusion (from RA spasm) rarely occurs.[29,46–49] The incidence of inotrope use and intra-aortic balloon pump support has been extremely low. Particularly gratifying have been low rates of deep sternal infection (1.4%). The low incidence of sternal infection and the absence of Gram-negative organisms may be due to the avoidance of leg and thigh incisions and potential contamination of the sternal and cardiac operative field. Re-operation for excessive bleeding is low (0.9%). There was no incidence of bleeding from an RA branch, and indeed the small size of the RA branches may protect against sudden catastrophic bleeding.[29,46] In general, the perioperative clinical results are similar to or better than those for the use of saphenous vein grafts in combination with the ITA.

Considering the numbers of RAs harvested, there have been few donor site problems. The incidence of forearm infection and hematoma is less than 1%. Finger or hand ischemia is rare. The commonest problem is that of lower forearm and thumb parasthesia, which occurs in 5–30% of patients and in most completely resolves over 3 months. Motor function of the hand and forearm and functional ability and power are not affected.[28,29,48,49]

MEDIUM AND LONG TERM

Although some workers have used the RA since the early 1990s (Acar, Calafiore, Dietl[50]), most groups have a 5–6-year experience with the RA. Actuarial survival rates of 97% at 1 year and 92% at 5 years have been published.[47–49] However, the survival rates may more specifically relate to the initial patient cohort, case selection, the number of arterial grafts and the completeness of revascularization. Calafiore reported an 8-year survival of 83%, and a cardiac event-free survival of 80% over the same 8-year period.[47] Freedom from angina rates are excellent: Acar and Calafiore have separately published 5-year freedom from angina rates of 89% and 90% respectively.[47,49]

Patency

The RA patency is superior to that of saphenous vein grafts, probably equal to that of free RITA grafts and, although similar to LITA grafts in the short term, inferior to those in the medium to long term (Figure 16.10).

Early patency rates (1–3 months) are reported at 96–99%,[31,47,51] at 1 year, 90–94%,[29,31,46–49,52,53] and up to 95% at 4–5 years.[47,49] Patency results are summarized in Table 16.2. The RA patency was not affected by the site of

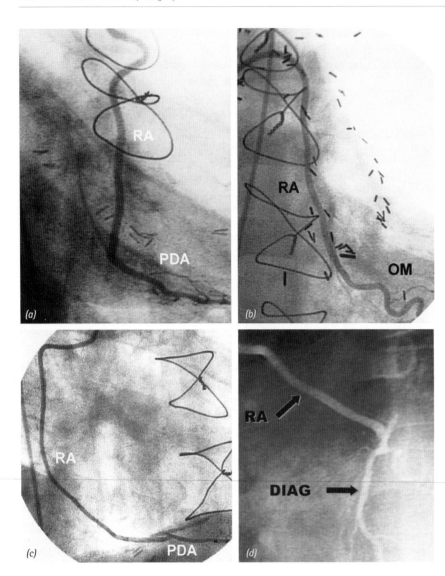

Figure 16.10 *Angiograms of radial arteries. (a) Radial artery to the posterior descending (PDA) – 4 years postoperatively. (b) Aortocoronary radial artery to the inferior circumflex marginal – 5 years postoperatively. (c) Aortocoronary radial artery to the posterior descending – 18 months postoperatively. (d) Aortocoronary radial artery to the diagonal/ intermediate artery – 5 years postoperatively. Note the uniform appearance of the radial artery, and excellent size match with the target coronary artery. DIAG, diagonal; OM, obtuse marginal; RA, radial artery.*

the proximal anastomosis, indeed there was a tendency for higher patency for aortocoronary RA grafts.[47] In 369 RA to coronary graft anastomoses studied angiographically at a mean of 14 months postoperatively, the cumulative patency was 91%, with a trend for lower patency for RA grafts to the right coronary artery system.[46] There is a lower patency for RA grafts anastomosed to coronary vessels with a low-grade (less than 60%) native stenosis, and also for the last segment to the posterior descending artery of an LITA/RA Y-graft.[17,45,52] The last two phenomena may be due to a competitive flow. Early RA graft failure may occur for technical reasons. Competitive flow is probably the cause of failure in the medium to long term.[45,46,49,52]

It is inappropriate to compare RA graft patency to that of the LITA to the LAD, as the RA grafts are deployed to more distal, often smaller and less suitable vessels in the same way that saphenous vein grafts to the LAD have

Table 16.2 *Radial artery (RA) graft patency*

Report	Percentage RA graft patent		
	1–3 months	1–2 years	4–5 years
Acar[49] (*n* = 102)	99	92	83
Calafiore[47] (*n* = 89)	99	–	–
Trehan[48] (*n* = 104)	–	92.5	–
Tatoulis[46] (*n* = 369)	–	91	–
Calafiore[47] (*n* = 91)	–	–	96

higher patency rates compared with saphenous vein grafts to the right coronary artery or circumflex systems.

Some workers have expressed concern about the construction of LITA/RA Y-grafts, as they may compromise the LITA to the LAD – either because of technical problems, or a steal phenomenon into the RA portion of the

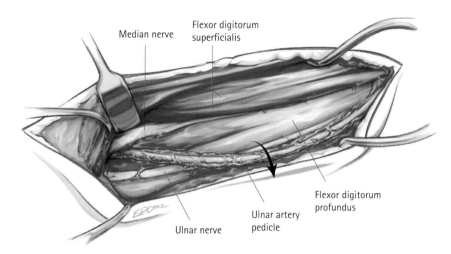

Figure 16.11 *Ulnar artery harvest. In the upper third of the forearm the ulnar artery lies in a 'tunnel' between the flexor digitorum superficialis and profundus after separating from the ulnar nerve. It can be removed up to a point distal to where it is crossed by the median nerve and the origin of the common interosseus artery.*

Y-graft.[38] There is one report of a reduction of LITA to LAD patency from 98% to 94% when a RA Y-graft was used.[52]

ULNAR ARTERY

The ulnar artery has been used in our unit since 1997 when other conduits were not available. Approximately half of the patients with a dominant RA as judged by an abnormal Allen test have had a satisfactory ulnar artery. The proximity of the ulnar artery to the ulnar nerve and the blood supply of the ulnar nerve from the ulnar artery may subject the nerve to ischemic damage after harvesting of the artery. Removal of the ulnar artery for use as a CABG is usually confined to the small number of patients in whom the RA, or other conduits, cannot be harvested.

Mobilization and harvest

The artery is approached through an incision on the medial aspect of the arm in the line of the medial condyle of the humerus and pisiform bone. Commencing the harvest distally, the fascia is divided lateral to the flexor carpi ulnaris tendon to display the artery and collateral veins. In the distal two-thirds of the forearm, the vascular pedicle consisting of the ulnar artery and veins is closely applied to the ulnar nerve, and division of branches of the ulnar artery to the nerve, the arteriae nervorum, cannot be avoided. This is not associated with neurological dysfunction in the majority of patients, presumably because of well-formed arterial connections throughout the length of the ulnar nerve. Mobilization is extended proximally, separating the humero-ulnar head of the flexor digitorum superficialis from the flexor carpi radialis until the artery disappears beneath the muscles arising from the medial epicondyle. The ulnar artery and veins are divided distally, leaving a stump of 2–3 cm above the level of the

wrist joint (Figure 16.11). The cut artery is injected with a solution of papaverine mixed with equal parts of blood and Ringer's lactate solution with a final concentration of $1 \, \mathrm{mmol} \, L^{-1}$ (40 mg/100 mL). The upper third of the ulnar artery separates from the ulnar nerve and passes beneath the flexor digitorum superficialis and overlying palmaris longus and flexor carpi radialis. The artery lies posterior to the flexor digitorum profundus, which separates it from the upper part of the ulna. The ulnar artery passes deep to the pronator teres muscle. The median nerve can be seen between the origins of the pronator teres where it crosses the ulnar artery from its medial to lateral side. The ulnar artery disappears from view passing under the (fibrous) arch between the humero-ulnar origin and the radial origin of the flexor digitorum superficialis. The artery is divided proximally at the level of the median nerve, usually distal to the common interosseous artery, thereby preserving an important collateral supply to the forearm.[54]

Clinical results

We have used the ulnar artery in 27 patients, anastomosed proximally with the aorta, as a Y-graft from the LITA or an extension graft on the right side in patients for whom no other conduit was available.

There have been few graft angiograms. One of the 27 patients developed neuralgic pain in the distribution of the ulnar nerve, which has remained. No patient had a residual motor deficit in the ulnar distribution.

INFERIOR EPIGASTRIC ARTERY

Harvesting of the IEA for use as a coronary artery graft was first reported by Puig in 1990.[55] The size and length of the IEA vary. The artery has been found useful for grafting proximal left-sided lesions such as the diagonal or intermediate coronary artery and also as a composite graft, for example as a Y-graft with the LITA or an extension graft from the RITA.[56]

The artery is removed through a midline subumbilical incision or more directly through a lateral incision with the rectus muscle retracted medially to expose the IEA at the level of the umbilicus. This lateral approach, however, will result in denervation of a segment of the rectus muscle. A length of 10–12 cm can be removed from some patients, but usually only half this vessel is useable. Frequently the IEA is affected by arteriosclerosis near its origin from the external iliac artery. The artery is harvested with its collateral veins.

Buche, in 1995, reported a clinical series of 200 IEA grafts, 95% of which were anastomosed proximally to the ascending thoracic aorta, either directly or via a saphenous vein patch or graft.[57] One hundred and forty-two (71%) patients consented to angiography within 2 weeks of operation; 86% had a perfect angiographic appearance, the remainder had anastomotic or focal narrowings. Califiore *et al.* reported a series of 70 IEA grafts attached to the ITA as a Y-graft.[31] Patency at 12 months was 93%.

RIGHT GASTRO-EPIPLOIC ARTERY

The right gastro-epiploic artery (RGEA) was first used as an intramural graft to collateralize the inferior myocardial wall (1966 to 1970).[58] It was first used as a pedicled graft with a direct graft to coronary artery anastomosis by Pym and co-workers in 1984,[59] and concurrently by Suma and associates.[60] This was followed by its use by a number of groups in the development of total arterial revascularization and beating-heart coronary surgery. Pym and Suma have reported the largest experiences.

Anatomy

The RGEA is a branch of the gastroduodenal artery, which is in turn a branch of the common hepatic artery, which arises from the celiac axis. The gastroduodenal artery passes behind the first part of the duodenum. At the lower border, it divides into the superior pancreatico-duodenal artery and RGEA. The RGEA then runs superiorly and to the left, following the greater curve of the stomach, between the layers of the greater omentum, accompanied by small satellite veins. It ends by anastomosing with the left gastro-epiploic branch of the splenic artery. Near the pylorus it is adjacent to the stomach, but in general it lies approximately 1.5–2.5 cm from and parallel to the greater curve of the stomach. At its origin, the RGEA is relatively large (3 mm). It tapers significantly and reduces to approximately 1.5–2 mm (luminal size) distally, before terminating in a leash of branches to the upper body of the stomach.

From right to left, there are several small branches to the head of the pancreas and duodenum, and several slightly larger branches to the pylorus. In its omental location along the greater curve, there are smaller inferior branches (usually single, every 2–3 cm) to the greater omentum, and larger superior branches (often paired) that run between the omental layers to the body of the stomach at intervals of approximately 1.5–2 cm. On the left and upper portion of the body of the stomach, multiple gastric branches arise, and the RGEA becomes significantly smaller before finally anastomosing with the left gastro-epiploic artery (LGEA) (branch of the splenic artery). Anatomical abnormalities can occur, the most common and important being an origin from the superior mesenteric artery (5%). The practical useable length (from the gastroduodenal artery to just beyond the midpoint of the stomach) is approximately 20 cm.

The RGEA is a muscular artery with an endothelium and a thin intimal layer (50 μm). It has a thin, internal elastic lamina, which is fenestrated. There is a well-developed media (200–350 μm) with many smooth muscle cells, but which is relatively lacking in elastic fibers (by comparison to the ITA). There is also a fenestrated external elastic lamina and a thin adventitia. The thickness of the respective layers reduces to approximately 50% towards the distal end of the RGEA.[35,61]

The RGEA is usually free from atherosclerosis and calcification. A normal to mildly thickened intima and normal wall are seen in more than 92% of cases. However, in patients with extensive arterial disease, the RGEA may be compromised by atherosclerotic disease in the abdominal aorta and celiac axis. The histology of the RGEA wall is more akin to the RA and IEA.[61]

Harvesting

EVALUATION OF SUITABILITY

Angiography of the celiac axis can be performed at the time of coronary angiogram. This is not routine, but can be important if planning a re-operation in which the inferior surface of the left ventricle is to be revascularized by the RGEA. Aberrant origins from the superior mesenteric artery should also be considered.[16]

MOBILIZATION

The lower part of the sternotomy incision is extended 5–7 cm beyond the xiphisternum. The RGEA is harvested after ITA is completed. The sternal retractor is left in place; an abdominal retractor is used to retract laterally and inferiorly. A nasogastric tube is passed after induction decompresses the stomach, and for the first 48 hours postoperatively.

The RGEA is located and assessed visually and by palpation for the presence of pulsation. The mobilization is commenced opposite the midpoint of the body of the stomach, dividing omental tissues and small omental branches on the inferior border, entering the lesser sac, and dividing adjacent gastric branches to free the pedicle circumferentially.

The mobilization extends proximally, towards the pylorus and duodenum, separating omentum and dividing the small omental branches along the inferior border. Mobilization is performed with low-power cautery and the use of metal clips. Alternatively, the Harmonic scalpel (Ethicon) can be used. Any adhesions within the lesser sac are divided. The mobilization ceases at the pylorus. Distally, the mobilization, according to the length required, extends to just beyond the mid-section of the greater curve and body of the stomach to the leash of branches in the proximal stomach.

The gastric side of the pedicle is mobilized from the fat. A small amount of adipose tissue (approximately 1.5 cm wide) is retained around the RGEA to protect the artery. Alternatively, the RGEA is skeletonized, extending the length of the pedicle by an extra 2–3 cm of length.[62] There is usually an avascular area between the RGEA and the pylorus, before the RGEA assumes a close relationship to the pylorus and duodenum. The branches to the pylorus are left intact, as mobilization of this part does not greatly contribute to the length of the pedicle, and because it is important to maintain the vascularity of the pylorus, duodenum and head of pancreas. The mobilization of the RGEA typically takes 15–20 minutes. The techniques used for prevention of spasm are similar to those for the RA and ITA.[29,40,41,46] The RGEA is clipped at its tip and allowed to pulsate against its occluded distal end at arterial pressure. It is wrapped in a warm (37 °C) papaverine-soaked gauze. Anti-spasm strategies are essential for this muscular artery. Maximum dilatation facilitates the construction of the RGEA anastomoses, ensures optimal myocardial perfusion and avoids the hypoperfusion syndrome.[63] After harvesting, but before use, the free flow of blood is assessed (usually 60–120 mL min^{-1}).

Grafting techniques

ENTRY INTO THE PERICARDIUM

The RGEA is the last conduit to be used. It is passed anterior to the stomach and anterior to the left lobe of the liver, and care is taken to avoid rotation. The gastric side is oriented to the right and the anastomosis constructed on the posterior side of the pedicle so that orientation and bleeding can be checked (Figure 16.12).

The RGEA can be taken posterior to the stomach. Some workers prefer this route to the postero-lateral branches of the circumflex.[64,65] There does not appear to

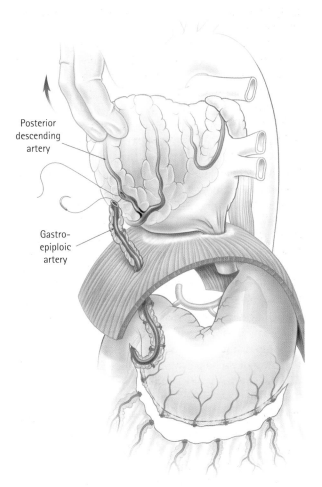

Figure 16.12 *The gastro-epiploic artery has been harvested from the greater curve. It passes anterior to the pylorus through an opening created in the diaphragm to be anastomosed directly to the posterior descending coronary artery.*

be a clear advantage, as in most instances the RGEA is anastomosed to the posterior descending coronary artery. The RGEA is brought into the pericardium through a wide cruciate incision (3 cm diameter) just anterior to the inferior vena cava, directly opposite to the atrioventricular groove. The left lobe of the liver protects the diaphragmatic incision so that intra-abdominal contents do not herniate into the pericardium. In the rare situation in which the RGEA is anastomosed retrogradely to the LAD, it is brought through the diaphragm anteriorly.

TARGET ARTERIES

The RGEA is most commonly anastomosed to the posterior descending artery, distal to all stenotic lesions, as this allows the best lie and size match.

The heart is retracted vertically, thus lining up the posterior descending artery and RGEA; the anastomosis starts at the heel and, on completion, the small residual pedicle is secured to the epicardium to maintain orientation and avoid kinking. The RGEA can also be anastomosed to the main right coronary artery before the crux – in a retrograde fashion to ensure the best lie – or to the right coronary artery/left ventricular branch beyond the crux – in an antegrade fashion. These techniques are suitable for both on-pump and off-pump surgery.

Inferior circumflex marginal branches can be grafted (antegrade), and even the distal LAD artery (in a retrograde fashion).[66] Sequential grafting may be used, providing the RGEA is greater than 2 mm at the site for a distal anastomosis and preferably greater than 2.5 mm for a sequential anastomosis. Separate stenoses in the posterior descending artery and the left ventricular branch of right coronary artery or even in an inferior circumflex marginal are bypassed sequentially. Parallel side-to-side anastomoses are preferred. Diamond-shaped sequential anastomoses should be avoided unless the RGEA is at least 2.5–3 mm internal diameter at that point, to avoid distorting and 'flattening out' the RGEA at that site.[16] After grafting, the redundant pedicle is returned to the abdomen.

Large-diameter GEA grafts are necessary because of the lower diastolic pressure by comparison with the ITA or aortocoronary grafts. Residual ischemia is seen in patent but small RGEA grafts.[16] The RGEA can also be used as a free graft or as a Y-graft (as for the RA) – although these configurations would only be used in exceptional circumstances such as disease in the aorta or the celiac axis. For proximal anastomosis of a free RGEA graft to the aorta, saphenous vein patch is used.[64] The greatest value of the RGEA is its availability as an *in situ* graft for the inferior or infero-lateral aspect of the heart.[60,64,67]

Special technical issues

RE-OPERATIONS

The RGEA is ideally suited to re-operations, particularly if only the inferior or infero-lateral aspect of the heart needs to be revascularized. The incision can be confined to the linea alba and the lower third of the sternum. The RGEA can be readily harvested, and the posterior descending artery exposed by upward retraction on the sternum and inferior retraction on the diaphragm. Repeat sternotomy can be avoided; the LITA and atheromatous grafts and the ascending aorta can be left undisturbed. The posterior descending artery or other infero-lateral branches can be grafted using off-pump techniques.[68]

Grafting techniques

COMPOSITE

Extensive revascularization of the inferior and lateral walls of the heart can be achieved by an RGEA/RA U-graft,

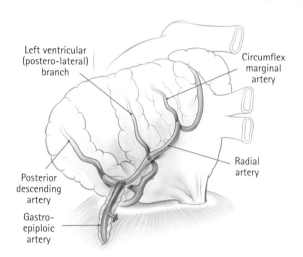

Figure 16.13 *A composite gastro-epiploic, radial artery U graft. The proximal limb of the radial artery is anastomosed to the posterior descending. The distal limb is anastomosed sequentially to the left ventricular branch of the right coronary artery and then end-to-side to the circumflex marginal.*

with the RGEA providing the inflow, end-to-side to the RA, and one limb (shorter) of the RA graft supplying the posterior descending artery, and the other (longer) limb passing sequentially to the left ventricular branch of the right coronary artery and circumflex marginal vessels up as far as a first marginal or intermediate artery (Figure 16.13).[69,70]

OFF-PUMP CORONARY SURGERY

The RGEA is an ideal *in situ* arterial graft to the posterior descending artery or other infero-lateral branches. Used in conjunction with the *in situ* LITA to LAD and *in situ* RITA to circumflex, total arterial revascularization with these three grafts can be achieved without cardiopulmonary bypass and without manipulation of the ascending aorta.[70]

Clinical results

PERIOPERATIVE

The operative and 30-day mortality is similar to that for other primary coronary operations, at 1.5–2%. Consistent results have been reported from many large series.[71–74]

Perioperative morbidity is also low. Perioperative myocardial infarction rates are 1–2%, intra-aortic balloon pump use 2–3%. Hospital length of stay is typically 7 days.[71] In coronary re-operations in which the posterior descending artery was the most significant target vessel, use of the RGEA in an off-pump fashion may be extremely beneficial, with some groups reporting a 1% perioperative mortality, compared with up to 10% mortality using conventional sternotomy and cardiopulmonary bypass techniques.[75] With use of RGEA, rates of stroke or major neurological impairment are 1–2%, and deep sternal infection 1.5–2%. Again, these results of perioperative morbidity are totally consistent with contemporary reports of coronary artery grafting.[66,71,73] No gastric ischemic events have been recorded.[71]

MEDIUM AND LONG TERM

Actuarial survival of 95% at 3 years, 88–92% at 5 years, and 84% at 10 years (mean age at first operation 60 years) is reported. Freedom from cardiac events including angina was 85% at 5 years and 80% at 10 years.[16,71,76]

Patency

Early patency is excellent, and patency results improved over time with experience with the technique.[16,64,66,73,76]

The largest reported experience is that of Suma and colleagues.[76] In 685 RGEA grafts studied in symptomatic patients with the first year (mean 2.2 months), patency was 94%; in 102 patients studied between 1 and 5 years (mean 2.3 years), patency was 88%; in 52 patients studied between 5 and 10 years (mean 7.8 years), patency was 83%. The authors have estimated cumulative patency rates (Kaplan–Meier) to be 96.6%, 91.4%, 80.5% and 62.5% at 1 month, 1 year, 5 years and 10 years respectively.

Other reports involve smaller numbers and shorter follow-up: 100% patency at a mean of 6.8 months (30 patients),[16] 93% at a mean of 10.6 months (44 patients),[71] 88% patency at a mean of 16 months (56 patients),[73] and estimated 82% at 5 years (27 patients).[77]

It should be noted that these patency results are generally from studies undertaken in symptomatic patients, and probably represent the least optimistic values. It is likely that the true patency results in the general asymptomatic postoperative cohort of patients are superior to these. True patency may also be under-represented, as the celiac axis and RGEA may not always be defined at postoperative angiography.

MODES OF GRAFT FAILURE

Early graft failure is most likely to be due to technical errors. Medium-term graft failure may occur in those grafts anastomosed to coronary arteries with only mild to moderate (less than 75%) stenoses, or where there was poor run-off. Failure is in the form of progressive luminal reduction (string sign) and not by an atherosclerotic–thrombotic process as occurs in vein grafts. Hence, interventions in patients with failed arterial grafts do not suffer the same hazard of atheromatous coronary embolism when manipulating the heart with diseased vein grafts.[71,76]

SAPHENOUS VEIN

Saphenous vein graft is still arguably the most commonly used conduit for coronary bypass surgery. After implantation, vein grafts are affected by fibrointimal hyperplasia and severe atherosclerosis with ulceration and thrombosis, which lead to graft stenosis and occlusion in approximately 50% of patients over the 10–12 years following surgery. The saphenous vein has different physiological properties from the ITA. The saphenous vein releases less nitric oxide in response to vascular endothelial growth factor compared with the ITA.[78] In recent years, aggressive treatment by diet, lipid-lowering agents and control of hypertension may have ameliorated these changes. Despite these preventative strategies, continued progression of disease in saphenous vein grafts has led surgeons to examine the use of arterial grafts.

Harvesting

The basic technique for harvesting a long saphenous vein is well known. The lower end of the long saphenous vein is used commonly, because the diameter is similar to that of the native coronary artery. Changes in the wall of the saphenous vein increase with age. In elderly patients, some saphenous veins are dilated and diseased; these grafts should be discarded. Peripheral vascular disease increases with age and is often associated with coronary artery disease and may cause poor wound healing and ulceration after removal of the long saphenous vein.

A vein stripper can be used to isolate the vein. It is passed distally to identify the valves and side branches, which are ligated through a small incision. Videoscopic harvesting of the saphenous vein is increasing in popularity and has the advantage of minimizing the risk of skin necrosis and causing minimal damage to the long saphenous vein.[79]

The number of saphenous veins harvested for CABG has progressively reduced in our program because of increasing satisfaction with internal thoracic, radial and other arterial conduits. However, the long saphenous vein is used in some patients who have atherosclerotic disease or calcification of the RAs, and in whom other arterial conduits are not readily available. Saphenous vein grafts are also used in some patients who are unstable, because of the ease and rapidity of harvesting, thereby reducing the ischemic time. If the saphenous vein is required, it is harvested below the knee. If the long saphenous vein is not available, the short saphenous vein may be removed.

PROTECTION OF THE ENDOTHELIUM

Avoidance of distension improves the quality and future function of the endothelium and may increase the late patency in humans and animal models.[80,81] Rosenfeldt recommends vasodilator therapy in a fashion similar to that described for the RA when harvesting all saphenous vein grafts.[80]

Deployment

This vein is usually delegated to grafting less important vessels such as the circumflex and right coronary arteries. Preference may be given to the use of saphenous vein grafts for a native coronary artery with a low-grade stenosis where competitive flow may cause graft failure if an arterial graft is used.

Patency

Some saphenous vein grafts fail early because of surgical technique and the early onset of fibrointimal hyperplasia. The majority of grafts fail between 5 and 15 years following bypass surgery, resulting in loss of about 85% of the grafts. The 20-year patency is approximately 10%. Interestingly, some vein grafts even at 20 years look normal, and these have been described as 'biologically privileged'. The late results of saphenous vein grafts in the University of Melbourne database (J Fuller, unpublished data) are shown in Figure 16.14.

SUMMARY

Our unit has adopted a policy of extensive and, subsequently, complete arterial grafting. This is achieved by using combinations of ITA, RA and GEA grafts and different techniques of proximal and distal anastomoses.

Preference is given to using *in situ* grafts because of their proven durability and excellent late patency results.

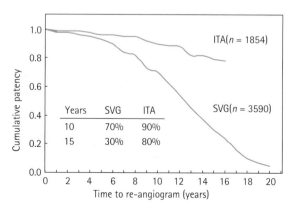

Figure 16.14 *Twenty-year patency of the saphenous vein coronary artery bypass grafts. ITA, internal thoracic artery; SVG, saphenous vein graft.*

If harvesting more than one *in situ* graft is undesirable, free arterial grafts are used. A free arterial graft is attached to the aorta. If the aorta is poor, or graft length is insufficient, the inflow may be from another arterial conduit using a T, Y or U configuration. This is known as a composite graft.

Distal anastomoses are single or sequential. Sequential grafts are used when there are multiple targets, usually in the same territory. A sequential graft, when combined with a composite graft, is a complex reconstruction. This is the most efficient technique of using arterial conduits, but late results need further assessment. Arterial grafting techniques can be applied to off-pump or conventional cardiopulmonary bypass.

The optimal treatment of a low-grade stenosis in a native coronary artery graft remains unresolved. Free arterial grafts to vessels with a poor run-off are also prone to failure. Low arterial graft flow is common to both situations. The use of an *in situ* artery, a saphenous vein graft or percutaneous intervention may be preferable.

KEY REFERENCES

Acar C, Ramsheyi A, Pagny JY, Jebara V, Barrier P, Fabiabi JN, *et al.* The radial artery for coronary artery bypass grafting: clinical and angiographic results at five years. *J Thorac Cardiovasc Surg* 1998; **116**:981–9.
The French surgeons have demonstrated the feasibility of using the RA as a coronary bypass graft and have provided 5-year patency data using the RA as an aorta coronary bypass graft. Their results suggest that the patency of the RA is superior to that of the saphenous vein. This is an uncontrolled and non-matched study, but nonetheless provides us with the best long-term data on radial graft patency.

Buxton BF, Ruengsakulrach P, Fuller J, Rosalion A, Reid CM, Tatoulis J. The right internal thoracic artery graft – benefits of grafting the left coronary system and native vessels with a high grade stenosis. *Eur J Cardiothorac Surg* 2000; **18**:255–61.
This series of 400 ITA graft angiograms over a period of 10 years confirms the excellent patency of using the *in situ* RITA graft to the left system when the RITA is anastomosed to the LAD. The patency is identical with that of the LITA. The paper quantitates the increased failure rates when grafting non-LAD vessels, especially the distal right coronary branches. This study demonstrates a near-fourfold increase in graft failure when the RITA graft is subjected to competitive flow, and a twofold increase in graft failure when using as a free graft compared with being left *in situ*.

Calafiore AM, Di Giammarco G, Teodori G, D'Annunzio E, Vitolla G, Fino C, *et al.* Radial artery and inferior epigastric artery in composite grafts: improved mid-term angiographic results. *Ann Thorac Surg* 1995; **60**: 517–24.

Calafiore and colleagues have demonstrated the reliability of attaching an arterial free graft to the *in situ* LITA in a large series of patients. The paper confirms the safety and minimal risk to the LITA itself and also the high patency rates of both the radial and inferior epigastric artery used in a 'Y' configuration.

Lytle BW, Blackstone EH, Loop FD, Houghtaling PL, Arnold JH, Akhrass R, *et al*. Two internal thoracic artery grafts are better than one. *J Thorac Cardiovasc Surg* 1999; **117**:855–72.

This large retrospective series of patients from the Cleveland Clinic demonstrates the benefits of bilateral compared with single internal thoracic grafting over a long follow-up for a period between 10 and 20 years. The patients were matched retrospectively and the authors demonstrated an improved survival and a lower re-operation rate in patients having bilateral compared with single internal thoracic grafts.

Maniar H, Sundt T, Barner H, Prasad S, Peterson L, Absi T, *et al*. Impact of target stenosis and location on radial artery graft patency. *J Thorac Cardiovasc Surg* 2002; **123**:45–52.

The RA is being used as a Y-graft increasingly frequently with or without cardiopulmonary bypass. Maniar's group has confirmed the safety of anastomosing the RA to the side of the LITA. The high patency of the distal LITA and the proximal RA graft used in this fashion is confirmed. The authors draw attention to the high failure rate of the post-sequential anastomotic segment of the RA, particularly grafted to the right-sided vessels and in situations where there is competitive flow.

REFERENCES

1. Spencer FC, Yong NK, Prachuabmoh K. Internal mammary– coronary artery anastomosis performed during cardiopulmonary bypass. *J Cardiovasc Surg* 1964; **5**:292–7.
2. Goetz RH, Rohman M, Haller JD, Dee R, Rosanak SS. Internal mammary–coronary artery anastomosis – a nonsuture method employing tantalum rings. *J Thorac Cardiovasc Surg* 1961; **41**:378–86.
3. Longmire WP, Cannon JA, Kattus AA. Direct vision coronary endarterectomy for angina pectoris. *N Engl J Med* 1958; **259**:993–9.
4. Green GE, Spencer FC, Tice DA, Stertzer SH. Arterial and venous micro-surgical bypass grafts for coronary artery disease. *J Thorac Cardiovasc Surg* 1970; **60**:491–503.
5. Kolessov VI. Mammary artery coronary artery anastomosis as method of treatment for angina pectoris. *J Thorac Cardiovasc Surg* 1967; **54**:535–44.
6. De Jesus RA, Acland RD. Anatomic study of the collateral blood supply of the sternum. *Ann Thorac Surg* 1995; **59**:163–8.
7. Lytle BW. Skeletonized internal thoracic artery grafts and wound complications. *J Thorac Cardiovasc Surg* 2001; **121**:625–7.
8. Matsa M, Paz Y, Gurevitch J, Shapira I, Kramer A, Pevny D, *et al*. Bilateral skeletonized internal thoracic artery grafts in patients with diabetes mellitus. *J Thorac Cardiovasc Surg* 2001; **121**:668–74.
9. Noyez L, van Druten JA, Mulder J, Schroën A, Skotnicki SH, Brouwer RM. Sternal wound complications after primary isolated myocardial revascularization: the importance of the post-operative variables. *Eur J Cardiothorac Surg* 2001; **19**:471–6.
10. Casha A, Gauci M. Sternal vascularity after harvesting of the internal thoracic artery. *J Thorac Cardiovasc Surg* 2001; **121**:1219.
11. Ascione R, Underwood MJ, Lloyd CT, Jeremy JY, Bryan AJ, Angelini GD. Clinical and angiographic outcome of different surgical strategies of bilateral internal mammary artery grafting. *Ann Thorac Surg* 2001; **72**:959–65.
12. Lev-Ran O, Pevni D, Matsa M, Paz Y, Kramer A, Mohr R. Arterial myocardial revascularization with *in situ* crossover right internal thoracic artery to left anterior descending artery. *Ann Thorac Surg* 2001; **72**:798–803.
13. Buxton B, Knight S. Retrophrenic location of the internal mammary artery graft. *Ann Thorac Surg* 1990; **49**:1011–12.
14. Prifti E, Bonacchi M, Frati G. A graft with the radial artery or free left internal mammary artery anastomosed to the right internal mammary artery: flow dynamics. *Ann Thor Surg* 2001; **72**:1275–81.
15. Buxton BF, Ruengsakulrach P, Fuller J, Rosalion A, Reid CM, Tatoulis J. The right internal thoracic artery graft – benefits of grafting the left coronary system and native vessels with a high grade stenosis. *Eur J Cardiothorac Surg* 2000; **18**:255–61.
16. Ochi M, Hatori N, Fujii M, Yoshiaki S, Tanaka S, Honma H. Limited flow capacity of the right gastro-epiploic artery graft: postoperative echocardiographic and angiographic evaluation. *Ann Thorac Surg* 2001; **71**:1210–14.
17. Maniar H, Sundt T, Barner H, Prasad S, Peterson L, Absi T, *et al*. Impact of target stenosis and location on radial artery graft patency. *J Thorac Cardiovasc Surg* 2002; **123**:45–52.
18. Markwith T, Hennen B, Scheller B, Schäfers H-J, Wendler O. Flow wire measurements after complete arterial coronary revascularizatuion with T-grafts. *Ann Thorac Surg* 2001; **71**:788–93.
19. Vitolla G, Di Giammarco G, Teodori G, Mazzei V, Canosa C, Di Mauro M, *et al*. Composite lengthened arterial conduits: long-term angiographic results of an uncommon surgical strategy. *J Thorac Cardiovasc Surg* 2001; **122**:687–90.
20. Dion R, Glineur D, Derouck D, Verhelst R, Noirhomme P, El Khoury G, *et al*. Long-term clinical and angiographic follow-up of sequential internal thoracic artery grafting. *Eur J Cardiothorac Surg* 2000; **17**:407–14.
21. Lytle BW, Blackstone EH, Loop FD, Houghtaling P, Arnold J, Akhrass R, *et al*. Two internal thoracic artery grafts are better than one. *J Thorac Cardiovasc Surg* 1999; **117**:855–72.
22. Buxton BF, Komeda M, Fuller JA, Gordon I. Bilateral internal thoracic artery grafting may improve outcome of coronary artery surgery. Risk-adjusted survival. *Circulation* 1998; **98**(19 Suppl.):II1–6.
23. Calafiore AM, Contini M, Vitolla G, Di Mauro M, Mazzei V, Teodori G, *et al*. Bilateral internal thoracic artery grafting: long-term clinical and angiographic results of *in situ* versus Y-grafts. *J Thorac Cardiovasc Surg* 2000; **120**:990–6.
24. Carpentier A, Guermontrez JL, Deloche A, Frechette C, DuBost C. The aorta-to-coronary radial artery bypass graft: a technique avoiding pathological changes in grafts. *Ann Thorac Surg* 1973; **16**:111–21.
25. Curtis JJ, Stoney WS, Alford WC, Burrus GR, Thomas CS Jr. Intimal hyperplasia: a cause of radial artery aorto-coronary bypass graft failure. *Ann Thorac Surg* 1975; **20**:628–35.

26. Acar C, Jebara V, Portoghese M, Beyssen B, Pagny JY, Grare P, et al. Revival of the radial artery for coronary artery bypass grafting. Ann Thorac Surg 1992; 54:652–9.

27. Calafiore A, Teodori G, Di Giammarco G, D'Annunzio E, Angelini R, Vitolla G, et al. Coronary revascularization with the radial artery: new interest for an old conduit. J Card Surg 1995; 10:140–6.

28. Royse A, Royse C, Shah P, Williams A, Kaushik S, Tatoulis J. Radial artery harvest technique, use and functional outcome. Eur J Cardiothorac Surg 1999; 15:186–93.

29. Tatoulis J, Buxton BF, Fuller JA, Royse AG. The radial artery as a graft for coronary revascularization: techniques and follow-up. In: Advances in Cardiac Surgery, Vol. 11, Karp R, Lacks H, Weschler A (eds). St Louis, MI: Mosby, 1999, 99–128.

30. Fremes SE, Christakis GT, Del Rizzo DF, Musiani A, Mallidi H, Goldman BS. The technique of radial artery bypass grafting and early clinical results. J Card Surg 1995; 10:537–44.

31. Calafiore AM, Di Giammarco G, Teodori G, D'Annunzio E, Vitolla G, Fino C, et al. Radial artery and inferior epigastric artery in composite grafts: improved mid-term angiographic results. Ann Thorac Surg 1995; 60:517–24.

32. Brodman RF, Frame R, Camacho M, Hu E, Chen A, Hollinger I. Routine use of unilateral and bilateral radial arteries for coronary bypass graft surgery. J Am Coll Cardiol 1996; 28:959–63.

33. McCormack LJ, Cauldwell EW, Anson BJ. Brachial and antebrachial arterial patterns: a study of 750 extremities. Surg Gynecol Obstet 1953; 96:43–54.

34. Little JM, Zylstra PL, West J, May J. Circulatory patterns in the normal hand. Br J Surg 1973; 60:652–5.

35. Van Son JAM, Vincent JG, Van Lier HJ, Kubat K. Comparative anatomic studies of various arterial conduits for myocardial revascularization. J Thorac Cardiovasc Surg 1990; 99:703–7.

36. Kaufer E, Factor SM, Frame R, Brodman RF. Pathology of the radial and internal thoracic arteries used as coronary artery bypass grafts. Ann Thorac Surg 1997; 63:1118–22.

37. Buxton BF, Fuller JA, Gaer J, Liu JJ, Mee J, Sinclair R, et al. The radial artery as a bypass graft. Curr Opin Cardiol 1996; 11:591–8.

38. Acar C, Buxton BF, Notsworthy C, Eisenberg N, Liu JJ, Taggart D. Radial artery. In: Ischaemic heart disease. Surgical management, Buxton B, Frazier OH, Westaby S (eds). London: Mosby, 1999, 151–8.

39. Reyes AT, Frame R, Brodman RF. Technique for harvesting the radial artery as a coronary bypass graft. Ann Thorac Surg 1995; 59:118–26.

40. Chardigny C, Jebara VA, Acar C, Descombes JJ, Verbeuren TJ, Carpentier A, et al. Vaso-reactivity of the radial artery: comparison with the internal mammary and gastro-epiploic arteries, with implications for coronary artery surgery. Circulation 1993; 88:115–27.

41. He GW, Yang CQ. Radial artery has higher receptor mediated contractility, but similar endothelial function compared with mammary artery. Ann Thorac Surg 1997; 63:1346–52.

42. Cable DG, Caccitolo JA, Pearson PJ, O'Brien T, Mullany CJ, Daly RC, et al. Approaches to prevention and treatment of radial artery graft vasospasms. Circulation 1998; 98:15S–22S.

43. Tatoulis J, Buxton BF, Fuller JA. Bilateral radial artery grafts in coronary reconstruction: technique and early results in 261 patients. Ann Thorac Surg 1998; 66:714–19.

44. Tatoulis J, Buxton BF, Fuller JA. The radial artery in coronary re-operation. Eur J Cardiothorac Surg 2001; 19:266–73.

45. Sundt TM 3rd, Barner HB, Camillo CJ, Gay WA Jr. Total arterial revascularization with an internal thoracic artery and radial artery T-graft. Ann Thorac Surg 1999; 68:399–404.

46. Tatoulis J, Royse AG, Buxton BF, Fuller JA, Skillington PD, Goldblatt JG, et al. The radial artery in coronary surgery – a 5 year experience: clinical and angiographic results. Ann Thorac Surg 2002; 73:143–8.

47. Iaco AL, Teodori G, Di Giammarco G, Di Mauro M, Storto L, Mazzi V, et al. Radial artery for myocardial revascularization: long-term clinical and angiographic results. Ann Thorac Surg 2001; 72:464–9.

48. Meharwal ZS, Trehan N. Functional status of the hand after radial artery harvesting: results in 3977 cases. Ann Thorac Surg 2001; 72:1557–61.

49. Acar C, Ramsheyi A, Pagny JY, Jebara V, Barrier P, Fabiani J-N, et al. The radial artery for coronary artery bypass grafting: clinical and angiographic results at five years. J Thorac Cardiovasc Surg 1998; 116:981–9.

50. Dietl CA, Benoit CH. Radial artery graft for coronary revascularization. Ann Thorac Surg 1995; 60:102–10.

51. Chen AH, Nakao T, Brodman RF, Greenberg M, Charney R, Menegus M, et al. Early postoperative angiographic assessment of radial artery grafts used for coronary artery bypass grafting. J Thorac Cardiovasc Surg 1996; 111:1208–12.

52. Royse AG, Royse CF, Tatoulis J, Grigg LE, Shah P, Hunt D, et al. Postoperative radial artery angiography for coronary artery bypass surgery. Eur J Cardiothorac Surg 2000; 17:294–304.

53. Possati G, Gaudino M, Alessandrini F, Luciani N, Glieca F, Trani C, et al. Midterm clinical and angiographic results of radial artery grafts used for myocardial revascularization. J Thorac Cardiovasc Surg 1998; 116:1015–21.

54. Buxton BF, Chan AT, Dixit AS, Eizenberg N, Marshall RD, Raman JS. Ulnar artery as a coronary bypass graft. Ann Thorac Surg 1998; 65:1020–4.

55. Puig LB, Ciongolli W, Cividanes GVL, Dontos A, Kopel L, Bittencourt D, et al. Inferior epigastric artery as a free graft for myocardial revascularization. J Thorac Cardiovasc Surg 1990; 99:25–55.

56. Mills NL, Everson CT. Technique for use of the inferior epigastric artery as a coronary bypass graft. Ann Thorac Surg 1991; 51:208–14.

57. Buche M, Schroeder E, Gurné O, Chenu P, Paquay J-L, Marchandise B, et al. Coronary artery bypass grafting with the inferior epigastric artery: midterm clinical and angiographic results. J Thorac Cardiovasc Surg 1995; 109:553–60.

58. Bailey CP, Hirose T, Aventura A, Yamamoto N, Brancato R, Vera C, et al. Revascularization of the ischemic posterior myocardium. Dis Chest 1966; 52:273–85.

59. Pym J, Brown PM, Charrette EJP, Parker JO, West RO. Gastro-epiploic to coronary anastomosis: a viable alternative bypass graft. J Thorac Cardiovasc Surg 1987; 94:256–9.

60. Suma H, Fukumoto H, Takeuchi A. Coronary artery bypass grafting by using the in situ right gastro-epiploic artery: basic study and clinical application. Ann Thorac Surg 1987; 44:394–7.

61. Van Son JAM, Smeldts FM, Yang CQ, Mravunac M, Falk V, Mohr FW, et al. Morphometric study of the right gastro-epiploic and inferior epigastric arteries. Ann Thorac Surg 1997; 63:709–15.

62. Ochi M, Bessho R, Saji Y, Fujii M, Hatori N, Tanaka S. Sequential grafting of the right gastro-epiploic artery in coronary bypass surgery. Ann Thorac Surg 2001; 71:1205–9.

63. Suma H, Wanibuchi Y, Furuta S, Isshiki T, Yamaguchi T, Takanashi R. Comparative study between the gastro-epiploic and the internal thoracic artery as a coronary bypass graft. Size, flow, patency, histology. Eur J Cardiothorac Surg 1991; 5:244–7.

64. Lytle BW, Cosgrove DM, Ratliff NB, Loop FD. Coronary artery bypass grafting with the right gastro-epiploic artery. J Thorac Cardiovasc Surg 1989; 97:826–31.

65. Dietl CA, Deitrick JE, West JC, Pagana TJ. Laparotomy after using the gastro-epiploic artery graft: retrogastric versus antegastric route. Ann Thorac Surg 1995; 60:382–6.

66. Suma H, Wanibuchi Y, Terada Y, Fukuda S, Takayama T, Furuta S. The right gastro-epiploic artery graft: clinical and angiographic

mid-term results in 200 patients. *J Thorac Cardiovasc Surg* 1993; **105**:615–23.

67. Dietl CA, Benoit CH, Gilbert CL, Woods EL, Pharr WF, Berkheimer MD, *et al.* Which is the graft of choice for the right coronary artery and the posterior descending arteries? Comparison of the right internal mammary artery and the right gastro-epiploic artery. *Circulation* 1995; **92**(Suppl. 2):96–7.

68. Grandjean JG, Mariani MA, Ebels T. Coronary re-operation via small laparotomy using the right gastro-epiploic artery without cardiopulmonary bypass. *Ann Thorac Surg,* 1996; **61**:1853–5.

69. Sato T, Isomura T, Suma H, Horii T, Kikuchi N. Coronary artery bypass grafting with gastro-epiploic artery composite graft. *Ann Thorac Surg* 2000; **69**:65–9.

70. Quigley RL, Weiss SJ, Highbloom RY, Pym J. Creative arterial bypass grafting can be performed on the beating heart. *Ann Thorac Surg* 2001; **72**:793–7.

71. Pym J, Brown PM, Pearson M, Parker JO. Right gastro-epiploic to coronary artery bypass graft: the first decade of use. *Circulation* 1995; **92**:II45–9.

72. Jegaden O, Eker A, Montagna P, Ossette J, DeGevigney G, Finet G, *et al.* Risk and results of bypass grafting using bilateral internal mammary and right gastro-epiploic arteries. *Ann Thorac Surg* 1995; **59**:955–60.

73. Grandjean JG, Voors AA, Boonstra PW, den Heyer P, Ebels T. Exclusive use of arterial grafts in coronary artery bypass operations for three-vessel disease: use of both thoracic arteries and the gastro-epiploic artery in 256 consecutive patients. *J Thorac Cardiovasc Surg* 1996; **112**:935–42.

74. Suma H, Wanibuchi Y, Furuta S, Takeuchi A. Does use of gastro-epiploic artery graft increase surgical risk? *J Thorac Cardiovasc Surg* 1991; **101**:121–5.

75. Stamou SC, Pfister AJ, Dangas G. Beating heart versus conventional single vessel reoperative coronary bypass. *Ann Thorac Surg* 2000; **69**:728–31.

76. Suma H, Isomura T, Horii T, Sato T. Late angiographic results of using the right gastro-epiploic artery as a graft. *J Thorac Cardiovasc Surg* 2000; **120**:496–8.

77. Voutilainen S, Varkkala K, Jarvinen A, Keto P. Angiographic 5-year follow-up study of right gastro-epiploic artery grafts. *Ann Thorac Surg* 1996; **62**:501–5.

78. Broeders MA, Doevendans PA, Maessen JG, van Gorsel E, Oude Egbrink M, Daemen M, *et al.* The human internal thoracic artery releases more nitric oxide in response to vascular endothelial growth factor than the human saphenous vein. *J Thorac Cardiovasc Surg* 2001; **122**:305–9.

79. Black A, Guzik T, West N, Campbell K, Pillai R, Ratnatunga C, *et al.* Minimally invasive saphenous vein harvesting: effects on endothelial and smooth muscle function. *Ann Thorac Surg* 2001; **71**:1503–7.

80. Roubos N, Rosenfeldt FL, Richards SM, Conyers RA, Davis BB. Improved preservation of saphenous vein grafts by the use of glyceryl trinitrate-verapamil solution during harvesting. *Circulation* 1995; **92**(9):II31–6.

81. Rosenfeldt F, Meldrum-Hanna W, Raman J. Vein grafts. In: *Ischemic Heart Disease Surgical Management*, Buxton BF, Frazier OH, Westaby S (eds). London: Mosby International Ltd, 1999, 169–77.

17

The role of coronary endarterectomy

THORALF M SUNDT AND HENDRICK B BARNER

BACKGROUND

Within a decade of the introduction of cardiopulmonary bypass, coronary endarterectomy was developed as a direct surgical approach to relieving coronary occlusive disease. Early clinical successes were reported, with improvements in angina pectoris.[1–5] The newly developed techniques for coronary angiography were advocated for preoperative evaluation of candidates for the procedure,[4] and postoperatively demonstrated patency of endarterectomized vessels for up to 2 years.[5] The successful development of coronary artery bypass grafting (CABG), a more expeditious and straightforward procedure with reproducibly good results, relegated endarterectomy to a position of secondary importance. Although endarterectomy was shown to yield satisfactory late patency at low operative risk,[6,7] results were generally felt to be somewhat inferior to CABG to more distal targets. This view continues to be widely held today by others as well as ourselves. Still, endarterectomy has been championed by a cadre of loyal enthusiasts over the years, albeit as an adjunct to CABG for the preparation of a distal anastomotic site rather than as a means of restoring flow via the native circulation as originally described. In the 1980s, there was a resurgence of interest in the technique as surgeons were challenged to care for patients with increasingly extensive, diffuse, end-stage coronary atherosclerosis.[8] With no end to this trend in sight, coronary endarterectomy will probably continue to have a place in our surgical armamentarium for some years to come.

INDICATIONS

The majority of published reports and the bulk of clinical experience suggest at least modestly increased operative risk and decreased late graft patency with endarterectomy as compared with direct coronary bypass.[9–13] As a consequence, we agree with the notion that endarterectomy should be reserved for cases in which bypass to distal vessels of acceptable quality and at least 1.5 mm diameter is not otherwise possible. This is true even if multiple distal anastomoses are required, such as grafting the posterior descending and a postero-lateral branch rather than endarterectomy of the distal right coronary artery (RCA), or sequential anastomoses to several sites on the left anterior descending (LAD) above and below segmental disease.

Occasionally, however, the occlusive disease may be sufficiently diffuse that no satisfactory targets are apparent angiographically (typically in a young, insulin-dependent diabetic individual with hypercholesterolemia and disabling angina pectoris). The patient's operability may then be questioned. The choice of operation may be between extensive endarterectomy and transplantation. In the presence of well-preserved left ventricular function, we have advocated the former, with good results.[14]

In our experience, the issue is more often raised intra-operatively when angiography has under-represented the extent of the atherosclerotic disease and no soft site can be identified for arteriotomy or a vessel has been inadvertently opened in a diseased area. When a rigid calcific plaque is encountered, the adventitia may begin to separate itself from the core, presenting an endarterectomy plane. At this point the surgeon may choose to close the adventitia and attempt another site, or to extend the arteriotomy proximally and distally in the hope of encountering soft vessel wall (permitting the construction of an anastomosis spanning the plaque) while tacking the plaque back to the vessel wall, or to commit to endarterectomy. This choice is influenced by the quality and size of the vessel more distally and of the adjacent vessel wall. Often the more distal vessel is small or diseased. If the plaque appears segmental, an extended arteriotomy and long anastomosis is preferable. Frequently, however, the effort to find a soft site distally yields none, and endarterectomy is the only alternative to leaving the territory ungrafted.

TECHNIQUES

The success of the endarterectomy is dependent upon adequate relief of the obstruction of the branch vessels, not merely extraction of the central core, as Effler graphically illustrated with his analogy to the ineffectiveness of a snowplow that clears the roadway but obstructs each driveway in so doing.[4] Achieving such results demands meticulous technique and patience, as graft patency is contingent upon distal run-off. We therefore make provisions for retrograde delivery of cardioplegia if endarterectomy is anticipated. Distal endpoints of the endarterectomy core must be smoothly tapered or 'feathered' rather than fractured. The importance of such an endpoint was demonstrated angioscopically by Keogh and associates.[15] In their intraoperative study of 30 endarterectomized coronary vessels, 22 endpoints were well tapered and 8 were not. Of those vessels with poorly tapered cores, all had major intraluminal flaps, while only 6 of 21 evaluable vessels with well-tapered cores had flaps. If fracture occurs, therefore, a distal counter-incision must be made to extract the remaining core.

A variety of techniques for endarterectomy have been advocated, including the injection of cardioplegia solution[16] or forced carbon dioxide[17,18] in the plane between the adventitia and the atherosclerotic core. More commonly, manual eversion endarterectomy or open dissection via an extended arteriotomy has been advocated, and we have found these simple approaches to be satisfactory. The optimal technique is dependent upon the target vessel, as each has a different pattern of arborization.

Right coronary artery

In most series in the literature the RCA is the vessel most frequently endarterectomized. Its usual configuration at the crux with bifurcation into two relatively large branches – the posterior descending and the left ventricular branch of the right – makes it amenable in most circumstances to eversion endarterectomy. The disease here is also frequently localized to the region of the crux itself.

The technical aspects of right coronary endarterectomy are illustrated in Figure 17.1. The RCA may be entered at least 1 cm proximal to the crux, permitting the development of a circumferential plane before encountering any branches. The vessel is opened for a distance of approximately 1 cm. A fine coronary spatula is used to separate the core from the adventitia circumferentially. The core is then transected sharply at the heel of the arteriotomy such that there is no blind pouch. Gentle traction is applied to the core with DeBakey forceps or a mosquito clamp, while the spatula is used 180° opposite to push the distal vessel wall off the core. It is critical that the wall be pushed off the core rather than the core being pulled out of the vessel, as excessive traction on the core will cause it to fracture prematurely.

The core must be regrasped hand-over-hand as distally as possible to minimize the risk of fracture. Once the crux has been reached, each branch vessel must be endarterectomized separately, first the posterior descending artery and then the continuation of the right. The distal end should be tapered or 'feathered', indicating that the end of the plaque has been reached. If the core does fracture, an attempt to recover it should be made even if a counter-incision in the distal vessel is required. The remainder of the core can then be extracted and the arteriotomy closed primarily or, as is our preference, with a small vein patch. We have not used intraoperative angioscopy.

In contrast to some other authors,[19] we do not advocate retrograde endarterectomy of the proximal RCA. Run-off is critical to prevent thrombosis of the endarterectomized segment. Therefore, unless the entire vessel is opened sufficiently to permit antegrade flow via the native vessel, patency of the proximal segment is dependent upon adequate opening of the origins of the acute marginal vessels. This can be difficult to accomplish with certainty in a retrograde manner. We have had the experience of early thrombosis of such a segment, with resulting ventricular dysrhythmias and right ventricular dysfunction in a patient in whom occlusion of this segment was confirmed by postoperative angiography. Therefore, when there are acute marginal branches that we wish to open, we extend the arteriotomy proximally and access this portion of the core directly via an 'open' technique.

Left anterior descending

Early experience suggested that the risk associated with endarterectomy of the LAD was higher than that for the RCA.[11,20] This has not been our experience,[14] or that of

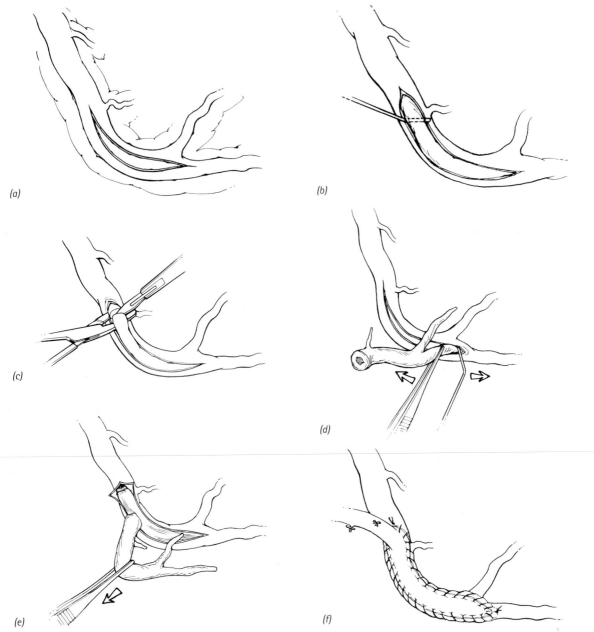

Figure 17.1 *Endarterectomy of the RCA is most often accomplished via an arteriotomy beginning at the acute margin 1 to 2 cm proximal to the crux (a). This permits a circumferential plane to be developed with an endarterectomy spatula before the posterior descending branch is encountered (b). The core can then be transected with a No.15 blade knife (c). Gentle traction is applied to the core with DeBakey forceps or a mosquito clamp while the vessel wall is pushed off the core with the spatula (d) – the core is not pulled out of the distal vessel.*

    Once the crux has been reached, each vessel is endarterectomized separately, taking care to obtain a complete specimen with a 'feathered' endpoint (e). The vessel wall is reconstructed by creating a long hood with the bypass conduit of saphenous vein, radial artery or internal thoracic artery (f).

authors of several other series.[12,21,22] We are, therefore, not reluctant to endarterectomize this vessel when we feel the alternatives are unappealing. Some authors have advocated endarterectomy of this vessel through a small arteriotomy.[23] However, because of the large number of diagonal and septal branches, many of which are small in diameter, we, like others,[12,22,24] are careful always to perform this endarterectomy 'open' via an extended

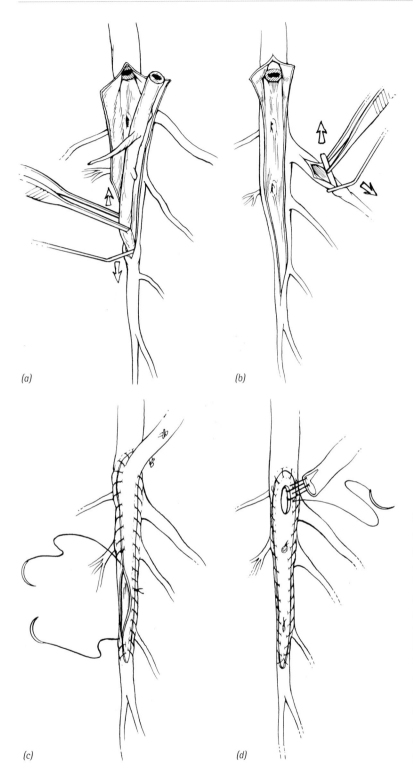

(a)

(b)

(c)

(d)

Figure 17.2 *In contrast to the 'closed' endarterectomy of the RCA, the LAD endarterectomy is performed 'open' via an arteriotomy, which may measure 6–8 cm in length. This permits careful extraction of core material from the origins of septal perforators and diagonal branches (a). If the core fractures prematurely, the arteriotomy must be extended or a counter-incision made in the distal vessel to re-grab the specimen, permitting completion of the endarterectomy (b). The vessel may be reconstructed with a long hood of saphenous vein or internal thoracic artery (c). Alternatively, a saphenous vein patch may be placed into which the internal thoracic artery graft is anastomosed (d).*

arteriotomy. This difference in technique may account, in part, for the differences in reported clinical results.

Figure 17.2 illustrates the important elements for successful endarterectomy of the LAD. If endarterectomy is anticipated, we open the vessel as far proximally as possible. If the vessel has been opened in its mid-portion

before it is apparent that endarterectomy is necessary, we extend the incision in the adventitia proximally before developing the endarterectomy plane. The removal of the core with its delicate branch vessels is always easier antegrade than retrograde because of the angle of their take-off. Once separated from the adventitia, the core is divided proximally at the heel of the arteriotomy. Distally the vessel is opened for 4–6 cm extending beyond the origins of the major diagonals, thereby permitting individual eversion endarterectomy of branch septals and diagonals. The eversion of the core from the distal LAD to the apex is usually possible. If the core fractures in a major diagonal, a separate arteriotomy to recover it is indicated. As mentioned above, such counter-incisions may be closed primarily or with a vein patch.

Circumflex coronary artery

The obtuse marginal branches of the circumflex coronary artery often arborize quickly into multiple branches, much like an oak tree. This makes eversion endarterectomy difficult, because it is impractical to follow each core, as is possible with the RCA. It also complicates open endarterectomy since there is often no central core to follow, as is the case for the LAD (Figure 17.3). The circumflex is, therefore, the most difficult, and consequently the least commonly endarterectomized, vessel in most series. We tend to begin by using an eversion technique to the extent possible, focusing our efforts on opening the largest distal branches. Unfortunately, the rapid branching pattern into small vessels makes it difficult to recover a fractured core.

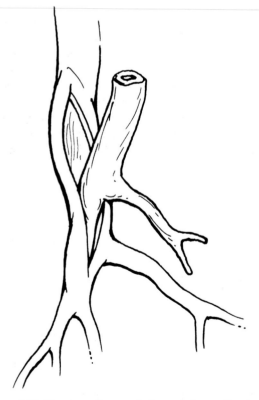

Figure 17.3 *The circumflex marginal vessels frequently arborize extensively, making satisfactory endarterectomy difficult.*

Reconstruction

Most commonly, the bypass conduit itself is opened sufficiently to restore vessel integrity with a long, onlay patch. We often start separate sutures at the heel and toe to hold the conduit in position as the mid-portion is closed expeditiously. It is our preference to place the internal thoracic artery (ITA) to the LAD, as has been previously advocated by others.[24–26] Use of an ITA has been associated with reduced operative risk and improved early and late patency.[25] We prefer to spatulate the ITA itself when grafting the LAD, although initial closure with a patch of saphenous vein into which the ITA may be sewn has been described.[27,28] This approach is particularly useful when the arteriotomy extends quite far proximally, making the angle of entry for the ITA awkward. Occasionally the right ITA will be used to reconstruct the endarterectomized RCA, although, more commonly, saphenous vein or radial artery is used to this target, as they are for reconstruction of the circumflex marginal.

PERIOPERATIVE CARE

Our experience supports the notion that the risk of ventricular arrhythmias is increased in this population.[14] We therefore routinely begin intravenous anti-arrhythmics (lidocaine) intraoperatively and continue them into the first postoperative day. Neither coumadin[20] nor platelet inhibitors[29] postoperatively have been shown to improve graft patency, but both are used by many authors, including ourselves. Based on experimental work in carotid endarterectomy,[30] we initiate intravenous heparin at low dose (500 units h^{-1}) 6–8 hours postoperatively, provided mediastinal tube output is acceptable. Oral coumadin is begun on the first day postoperatively and continued for 3 months. We have used aspirin, but no other antiplatelet agents. Antifibrinolytics and aprotinin are avoided intraoperatively if endarterectomy is anticipated, or discontinued when it becomes apparent that endarterectomy is necessary.

RESULTS

Perioperative risk

Most studies comparing the operative risk of patients undergoing endarterectomy and CABG with that of patients undergoing CABG alone indicate a somewhat higher risk for the endarterectomy group, although the difference usually fails to reach statistical significance (Table 17.1). At Washington University, of 177 patients undergoing single-vessel or multivessel endarterectomy, the operative mortality rate of 6% was not statistically different from the 4.5% for patients undergoing CABG alone during the same time interval. However, the trend for higher operative risk is present in most series, suggesting that this is a real phenomenon. It may simply reflect the more advanced disease of the patients requiring endarterectomy rather than an increased risk actually imposed by the procedure itself. Nonetheless, we adhere to the principle that primary grafting to more distal, non-diseased vessel is preferable when possible. It should be noted, however, that in their study of more than 1200 patients undergoing CABG, a quarter of whom had endarterectomy, Christakis and associates observed no increase in operative risk.[31]

There is some evidence to suggest that the perioperative mortality is increased when the LAD is endarterectomized as compared with the RCA.[11,32,33] Our experience has been contrary to this, as has that of other authors.[21,22,31] Among 52 patients undergoing endarterectomy of the LAD, we observed no perioperative deaths. We are, therefore, not reluctant to approach this vessel, although there is no doubt that it demands more patience and attention to detail. There was, however, a trend in our series towards higher perioperative mortality among those undergoing endarterectomy of the circumflex marginal system (17%) or multivessel endarterectomy (14%). Given the technical complexity of circumflex endarterectomy, we feel this increased risk may be reflective of an incomplete surgical result. Others have also observed an increased risk of mortality with multiple endarterectomy.[11,21,22]

The incidence of perioperative myocardial infarction is probably higher among endarterectomy patients (Table 17.1). This may be due to thrombosis of endarterectomized side branches or, possibly, the entire endarterectomized vessel in some cases. The incidence of this complication will be influenced dramatically by diagnostic criteria. Djalilian and Shumway have suggested that this risk is increased if the target vessel is not 100% occluded.[32] The risk of late infarction is also likely to be elevated somewhat among patients undergoing endarterectomy.[34]

Late clinical outcome: angina relief, ventricular function and survival

Initial angina relief has been excellent in most series, although the rate of recurrent angina may be somewhat higher than that after uncomplicated CABG. Walter and associates reported resolution or marked improvement in angina pectoris in 93% of patients following endarterectomy.[35] In our series, 27% of patients had recurrent angina at approximately 5 years after surgery.[14] Gill has reported a 15% incidence of recurrent angina at 36 ± 16 months,[26] and Christakis a 35% incidence at 5 years.[31] In contrast, only 9% of the patients studied by Djalilian and Shumway were experiencing angina at 46 ± 19 months.[32] The difficulty in evaluating this outcome, of course, is the accurate identification of the symptom as true angina pectoris. This problem is shared by all studies of revascularization techniques whether catheter based, utilizing laser technology or conventional surgery. Interestingly, the study by Minale and colleagues indicated that clinical improvement was unrelated to postoperative graft patency.[21]

The impact of endarterectomy on ventricular function is a matter of some dispute. Gill reported 'preservation' of anterior wall function after endarterectomy,[26] but Minale observed an equal chance of improvement or deterioration in regional wall function.[21] Unfortunately, it appeared that the better the contractility was preoperatively, the greater the deterioration postoperatively.[21] These authors therefore recommended that endarterectomy be reserved for walls with reduced contractility.

Table 17.1 *Outcome of coronary endarterectomy*

Authors	Mortality CABG + EA	CABG	Perioperative MI CABG + EA	CABG	Patient survival	Graft patency Early	Late
Brenowitz[22]	6.3% (n = 1255)	4.0% (n = 2504)	9.8%	5.6%	78.8% (5 years)	88.9%	71.7%
Asimakopoulos[44]	3.6% (n = 56)	0% (n = 56)	5.3%	0%	90% (4 years)		
Goldstein[36]	2% (n = 51)		8% (n = 51)			90%	64%
Beretta[25]	5.2% (n = 96)		6.3%				
Saphenous reconstruction (n = 50)					70% (5 years)	85%	67%
ITA reconstruction (n = 46)					87% (5 years)	93%	82%
Sundt[14]	6.2% (n = 177)	4.5% (n = 7096)	5.6%	3.0%	75% (5 years)		

CABG, coronary artery bypass grafting; EA, endarterectomy; ITA, internal thoracic artery; MI, myocardial infarction.

This has not been our practice, although we have not undertaken a rigorous study of regional wall motion in our patient population.

Despite the co-morbidities frequently present among the patients requiring endarterectomy, late survival has been encouraging as well. Patient survival at 5 years has been reported between 71%[32] and 90%.[31] Our results and those of others are consonant with these.[14]

Graft patency

It is likely that the patency of grafts to endarterectomized vessels is inferior to that of grafts to less diseased targets. As shown in Table 17.1, Beretta and colleagues[25] demonstrated patency of the ITA to the LAD at 90% when evaluated in the early postoperative period, falling to approximately 80% between 30 and 36 months postoperatively. Gill and co-workers[26] reported a 74% patency for the same reconstruction at 36 ± 16 months, while Goldstein et al.[36] observed a similar patency for 68 endarterectomy vessels among which RCA targets predominated. This patency fell to 65% at a mean of 19 months, with evidence of late fibrosis of the target vessels. While these patencies fall below those expected for primary CABG, they are sufficiently encouraging to warrant endarterectomy as an alternative to leaving the target region ungrafted. Furthermore, it is likely that comparison of graft patency in individuals whose disease is sufficiently severe as to require endarterectomy with non-endarterectomy patients with less severe disease is unfair. The recent findings from Ferraris and colleagues support this position: graft patency for 132 endarterectomized vessels was 40% at 7.1 years mean follow-up as compared with 58% for non-endarterectomized vessels in study patients, while graft patency was 65% among control, non-endarterectomy patients.[33] In this study, the only statistically significant risk factor for graft occlusion was lower body surface area.

CONTROVERSIES: ENDARTERECTOMY, TRANSMYOCARDIAL LASER REVASCULARIZATION OR ANGIOGENIC FACTOR THERAPY?

The recent development of new technologies such as transmyocardial laser revascularization (TMR) and the delivery of angiogenic growth factors provide other options for the treatment of diffusely diseased vascular beds. The results of clinical trials of TMR have been encouraging, at least with respect to the relief of angina pectoris.[37,38] There is mounting evidence to suggest at least some improvement in regional perfusion[39,40] and even regional wall motion[41] with this therapy. Unfortunately, there is also some evidence that angina may recur late after TMR.[42] Initial trials of angiogenic growth factors are beginning to be reported.[43] As the most frequently proposed mechanism of action of TMR is the stimulation of angiogenesis, however, it seems logical that this modality will supersede TMR once the appropriate factors have been identified. It is likely that at some point in the future these technologies will replace endarterectomy (if not all of coronary bypass surgery). Until that time, however, coronary endarterectomy will continue to play a small but significant role in the management of advanced coronary artery disease.

KEY REFERENCES

Asimakopoulos G, Taylor KM, Ratnatunga CP. Outcome of coronary endarterectomy: a case control study. *Ann Thorac Surg* 1999; **67**:989–93.
A study comparing clinical outcomes after coronary endarterectomy with a contemporary control group of patients having CABG surgery.

Beretta L, Lemma M, Vanelli P, DiMattia D, Bozzi G, Broso P, et al. Coronary 'open' endarterectomy and reconstruction: short- and long-term results of the revascularization with saphenous vein versus ITA-graft. *Eur J Cardiothorac Surg* 1992; **6**:382–7.
Focuses on the use of ITA grafts to revascularize endarterectomized vessels and the improved outcomes associated with this type of reconstruction.

Brenowitz JB, Kayser KL, Johnson WD. Results of coronary endarterectomy and reconstruction. *J Thorac Cardiovasc Surg* 1988; **95**:1–10.
A classic paper by pioneers in the development of this technique that reviews their experience with over 5000 patients undergoing surgery during a 10-year period.

Goldstein J, Cooper E, Saltups A, Boxall J. Angiographic assessment of graft patency after coronary endarterectomy. *J Thorac Cardiovasc Surg* 1991; **102**:539–45.

Ferraris VA, Harrah JD, Moritz DM, Striz M, Striz D, Ferraris SP. Long-term angiographic results of coronary endarterectomy. *Ann Thorac Surg* 2000; **69**:1737–43.
Two more recent papers that focus on short-term and long-term angiographic evaluation of endarterectomized vessels, respectively.

Sundt TM, Camillo CJ, Mendeloff EN, Barner HB, Gay WA. Reappraisal of coronary endarterectomy for the treatment of diffuse coronary artery disease. *Ann Thorac Surg* 1999; **68**:1272–7.
This review of the experience at Washington University discusses the clinical results of coronary endarterectomy as compared with novel techniques such as TMR, and attempts to

define the place of each in the management of end-stage coronary artery disease.

REFERENCES

1. Bailey CP, May A, Lemmon WM. Survival after coronary endarterectomy in man. *JAMA* 1957; **164**:641–6.

2. Longmire WP, Cannon JA, Kattus AA. Direct-vision coronary endarterectomy for angina pectoris. *N Engl J Med* 1958; **259**:993–9.

3. Senning A. Strip grafting in coronary arteries. Report of a case. *J Thorac Cardiovasc Surg* 1961; **41**:542–9.

4. Effler DB, Groves LK, Sones FM Jr, Shirley EK. Endarterectomy in the treatment of coronary artery disease. *J Thorac Cardiovasc Surg* 1961; **47**:98–108.

5. Hallen A, Bjork L, Bjork VO. Coronary thromboendarterectomy. *J Thorac Cardiovasc Surg* 1963; **45**:216–23.

6. Cheanvechai C, Groves LK, Reyes EA, Shirey EK, Sones FM Jr. Manual coronary endarterectomy. Clinical experience in 315 patients. *J Thorac Cardiovasc Surg* 1975; **70**:524–8.

7. Wallsh E, Franzone AJ, Clauss RH, Armellini C, Steichen F, Stertzer SH. Manual coronary endarterectomy with saphenous bypass: experience with 263 patients. *Ann Thorac Surg* 1981; **32**:451–7.

8. Loop FD. Resurgence of coronary endarterectomy. *J Am Coll Cardiol* 1988; **11**:712–13.

9. Keon WJ, Hendry P, Boyd WD, Walley VM. Long term follow-up of coronary endarterectomy. *Adv Cardiol* 1988; **36**:19–26.

10. Eschenbruch E, Tollenaere P, Gornandt L, Schmuziger M. Endarterectomy in coronary surgery. *Adv Cardiol* 1988; **36**:1–7.

11. Livesay JJ, Cooley DA, Hallman GL, Reul GJ, Ott DA, Duncan JM, *et al.* Early and late results of coronary endarterectomy. *J Thorac Cardiovasc Surg* 1986; **92**:649–60.

12. Quershi SA, Halim MA, Pillai R, Smith P, Yacoub MH. Endarterectomy of the left coronary system. Analysis of a 10 year experience. *J Thorac Cardiovasc Surg* 1985; **89**:852–9.

13. Hochberg MS, Merril WH, Michaelis LL, McIntosh CL. Results of combined coronary endarterectomy and coronary bypass for diffuse coronary artery disease. *J Thorac Cardiovasc Surg* 1978; **75**:38–46.

14. Sundt TM, Camillo CJ, Mendeloff EN, Barner HB, Gay WA. Reappraisal of coronary endarterectomy for the treatment of diffuse coronary artery disease. *Ann Thorac Surg* 1999; **68**:1272–7.

15. Keogh BE, Bidstrup BP, Taylor KM, Sapsford RN. Angioscopic evaluation of intravascular morphology after coronary endarterectomy. *Ann Thorac Surg* 1991; **52**:766–71.

16. Harrer J, Zacek P, Lonsky V, Dominik J, Brzek V Sr, Knap J, *et al.* Contribution to technique of endarterectomy of the right coronary artery. *Acta Med (Hradec Kralove)* 1996; **39**:155–8.

17. Barmada B, Detrich EB. Gas endarterectomy with distal bypass of the coronary arteries. *Heart Lung* 1975; **4**:397–401.

18. Urschel HC, Razzuk MA, Wood RE, Paulson DL. Distal CO_2 coronary endarterectomy and proximal vein bypass graft. *Ann Thorac Surg* 1972; **14**:10–15.

19. Mills NL. Coronary endarterectomy. *Adv Card Surg* 1998; **10**:197–227.

20. Ivert T, Welti R, Forsell G, Landou C. Coronary endarterectomy – angiographic and clinical results. *Scand J Thorac Cardiovasc Surg* 1989; **23**:95–102.

21. Minale C, Nikol S, Zander M, Uebis R, Effert S, Messmer BJ. Controversial aspects of coronary endarterectomy. *Ann Thorac Surg* 1989; **48**:235–41.

22. Brenowitz J, Kayser KL, Johnson WD. Results of coronary artery endarterectomy and reconstruction. *J Thorac Cardiovasc Surg* 1988; **95**:1–10.

23. Huysmans HA, Aytug Z, Buis B, Verwey H. Treatment of peripheral coronary artery disease by endarterectomy. *Adv Cardiol* 1988; **36**:13–18.

24. Harjola P-T, Harjula ALJ, Jarvinen A. Coronary bypass grafting with multiple coronary endarterectomies. *Adv Cardiol* 1988; **36**:8–12.

25. Beretta L, Lemma M, Vanelli P, DiMattia D, Bozzi G, Broso P, *et al.* Coronary 'open' endarterectomy and reconstruction: short- and long-term results of the revascularization with saphenous vein versus ima-graft. *Eur J Cardiothorac Surg* 1992; **6**:382–7.

26. Gill IS, Beanlands DS, Boyd WD, Finlay S, Keon WJ. Left anterior descending endarterectomy and internal thoracic artery bypass for diffuse coronary disease. *Ann Thorac Surg* 1998; **65**:659–62.

27. Fundaro P, Di Biasi P, Santoli C. Coronary endarterectomy combined with saphenous vein patch reconstruction and internal mammary artery grafting. *Tex Heart Inst J* 1987; **14**:389–94.

28. Ladowski JS, Schatzlein MH, Underhill DJ, Peterson AC. Endarterectomy, vein patch, and mammary bypass of the anterior descending artery. *Ann Thorac Surg* 1991; **52**:1187–9.

29. Limet R, David J-L, Magotteaux, Larock M-P, Rigo P. Prevention of aorta-coronary bypass graft occlusion. Beneficial effect of ticlopidine on early and late patency rates of venous coronary bypass grafts: a double-blind study. *J Thorac Cardiovasc Surg* 1987; **94**:773–83.

30. Dirrenberger RA, Sundt TM Jr. Carotid endarterectomy. Temporal profile of the healing process and effects of anticoagulation therapy. *J Neurosurg* 1978; **48**:201–19.

31. Christakis GT, Rao V, Fremes SE, Chen E, Naylor CD, Goldman BS. Does coronary endarterectomy adversely affect the results of bypass surgery? *J Card Surg* 1993; **8**:72–8.

32. Djalilian AR, Shumway SJ. Adjunctive coronary endarterectomy: improved safety in modern cardiac surgery. *Ann Thorac Surg* 1995; **60**:1749–54.

33. Ferraris VA, Harrah JD, Moritz DM, Striz M, Striz D, Ferraris SP. Long-term angiographic results of coronary endarterectomy. *Ann Thorac Surg* 2000; **69**:1737–43.

34. Abrahamov D, Tamaris M, Guru V, Fremes S, Christakis G, Bhatnagar G, *et al.* Clinical results of endarterectomy of the right and left anterior descending coronary arteries. *J Card Surg* 1999; **14**:16–25.

35. Walter PJ, Armbruster M, Amsel BJ, Scheld HH. Endarterectomy in patients with diffuse coronary artery disease. *Adv Cardiol* 1988; **36**:41–53.

36. Goldstein J, Cooper E, Saltups A, Boxall J. Angiographic assessment of graft patency after coronary endarterectomy. *J Thorac Cardiovasc Surg* 1991; **102**:539–45.

37. Burns SM, Sharples LD, Tait S, Caine N, Wallwork J, Schofield PM. The Transmyocardial Laser Revascularization International Registry Report. *Eur Heart J* 1999; **20**:31–7.

38. Landolfo CK, Landolfo KP, Hughes GC, Coleman ER, Coleman RB, Lowe JE. Intermediate-term clinical outcome following transmyocardial laser revascularization in patients with refractory angina pectoris. *Circulation* 1999; **100**(19 Suppl.):II128–33.

39. Horvath KA, Cohn LH, Cooley DA, Crew JR, Frazier OH, Griffith BP, *et al.* Transmyocardial laser revascularization: results of a multicenter trial with transmyocardial laser revascularization used as sole therapy for end-stage coronary artery disease. *J Thorac Cardiovasc Surg* 1997; **113**:645–53.

40. Frazier OH, Cooley DA, Kadipasaoglu KA, Pehlivanoglu S, Lindenmeir M, Barasch E, *et al.* Myocardial revascularization with laser. *Circulation* 1995; **92**(9 Suppl.):II58–65.

41. Hughes GC, Shah AS, Yin B, Shu M, Donovan CL, Glower DD, et al. Early postoperative changes in regional systolic and diastolic left ventricular function after transmyocardial laser revascularization: a comparison of holmium:YAG and CO_2 lasers. *J Am Coll Cardiol* 2000; **35**:1022–30.

42. Schneider J, Diegeler A, Krakor R, Walther T, Kluge R, Mohr FW. Transmyocardial laser revascularization with the holmium:YAG laser: loss of symptomatic improvement after 2 years. *Eur J Cardiothorac Surg* 2000; **19**:164–9.

43. Sellke FW, Laham RJ, Edelman ER, Pearlman JD, Simons M. Therapeutic angiogenesis with basic fibroblast growth factor: technique and early results. *Ann Thorac Surg* 1998; **65**:1540–4.

44. Asimakopoulos G, Taylor KM, Ratnatunga CP. Outcome of coronary endarterectomy: a case control study. *Ann Thorac Surg* 1999; **67**:989–93.

18

Management of the atherosclerotic ascending aorta

PAOLO MASETTI AND NICHOLAS T KOUCHOUKOS

THE PROBLEM

Despite important advances in the surgical treatment of coronary artery disease, postoperative neurological deficits remain a serious complication of operative procedures that involve coronary artery bypass grafting (CABG).[1,2] Important neurological injury occurs in up to 5–6% of patients who undergo CABG employing cardiopulmonary bypass (CPB).[1–3] Of the patients who sustain a major perioperative neurological injury, one-third die, and only about one-third of the survivors recover substantial neurological function.[4–6] Although there are multiple causes for these postoperative neurological deficits, atheroembolism associated with a severely atherosclerotic ascending aorta and aortic arch is widely recognized as the principal pathophysiological mechanism for the development of frank stroke, and may be responsible for other abnormalities such as impaired cognitive function.[1,7–11] In large clinical studies, ascending aortic atherosclerosis has been identified as an independent predictor of postoperative stroke.[1,5,10,12,13]

The prevalence and severity of ascending aortic and aortic arch atherosclerosis increase with increasing age of the patient.[11,13,14] In a prospective study of 1200 patients undergoing cardiac surgical procedures, 88% of whom had coronary artery disease, epi-aortic ultrasonography was used to detect the presence of ascending aortic atherosclerosis.[14] Moderate or severe atherosclerosis was present in 9% of the patients between 50 and 59 years of age, in 18% of the patients between 60 and 69 years, in 22% of those between 70 and 79 years, and in 33% of those 80 years of age and older. Since the mean age of patients undergoing CABG is steadily increasing,[11] the number of patients with aortic atherosclerosis has also increased, thus increasing the substrate of patients who are at risk for neurological injury from this condition.

Accurate detection of the presence of ascending aortic atherosclerosis is essential in order to minimize the occurrence of perioperative neurological injury from embolization of atherosclerotic debris following surgical myocardial revascularization. This will permit the formulation and evaluation of protocols to modify surgical techniques, so that embolization can be avoided.

METHODS FOR DETECTION

A number of diagnostic studies, both preoperative and intraoperative, have been used to detect the presence of atherosclerosis in the ascending aorta.

Chest radiography and cineangiography

The presence of calcification in the ascending aorta and the aortic arch that is noted on a chest radiograph or during cineangiography does not correlate with the presence of substantial atherosclerosis that can be detected by more sensitive methods such as intraoperative epi-aortic ultrasonography (see below).[14–16] In a series of 500 patients

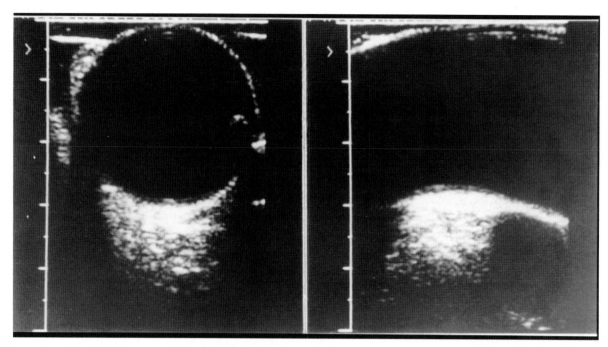

Figure 18.1 *Epi-aortic ultrasonographic images in transverse and longitudinal views of normal ascending aorta. Reproduced from Wareing et al.,[17] with permission from Harcourt Health Sciences.*

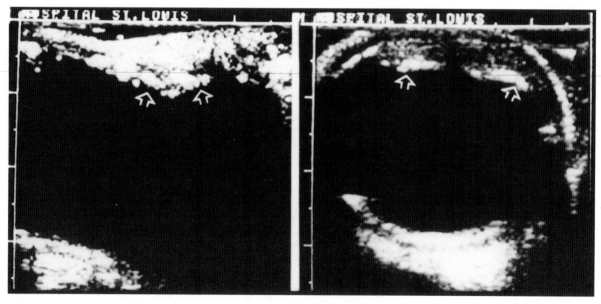

Figure 18.2 *Epi-aortic ultrasonographic images in longitudinal and transverse views of severe atherosclerosis in the ascending aorta. The arrows indicate areas of calcification and projection of atheroma into the lumen.*

evaluated intraoperatively with epi-aortic ultrasonographic scanning of the ascending aorta, we observed that among the 68 patients in whom severe atherosclerosis of the ascending aorta was detected by epi-aortic scanning, calcification was present in only 19% of the chest radiographs and in only 10% of the cineangiograms of these patients.[17] Calcification was present in both studies in only 4.4% of the patients.

Intraoperative inspection and palpation

Intraoperative evaluation of the ascending aorta begins with careful inspection. Discrete areas of discoloration and non-uniform distribution of the vasa vasorum on the surface of the aorta suggest the presence of severe atherosclerosis. Direct palpation identifies only firm atheromatous plaque.[14,18,19] More often, the atheromatous

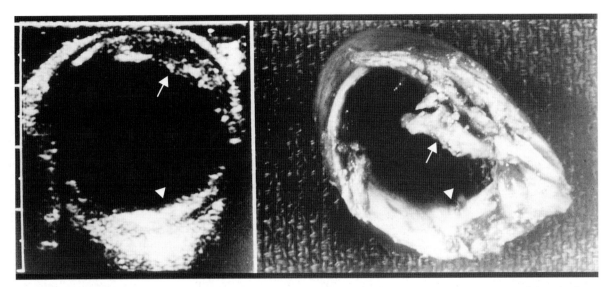

Figure 18.3 *Transverse epi-aortic ultrasonographic image of the ascending aorta and the corresponding segment of the aorta in a patient with severe atherosclerosis. Note the calcification (triangles) and the projection of atheroma (arrows) into the lumen. Reproduced by permission from Wareing et al.[17]*

lesions that are prone to embolization are soft in consistency. In this setting, vigorous palpation may result in dislodgement of atheromatous material from the wall of the aorta. For this reason, palpation should be done gently or, preferably, avoided altogether. In the series of Wareing and associates,[17] palpation of the aorta identified sites with substantial atheromatous changes in only 38% of the 68 patients with severe atherosclerosis that were detected by epi-aortic scanning. Furthermore, the sites identified by palpation did not correlate completely with the sites identified by ultrasonography.

Transthoracic echocardiography

Preoperative transthoracic echocardiography (TTE) has been used to evaluate the ascending aorta prior to cardiac surgical procedures, but does not consistently provide useful information. One retrospective study using TTE correctly identified atherosclerosis of the sino-tubular area of the ascending aorta in 60 patients, but could not define the structural details of the plaques.[20] In another study of 20 patients, comparing TTE and transesophageal echocardiography (TEE), the TTE findings compared favorably with those by TEE in the distal ascending aorta and aortic arch, but not in the proximal ascending aorta.[21]

Transesophageal echocardiography

Transesophageal echocardiography is currently widely used during cardiac surgical procedures and provides important information to the surgeon.[18,22] Although TEE can accurately detect the presence of severe atherosclerosis in

the aortic arch and the descending thoracic aorta, it is far less sensitive than direct epi-aortic scanning for identifying disease in the ascending aorta.[10,23,24] An important limitation of TEE is that the distal ascending aorta, the area that is usually cannulated and clamped during CABG procedures, and thus is most susceptible to dislodgement and embolization of atheroma, cannot be adequately visualized because of interference from the column of air in the trachea and the major bronchi that is positioned between the aorta and the ultrasonographic probe in the esophagus.[22,23,25] Nevertheless, TEE is currently widely used for the intraoperative detection of aortic atherosclerosis in cardiac surgical patients.[24,26]

Intraoperative epi-aortic ultrasonographic imaging

Direct intraoperative epi-aortic ultrasonographic imaging using a surface probe is a sensitive, rapid and safe technique for the detection of atherosclerotic changes in the entire ascending aorta and the proximal aortic arch (Figures 18.1, 18.2 and 18.3).[27,28] In comparative studies against TEE, it has been shown to be a more accurate method for the detection of ascending aortic atherosclerosis (Tables 18.1 and 18.2).[23,29,30] Because the epi-aortic transducer has a higher frequency (7 MHz) than the TEE transducer (5 MHz) that is used for biplane studies, and because attenuation of the ultrasound wave is eliminated by placing the transducer directly over the aorta, image resolution is optimized. With epi-aortic imaging, multiple views of the entire ascending aorta and proximal aortic arch can be obtained, whereas with biplane TEE only a thin

Table 18.1 *Comparison of transesophageal versus epi-aortic scanning in 44 patients having cardiac surgical procedures*[a]

	Proximal ascending aorta (n = 44)	Distal ascending aorta (n = 44)	Both segments (n = 88)
TEE findings more severe	2 (5%)	2 (5%)	4 (5%)
Agreement between TEE and epi-aortic ultrasound	25 (57%)	13 (30%)	38 (43%)
Epi-aortic ultrasound findings more severe	17 (39%)	29 (66%)	46 (52%)
P value	0.0006	<0.0001	<0.00001

[a]84% of patients underwent CABG.
TEE, transesophageal echocardiography; CABG, coronary artery bypass grafting.
Data presented are number (%) of segments.
Reprinted from Davila-Roman and colleagues,[23] with permission from the American College of Cardiology.

Table 18.2 *Detection of severe atheroma in 28 subjects (38 segments): comparison of palpation, TEE and epi-aortic imaging*[a]

Technique	Number of segments	P value (versus linear array)
Palpation	2	<0.0001
TEE	3	<0.0001
Epi-aortic imaging (phased array)	35	NS
Epi-aortic imaging (linear array)	36	

[a]90% of patients underwent CABG.
CABG, coronary artery bypass grafting; TEE, transesophageal echocardiography.
Reprinted from Sylivris and colleagues,[29] with permission from WB Saunders.

Table 18.3 *A classification for ascending aortic atherosclerosis using ultrasonic epi-aortic imaging*

Severity of atherosclerosis	Criteria
None	Normal aortic image in transversal and longitudinal planes
Mild	Focal intimal thickening <3 mm in height, no calcification
Moderate	Diffuse intimal thickening 3–5 mm in height, with or without calcification
Severe	Diffuse intimal thickening >5 mm in height, sessile, mobile or protruding atheroma, circumferential involvement with or without calcification

Reprinted from Wareing et al.,[17] with permission from Harcourt Health Sciences.

slice of the ascending aorta is seen in the longitudinal plane.[23,26]

CLASSIFICATION OF AORTIC ATHEROSCLEROSIS

Several classifications of the severity of atherosclerosis in the ascending aorta have been proposed. These have involved inspection and palpation of the aorta,[15,16,31] use of TEE,[26,32] and use of ultrasonographic epi-aortic imaging.[14,23,33] Since ultrasonographic epi-aortic imaging is currently the most accurate method for the detection of ascending aortic atherosclerosis, we favor and utilize this classification (Table 18.3). Examples of some of the degrees of aortic atherosclerosis are shown in Figures 18.1, 18.2 and 18.3.

STRATEGIES FOR MANAGEMENT

During CABG procedures, dislodgement of atheromatous material from an atherosclerotic aorta can occur at the time of insertion of the cannula into the ascending aorta for CPB,[34,35] from the effect of the jet of blood from the aortic cannula on the opposite wall of the aorta ('sandblast effect'),[36–38] when the aortic occlusion or partially occluding clamps are applied and released, and when needles or cannulas are inserted into the ascending aorta for venting or for delivery of cardioplegic solution.[34] Vigorous palpation or other manipulation of a severely atherosclerotic aorta, particularly if it is shown to contain soft atheromatous material, should be avoided, since this may result in dislodgement of atheromatous material.

Patients with normal aortas or with only mild atherosclerotic disease detected by epi-aortic imaging can undergo a standard CABG procedure with little if any risk of neurological injury;[17] thus, modifications in operative technique are not necessary. In patients in whom moderate or severe ascending aortic atherosclerosis is present, modifications in the conventional operative techniques should be made whenever possible, to reduce or eliminate the possibility for embolization.

A number of options for modification of the operative procedure have been utilized, and they are summarized in Table 18.4.

Table 18.4 *Surgical options for management of the moderately or severely atherosclerotic ascending aorta*

Modifications in technique
Arterial cannulation for CABG
  Alternative aortic site – ascending aorta or aortic arch
  Femoral or external iliac artery
  Axillary artery
  Innominate artery
Aortic clamping (CPB or OPCAB)
  Alternative site on ascending aorta (CPB or OPCAB)
  No aortic clamping
  – Hypothermic ventricular fibrillation (CPB)
  – Beating-heart CABG with pedicled grafts (OPCAB)
Proximal graft anastomoses
  Use of aortic cross-clamp only (CPB)
  Attachment to IMA graft (CPB or OPCAB)
  Attachment to innominate, subclavian or axillary artery (CPB or OPCAB)
  Use of only pedicled grafts (IMA, RGEPA) (CPB or OPCAB)
  Attachment to aortic graft patch (CPB or OPCAB)

Direct management of the atherosclerotic ascending aorta
Aortic endarterectomy with hypothermic circulatory arrest
Graft replacement of ascending aorta with hypothermic circulatory arrest

CABG, coronary artery bypass grafting; CPB, cardiopulmonary bypass; OPCAB, off-pump coronary artery bypass grafting; IMA, internal mammary artery; RGEPA, right gastroepiploic artery.

Implementation of one or more of these techniques is advisable, because previous studies have shown that failure to implement modifications in technique in patients with severe aortic atherosclerosis undergoing CABG is associated with a high prevalence of neurological injury.[4,10,14,17] Many of these modifications can be easily implemented with little or no risk to the patient. They are designed to avoid dislodgement of atherosclerotic material. Other modifications are more complex, and they involve removal of the atherosclerotic disease by endarterectomy or removal and replacement of the ascending aorta.

Modifications in technique

ARTERIAL CANNULATION FOR CARDIOPULMONARY BYPASS

If the CABG procedure is performed with CPB, and if the usual site for aortic cannulation is diseased, alternative sites can be used. These include the distal aortic arch, the common femoral or external iliac artery, the axillary artery or the innominate artery.[14,17,39–41] If the distal aortic arch is used, the tip of the aortic cannula should be positioned at or distal to the origin of the left subclavian artery,

so that if atheromatous material is dislodged by a sandblast effect, it will be directed into the descending thoracic aorta. If intraoperative TEE demonstrates moderate or severe atherosclerosis in the aortic arch or the descending thoracic aorta, the arch should not be cannulated. Femoral or external iliac artery cannulation should be avoided if intraoperative TEE demonstrates severe atherosclerosis in the descending aorta, so that retrograde embolization of atheromatous material into the brachiocephalic arteries is avoided. Femoral or external iliac artery cannulation should also be avoided if there are severe atherosclerotic changes at the site of proposed cannulation, or if an abdominal aortic aneurysm is present. In these situations, cannulation of the axillary artery is an appropriate alternative.[41]

AORTIC CLAMPING

If the usual site for aortic clamping is diseased, the clamp can be applied at alternative sites that are free of atheroma, as determined by epi-aortic scanning. Commonly, the very proximal portion of the ascending aorta just above the valve is free of atheromatous disease when the most distal portion is diseased. If no disease is present, the clamp can be applied easily and safely in this position. If this is done, it is often not possible to infuse cardioplegic solution into the aortic root, and thus cardioplegic solution must be retrogradely infused into the coronary sinus. If aortic clamping is not possible, the CABG procedure can be performed using hypothermic ventricular fibrillation, which does not require clamping of the ascending aorta.[42] Another alternative is to perform the procedure without CPB.[43,44]

SITE OF PROXIMAL CORONARY GRAFT ANASTOMOSES

Whether the CABG procedure is performed with or without CPB, a partially occluding clamp is commonly placed on the ascending aorta to perform the proximal anastomoses to vein grafts or other conduits. This may not be possible or safe if the aorta is severely diseased. If, using CPB, the more distal ascending aorta has been occluded with a clamp, the proximal anastomoses can be performed with the heart arrested. Even when moderate or severe atherosclerosis is present in the distal half of the ascending aorta, the proximal half may be free of important disease, and this area of the aorta can sometimes be used for performance of the proximal anastomoses. If, with or without the use of CPB, the grafts cannot be attached to the ascending aorta, they can be attached to the internal mammary artery graft,[15] to the innominate artery,[45] or to the distal subclavian or proximal axillary artery.[46,47] Occasionally it may be possible to use only pedicled grafts, with one or both internal mammary arteries and the gastro-epiploic artery.[48] If, when using CPB, the atherosclerosis is confined to the anterior half of the ascending aorta, this portion of the aorta can be resected and replaced with a portion of graft or a patch of bovine pericardium.[49] The vein grafts or other conduits can then be anastomosed to the aortic patch graft. When using CPB, it may not be possible to occlude the ascending aorta with a clamp or to place a partially occluding clamp on it. If there is a segment of the ascending aorta that is free of important atherosclerosis to which one or more grafts could be attached, the technique of hypothermic fibrillation with venting of the heart through the right superior pulmonary vein can be used.[42] While the distal coronary graft anastomoses are being completed, systemic cooling is continued to a nasopharyngeal temperature of 16–18 °C. Perfusion flow is reduced to almost zero, and one or more openings are made in the ascending aorta with a standard punch. With gentle aspiration of blood away from these openings, the proximal anastomoses to the grafts can be completed. Perfusion flow is then increased, rewarming is begun and, when complete, CPB is discontinued.[33]

Direct management of the ascending aorta

If the ascending aortic atherosclerosis is severe, and especially if there is protruding atheroma, repair or replacement of the diseased aortic segment may be advisable to prevent embolization of the atheroma. This can be accomplished by aortic endarterectomy, or by resection and graft replacement of all or a part of the ascending aorta and, when indicated, the adjacent aortic arch.

AORTIC ENDARTERECTOMY

Endarterectomy of the ascending aorta and the aortic arch, with removal of the intimal layer and a portion of the media during an interval of hypothermic circulatory arrest, has been used as a method to prevent stroke during and after cardiac operations.[50–54] Satisfactory early results were reported by Koul and colleagues in 10 patients,[51] by Svensson and colleagues in 6 patients,[53] and by Vogt and colleagues in 22 patients,[54] all of whom had severe calcification of the ascending aorta. Follow-up studies of the aorta were only obtained by Vogt and colleagues.[54] After a mean follow-up of 21.5 months, no increase in the diameter of the aorta was observed by magnetic resonance imaging or TTE studies. The results from a large series of 268 patients with protruding or mobile atheromas in the aortic arch reported by Stern and colleagues were disappointing.[52] Among the 43 patients in this series who underwent endarterectomy to remove the atheroma, the prevalence of postoperative stroke was 34.9%, while among the remaining patients the stroke rate was 11.6% ($P < 0.001$). By multivariate analysis, older age (odds

ratio 3.9, $P = 0.01$) and arch endarterectomy (odds ratio 3.6, $P = 0.001$) were independently predictive of postoperative stroke.

When extensive endarterectomy of the intimal and medial layers is performed, the potential for progressive dilatation of the endarterectomized aorta and recurrence of atherosclerosis remains. Occasionally, solitary, sessile or pedunculated masses of atheroma that are surrounded by normal or minimally diseased aorta can be safely removed at the time of CABG or valve replacement using a short interval of hypothermic circulatory arrest.[19]

REPLACEMENT OF THE ATHEROSCLEROTIC AORTA

An alternative method of management of the severely atherosclerotic aorta is resection of the diseased segment and replacement with a polyester graft during an interval of hypothermic circulatory arrest. We favor this approach when multiple areas of severe atherosclerosis or circumferential disease are present, when there is extensive involvement of the distal half of the ascending aorta, and when extensive protruding atheroma is present in the ascending aorta or the aortic arch. During an 11-year period, 81 patients (mean age 71 years) who underwent CABG were found by epi-aortic scanning to have severe aortic atherosclerosis. This represented approximately 2% of the patients over the age of 50 years who underwent operation during this period. Eighty of the patients had complete (75) or partial (5) replacement of the ascending aorta with a polyester graft. One patient had resection of a solitary protruding atheroma. In addition to total or partial ascending aortic replacement, 34 of these patients had replacement of all or a part of the aortic arch, 19 had valve replacement, and six had carotid endarterectomy.[19] The 30-day mortality was 8.6% (seven patients). Four patients (4.9%) sustained perioperative strokes, and two (2.5%) had transient ischemic neurological deficits. Gillinov and colleagues have also reported an experience with hypothermic circulatory arrest for the management of 62 patients with severe atherosclerosis of the ascending aorta who underwent aortic valve replacement.[55] Several different strategies were used to manage the ascending aorta. These included aortic valve replacement during a single period of circulatory arrest, ascending aortic endarterectomy, ascending aortic replacement, aortic inspection and clamping during the arrest interval, and balloon occlusion of the ascending aorta. The hospital mortality was 14%, and 10% of the patients sustained a stroke. The choice of operative technique (all operations were performed with an interval of circulatory arrest) did not influence patient outcome. However, no patient who underwent aortic replacement sustained a stroke. King and colleagues have reported less satisfactory results with ascending aortic replacement in patients undergoing elective CABG.[56] Among 17 patients who had tube graft replacement during an interval of hypothermic circulatory arrest, the hospital mortality was 24%, and 18% of the patients sustained a stroke.

EMERGING STRATEGIES

Intra-aortic filtration

During cardiac operations performed with CPB, substantial numbers of emboli, both gaseous and particulate, may be released following release of the aortic occlusion clamps.[34,57] An intra-aortic filter has been developed (EMBOL-X©Inc., Mountain View, CA) that is attached to the aortic perfusion cannula and is deployed in the aorta just proximal to the cannula before release of the aortic clamp (Figure 18.4). This filter has a pore size of 120 μm and has been designed to capture particulate emboli that may be generated during the procedures. There is the potential for atheromatous debris to be dislodged by the filter during deployment. In a study by Reichenspurner and colleagues[58] evaluating this cannula in 77 patients, 74% of whom underwent CABG, visual inspection of the filter showed granular particles or soft material in 74 (96%) of the 77 filters (Figure 18.5). Histologic evaluation of 44 of the filters demonstrated fibrous atheroma or fibrous cap in 29 (66%), platelet-fibrin aggregates in 16 (36%), thrombus or blood clot in 11 (25%), and normal vessel wall, grumous plaque-cholesterol and hyaline cartilage in five of the filters. None of the 77 patients sustained a stroke. A similar filter has been developed for use during off-pump CABG. A prospective, randomized, multicenter clinical trial is currently underway to assess the effectiveness of the filter in reducing the prevalence of neurological dysfunction after isolated CABG and isolated valve replacement procedures.

Pre-bypass and post-bypass epi-aortic scanning

Ura and colleagues have performed epi-aortic ultrasonographic scanning before and after cannulation in 472 patients having cardiac operations with CPB.[59] Seventy-four percent of the patients had CABG procedures. New lesions in the intimal layer of the ascending aorta were identified in 16 (3.4%) of the 472 patients. The maximal thickness of the aorta was a predictor of the development of new lesions, which were severe in 10 patients with mobile atheroma or disruption of the intima. The new lesions were attributed to aortic clamping in six patients, and to aortic cannulation in the remaining four patients. Three of the 16 patients with new lesions sustained a postoperative stroke. In the entire series, arteriosclerosis obliterans, atherosclerosis of the aorta, and new mobile lesions were identified as predictors of stroke. This important study suggests that the creation of new lesions in the aorta, even in those without demonstrable atherosclerosis, may be an important cause of postoperative neurological injury, and that modifications in the design of the aortic cannulas and clamps and in surgical technique may prevent the creation of new lesions.

Off-pump coronary artery bypass grafting (OPCAB)

Because CPB, aortic cannulation and, in some instances, aortic clamping are not utilized during OPCAB procedures, it has been hypothesized that the risks of neurological

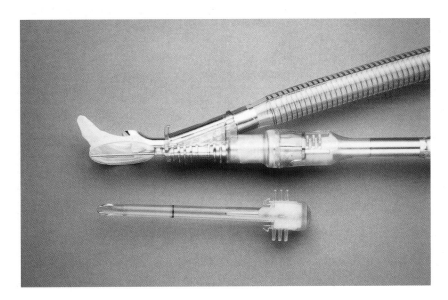

Figure 18.4 *Intra-aortic filtration system consisting of a 24 F arterial cannula and a 120 μm filter that is extruded into the aortic lumen (EMBOL-X©).*

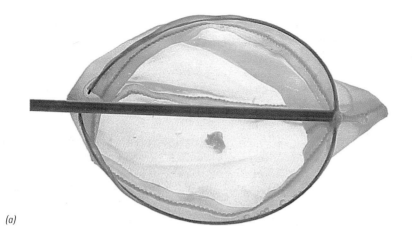

(a)

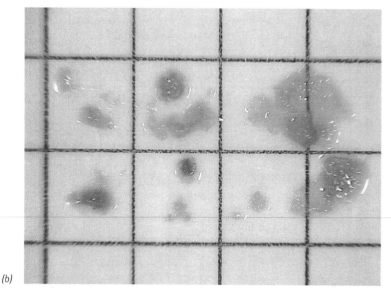

(b)

Figure 18.5 *(a) Grossly visible atheromatous debris removed from the ascending aorta with the intra-aortic filter. (b) Debris in the filter visible with magnification after removal from the ascending aorta. The distance between the horizontal and vertical grid lines is 3 mm.*

injury, both from focal neurological deficits and from neurocognitive dysfunction, would be lower than when CPB is used, primarily because the risk of embolization of atherosclerotic debris would be reduced. Although this hypothesis may be correct, it remains unproven at the present time. Large, prospective, randomized, blinded clinical trials that systematically assess neurological outcome in truly comparable patients undergoing CABG procedures with or without the use of CPB are required before it can be concluded that CPB is an independent risk factor for neurological injury.[60]

CONCLUSIONS

Ideally, the presence of moderate or severe ascending aortic atherosclerosis should be detected preoperatively in patients who are to undergo CABG. This would permit a more accurate assessment of operative risk, and proper planning or even avoidance of the proposed operative procedure. Unfortunately, this is not possible for the majority of patients. Transesophageal echocardiography, which can be performed preoperatively, is not routinely utilized in patients with coronary artery disease, and lacks the sensitivity for the diagnosis of ascending aortic atherosclerosis that can be obtained with intraoperative epi-aortic ultrasonography. Epi-aortic scanning is currently the most reliable technique for the diagnosis of ascending aortic disease. At the present time, no single maneuver or intervention has proven entirely effective for the intraoperative management of the atherosclerotic ascending aorta. Thus, the treatment of this disorder must be individualized.

In many instances, relatively simple modifications in technique, based upon the accurate identification and location of the atherosclerotic disease, can be implemented that should prevent dislodgement and embolization of atherosclerotic debris. In patients with severe disease, more aggressive measures may be necessary, but they may be associated with increased operative risk.

Critical, ongoing assessment of the outcomes following operations in patients with atherosclerosis of the ascending aorta is essential, so that optimal strategies for management can be formulated that will reduce the prevalence of neurological and other organ system injury following CABG.

KEY REFERENCES

The problem

Amarenco P, Cohen A, Tzourio C, Bertrand B, Hommel M, Besson G, *et al.* Atherosclerotic disease of the aortic arch and the risk of ischemic stroke. *N Engl J Med* 1994; **331**:1474–9.

In this study of 250 patients with ischemic stroke who underwent TEE, a strong, independent association between atherosclerotic disease of the aortic arch and the risk of ischemic stroke was identified.

Blauth CI, Cosgrove DM, Webb BW, Ratliff NB, Boylan M, Piedmonte MR, *et al.* Atheroembolism from the ascending aorta. An emerging problem in cardiac surgery. *J Thorac Cardiovasc Surg* 1992; **103**:1104–12.

This landmark study documented, in patients dying after cardiac operations, a high correlation between atheroembolism to the brain and other organs and the presence of severe atherosclerosis in the ascending aorta. Atheroemboli were more common in patients undergoing coronary artery procedures than in those undergoing valve procedures.

Methods for detection

Wareing TH, Davila-Roman VG, Barzilai B, Murphy SF, Kouchoukos NT. Management of the severely atherosclerotic ascending aorta during cardiac operations. A strategy for detection and treatment. *J Thorac Cardiovasc Surg* 1992; **103**:453–62.

Using epi-aortic ultrasonographic imaging in 500 patients undergoing cardiac surgical procedures, the authors describe a classification for ascending aortic atherosclerosis and an algorithm for management of the atherosclerotic aorta based upon the ultrasonographic findings.

Emerging strategies

Reichenspurner H, Navia JA, Berry G, Robbins RC, Barbut D, Gold JP, *et al.* Particulate emboli capture by an intra-aortic filter device during cardiac surgery. *J Thorac Cardiovasc Surg* 2000; **119**:233–41.

Using an intra-aortic filter attached to an aortic perfusion cannula in patients undergoing cardiac operations with CPB, the authors captured atheromatous material, platelet-fibrin, thrombus or clot, aggregates of cholesterol or grumous

atheroma, or normal aortic wall in 96% of the 77 patients in whom the filter was used.

Ura M, Sakata R, Nakayama Y, Miyamoto TA, Goto T. Extracorporeal circulation before and after ultrasonographic evaluation of the ascending aorta. *Ann Thorac Surg* 1999; **67**:478–83.

Using intraoperative epi-aortic ultrasonographic imaging of the ascending aorta before and after cardiac operations employing CPB, the authors identified new intimal lesions resulting from clamping or cannulation of the aorta in 10 (5.3%) of 188 patients. Three of the 10 patients sustained a stroke. Only 2 (1.1%) of the 178 patients in whom no new intimal changes were observed sustained a stroke.

REFERENCES

1. Roach WR, Kanchuger M, Mangano CM, Newman M, Nussmeier N, Wolman R, *et al.* Adverse cerebral outcomes after coronary bypass surgery. *N Engl J Med* 1996; **335**:1857–63.
2. Wolman RL, Nussmeier NA, Aggarwal A, Kanchuger MS, Roach GW, Newman MF, *et al.* Cerebral injury after cardiac surgery. Identification of a group at extraordinary risk. *Stroke* 1999; **30**:514–22.
3. Cronin L, Shamit RM, Zhao F, Pogue J, Budaj A, Hunt D, *et al.* for the OASIS Investigators. Stroke in relation to cardiac procedures in patients with non-ST-elevation acute coronary syndrome. A study involving >18000 patients. *Circulation* 2001; **104**:269–74.
4. Mills SA. Risk factors for cerebral injury in cardiac surgery. *Ann Thorac Surg* 1995; **59**:1296–9.
5. Gardner TJ, Horneffer PJ, Manolio TA, Pearson TA, Gott VL, Baumgartner WA, *et al.* Stroke following coronary artery bypass grafting: a ten-year study. *Ann Thorac Surg* 1985; **40**:574–81.
6. Mills SA. Cerebral injury and cardiac operations. *Ann Thorac Surg* 1993; **56**:S86–91.
7. Amarenco P, Cohen A, Tzourio C, Bertrand B, Hommel M, Besson G, *et al.* Atherosclerotic disease of the aortic arch and the risk of ischemic stroke. *N Engl J Med* 1994; **331**:1474–9.
8. Amarenco P, Duyckaerts C, Tzourio C, Henin D, Bousser MG, Hauw JJ. The prevalence of ulcerated plaques in the aortic arch in patients with stroke. *N Engl J Med* 1992; **326**:221–5.
9. Atherosclerotic disease of the aortic arch as a risk factor for recurrent ischemic stroke. The French study of aortic plaques in stroke group. *N Engl J Med* 1996; **334**:1216–21.
10. Hartman GS, Yao FS, Bruefach M 3rd, Barbut D, Peterson JC, Purcell MH, *et al.* Severity of aortic atheromatous disease diagnosed by transesophageal echocardiography predicts stroke and other outcomes associated with coronary artery surgery: a prospective study. *Anesth Analg* 1996; **83**:701–8.
11. Blauth CI, Cosgrove DM, Webb BW, Ratliff NB, Boylan M, Piedmonte MR, *et al.* Atheroembolism from the ascending aorta. An emerging problem in cardiac surgery. *J Thorac Cardiovasc Surg* 1992; **103**:1104–12.
12. Davila-Roman VG, Barzilai B, Wareing TH, Murphy SF, Schechtman KB, Kouchoukos NT. Atherosclerosis of the ascending aorta. Prevalence and role as an independent predictor of cerebrovascular events in cardiac patients. *Stroke* 1994; **25**:2010–16.
13. Davila-Roman VG, Murphy SF, Nickerson NJ, Kouchoukos NT, Schechtman KB, Barzilai B. Atherosclerosis of the ascending aorta

is an independent predictor of long-term neurologic events and mortality. *J Am Coll Cardiol* 1999; 33:1308–16.

14. Wareing TH, Davila-Roman VG, Daily BB, Murphy SF, Schechman KB, Barzilai B, *et al.* Strategy for the reduction of stroke incidence in cardiac surgical patients. *Ann Thorac Surg* 1993; 55:1400–8.

15. Mills NL, Everson CT. Atherosclerosis of the ascending aorta and coronary artery bypass. Pathology, clinical correlates, and operative management. *J Thorac Cardiovasc Surg* 1991; 102:546–53.

16. Bonatti J. Ascending aortic atherosclerosis. A complex and challenging problem for the cardiac surgeon. *Heart Surg Forum* 1999; 2:125–35.

17. Wareing TH, Davila-Roman VG, Barzilai B, Murphy SF, Kouchoukos NT. Management of the severely atherosclerotic ascending aorta during cardiac operations. A strategy for detection and treatment. *J Thorac Cardiovasc Surg* 1992; 103:453–62.

18. Tunick PA, Krinsky GA, Lee VS, Kronzon I. Diagnostic imaging of thoracic aortic atherosclerosis. *Am J Radiol* 2000; 174:1119–25.

19. Rokkas CK, Kouchoukos NT. Surgical management of the severely atherosclerotic ascending aorta during cardiac operations. *Semin Thorac Cardiovasc Surg* 1998; 10:240–6.

20. Barasch E, Kaushik V, Ahn C. Aortic sinotubular atherosclerotic debris associated with cerebral embolic events can be identified by transthoracic echocardiography. *Cardiology* 1998; 90:253–7.

21. Weinberger J, Azhar S, Danisi F, Hayes R, Goldman M. A new noninvasive technique for imaging atherosclerotic plaque in the aortic arch of stroke patients by transcutaneous real-time B-mode ultrasonography. *Stroke* 1998; 29:673–6.

22. Bryan AJ, Barzilai B, Kouchoukos NT. Transesophageal echocardiography and adult cardiac operations. *Ann Thorac Surg* 1995; 59:773–9.

23. Davila-Roman VG, Phillips KJ, Daily BB, Davila RM, Kouchoukos NT, Barzilai B. Intraoperative transesophageal echocardiography and epiaortic ultrasound for assessment of atherosclerosis of the thoracic aorta. *J Am Coll Cardiol* 1996; 28:942–7.

24. Mishra M, Chauhan R, Sharma KK, Dhar A, Bhise M, Dhole S, *et al.* Real-time intraoperative transesophageal echocardiography. How useful? Experience in 5016 cases. *J Cardiothorac Vasc Anesth* 1998; 12:625–32.

25. Konstadt SN, Reich DL, Quintana C, Levy M. The ascending aorta: how much does transesophageal echocardiography see? *Anesth Analg* 1994; 78:240–4.

26. Ribakove GH, Katz ES, Galloway AC, Grossi EA, Esposito RA, Baumann G, *et al.* Surgical implications of transesophageal echocardiography to grade the atheromatous aortic arch. *Ann Thorac Surg* 1992; 53:758–63.

27. Beique FA, Joffe D, Tousignant G, Konstadt S. Echocardiography-based assessment and management of atherosclerotic disease of the thoracic aorta. *J Cardiothorac Vasc Anesth* 1998; 12:206–20.

28. Nicolosi AC, Aggarwal A, Almassi H, Olinger GN. Intraoperative epiaortic ultrasound during cardiac surgery. *J Card Surg* 1996; 11:49–55.

29. Sylivris S, Calafiore P, Matalanis G, Rosalion A, Yuen HP, Buxton BF, *et al.* The intraoperative assessment of ascending aortic atheroma: epiaortic imaging is superior to both transesophageal echocardiography and direct palpation. *J Cardiothorac Vasc Anesth* 1997; 11:704–7.

30. Grigore AM, Grocott HP. Pro: epiaortic scanning is routinely necessary for cardiac surgery. *J Cardiothorac Vasc Anesth* 2000; 14:87–90.

31. Landymore R, Spencer F, Colvin S, Culliford A, Trehan N, Cartier P, *et al.* Management of the calcified aorta during myocardial revascularization. *J Thorac Cardiovasc Surg* 1982; 84:455–6.

32. Choudhary SK, Bhan A, Sharma R, Reddy SCB, Airan B, Narang S, *et al.* Aortic atherosclerosis and perioperative stroke in patients undergoing coronary artery bypass: role of intra-operative transesophageal echocardiography. *Int J Cardiol* 1997; 61:31–8.

33. Kouchoukos NT, Wareing TH, Daily BB, Murphy SF. Management of the severely atherosclerotic aorta during cardiac operations. *J Card Surg* 1994; 9:490–4.

34. Barbut D, Yao FS, Hager DN, Kavanaugh P, Trifiletti RR, Gold JP. Comparison of transcranial Doppler ultrasonography and transesophageal echocardiography to monitor emboli during coronary artery bypass surgery. *Stroke* 1996; 27:87–90.

35. Brown WR, Moody DM, Challa VR, Stump DA, Hammon JW. Longer duration of cardiopulmonary bypass is associated with greater numbers of cerebral microemboli. *Stroke* 2000; 31:707–13.

36. Grossi EA, Kanchuger MS, Schwartz DS, McLoughlin DE, LeBoutillier M, Ribakove GH, *et al.* Effect of cannula length on aortic arch flow: protection of the atheromatous aortic arch. *Ann Thorac Surg* 1995; 59:710–12.

37. Benarola M, Baker AJ, Mazer D, Erretti L. Effect of aortic cannula characteristics and blood velocity on transcranial Doppler-detected microemboli during cardiopulmonary bypass. *J Cardiothorac Vasc Anesth* 1998; 12:265–9.

38. Mullges W, Franke D, Reents W, Babin-Ebell J. Brain microembolic counts during extracorporeal circulation depend on aortic cannula position. *Ultrasound Med Biol* 2001; 27:933–6.

39. Rokkas CK, Kouchoukos NT. The severely atherosclerotic ascending aorta: detection and surgical options. *ACC Current Journal Review* 1999; 8 Dec:33–6.

40. Sabik JF, Lytle BW, McCarthy PM, Cosgrove DM. Axillary artery: an alternative site of arterial cannulation for patients with extensive aortic and peripheral vascular disease. *J Thorac Cardiovasc Surg* 1995; 109:885–91.

41. Baribeau YR, Westbrook BM, Charlesworth DC, Maloney CT. Arterial inflow via an axillary artery graft for the severely atheromatous aorta. *Ann Thorac Surg* 1998; 66:33–7.

42. Akins CW. Hypothermic fibrillatory arrest for coronary artery bypass grafting. *J Card Surg* 1992; 7:342–7.

43. Murkin JM, Boyd WD, Ganapathy S, Adams SJ, Peterson RC. Beating heart surgery: why expect less central nervous system morbidity? *Ann Thorac Surg* 1999; 68:1498–501.

44. Bonatti J, Hangler H, Oturanlar D, Posch L, Muller LC, Voelckel W, *et al.* Beating heart axillocoronary bypass for management of the untouchable ascending aorta in coronary artery bypass grafting. *Eur J Cardiothorac Surg* 1999; 16(Suppl. II):II18–23.

45. Ricci M, Karamanoukian HL, Jajkowski MR, D'Ancona G, Bergsland J, Salerno TA. The innominate artery as an inflow site in coronary reoperations without cardiopulmonary bypass. *Ann Thorac Surg* 2000; 69:1606–8.

46. Suma H. Innominate and subclavian arteries as an inflow of free arterial graft. *Ann Thorac Surg* 1996; 62:1865–6 .

47. Bonatti J, Coulson AS, Bakhshay SA, Posch L, Sloan TJ. The subclavian and axillary arteries as inflow vessels for coronary artery bypass grafts: combined experience from three cardiac surgery centers. *Heart Surg Forum* 2000; 3:307–11.

48. Nishida H, Tomizawa Y, Endo M, Koyanagi H, Kasanuku H. Coronary artery bypass with only *in situ* bilateral internal thoracic arteries and right gastroepiploic artery. *Circulation* 2001; 104(Suppl. I):I76–80.

49. Robicsek F, Rubenstein RB. Calcification and thickening of the aortic wall complicating aortocoronary grafting: a technical modification. *Ann Thorac Surg* 1980; 29:84–5.

50. Culliford TA, Colvin SB, Rohrer K, Baumann FG, Spencer FC. As originally published in 1986. The atherosclerotic ascending aorta and transverse arch: a new technique to prevent cerebral injury during bypass: experience with 13 patients. *Ann Thorac Surg* 1994; 57:1051–2.

51. Koul B, Wierup P, Englund E, Lundin A. Radical endarterectomy of severely calcified ascending aorta prevents stroke during open heart surgery. *Scand Cardiovasc J* 1997; **31**:33–7.

52. Stern A, Tunick PA, Culliford AT, Lachmann J, Baumann FG, Kanchuger MS, *et al*. Protruding aortic arch atheromas: risk of stroke during heart surgery with and without aortic arch endarterectomy. *Am Heart J* 1999; **138**:746–52.

53. Svensson LG, Sun J, Cruz HA, Shahian DM. Endarterectomy for calcified porcelain aorta associated with aortic valve stenosis. *Ann Thorac Surg* 1996; **61**:149–52.

54. Vogt PR, Hauser M, Schwarz U, Jenni R, Lachat ML, Zund G, *et al*. Complete thromboendarterectomy of the calcified ascending aorta and aortic arch. *Ann Thorac Surg* 1999; **67**:457–61.

55. Gillinov AM, Lytle BW, Hoang V, Cosgrove DM, Banbury MK, McCarthy PM, *et al*. The atherosclerotic aorta at aortic valve replacement: surgical strategies and results. *J Thorac Cardiovasc Surg* 2000; **120**:957–65.

56. King RC, Kanithanon RC, Shockey KS, Spotnitz WD, Tribble CG, Kron IL. Replacing the atherosclerotic ascending aorta is a high-risk procedure. *Ann Thorac Surg* 1998; **66**:396–401.

57. Barbut D, Hinton RB, Szatrowski TP, Hartman GS, Bruefach M, Williams-Russo P, *et al*. Cerebral emboli detected during bypass surgery are associated with clamp removal. *Stroke* 1994; **25**:2398–402.

58. Reichenspurner H, Navia JA, Berry G, Robbins RC, Barbut D, Gold JP, *et al*. Particulate emboli capture by an intra-aortic filter device during cardiac surgery. *J Thorac Cardiovasc Surg* 2000; **119**:233–41.

59. Ura M, Sakata R, Nakayama Y, Miyamoto TA, Goto T. Extracorporeal circulation before and after ultrasonographic evaluation of the ascending aorta. *Ann Thorac Surg* 1999; **67**:478–83.

60. Stump DA, Rorie KD, Jones TJJ. Does off-pump coronary artery bypass surgery reduce the risk of brain injury? *Heart Surg Forum* 2001; **4**(Suppl. I):S14–18.

19

Repeat coronary surgery

MICHAEL M MADANI AND STUART W JAMIESON

INTRODUCTION

With the knowledge that coronary disease is progressive in nature, and that coronary bypass conduits, especially veins,[1] are prone to disease, it is only to be anticipated that symptoms will recur following surgery, and the need for repeat intervention will arise.[2] The need for re-intervention becomes commoner in the second decade after initial operation. Sergeant's group report 89% freedom from re-intervention at 10 years, and 72% freedom at 15 years.[3]

Despite the growth in percutaneous coronary interventions (PCI), which are increasingly being applied to patients who would have been erstwhile candidates for coronary artery bypass grafting (CABG), coronary surgery remains one of the commonest operative procedures (in 2000, 314 000 CABG procedures were performed in the USA).[4] The Society of Thoracic Surgeons (STS) database documents a peak in the level of redo coronary surgery in 1992/93 at 10% of CABG reported by its contributing centers, dropping to 8% in 1995 and to 7% by the year 2000.[5] This decrease can be attributed to several factors, among them the use of PCI for re-intervention,[6,7] as well as improvements in preventative strategies. It is likely that those patients who *are* referred for repeat surgery will have more risk factors[8,9] and suboptimal distal vasculature and target vessels.

Repeat CABG imposes a morbidity and mortality that is greater than that of the initial operation.[8,10,11] Data from the STS database suggest an odds ratio for operative mortality of just over 2 for redo coronary surgery.[5]

Although the long-term results following repeat coronary surgery are encouraging,[10,12] the need for urgent surgery, unstable angina, poor left ventricular function and an interval of less than 1 year between initial operation and repeat operation have all been identified as important, independent risk factors for hospital mortality.[8]

Repeat operations pose difficulties not encountered with first-time operations. Generally, reoperation candidates are older and have more advanced coronary disease and more co-morbidity. Reopening of the sternotomy wound carries risks. Patent, diseased vein grafts pose a risk of atheroembolism. Adhesions make it more difficult to gain access to the heart and aorta, and are a source of bleeding. The coronary targets are likely to be smaller and more diseased, and the best conduits have often been used for the first operation, leaving a restricted choice of less satisfactory conduit. In the presence of previous aortocoronary grafts, the ascending aorta may offer little space for siting new conduits. In this chapter we discuss causes of recurrent angina, the techniques of redo coronary surgery, including re-sternotomy, myocardial protection, conduit availability, and the results and outcome of repeat surgery.

CAUSES OF RECURRENT ANGINA AND RISK FACTORS

Recurrent angina may be due to graft failure, either early or late, progression of disease, either in grafted or ungrafted vessels, incomplete primary operation, or a combination of all of these factors. Graft failure is the major cause of recurrent angina and can occur early or late. [10,12] Early graft failure is generally thrombotic in nature. By and large, this failure occurs within 10 days of operation and may be due to technical complications, such as graft kinking, suboptimal vein graft quality, the vein being too large, too small or varicose, or poor distal cardiac vasculature with a resultant low flow through the graft.[2] The use of arterial grafts should reduce the risk of late conduit occlusion; this has long been shown to be so for the internal thoracic artery as a conduit to the anterior descending artery.[13,14] Late vein graft failure is generally due to a form of progressive fibrosis, with fibromuscular intimal proliferation and eventually atheromatous plaque formation within the vessel wall. Increased vein graft patency can be obtained by careful surgical handling at the time of operation and the use of antiplatelet agents.[2]

In addition to failure of the grafts, recurrence of angina may be the result of progression of disease in the native vasculature, either in ungrafted vessels because of insignificant disease at the time of the original operation, or in grafted vessels. Though the incidence of this can be reduced with the avoidance of known risk factors (such as smoking or obesity) and the use of antiplatelet and statin therapy, current preventative measures will not eradicate the problem.

Recurrence of angina occurs earlier in those having their first operation at a young age, this being a reflection of the more aggressive and ruthless nature of the atherosclerosis that develops early in life. Early recurrence of angina is also seen in those who had inadequate initial revascularization, and in those patients with diffuse disease and small vessels. Included in the latter group are diabetic patients and those with hyperlipidemia.

PREOPERATIVE CONSIDERATIONS

The improving outcome and the potential for full rehabilitation in patients with recurrent angina warrant invasive investigation. The surgeon will probably not be the first port of call for most patients experiencing return of angina. If investigations indicate graft stenosis or progression of native disease, the interventional cardiologist will undertake PCI in many cases. Surgeons nowadays are usually presented with a pre-selected group of patients for whom PCI may not be feasible.

It has been shown that late survival and relief of angina following re-operation can rival that after first-time CABG. As with first-time candidates for CABG, investigations will indicate the appropriateness of surgery as well as the risk imposed by any co-morbidity or state of left ventricular function. It is of particular

importance to demonstrate that the internal mammary artery is patent and disease free in those patients in whom it was not used as a conduit at first CABG. Unrecorded damage to the artery at first operation, and injury from sternal wires, are occasional pitfalls. Where there is a previously placed functioning internal thoracic artery conduit, an effort should be made to assess its anatomical position relative to the sternum (e.g. from an angiogram or from a lateral chest x-ray, using the metal clips on the graft as a guide to its course).

Assessment of the coronary vasculature, as with first-time surgery, is aimed at identification of suitable target vessels supplying viable myocardium (the basic principles of bypass surgery still apply). However, candidates for repeat surgery, in general, have more extensive disease, which may not represent the best surgical prospect. In this case, judgment is required about the likely success of endarterectomy in creating suitable targets. Conversely, it should also be borne in mind that PCI may be a more acceptable treatment option (avoiding the operative hazards of repeat surgery), and less than full revascularization by this method may produce a good outcome. The danger of thromboembolism and atheroembolism from dilating stenoses in patent grafts is well recognized,[15] but not an absolute contraindication. Similarly, left ventricular function may often be severely impaired and in some patients may be of an extent that precludes 'conventional' revascularization alone. Left ventricular reconstruction combined with coronary surgery, and at times with mitral valve repair (the 'Dor procedure'), may have a role in some of these patients. Exceptionally, transplantation may be an option.

TECHNICAL CONSIDERATIONS

The principles of anesthetic technique and monitoring are no different for repeat surgery. All patients have a pulmonary artery catheter, and almost all our patients have a transesophageal echocardiogram throughout the procedure. It is important that both groins are prepared and draped and readily available for urgent access to the femoral vessels if needed, but it is unnecessary to expose or cannulate them prophylactically. External defibrillating paddles should be positioned appropriately on the patient's chest and back. The use of aprotinin (Trasylol) is advantageous in redo coronary operations.[16]

Repeat sternotomy

Repeat sternotomy can be performed safely with adequate preparation and careful planning.[17–19] The outer table of the sternum is divided with an oscillating saw, and the inner table with heavy scissors, beginning at the xiphoid process. Adhesions to the underlying surface of the sternum are divided with electrocautery at a low setting. An extra few minutes spent here greatly increases the safety of the operation. Some authors have advocated the addition of thoracoscopic substernal visualization as an aid to risk reduction.[20,21]

Dissection of the heart and cardiopulmonary bypass

The right atrium, ascending aorta and anterior ventricular surface are exposed with electrocautery. There is no place for blunt dissection. The innominate vein should be freed from the undersurface of the sternum to prevent its avulsion when the sternum is retracted.

We perform most of the dissection with electrocautery; this increases visualization and reduces bleeding from raw surfaces. It is important to avoid excessive dissection around patent grafts and particularly to avoid mobilizing these until bypass has been fully established. The risk of embolism from patent and diseased grafts is ever present,[10,12] and surgery is safer if all grafts have closed. If the internal mammary artery is to be used, it is dissected free early during mobilization.

The aorta and the right side of the heart are dissected free first. Cardiopulmonary bypass should be initiated as soon as dissection about the heart on the left side can no longer be carried out without undue traction and hemodynamic compromise, as dissection and visibility are greatly enhanced once ventilation has been discontinued and the heart emptied of blood. A pulmonary artery vent is inserted as soon as bypass is initiated. An empty beating heart makes identification of the dissection planes easier, and allows the heart to fall away from the pericardium on the left side. Early institution of bypass and decompression of the heart also allows the avoidance of excessive manipulation with distension of the ventricles, and makes undue handling of patent grafts less likely. After bypass has been initiated, previously placed grafts are dissected free and the heart entirely mobilized. It has been suggested that the distal end of patent and diseased grafts should be ligated early in the course of the dissection.[10,12] As the success of this maneuver will depend upon the status of the collateral circulation and the myocardium perfused by the ligated grafts, we feel that it is probably not necessary to do this provided that care is taken to avoid manipulation of patent grafts and the aorta during the dissection and exposure.

With the wide use of the left internal thoracic artery as a pedicled graft to the left anterior descending artery because of its superior patency rate, it is not uncommon to perform a second operation on a patient with a patent and disease-free internal thoracic artery graft. This

provides a challenge for the surgeon. This is particularly true when this vessel supplies a large territory, and on occasion may be the only disease-free blood supply that sustains the heart. Careful dissection and approach to this vessel concentrate on isolating it free from the surrounding adhesions and tissues, so that it can be gently occluded during the aortic cross-clamp time. Once the patient is on cardiopulmonary bypass, with the heart decompressed, the left internal thoracic artery can be isolated with careful and meticulous dissection. We have found it quite helpful first to dissect out the apex of the heart while on bypass, and then continue the dissection in a retrograde fashion towards the base of the heart over the anterior surface to identify the site of the anastomosis, and then work back to free up the pedicle circumferentially. Depending on the severity of the disease, the number of grafts required and the sites of the anastomoses, it may be unnecessary, or on occasion unsafe, to dissect out the left side of the heart for the sole purpose of isolating the internal thoracic artery graft. In these rare situations, an option would be to cool the systemic temperature further and perform the distal anastomosis with fibrillatory arrest, leaving the left internal thoracic artery pedicle intact and undissected.

The aorta is now cross-clamped. Our preference is to use a single dose of cold crystalloid cardioplegia solution infused into the aortic root, followed by the continued placement of topical cold saline for myocardial protection. The internal thoracic artery is also occluded with a non-traumatizing bulldog clamp. The grafts are now divided, and all distal anastomoses are then constructed during a single aortic cross-clamp interval. Others have advocated the use of retrograde cardioplegic solution, the rationale being that atheromatous debris may be flushed away from the coronary vasculature, provided the grafts are divided.

Placement of grafts

The optimal site for the insertion of a new graft is immediately distal to the previous distal anastomosis (Figure 19.1). This aids in the identification of the artery, and provides a good margin for sutures in the superior part of the anastomosis (Figure 19.2). The identification of non-grafted vessels can be difficult at the time of surgery if they are embedded in epicardial adhesions, or if the reason they were not grafted at the original operation was that they could not be identified within muscle or fat. Knowledge of the angiograms will generally allow the identification of these vessels.

It is important to replace grafts, rather than to attempt to endarterectomize these vessels or to merely replace a segment. If a sequential graft is to be constructed, the largest artery should be selected for the most distal

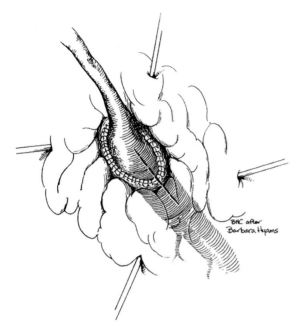

Figure 19.1 *The optimal site for re-implantation is over the distal end of a previously placed graft.*

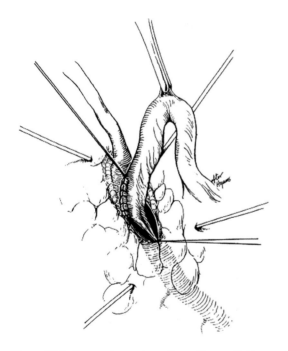

Figure 19.2 *The previous vein graft provides a suitable margin for anastomosis of the superior segment to the new conduit.*

anastomosis. This maximizes the flow through the graft, with the greatest possibility for long-term patency. Suitable sites for sequential grafting are left anterior descending–diagonal-diagonal, obtuse marginal–obtuse

marginal, obtuse marginal–posterior descending or right, or posterior descending–obtuse marginal. In every case the largest vessel should be the most distal target, and the venotomy for intermediate targets is always made longitudinally. The venotomy should be small, and is sewn to a longitudinal arteriotomy. Whether the anastomosis is made in parallel or at right angles depends upon the vessel: an obtuse marginal or posterior descending intervening anastomosis is made at right angles, whereas the diagonal or right is made in parallel. In addition to increasing patency rates, sequential coronary artery grafts have the advantage that less vein and only one proximal anastomosis are required.

A patent but stenotic internal thoracic artery can be re-used in several different ways. In most circumstances, the stenotic lesion is the site of the anastomosis, at which point this can be disconnected and a re-anastomosis can be performed elsewhere. Alternatively, a jump-graft using either a venous or an arterial conduit can be performed from the internal thoracic artery to an appropriate site either distally or to a different coronary branch.

Once the distal anastomoses have been completed, the aortic cross-clamp and the internal thoracic artery clamp are released and the proximal anastomoses are performed. These are performed using partial occluding clamps and may be more difficult because of inadequate areas for implantation of the vein into the aorta or severe and diffuse disease of the ascending aorta. The proximal anastomosis is generally conveniently made into the site of the previous vein graft, after removing previous venous material. If insufficient vein is available for grafting, the proximal anastomosis may be placed into another vein graft. Veno-venous anastomoses, if performed, should be constructed with wide ostia. Should the ascending aorta be severely diseased with diffuse atheroma, the proximal anastomosis may be performed with the aorta cross-clamped. Although this is rarely necessary, it prevents the dislodging of atheromatous material from within the aorta by the placement of a side-biting clamp.

Choice of conduits

Every effort should be made to use arterial conduits. The internal thoracic artery on the left side should certainly be used if available. The right internal thoracic artery and the radial arteries offer alternative sources of arterial conduit. Use of these conduits in a sequential fashion or as free grafts anastomosed to the left internal thoracic artery may greatly extend their applicability. Whatever saphenous vein is available should be used, provided that it is healthy. The use of unsatisfactory venous conduit will give a poor outcome.

ALTERNATIVE SURGICAL OPTIONS

Beating-heart surgical techniques have been advocated in high-risk patients, including those undergoing repeat CABG.[22–24] Good results have been obtained with this approach in centers where there is experience of this technique, or a policy promoting its use.[25] Avoidance of repeat sternotomy by a left thoracotomy approach, particularly in combination with beating-heart techniques, can make revascularization of the left side of the heart[26] a safe and successful procedure.

RESULTS

Redo coronary surgery is more complicated than the first operation and carries a higher risk and mortality rate. There are several risk factors that contribute to its high mortality rate, estimated at about 8–10% for elective procedures, with an increase to about 17% for emergency cases.[27] The mortality for urgent re-operations has been estimated to be about 11%. There has been a comprehensive list of risk factors reported in the literature, including increased age, shorter interval between first operation and re-operation, evidence of generalized atherosclerotic disease, higher grade Canadian Cardiovascular Society or New York Heart Association classifications, greater ventricular dysfunction, renal insufficiency, female gender, left main disease, and emergency operation.[10,28,29] Of these, the most significant risk factors are the urgency of the operation and interval between the first and second operations. The mortality rate for patients who require a second operation within 1 year of the first operation has been reported at 18% compared to 9% more than 1 year after the first operation.[8]

Redo coronary bypass surgery is associated with complications similar to those of first operations. However, some have been described to be more common and specifically related to repeat surgery. According to Christenson,[8] postoperative low cardiac output syndrome, intra-aortic balloon pump support, prolonged ventilatory support (>24 hours), hemorrhage and gastrointestinal complications were prominent features of the redo group.

In a large retrospective study involving 1300 patients undergoing redo coronary bypass surgery, Kaul et al.[11] found that the majority of patients were male (75%) and less than 70 years of age (83%). In this study, the actuarial survival at 10 years for patients who received an internal thoracic artery bypass was found to be higher than for those who received saphenous vein grafts only (86% vs 76%, P <0.05). Patients with left ventricular ejection fractions of less than 20% had worse outcomes and a poor survival after 2 years. Overall, after 10 years, the cardiac-related event-free survival after the first re-operation was 53%.

Ninety-four of the 1300 patients in this study required subsequent second or third re-operations for recurrent angina, and 125 underwent saphenous vein angioplasty. Patients who underwent multiple re-operations enjoyed a superior cardiac event-free survival compared to those who had angioplasty (45% vs 35%, P <0.05). In this study it was concluded that the survival and quality of life were significantly improved by the use of the internal thoracic artery, as well as by choosing second or third re-operations over angioplasty for patients with recurrent angina who were candidates for surgery.

Beating-heart techniques for repeat coronary surgery in selected patients have been shown by some authors to give comparable or possibly better early outcome than conventional techniques.[22,24,30–32] Long-term outcomes are not yet available for this alternative approach.

KEY REFERENCES

Fitzgibbon GM, Kafka HP, Leach AJ, Keon WJ, Hooper GD, Burton JR. Coronary bypass graft fate and patient outcome: angiographic follow-up of 5,065 grafts related to survival and re-operation in 1,388 patients during 25 years. *J Am Coll Cardiol* 1996; **28**:616–26.

An excellent account of the natural history of saphenous vein bypass conduits and the hazards and outcomes of repeat surgery.

Mack MJ, Dewey TM, Magee MJ. Facilitated anastomosis for reoperative circumflex coronary revascularization on the beating heart through a left thoracotomy. *J Thorac Cardiovasc Surg* 2002; **123**:816–17.

This report draws attention to the value of two alternatives to conventional redo CABG – an approach avoiding sternotomy combined with a beating-heart technique to circumvent the problems of cardiopulmonary bypass and aortic manipulation.

Motwani JG, Topol EJ. Aortocoronary saphenous vein graft disease: pathogenesis, predisposition, and prevention. [Review – 133 refs.] *Circulation* 1998; **97**:916–31.

A comprehensive review of the commonest cause for repeat CABG, with an update on preventative strategies for optimizing outcome with vein grafts.

Stephan WJ, O'Keefe JH Jr, Piehler JM, McCallister BD, Dahiya RS, Shimshak TM, *et al.* Coronary angioplasty versus repeat coronary artery bypass grafting for patients with previous bypass surgery. *J Am Coll Cardiol* 1996; **28**:1140–6.

A reminder of the alternative treatment for recurrent angina. Percutaneous coronary intervention, though associated with less complete revascularization, has been shown to reduce the procedure-related mortality and morbidity.

REFERENCES

1. Grondin CM, Campeau L, Thornton JC, Engle JC, Cross FS, Schreiber H. Coronary artery bypass grafting with saphenous vein. [Review – 62 refs.] *Circulation* 1989; **79**:I24–9.

2. Motwani JG, Topol EJ. Aortocoronary saphenous vein graft disease: pathogenesis, predisposition, and prevention. [Review – 133 refs.] *Circulation* 1998; **97**:916–31.

3. Sergeant P, Blackstone E, Meyns B, Stockman B, Jashari R. First cardiological or cardiosurgical reintervention for ischemic heart disease after primary coronary artery bypass grafting. *Eur J Cardiothorac Surg* 1998; **14**:480–7.

4. Hall MJ, Owings MF. *2000 National Hospital Discharge Survey. Advance Data from Vital and Health Statistics No. 329.* Hyattsville, MD: National Center for Health Statistics, 2002.

5. Keogh BE, Kinsman R. *National Adult Cardiac Surgical Database Report 2000–2001. Society of Cardiothoracic Surgeons of Great Britain and Ireland.* Henley-on-Thames: Dendrite Clinical Systems Ltd, 2002.

6. Stephan WJ, O'Keefe JH Jr, Piehler JM, McCallister BD, Dahiya RS, Shimshak TM, *et al.* Coronary angioplasty versus repeat coronary artery bypass grafting for patients with previous bypass surgery. *J Am Coll Cardiol* 1996; **28**:1140–6.

7. Mathew V, Clavell AL, Lennon RJ, Grill DE, Holmes DR Jr. Percutaneous coronary interventions in patients with prior coronary artery bypass surgery: changes in patient characteristics and outcome during two decades. *Am J Med* 2000; **108**:127–35.

8. Christenson JT, Schmuziger M, Simonet F. Re-operative coronary artery bypass procedures: risk factors for early mortality and late survival. *Eur J Cardiothorac Surg* 1997; **11**:129–33.

9. Brener SJ, Loop FD, Lytle BW, Ellis SG, Cosgrove DM, Topol EJ. A profile of candidates for repeat myocardial revascularization: implications for selection of treatment. *J Thorac Cardiovasc Surg* 1997; **114**:153–61.

10. Fitzgibbon GM, Kafka HP, Leach AJ, Keon WJ, Hooper GD, Burton JR. Coronary bypass graft fate and patient outcome: angiographic follow-up of 5,065 grafts related to survival and re-operation in 1,388 patients during 25 years. *J Am Coll Cardiol* 1996; **28**:616–26.

11. Kaul TK, Fields BL, Wyatt DA, Jones CR, Kahn DR. Re-operative coronary artery bypass surgery: early and late results and management in 1,300 patients. *J Cardiovasc Surg (Torino)* 1995; **36**:303–12.

12. Loop FD, Lytle BW, Cosgrove DM, Woods EL, Stewart RW, Golding LA, *et al.* Re-operation for coronary atherosclerosis. Changing practice in 2,509 consecutive patients. *Ann Surg* 1990; **212**:378–85.

13. Loop FD, Lytle BW, Cosgrove DM, Stewart RW, Goormastic M, Williams GW, *et al.* Influence of the internal-mammary-artery graft on 10-year survival and other cardiac events. *N Engl J Med* 1986; **314**:1–6.

14. Loop FD. Internal-thoracic-artery grafts. Biologically better coronary arteries. *N Engl J Med* 1996; **334**:263–5.

15. Holmes DR Jr, Berger PB. Percutaneous revascularization of occluded vein grafts: is it still a temptation to be resisted? *Circulation* 1999; **99**:8–11.

16. Levy JH, Pifarre R, Schaff HV, Horrow JC, Albus R, Spiess B, *et al.* A multicenter, double-blind, placebo-controlled trial of aprotinin for reducing blood loss and the requirement for donor-blood transfusion in patients undergoing repeat coronary artery bypass grafting. *Circulation* 1995; **92**:2236–44.

17. Follis FM, Pett SB Jr, Miller KB, Wong RS, Temes RT, Wernly JA. Catastrophic hemorrhage on sternal reentry: still a dreaded complication? *Ann Thorac Surg* 1999; **68**:2215–19.

18. Kulshrestha P, Garb JL, Rousou JA, Engelman RM, Wait RB. Reoperative median sternotomy using a cast spreader. *J Card Surg* 1999; **14**:185–6.

19. Machiraju VR. How to avoid problems in redo coronary artery bypass. *J Card Surg* 2002; **17**:20–5.

20. Athanasiou T, Stanbridge R De L, Kumar P, Cherian A. Video-assisted resternotomy in high-risk redo operations – the St Mary's experience. *Eur J Cardiothorac Surg* 2002; **21**:932–4.

21. Gazzaniga AB, Palafox BA. Substernal thoracoscopic guidance during sternal re-entry. *Ann Thorac Surg* 2001; **72**:289–90.

22. Bergsland J, Hasnain S, Lajos TZ, Salerno TA. Elimination of cardiopulmonary bypass: a prime goal in re-operative coronary artery bypass surgery. *Eur J Cardiothorac Surg* 1998; **14**:59–62.

23. Stamou SC, Corso PJ. Coronary revascularization without cardiopulmonary bypass in high-risk patients: a route to the future. [Review – 76 refs.] *Ann Thorac Surg* 2001; **71**:1056–61.

24. Hart JC, Puskas JD, Sabik JF III. Off-pump coronary revascularization: current state of the art. [Review – 50 refs.] *Semin Thorac Cardiovasc Surg* 2002; **14**:70–81.

25. Stamou SC, Pfister AJ, Dullum MK, Boyce SW, Bafi AS, Lomax T, *et al.* Late outcome of re-operative coronary revascularization on the beating heart. *Heart Surg Forum* 2001; **4**:69–73.

26. Mack MJ, Dewey TM, Magee MJ. Facilitated anastomosis for re-operative circumflex coronary revascularization on the beating heart through a left thoracotomy. *J Thorac Cardiovasc Surg* 2002; **123**:816–17.

27. Weintraub WS, Jones EL, Craver JM, Grosswald R, Guyton RA. In-hospital and long-term outcome after re-operative coronary artery bypass graft surgery. *Circulation* 1995; **92**:II50–7.

28. Yamamuro M, Lytle BW, Sapp SK, Cosgrove DM III, Loop FD, McCarthy PM. Risk factors and outcomes after coronary re-operation in 739 elderly patients. *Ann Thorac Surg* 2000; **69**:464–74.

29. Yau TM, Borger MA, Weisel RD, Ivanov J. The changing pattern of re-operative coronary surgery: trends in 1,230 consecutive re-operations. *J Thorac Cardiovasc Surg* 2000; **120**:156–63.

30. Mishra Y, Wasir H, Kohli V, Meharwal ZS, Bapna R, Mehta Y, *et al.* Beating heart versus conventional re-operative coronary artery bypass surgery. *Indian Heart J* 2002; **54**:159–63.

31. Trehan N, Mishra YK, Malhotra R, Sharma KK, Mehta Y, Shrivastava S. Off-pump redo coronary artery bypass grafting. *Ann Thorac Surg* 2000; **70**:1026–9.

32. Mack M, Bachand D, Acuff T, Edgerton J, Prince S, Dewey T, *et al.* Improved outcomes in coronary artery bypass grafting with beating-heart techniques. *J Thorac Cardiovasc Surg* 2002; **124**:598–607.

20

Surgical interventions in acute ischemia

JAMES J LIVESAY AND ROSS M REUL

Despite the well-known benefits and low risk of coronary bypass surgery in most patients, there are some groups of patients with coronary disease who are at increased risk because of acute ischemia and infarction, often with associated left ventricular failure. Controversy exists as to the selection of medical or surgical interventions, timing of treatment, and even the optimal methods of surgical repair in these patients. A clearer understanding of the natural history of acute myocardial infarction, the pathophysiology of ischemia and reperfusion, and current methods to combat ischemia and enhance reperfusion is necessary to achieve successful results. Dramatic improvement in myocardial recovery and patient survival can be achieved by thoughtful application of newer surgical methods of reperfusion and circulatory support for patients with acute myocardial infarction. Despite the improvements in overall perioperative management, mechanical complications of acute myocardial infarction continue to present a formidable challenge to successful surgical repair. In this setting, ventricular septal rupture and acute mitral regurgitation are life-threatening events. The surgical approach to these problems has been modified in recent years.

CONCEPTS OF ISCHEMIA AND REPERFUSION

Myocardial ischemia and infarction represent a continuum of a pathophysiological process initiated by an oxygen supply that is inadequate to meet myocardial metabolic demands.[1] The severity and duration of ischemia determine, if limited, the reversibility of the process and, if untreated, the magnitude of the resulting myocardial infarction. Severe ischemia interrupts energy supply and metabolism, suspends regional contractile function, and affects ion pumps necessary for cellular homeostasis. Prolonged ischemia leads to anaerobic cellular metabolism and acidosis, loss of ionic gradients, accumulation of intracellular calcium and sodium, loss of membrane integrity, release of toxic metabolites, production of oxygen free radicals, and ultimately to cellular swelling, membrane rupture and cell death. Ischemia may be thought of as an imbalance between myocardial oxygen supply and oxygen demand. Consideration of this supply/demand imbalance in patient management is very useful in reducing ischemia, especially prior to revascularization. Therapies that increase oxygen supply (i.e. intra-aortic balloon pump [IABP] support to augment diastolic pressure) or therapies that decrease oxygen demands (i.e. vasodilators and IABP to reduce afterload, beta-blockers to lower heart rate) have been shown to reduce ischemia and improve outcomes.

While revascularization affords the potential of restoring normal coronary blood flow, ischemic injury may not be reversed by reperfusion with normal blood alone. Studies have shown that reperfusion after short periods of ischemia (up to 15 minutes) may allow for correction of the biochemical and functional abnormalities induced by ischemia.[2] Intermediate periods of ischemia (20–30 minutes) with reperfusion may not be sufficient to produce cell death, but may result in the prolonged, yet reversible, impairment of contractile function known as 'myocardial stunning'.[3] After longer periods of ischemia (40–60 minutes), reperfusion with normal blood produces massive structural, biochemical and functional changes in the ischemic myocardium.[4] This reperfusion injury may paradoxically increase the abnormality produced by ischemia alone. Following prolonged ischemia (6 hours), normal blood reperfusion produces extensive transmural necrosis, with little possibility of myocardial salvage.

The mechanisms of reperfusion injury have been studied extensively.[1–4] Reperfusion produces explosive cellular swelling. An influx of intracellular calcium occurs, which precipitates, causing damage to the mitochondria. Despite the increased availability of oxygen with reperfusion, oxygen uptake is hampered and energy production is impaired. Calcium accumulation and a decreased energy supply result in irreversible ischemic contracture. Reoxygenation produces toxic reactive oxygen species. Complement activation releases pro-inflammatory mediators affecting vascular tone and leukocyte adherence, which may further compromise blood flow to an ischemic organ (the 'no-reflow' phenomenon). Activated neutrophils adhere to the endothelium, transmigrate, and release damaging lysosomal enzymes. Severe reperfusion injury results in increased microvascular permeability, edema, reduced blood flow, intravascular thrombosis, organ dysfunction and cell death.

SURGICAL METHODS TO COMBAT ISCHEMIA

A number of surgical methods have been used effectively in the past to combat ischemia by correcting the imbalance between myocardial oxygen supply and myocardial oxygen demand. Each method affords unique advantages as well as disadvantages that must be considered with application to the various subsets of ischemic patients undergoing coronary artery bypass grafting (CABG).

Intra-aortic balloon pump

The IABP improves ischemia by augmenting diastolic pressure (oxygen supply) while simultaneously reducing systolic pressure and afterload (oxygen demand). The IABP has been helpful in stabilizing hemodynamics in unstable patients, despite the fact that it contributes only 10% to the cardiac output. Its principal application has been in high-risk patients with acute ischemia or infarction, failed angioplasty, hemodynamic instability, left ventricular failure, cardiogenic shock and mechanical complications of myocardial infarction.[5] Peripheral arterial injury

and possible occlusion may complicate the use of IABP in 1–5% of patients.

Cardiopulmonary bypass

Cardiopulmonary bypass provides the most effective means of support of the ischemic myocardium. Myocardial oxygen consumption (demand) drops dramatically to 50% of the requirement of the normal beating working heart.[6] This energy saving is achieved only with full cardiopulmonary bypass diverting more than 95% of the systemic venous return from the beating empty heart. Cardiopulmonary bypass effectively supports the systemic circulation, while reducing left ventricular end-diastolic pressure, both of which are advantageous in ischemic, compromised patients with left ventricular failure and cardiogenic shock. It is not uncommon to see resolution of electrocardiographic (ECG) changes simply on commencement of cardiopulmonary bypass. The disadvantages of cardiopulmonary bypass in ischemic patients are found in the reduction of oxygen-carrying capacity with hemodilution and the often precipitous fall in blood pressure when non-pulsatile perfusion commences. Obligatory measures should be undertaken to maintain adequate hemoglobin (oxygen content) and mean blood pressure in a physiological range during the period of assisted circulation. Another disadvantage of cardiopulmonary bypass is that it activates the complement system, which may contribute to complications such as multi-organ dysfunction postoperatively.

Hemopump™, left ventricular assist devices and biventricular assist devices

These techniques have been used to support the circulation for CABG in high-risk patients.[7] They offer many of the advantages of circulatory support in unstable patients without the disadvantage of cardiopulmonary bypass activating a systemic inflammatory response.

Cardioplegia

Cardioplegia arrests the heart, reducing oxygen demand by 90% of that of the beating working heart. Cold cardioplegia further reduces the oxygen demands of the arrested heart (i.e. 97% reduction at 22 °C). This further reduces the basal metabolic demands of the myocardium. Blood cardioplegia provides sufficient oxygen delivery to the myocardium and buffers tissue acidosis. Cold blood cardioplegia affords additional protection during periods when coronary perfusion is interrupted for coronary anastomosis or intracardiac repair.[6] Intermittent cold blood cardioplegia provides complete protection of the

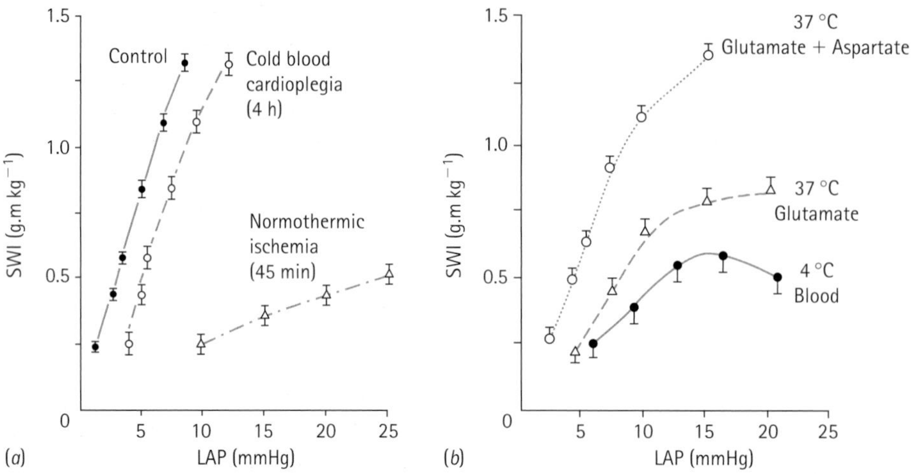

Figure 20.1 *Myocardial performance assessed by left ventricular function curves in normal and post-ischemic hearts. (a) Left ventricular function in normal hearts protected by multidose cold blood cardioplegia (4 °C) for 4 hours is similar to that in controls. (Note marked depression in function after 45 minutes of normothermic ischemia.) (b) Post-ischemic hearts protected by 2 hours of multidose cold blood cardioplegia show little recovery of left ventricular function, whereas ischemic hearts show significant recovery of left ventricular function after induction and reperfusion with warm glutamate and aspartate cardioplegia. SWI, stroke work index; LAP, left atrial pressure. Reprinted from Buckberg GD. Myocardial protection: an overview. Semin Thorac Cardiovasc Surg 1993; 5:98–106, with permission from Elsevier Science.*

normal heart for up to 4 hours, but does not resuscitate an ischemic injured heart with left ventricular dysfunction. Warm blood cardioplegia has been shown to enable ongoing metabolism while simultaneously reducing energy demands, which allows for resuscitation of ischemic-injured myocardium.[8] Functional recovery occurs if substrate-enhanced warm blood cardioplegia is used for the induction of cardioplegic arrest and terminal reperfusion (Figure 20.1).[6,8,9]

One of the theoretical disadvantages of cardioplegic arrest is that it superimposes the potential for global ischemia onto a heart with pre-existing severe regional ischemia.

The advantages of blood cardioplegia and controlled reperfusion may be lost unless the operator uses every means to ensure uniform delivery of cardioplegia to all regions of the myocardium and re-infuses oxygenated blood cardioplegia at frequent intervals to prevent ongoing ischemia. In the face of severe coronary occlusive disease, retrograde coronary sinus catheters, bypass grafts and the native coronary arteries can be utilized to ensure adequate and uniform delivery of blood cardioplegia for re-oxygenation of all areas of the myocardium (100–300 mL over 1–2 minutes every 15 minutes or after each distal anastomosis).

Controlled surgical reperfusion

Using methods of controlled surgical reperfusion, surgeons have the opportunity to control the reperfusion process

after acute myocardial infarction, to lessen reperfusion injury and to enable significant functional recovery, even in patients with severe left ventricular dysfunction and cardiogenic shock. Experimental studies have validated each of the concepts expressed; however, to achieve the maximum benefit, all components of the strategy must be applied consistently.[9] This method provides for control of the conditions of reperfusion and the components of the reperfusate. Cardiopulmonary bypass and cardioplegic arrest reduce oxygen demands to basal metabolic levels. Normothermia (37 °C) allows ongoing cellular metabolism and energy production for reparative processes.[10] The perfusion pressure is kept low (<50 mmHg) to reduce edema. Prolonged reperfusion of the infarct zone (20 minutes) with cardioplegic reperfusate has been shown to enhance functional recovery, reduce infarct size and improve clinical outcomes (Figure 20.2).[11]

Equally important is the composition of the reperfusion solution.[12] Oxygen is necessary to restore aerobic metabolism. Blood provides for oxygen delivery and protects against damage by oxygen free radicals. Potassium ensures electromechanical arrest, reducing energy demands. Hypocalcemia (150–250 μmol L^{-1}) is important to reduce calcium overload upon initial reperfusion. Magnesium and calcium channel blockers further limit calcium entry into ischemic cells. Diltiazem has been shown to reduce infarct size and enhance functional recovery after acute myocardial infarction.[13] Substrate enhancement with glutamate and aspartate improves post-ischemic contractile dysfunction and may reduce infarct size.[10] Intracellular acidosis is buffered. Hyperosmolarity decreases post-ischemic

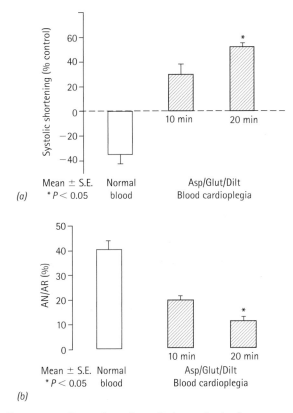

Figure 20.2 *Comparison of reperfusion methods after 2 hours of coronary occlusion. (a) Recovery of regional contractility is best after reperfusion by 20 minutes of substrate-enriched blood cardioplegia. Note absence of recovery and dyskinetic motion with normal blood reperfusion. (b) Extent of myocardial infarction measured by histochemical technique is greatest after normal blood reperfusion and is reduced by 20 minutes' reperfusion with substrate-enriched blood cardioplegia. Asp, aspartate; Glut, glutamate; Dilt, diltiazem; AN, area of non-staining; AR, area at risk. Reprinted from Allen BS, Okamoto F, Buckberg GD, Leaf J, Bugyi H. Studies of controlled reperfusion after ischemia. XII. Effects of 'duration' of reperfusate administration versus reperfusate 'dose' on regional functional, biochemical, and histochemical recovery. J Thorac Cardiovasc Surg 1986; 92:594–604, with permission from Elsevier Science.*

edema. Hyperglycemia provides substrate and counters edema. Leukocyte depletion may reduce reperfusion injury in ischemic hearts. Adenosine may enhance functional recovery.

ROLE OF PERIOPERATIVE ISCHEMIA AND UNSTABLE ANGINA

The impact of perioperative ischemia on outcomes following coronary bypass surgery was examined in the study by Slogoff and Keats.[14] In a prospective study of 1023 patients undergoing elective CABG surgery, silent ischemia was detected by ECG surveillance prior to the onset of cardiopulmonary bypass in 36.9% of patients, with almost half the episodes occurring before anesthetic induction. The severity of ischemia as judged by ST-segment depression correlated with the risk of postoperative myocardial infarction (a 2.5% risk with no ST depression vs a 9.3% risk with 3 mm ST depression). The presence of postoperative myocardial infarction increased the risk of hospital mortality from 0.9% (no myocardial infarction) to 12% (myocardial infarction present). This study demonstrates the frequent occurrence of perioperative ischemia in patients undergoing routine elective coronary bypass and the direct link of perioperative ischemia to postoperative myocardial infarction and death despite a technically satisfactory revascularization procedure.

Myocardial ischemia is uniformly present in patients presenting with unstable angina and a closely related condition, non-ST-segment elevation myocardial infarction (NSTEMI). These common manifestations of acute coronary syndromes represent an imbalance between myocardial oxygen supply and demand. Their etiology is reduced perfusion that results from a non-occlusive thrombus that forms after rupture of an atherosclerotic plaque. Both syndromes have common clinical presentations, differing only in the severity and presence of myocardial necrosis detected by biomarkers. Current medical practice provides for rapid clinical assessment and early risk stratification in patients with unstable angina.[15] Patients with unstable angina at high or intermediate risk of death or non-fatal myocardial infarction are often triaged to an early invasive strategy by any of the following indicators:

- new ST-segment depression,
- elevated biomarker (troponin T),
- recurrent angina at rest, despite therapy,
- angina plus symptoms of congestive heart failure,
- positive findings on stress tests,
- depressed left ventricular function,
- hemodynamic instability,
- ventricular tachycardia,
- percutaneous coronary intervention (PCI) within 6 months,
- prior CABG.

Initial treatment of unstable angina involves anti-ischemic therapy and anti-thrombotic therapy with aspirin, heparin and a platelet glycoprotein (GP) IIb/IIIa receptor antagonist. Coronary angiography is necessary to identify patients with high-risk coronary anatomy who are likely to benefit from revascularization by either PCI or CABG. The indications for each method of revascularization in patients with unstable angina or NSTEMI are similar to those applied in patients with stable angina.[15] High-risk patients with LV dysfunction, diabetes mellitus, two-vessel disease with severe left anterior descending (LAD) artery involvement, or three-vessel disease or left main disease should be considered for CABG. CABG (or PCI) may be indicated for one-vessel or two-vessel disease without proximal LAD involvement or if a large area of viable myocardium is at risk. Other patients at less risk of cardiac death may choose CABG to improve their quality of life or achieve better symptomatic relief.

High-risk subgroups with unstable angina have been identified. Diabetes is present in 25% of patients with unstable angina and is an independent predictor of adverse outcomes.[15] Diabetics have a reported mortality of 17% in the first year after unstable angina. Diabetes is associated with more extensive coronary artery disease, unstable lesions, other co-morbidities and worse long-term outcomes with revascularization. The Bypass Angioplasty Revascularization Investigation (BARI) trial demonstrated a striking advantage for CABG over percutaneous transluminal coronary angioplasty (PTCA) in diabetics.[16]

Unstable angina occurs in 20% of patients who have undergone a prior coronary bypass procedure during an average interval of 7.5 years, principally due to a thrombotic occlusion of vein grafts, but also due to progression of disease in native vessels. This high-risk subgroup has more frequent ischemic events, an increased risk for revascularization, and less symptomatic relief. Medical therapy and PCI are usually tried first in such patients, but afford less satisfactory control of symptoms than does redo coronary bypass.

Surgical treatment for unstable angina has progressed in the past decade because of aggressive treatment of perioperative ischemia and improved myocardial protective techniques. Recognition and treatment of preoperative ischemia are of primary importance in patients with unstable angina. Isom *et al.* observed that a maximum release of the cardiac isoenzyme CK-MB occurred in 93% of patients during the prebypass period after anesthetic induction.[17] Others observed that 67% of high-risk patients who had unstable angina within 2 days and an acute myocardial infarction within 2 weeks before operation (Braunwald class IIIC) had high levels of troponin T before operation and that 27% ultimately developed perioperative myocardial infarction.[18]

Preoperative treatment of ischemia using IABP insertion prior to surgery has been shown to improve postoperative cardiac performance, reduce mortality and benefit outcomes in high-risk patients with unstable angina, low ejection fraction, left main disease and redo procedures.[5] IABP improves hemodynamic instability, raises coronary perfusion pressure and reduces cardiac work, all of which are beneficial in reversing ischemia.

Improved outcomes for patients with unstable angina have been reported recently after CABG, with a decline in mortality from 5.9% to 2.6% and a decline in non-fatal infarctions from 13% to 6.2% between 1990 and 1995

due to improvements in perioperative management.[19] Warm blood cardioplegic induction has been shown to reverse the effects of ischemia in energy-depleted hearts.[8,20] Warm induction improves oxygen uptake, aerobic metabolism and functional recovery in ischemic hearts. Substrate enhancement by the addition of glutamate and aspartate to warm blood cardioplegia has resulted in dramatic improvement in post-ischemic ventricular function (see Figure 20.1).[10] Glucose–insulin–potassium (GIK) solutions given intraoperatively and continued postoperatively for 12 hours in patients with unstable angina have been shown to enhance myocardial performance and shorten recovery after urgent CABG.[21] Antegrade and retrograde cardioplegia enhances the delivery of cardioprotective solutions in spite of severe coronary occlusive disease. In our experience, strategies utilizing cardiopulmonary bypass, integrated cardioplegia, antegrade and retrograde delivery, and complete revascularization afford the optimal protection of the ischemic heart in patients with unstable angina.

Newer techniques of off-pump coronary artery bypass (OPCAB) surgery have been applied in patients with unstable angina.[22,23] Recent studies have utilized IABP for hemodynamic support and to improve ischemia during OPCAB procedures.[24] Some authors have reported good results using OPCAB without IABP support in unstable angina, but other studies have demonstrated ischemia using OPCAB methods that may be detrimental in patients with unstable angina and threatened infarction.[22,25]

ACUTE MYOCARDIAL INFARCTION

The initial trials of surgical revascularization for acute myocardial infarction demonstrated the importance of time to reperfusion.[26] Operative mortality was 5.8% if reperfusion was accomplished in less than 6 hours, but 7.1% if delayed more than 6 hours. Prompt reperfusion was believed to salvage ischemic border zones, limit infarct size and increase survival. From these early studies, the time to revascularization has been accepted as the primary determinant of myocardial salvage. The current medical approach to myocardial infarction is focused mainly on early reperfusion therapy using either thrombolysis or PCI.[27] Many studies have shown the benefits of early reperfusion for acute myocardial infarction, with a lower incidence of heart failure, hemodynamic shock and early mortality.[27] Current cardiological strategies reserve coronary artery bypass for failures of medical reperfusion. Despite these demonstrated improvements in care, many patients are not eligible for thrombolysis because of advanced age, prior stroke, or history of bleeding or anemia. In addition, many patients are not benefited by percutaneous reperfusion due to anatomic disease (such as left main or three-vessel disease), poor ventricular function or renal insufficiency. Indeed, these are the patients who face the greatest risk from acute myocardial infarction.

In a recent review of 163 000 Medicare patients in the USA (age 65 to over 85 years), the 30-day mortality for acute myocardial infarction rose from 10.9% to 31.2% with advancing age.[28] This represents an incremental mortality risk above 10.9% of approximately 1% risk for each year of age over 65. Following acute myocardial infarction, older patients frequently develop congestive heart failure or pulmonary edema (36–65%), hypotension (23–26%) or cardiogenic shock (6.5–8.9%). The 1-year mortality after myocardial infarction in the elderly is 20–43%. Despite the serious consequences of acute myocardial infarction, thrombolysis is used in only 2.1–12% of patients over 65 years, PCI in only 4–28% and CABG in only 1.5–20%. Despite the benefits of revascularization shown in randomized trials, in practice only a small minority of patients receive revascularization after acute myocardial infarction. Therefore, revascularization for acute myocardial infarction has not had an impact on overall outcome in large population studies. One-year mortality rates after myocardial infarction in elderly patients (over 65 years of age) were identical in the USA and Canada (34.3%), despite differences in frequency of catheterization (34.9% vs 6.7%) and revascularization by PTCA (11.7% vs 1.5%) or CABG (10.6% vs 1.4%).[29]

The appropriate timing of surgical intervention after acute myocardial infarction is controversial. Operative mortality is increased early after myocardial infarction: 11.8% (<6 hours), 9.5% (6 hours–1 day) and 2.8% (>1 day).[30] Transmural myocardial infarction poses twice the risk of non-transmural myocardial infarction (13.6% vs 6.2%). The increased risk drops after 24 hours, but remains elevated for 7 days. Despite the apparent reduction in operative risk conveyed by delayed revascularization, this strategy precludes many patients from the survival advantage of surgical revascularization. Furthermore, advances in the techniques of surgical revascularization have been shown to be associated with a reduction in reperfusion injury, diminished infarct size, enhanced recovery of ventricular function, reversed pump failure, reduced immediate mortality and improved long-term survival.[9,31–37] Controlled surgical reperfusion after acute coronary occlusion has been shown both experimentally and clinically to provide significant advantages over uncontrolled reperfusion with normal blood alone (i.e. thrombolysis or PCI), despite the longer duration of ischemia required for surgical reperfusion.[33–38] Uncontrolled reperfusion with normal blood after prolonged ischemia has been shown to accentuate severe damage in the ischemic zone, thus causing a reperfusion injury.[4,33–36]

Surgical control of the conditions and composition of the reperfusion has been shown to prevent reperfusion

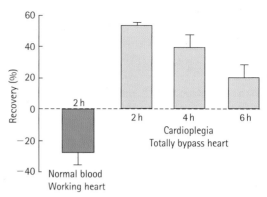

Figure 20.3 *Recovery of systolic shortening after coronary occlusion and reperfusion. Note failure of recovery after 2 hours of occlusion followed by normal blood reperfusion in working hearts, and immediate recovery after 2, 4 and 6 hours of occlusion followed by controlled reperfusion with substrate-enriched blood cardioplegia during total vented bypass. Reprinted from Allen BS, Okamoto F, Buckberg GD, Bagyi H, Young H, Leaf J, et al. Studies of controlled reperfusion after ischemia. XV. Immediate functional recovery after six hours of regional ischemia by careful control of conditions of reperfusion and composition of reperfusate. J Thorac Cardiovasc Surg 1986; 92:621–35, with permission from Elsevier Science.*

injury, enable recovery of cell function (up to 8 hours after myocardial infarction), resuscitate energy-depleted hearts, and enhance recovery of wall motion in the infarct zone in 86% of patients after acute myocardial infarction (Figure 20.3).[36,37] In light of these clear advantages, emergency surgical revascularization should be performed for acute coronary occlusion after failed PCI, in patients with large areas of myocardium threatened by transmural infarction, in patients with multivessel disease where the remote myocardium is ischemic or dysfunctional, and in patients likely to develop cardiogenic shock. If coronary occlusion occurs in the catheterization laboratory, and if it can be quickly remedied after a short ischemic interval by angioplasty or stenting, the advantages of prompt catheter reperfusion are clear; however, if prolonged ischemia (>1–2 hours) due to coronary occlusion is present, catheter-directed reperfusion with normal blood will result in severe reperfusion injury that cannot be reversed later by controlled reperfusion. In such patients, a better strategy of controlled surgical reperfusion should be considered.

The optimal strategy for surgical reperfusion utilizes total vented cardiopulmonary bypass and cardioplegic arrest to support the circulation and to reduce myocardial oxygen demands during aortic cross-clamping. Myocardial protection is provided with oxygenated blood cardioplegia delivered antegrade, retrograde and through vein grafts after each anastomosis to ensure global distribution. Warm substrate-enriched blood cardioplegia is used for cardioplegic induction and later for terminal reperfusion to enhance functional recovery of the ischemic myocardium.

Integrated cardioplegia combines the advantages of warm cardioplegia induction and terminal reperfusion with the advantages of cold multidose blood cardioplegia.[38] Reinfusion of blood cardioplegia (100–200 mL min[-1] for 1–2 minutes) delivered after each distal anastomosis or at least every 15 minutes maintains oxygen delivery during obligatory periods of interruptions of coronary blood flow. After completion of all distal anastomoses, terminal global reperfusion is applied for 2 minutes with warm blood cardioplegia enriched by glutamate and aspartate. Controlled reperfusion of the infarct zone using the bypass graft is continued for an additional 18 minutes to allow maximum recovery of cellular functions prior to reperfusion with normal blood.[11] Controlled reperfusion utilizes low flow (50 mL min[-1]) to prevent myocardial edema. The composition of the reperfusion solution is critical to avoid reperfusion injury.[12] Warm blood cardioplegia provides oxygen delivery and reduces oxygen debt. Hypocalcemia and calcium-channel blockers (e.g. diltiazem; 300 μg kg[-1] body weight) are used to decrease calcium overload, reduce infarct size and enhance recovery.[13] The proximal anastomosis may be completed using a partial occluding clamp on the aorta during the time required for regional reperfusion of the infarct (Figure 20.4). After completion of controlled surgical reperfusion, normal blood flow is restored through the bypass grafts. It is beneficial to maintain the heart in the beating empty state for 30 minutes to allow maximum recovery of jeopardized myocardium and to lower oxygen demands.[39] It is preferable to avoid inotropic drugs during this rest period.

Clinical reports have demonstrated the advantages of surgical revascularization in patients with acute coronary occlusion.[9,31–37] Initial reports comparing controlled surgical reperfusion to reperfusion with angioplasty demonstrated improved outcomes, better cardiac performance and less mortality in surgical patients, despite a longer duration of coronary occlusion, more severe coronary anatomy and worse ventricular function prior to treatment in the surgical patients.[33,37] In one multicenter trial of patients with acute evolving infarction, 156 patients were treated using methods of controlled surgical reperfusion.[33] Despite the long ischemic intervals (6.3 hours) and high incidence of LAD disease (61%), multivessel disease (42%) and cardiogenic shock (41%), surgical mortality was only 3.9%. Regional wall motion recovered significantly in 90% of patients. In contrast, in a consecutive series of 126 patients with acute coronary occlusion after PTCA failure who underwent uncontrolled reperfusion with normal blood after only 3.5 hours of ischemia, recovery of wall motion was incomplete and hospital mortality was 10.3%.[34] Additional studies have confirmed the reduction of hospital mortality (3.9–5.6%) using

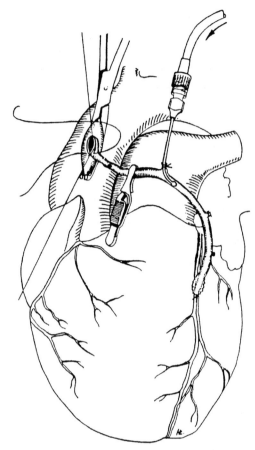

Figure 20.4 *Controlled reperfusion of the infarct zone is achieved through a side branch of the vein graft while the proximal aortic anastomosis is completed. Reprinted from Beyersdorf F, Buckberg GD. Myocardial protection in patients with acute myocardial infarction and cardiogenic shock. Semin Thorac Cardiovasc Surg 1993; 5:151–61, with permission from Elsevier Science.*

controlled surgical reperfusion for acute coronary occlusion.[9,32,40]

Early recovery of regional contractility occurs in 86% of patients after controlled reperfusion. Echocardiographic study 5–7 days after controlled surgical reperfusion demonstrates normokinesis in the infarct zone in 49% and only mild to moderate hypokinesis in 37%.[34] In contrast, after normal blood reperfusion, regional contractility recovers to normal in only 22–33% of patients, and the infarct zone remains non-functional in 39–52% of patients. Reperfusion arrhythmias commonly seen after normal blood reperfusion are infrequent after controlled reperfusion (20%).[34] Hemodynamic instability is seen in 55% of patients prior to surgical revascularization, but is usually reversed within 18–24 hours postoperatively.[9] Length of hospitalization is decreased in patients treated by controlled surgical reperfusion compared with those treated by reperfusion by angioplasty.[37]

Experimental and clinical studies have demonstrated that myocardial salvage with early recovery of contractile function after acute coronary occlusion is possible beyond 8 hours using controlled surgical reperfusion. The results of these studies suggest that the methods of reperfusion are more important in determining the fate of the myocardium at risk than how quickly blood flow is restored. Overall patient survival depends upon the size of the infarction and the functional recovery of the myocardium. Following acute myocardial infarction in patients with triple-vessel disease, ischemia of the remote myocardium may progress to heart failure and cardiogenic shock. Surgical techniques afford the benefits of circulatory support, controlled reperfusion of the infarct zone, and global myocardial protection and resuscitation, as well as complete revascularization of the remote myocardium to improve patient outcomes.

FAILED PTCA

With the advent of intracoronary stents, the complication of abrupt vessel closure seen with PTCA has been greatly reduced. The need for emergency CABG after failed PTCA has fallen from 2–7% to 0.6–1.5% in recent years.[41] Some have questioned whether surgical back-up is needed at all today for PTCA.[42] The broadening application of PCI in coronary artery disease has led to a changing profile of patients requiring emergency CABG after unsuccessful PCI. Compared with those in earlier series, patients requiring emergency CABG are now older and more likely to be female, have more advanced coronary disease, more cardiovascular risk factors and more frequent preoperative ischemia or evolving myocardial infarction.[43] In addition, many patients undergoing catheter-based interventions also receive potent anticoagulant, thrombolytic and antiplatelet drugs, which may increase the bleeding complications of emergency surgical procedures. As a consequence, the incidence of myocardial infarction and accompanying heart failure, and the perioperative morbidity and mortality of emergency CABG, have been steadily rising despite improvements in surgical management.[43,44]

After failed PTCA, ischemia is common in patients referred for urgent or emergency CABG. Even with the use of stents or perfusion catheters, more than 60% of patients referred for urgent CABG have either chest pain or unstable hemodynamics.[41] In one institution, unsuccessful PTCA occurred with coronary occlusion in 54%, chest pain in 78% and vasopressor use in 25%.[45] Even in the best centers, the time required for reperfusion is often prolonged – 2 hours or more. Cardiopulmonary resuscitation is required prior to surgery in up to 13% of patients. The results of emergency CABG after failed PTCA demonstrate an increased risk of perioperative myocardial infarction (9–51%) and hospital mortality (6–29%).[41–47] Perioperative myocardial infarction is associated with a reduced late survival (6 months or more) after CABG.[46,47] Patients requiring emergency CABG are less likely to have arterial grafts implanted and thus forgo the advantages internal mammary artery bypass confers on late survival. The optimal treatment of patients who require emergency surgery after unsuccessful PTCA requires a strategy that addresses the three key issues of concern in these patients:

1 perioperative ischemia/infarction,
2 hemodynamic instability,
3 bleeding complications.

The management of perioperative ischemia requires an understanding of the factors that influence ischemia and reperfusion. Perioperative ischemia can be influenced by a number of practical steps that decrease the severity of ischemia (decreased oxygen demand or increased oxygen supply) or shorten the duration of ischemia. The simple use of perfusion catheters, guide wires or stents can prevent total occlusion following coronary dissection after failed PTCA and provide maintenance of some level of coronary perfusion during transport to the operating room. Pre-procedure consultation in high-risk patients, effective communication between the catheterization laboratory and operating room personnel, and appropriate use of an acuity scale can improve the coordination of care and facilitate transfer to the operating room, reducing the duration of ischemia. Early institution of IABP support or cardiopulmonary bypass reduces ischemia, decreases myocardial oxygen demand, and provides hemodynamic support for patients with hypotension, heart failure or rhythm disturbances.

Strategies for myocardial protection and reperfusion are critically important in patients with severe ischemia or evolving infarction after failed PTCA. Although off-pump strategies have been employed in some patients who pose special risks for cardiopulmonary bypass, in general off-pump procedures do not afford optimal myocardial protection for ischemic patients because myocardial oxygen demands are not reduced and reperfusion with normal blood after prolonged ischemia may increase myocardial injury. Cardiopulmonary bypass with continuous coronary perfusion using warm blood and beta-blockade to reduce oxygen demand has potential advantages over cold crystalloid cardioplegia in some situations by avoiding global ischemia and reducing postoperative myocardial edema.[48] This approach presumes that coronary flow is evenly distributed and that coronary perfusion is not interrupted. This strategy has appeal in carefully selected patients with severe left ventricular dysfunction due to prior infarction, for revascularization of non-occluded coronary arteries, and for one-vessel or two-vessel disease. It has less appeal than integrated cardioplegia for patients with an acute coronary occlusion, evolving myocardial infarction, cardiogenic shock, multivessel disease or circumflex disease.

Integrated cardioplegia provides the best approach for patients with severe ischemia after failed PTCA.[49] Warm blood cardioplegia enables resuscitation of energy-depleted hearts after ischemia. With coronary occlusion, retrograde delivery has been shown to enhance cardioplegic protection and significantly reduce mortality in emergency CABG.[47] Controlled surgical reperfusion of the infarct zone with warm blood cardioplegia has been shown to significantly reduce infarct size, enhance functional recovery, improve clinical outcomes and reduce mortality in experimental and clinical settings.[9]

Beyersdorf demonstrated the importance of myocardial protection techniques in patients undergoing emergency CABG after failed angioplasty.[34] He examined the results of surgical revascularization after acute coronary occlusion in 163 patients. Over the time period studied (1977–1992), four techniques for protection were used:

1 crystalloid cardioplegia (1977–1980),
2 hypothermic fibrillation (1980–1986),
3 blood cardioplegia (1986–1989),
4 blood cardioplegia with controlled reperfusion (1989–1992).

During the period from 1989 to 1992, improvements in myocardial protection included preoperative insertion of IABP, warm blood cardioplegia induction, substrate-enhanced cardioplegia with amino acids, combined antegrade and retrograde delivery of cardioplegia, controlled reperfusion and prolonged vented bypass. Mortality was reduced by using warm blood cardioplegia with controlled reperfusion, despite a higher risk profile of patients in the latter half of the study. With controlled reperfusion as opposed to unmodified blood reperfusion, mortality was reduced from 11% to 5% and, for those patients in cardiogenic shock, from 50% to 15%. With controlled reperfusion, spontaneous sinus rhythm was restored in 81% versus 19% with unmodified reperfusion; arrhythmias were reduced to 22% versus 53%; and regional wall motion returned to normal or slight hypokinesis within 7 days postoperatively in 86% versus 34%. Bottner reported a reduction in perioperative myocardial infarction after emergency CABG for failed PTCA using warm blood cardioplegia for induction and terminal reperfusion and cold blood cardioplegia for maintenance of arrest.[40] This method reduced the incidence of myocardial infarction compared with cold blood cardioplegia from 65% to 26% and the incidence of Q-wave myocardial infarction from 38% to 16%.

For unstable patients in cardiac arrest after failed PTCA, rapid institution of cardiopulmonary bypass is necessary to restore the circulation, prevent neurological injury and avoid death. Percutaneous extracorporeal circulation is useful in patients refractory to conventional resuscitative measures.[50] After circulatory support is established, the myocardium should be resuscitated using warm blood cardioplegia enriched with glutamate and aspartate while emergency coronary revascularization is performed. Using this approach, intractable ventricular fibrillation has been reversed and cardiac function restored in 13 of 14 patients.[51]

BLEEDING COMPLICATIONS AFTER ANTI-THROMBOTIC THERAPY

Most cases of acute myocardial infarction are the result of thrombosis of the coronary artery supplying the infarcted region. A vast array of pharmacological therapies has targeted coronary arterial thrombi in an effort to restore blood flow to the ischemic myocardium rapidly and safely. As the diversity of anti-thrombotic agents used in acute coronary syndromes increases, the perioperative management of these patients becomes more complex.

Thrombolytic therapy initiated early after acute myocardial infarction has been shown to reduce both early and long-term mortality rates. Streptokinase and tissue-type plasminogen activator (t-PA, alteplase) are the most widely used thrombolytic agents. CABG surgery may be required early after thrombolytic therapy. The risk of postoperative hemorrhage has been shown to be higher in patients requiring surgery within 12 hours of thrombolytic therapy than in controls.[52] In addition, the Thrombolysis in Myocardial Infarction II (TIMI II) trial showed a significant increase in postoperative blood loss in patients operated on within 24 hours of thrombolysis compared with those operated on more than 24 hours after therapy.[53] Elective operations should be delayed at least 48 hours after thrombolysis, but urgent and emergency operations can be performed safely by utilizing aprotinin preoperatively and fresh frozen plasma and platelet transfusions when necessary to correct the coagulopathy. Fibrinogen levels below $100 \, mg \, dL^{-1}$ in the setting of microvascular bleeding should be treated with cryoprecipitate transfusion at a dose of 1 unit $10 \, kg^{-1}$ body weight.

The final common pathway of coronary artery platelet-rich thrombus formation is platelet aggregation mediated by cross-linking of platelet GPIIb/IIIa receptors and fibrinogen. Three inhibitors of platelet GPIIb/IIIa receptors – abciximab (ReoPro), eptifibatide (Integrilin) and tirofiban (Aggrestat) – have been shown to decrease the ischemic complications of acute myocardial syndromes in numerous large, multicenter, prospective, randomized trials.[54–56] Abciximab is a chimeric monoclonal antibody fragment that binds irreversibly to the GPIIb/IIIa receptor on the platelet surface. The standard intravenous dose blocks >90% of the GPIIb/IIIa receptors, resulting in defects in platelet aggregation and prolonged bleeding times. By 12 hours after discontinuing drug infusion, about 68% of the GPIIb/IIIa receptors are blocked, resulting in normalized bleeding times. Unbound antibodies are immediately eliminated from the plasma. Transfused platelets therefore do not encounter unbound abciximab in the plasma, but the antibody redistributes to the receptors on both native and transfused platelets, resulting in normalized platelet aggregation. Several trials, including the Evaluation of c7E3 in Preventing Ischemic Complications (EPIC), Evaluation of PTCA to Improve Long-Term Outcome by c7E3 GPIIb/IIIa Receptor Blockade (EPILOG), and Evaluation of Platelet IIb/IIIa Inhibition in Stenting (EPISTENT) trials, failed to show any statistically significant increase in bleeding complications or transfusion requirements in the subsets of patients requiring CABG after treatment with abciximab, but both placebo and treated groups did demonstrate a higher than expected transfusion requirement.[55,56] Several single-institution series report serious bleeding complications, especially when surgery is required within 12–24 hours of discontinuation of the drug.[57–59]

This experience has led surgeons to alter the perioperative management of these patients. Some have advocated delaying surgery when possible for 24 hours after discontinuing abciximab. Obviously, emergency operations should not be delayed, and the risk of potential excessive bleeding must be weighed against the urgency of the intervention. Others have suggested routine transfusions of platelets early after weaning from bypass.[58] This platelet 'antidote' approach may actually decrease the overall number of blood products required in patients with deficient platelet aggregation postoperatively. Owing to the variability in duration of inhibition of platelet aggregation and patient response characteristics, an individualized approach to perioperative management is advised. At the Texas Heart Institute, we use a rapid assay for platelet aggregation and platelet function as well as clinical evidence of microvascular bleeding to determine whether platelet transfusion is indicated.[57] Patients who have received abciximab and have moderate to severe platelet dysfunction preoperatively are transfused with platelets prior to surgery. Platelet function is then monitored after weaning from cardiopulmonary bypass and in the early postoperative period.

Eptifibatide (a cyclic heptapeptide) and tirofiban (a small non-peptide molecule) are smaller than abciximab and have a high specificity but low affinity for GPIIb/IIIa receptors, resulting in a rapid onset of action and short half-life of 1–2 hours. The shorter half-life may offer safety advantages over the longer-acting monoclonal antibody abciximab. The Integrilin to Minimize Platelet Aggregation and Coronary Thrombosis (IMPACT) II and Platelet Glycoprotein IIb/IIIa in Unstable Angina: Receptor Suppression Using Integrilin Therapy (PURSUIT) trials

reported no significant increase in major bleeding complications or transfusion requirements in patients requiring CABG early after treatment with Integrilin. Turina and colleagues also reported no increase in transfusion requirements in patients undergoing coronary artery bypass within 8 hours of discontinuation of tirofiban compared with those operated on more than 8 hours after treatment.[60] Our experience with patients requiring CABG early after tirofiban treatment is similar. Platelet transfusion requirements are determined by the presence of clinical microvascular bleeding along with evidence of platelet dysfunction on rapid platelet aggregometry and platelet function assays after bypass. Orally active GPIIb/IIIa receptor antagonists showed early promise, but phase III clinical trials reported increased bleeding complication rates and increased mortality.

Ticlopidine (Ticlid) and clopidogrel (Plavix) are orally active thienopyridines that selectively bind to adenylate cyclase-coupled adenosine diphosphate receptors on the surface of platelets and irreversibly inhibit platelet aggregation and activation. Clopidogrel has equivalent therapeutic effects but a more rapid onset of action when compared with ticlopidine. In addition, the side effects that have maligned the use of ticlopidine, including rash, diarrhea, neutropenia, aplastic anemia, thrombocytopenia and thrombotic thrombocytopenic purpura, are less prevalent with the use of clopidogrel. The Clopidogrel in Unstable Angina to Prevent Recurrent Ischemic Events (CURE) trial reported decreased risk of death, myocardial infarction and stroke but a slightly increased risk of major bleeding in patients treated with clopidogrel and aspirin compared with those receiving placebo and aspirin.[61] To date, there have been no published studies of patients undergoing CABG after treatment with clopidogrel. In our experience, patients treated with clopidogrel preoperatively were found to have significant increases in postoperative blood loss and transfusion requirements, especially for platelets. Platelet aggregation studies have identified a subset of patients with abnormal preoperative and postoperative platelet function that more often require transfusions. As use of these anti-thrombotic agents becomes more widespread, it is imperative that cardiac surgeons and cardiologists understand the implications of their use in the perioperative management and outcomes in patients who require surgical intervention.

CARDIOGENIC SHOCK

Cardiogenic shock due to left ventricular power failure occurs in 7–8% of patients following acute coronary occlusion and is the leading cause of in-hospital death after acute myocardial infarction.[62] Shock may occur on initial presentation, but usually develops more than

6 hours after the onset of symptoms due to extension of the infarction or dysfunction of the remaining myocardium. Without revascularization, the mortality for cardiogenic shock is 80–90%. In the past, a number of different approaches have been applied for the treatment of cardiogenic shock, with disappointing results.

In the SHOCK registry, cardiogenic shock was studied in 19 centers to reveal an overall mortality of 66%.[63] Mortality was lower in patients selected for cardiac catheterization (51%) than in those who were not (85%). Patients found to have an open infarct-related artery at catheterization (whether spontaneous or treatment induced) had improved survival.

Thrombolytic therapy has been applied in cardiogenic shock, but intracoronary streptokinase has a disappointing patency rate (43%) in cardiogenic shock due to hypotension.[64] In the Gruppo Italiano per lo Studio della Sopravvivenza nell'Infarto Miocardico (GISSI) I trial, streptokinase alone (without aspirin or heparin) did not reduce mortality for patients with cardiogenic shock (70%). In the Global Utilization of Streptokinase and Tissue Plasminogen Activator for Occluded Coronary Arteries (GUSTO) I trial, a more aggressive anticoagulation strategy was employed, resulting in a 30-day mortality of 58%.[65] The use of IABP support or vasopressors combined with t-PA may improve the reperfusion rate in experimental studies. Among 17 published series of patients undergoing PTCA for cardiogenic shock after acute myocardial infarction ($n = 453$), the combined hospital mortality was 46%,[66] but the overall rate of successful revascularization was only 73% and the mortality was even higher if PTCA was unsuccessful. The timing of PTCA varied and most patients underwent PTCA of the infarct-related artery only. The results of CABG in cardiogenic shock in 19 studies (323 patients) have been reported in the literature, revealing a combined hospital mortality rate of 32%.[66]

Intra-aortic balloon counterpulsation has been shown to be extremely helpful for circulatory support in patients with refractory cardiogenic shock. Early experience with IABP alone without revascularization did not reduce mortality rates. IABP has proven to be highly effective in the clinical stabilization of cardiogenic shock, allowing improved support for patients undergoing angiography and revascularization. Despite the observed survival advantages of early catheterization and revascularization in cardiogenic shock, few patients are selected for early invasive treatment. In the GUSTO I trial of 2600 patients with cardiogenic shock treated by thrombolysis, the rate of utilization of invasive procedures was low.[67] Among patients with myocardial infarction who arrived in shock, only 16% underwent PTCA, 7% CABG and 22% IABP support. Of those who developed shock later, only 20% had PTCA, 12% CABG and 25% IABP support. Despite the infrequent use of IABP in the GUSTO I trial, IABP-supported patients showed a trend towards lower

mortality at 30 days (48% vs 59%) and significantly reduced 1-year mortality (57% vs 67%).

At the present time, the current medical treatment of cardiogenic shock involves pharmacological support with occasional mechanical circulatory support if an early angiographic study is undertaken. Thrombolytic therapy is used mostly in patients who present early in infarction (less than 6 hours from onset) and rarely for a delayed presentation. Angioplasty is usually employed to re-open target vessels to the infarct zone, but little attention is paid to the timing of revascularization or the presence of critical disease in remote areas. Operation is generally delayed and reserved for patients whose condition does not improve with medical therapy or who survive long enough for semi-elective revascularization.[66]

Excluding other causes of shock after acute myocardial infarction, such as right ventricular failure, ventricular septal rupture, acute mitral insufficiency and cardiac tamponade, the pathophysiology of cardiogenic shock complicating myocardial infarction is well understood.[68] With coronary occlusion, the ischemic muscle develops immediate akinesis or dyskinesis and ceases to contribute to the cardiac output. If more than 40% of the left ventricle is involved, the heart is unable to provide an adequate cardiac output and shock occurs, leading to multi-organ failure and death. If less than 30% of the left ventricle is at risk, remote areas of the myocardium at a distance from the infarct region develop compensatory hyperkinesis to maintain the cardiac output. Failure of the remote muscle to increase contractility may occur due to prior infarction or ischemic dysfunction from coronary stenosis, or following failure of myocardial protective strategies. Since most patients develop cardiogenic shock 2–4 days after the acute myocardial infarction, there is little chance that reperfusion of the infarct zone will restore regional contractility. The primary focus of therapy is directed towards resuscitation and revascularization of the remote myocardium.[69] The aim of therapy is to restore contractile function to the remote myocardium sufficient to support the circulation and reverse pump failure.

In 1989, Allen and colleagues presented a comprehensive strategy for the management of cardiogenic shock that called for revascularization as a medical/surgical emergency.[70] In their study of 80 consecutive patients in cardiogenic shock after acute myocardial infarction receiving inotropic and IABP support, the authors performed emergency CABG an average of 3.4 days after acute myocardial infarction. Maximal protection of the remote myocardium was achieved by induction with warm blood cardioplegia enriched by glutamate and aspartate, maintenance of arrest with multidose cold blood cardioplegia, and terminal reperfusion by warm blood cardioplegia.

The primary focus of therapy was revascularization of all viable areas of remote myocardium necessary to sustain contractile function postoperatively. The first grafts

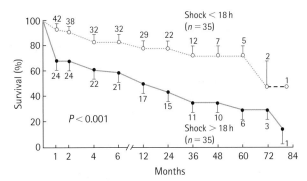

Figure 20.5 *Actuarial survival after coronary artery bypass grafting for cardiogenic shock. Note influence of time from onset of shock to operation (<18 hours or >18 hours) on patient survival. Reprinted from Allen BS, Rosenkranz E, Buckberg GD, et al. Studies on prolonged acute regional ischemia. VI. Myocardial infarction with left ventricular power failure: a medical/surgical emergency requiring urgent revascularization with maximal protection of the remote muscle.* J Thorac Cardiovasc Surg *1989; 98:691–703, with permission from Elsevier Science.*

were placed to the areas of 'greatest importance' (i.e. the largest vessels supplying viable, remote myocardium). The infarct zone was judged the 'least' important region during revascularization if the infarct was established or extending (>18 hours). However, in an evolving myocardial infarction, early recovery of function of the infarct muscle can be anticipated 6 hours or more after acute occlusion using the methods of controlled surgical reperfusion. Vein grafts are preferred to arterial conduits because the flow rate can vary in arterial grafts postoperatively, especially if vasopressors are required. In addition, vein grafts provide a conduit for the administration of warm blood cardioplegia that is beneficial for resuscitation of the ischemic heart. Prolonged cardioplegic reperfusion of the infarct zone was effective in patients with acute evolving infarction less than 18 hours old in this study. Regional wall motion in the infarct zone improved even after this extended period. Using this approach, left ventricular power failure was reversed in 94% of the patients, all of whom were successfully weaned from inotropic drugs and the IABP.

The importance of urgent revascularization before the effects of shock progress to multi-organ failure was emphasized.[70] If the operation was performed within 18 hours after the onset of shock, the 30-day mortality rate was only 7%. If, however, operation was delayed more than 18 hours, the 30-day mortality rose to 31% (Figure 20.5). A high late mortality (26%) was found in patients with late extending infarction (>18 hours after myocardial infarction), longer delay from shock to operation (>18 hours after onset of shock), preoperative organ failure, and a prior history of myocardial infarction.

Among late survivors, 67% were physically active. Other studies have confirmed the dramatic decrease in early mortality in patients with cardiogenic shock (3–16%) when using an aggressive approach of revascularization with CABG and surgical reperfusion techniques.[33,34,71]

Early and late mortality in cardiogenic shock are related to time from infarct to operation, time from shock to operation, preoperative organ failure and history of previous infarction.[70] Most late deaths are due to cardiac failure in patients with inadequate contractile reserve. Patients with only a small remnant of viable muscle in the remote myocardium are probably not good candidates for surgery. Preoperative criteria for revascularization in patients in cardiogenic shock include adequate target vessels to the remote myocardium as well as a mass of remote muscle sufficient to sustain contractility and circulation after surgery. Dramatic improvement in survival can be achieved by surgical revascularization using advanced cardioprotective techniques.

POST-INFARCTION VENTRICULAR SEPTAL RUPTURE

Although relatively rare, ventricular septal rupture (VSR) is a devastating complication of acute myocardial infarction. VSR occurs in about 1–2% of patients suffering an acute infarction, but accounts for up to one-third of deaths.[72,73] The results of non-surgical management are dismal.[74] Since Cooley performed the first successful repair of a post-infarction VSR in 1956,[75] the timing, indications and surgical techniques have evolved, resulting in significant improvements in operative mortality.

Ventricular septal rupture is more likely to occur in older patients, in female patients, in patients with hypertension and in patients suffering a first myocardial infarction (often transmural) with occlusion of a single vessel. Rupture of the anterior septum associated with occlusion of the LAD artery and rupture of the posterior septum associated with right coronary artery or dominant left circumflex artery occlusion occur with equal frequency, although a trend towards the increasing incidence of posterior VSR has been reported. Septal rupture can happen within hours to 2 weeks after acute myocardial infarction, but occurs most often 2–4 days after myocardial infarction.[76] Patients complain of sudden onset of severe chest pain hours to days following myocardial infarction. The association of a new, harsh, systolic murmur and rapid hemodynamic decompensation probably indicates post-infarction VSR or acute mitral regurgitation. Color-flow Doppler echocardiography has high sensitivity and specificity in this situation, approaching 100%. The diagnosis of post-infarction VSR with hemodynamic compromise requires emergency surgery.

Historically, surgery was postponed several weeks until the infarction matured and fibrosed, allowing sutures to hold better than in the acutely infarcted, friable myocardium. Only about 5% of patients survived the interim, most dying of cardiogenic shock and multiple system organ failure. Currently, most agree that surgery should not be delayed in patients with any evidence of hemodynamic instability because of the potential for rapid deterioration. Cardiogenic shock resulting in renal, respiratory and hepatic failure is the leading cause of morbidity and mortality in these patients. The use of IABP for afterload reduction can offer enough stability to obtain coronary catheterization prior to surgery, but will not usually improve the condition for more than 24 hours. Surgery should not be delayed after the diagnosis has been made. Several important advancements have allowed for earlier surgical intervention with acceptable risks. Improvements in perioperative management, pharmacological support and myocardial protection, as well as routine use of IABP and early diagnosis, have improved operative mortality.

As mentioned in the discussion of cardiogenic shock, advanced methods of myocardial protection are of the utmost importance to support and to resuscitate the failing heart in patients with VSR. However, over the last 45 years, surgical techniques have also evolved for the treatment of this high-risk population. The early procedures for repair of post-infarction VSR involved techniques used to repair congenital septal defects that approached the septum through a right ventriculotomy. This approach was replaced by a left ventriculotomy and initially involved an infarctectomy because of the recognized need to place sutures in healthy tissues. Buttressing pledgets and strips were used to secure an endocardial patch of glutaraldehyde-treated pericardium or Dacron.[76] The recognition of a 10–25% recurrence rate and the weakness of peri-infarct muscle led to an important technical modification of the endocardial septal patch.[77–79] Enlargement of the endocardial patch to exclude both the septal defect and the infarct from the high-pressure left ventricular chamber, as well as placement of the suture line in normal myocardium, provided a more secure repair (Figure 20.6). These modifications were adapted from previous techniques for the repair of left ventricular aneurysms. Secure closure of the left ventriculotomy requires wide suture placement reinforced by Teflon felt strips. While closure of the VSR is the primary goal of the operation, coronary revascularization may be necessary. It is reasonable to include expeditious bypass of several large stenotic arteries supplying significant areas of viable myocardium.

Although a high operative mortality of 60% is generally reported in patients with acute post-infarction VSR, several recent reports suggest that an improvement in mortality (14–20%) is possible with early surgical

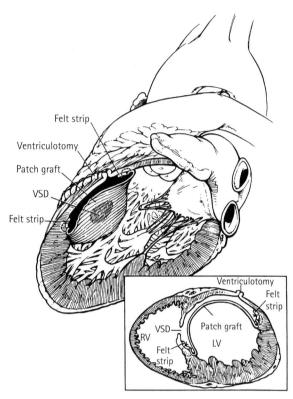

Figure 20.6 Repair of post-infarction ventricular septal rupture. Note the infarcted septum is excluded by a Dacron patch from ventricular pressure. Interrupted mattress sutures and felt pledgets are used to reinforce the repair. A continuous suture is used to secure the patch. LV, left ventricle; RV, right ventricle; VSD, ventricular septal defect. Reprinted from Cooley DA. Repair of postinfarction ventricular septal rupture. J Card Surg 1994; 9:427–9, with permission from Blackwell Publishing Ltd.

intervention.[78,79] Independent predictors of operative mortality include advanced age, cardiogenic shock, right ventricular dysfunction, posterior location of VSR and renal failure. Despite the high operative risk of VSR, long-term survival at 5 years (70%) and 10 years (50%) and late functional status are good. Late survival is better in patients with inferior VSR than in those with anterior VSR. Recurrent VSR is uncommon after repair using endocardial patch techniques with septal exclusion.[79]

ISCHEMIC MITRAL REGURGITATION

Ischemic mitral regurgitation (IMR) is a complex and potentially lethal complication of acute myocardial infarction. Management of patients with IMR requires an accurate understanding of its mechanism and of the outcomes of the various therapeutic options. IMR involves moderate to severe mitral regurgitation preceded by myocardial ischemia and excludes other etiologies of mitral valve pathology (i.e. rheumatic, degenerative or congenital).

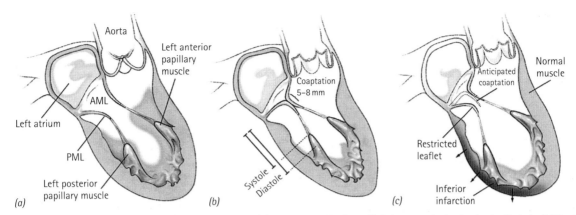

Figure 20.7 *Mechanisms of ischemic mitral regurgitation. (a) Diagrammatic view of left heart and mitral valve in diastole. (b) During systole, the distance is reduced between the base of the papillary muscle and the mitral annulus, allowing coaptation of the mitral leaflets. (c) After infero-basal myocardial infarction, the papillary muscle and inferior wall are displaced away from the mitral annulus during systole, restricting leaflet motion and preventing coaptation. Mitral regurgitation occurs in extreme cases. Annular dilatation produces further loss of coaptation. AML, anterior mitral leaflet; PML, posterior mitral leaflet. Reprinted from Tatoulis J. Ischemic mitral valve disease: surgical repair. In Ischemic Heart Disease. Surgical Management, Buxton B, Frazier OH, Westaby S (eds). London: Mosby International Ltd, 1999, 303–20, with permission from Elsevier Science.*

Several studies reporting the results of IMR treatment have included non-ischemic etiologies of mitral regurgitation associated with coronary artery disease. Operative mortality is significantly worse in patients with IMR than in those with non-ischemic mitral regurgitation.[80] This has added to the controversy concerning the optimal management strategies.

Ischemic mitral regurgitation occurs in less than 5% of patients undergoing coronary catheterization and in 10–20% of patients undergoing CABG. The mechanisms of IMR include papillary muscle dysfunction, severe left ventricular dysfunction and dilatation, and papillary muscle rupture. Patient presentation and therapeutic outcomes depend on the mechanisms of IMR and on the degree of ventricular dysfunction. Recent evidence from animal studies has improved our understanding of the dynamic changes in geometry involved in normal and pathological mitral valves.[81,82] These experimental studies may have important implications for selecting and developing surgical techniques to make repair of these valves more predictable.

Ischemic mitral regurgitation may be transient, with episodes of dyspnoea and pulmonary edema temporally associated with angina symptoms, or sudden, acute and progressive congestive heart failure associated with acute rupture of a papillary muscle. Rupture of a papillary muscle trunk carries a grim prognosis with a high mortality rate. Rupture of a papillary head may cause acute leaflet prolapse. Infarction and scarring may result in elongation of the papillary muscle with mitral leaflet prolapse, while atrophy of the papillary muscle after infarction may cause leaflet restriction and poor leaflet coaptation. Dysfunction of the left ventricular wall adjacent to a papillary muscle is associated with IMR due to restriction of leaflet motion (Figure 20.7). A severely dilated left ventricle can cause mitral regurgitation by papillary muscle displacement.

The operative mortality and survival rates following the surgical correction of IMR are worse than the results of non-ischemic mitral regurgitation, even when the latter is associated with coronary artery disease and concomitant CABG is performed.[83–87] However, several recent advances will probably improve outcomes. These include improved myocardial preservation techniques, a better understanding of the underlying mechanism of IMR, techniques to maintain or improve the integrity of the subvalvular apparatus by repairing the valve when appropriate or preserving chordae during mitral valve replacement, and expanded use of echocardiography.

Patients suspected of having IMR should undergo transthoracic or transesophageal echocardiography (TEE) to define the underlying pathology, followed by coronary angiography and percutaneous revascularization if possible. An IABP placed in the catheterization laboratory can be critical for resuscitation, to decrease left ventricular afterload and improve forward flow. If moderate to severe mitral regurgitation persists or adequate percutaneous revascularization is not feasible, the patient should be taken urgently to surgery for CABG and surgical correction of mitral regurgitation. Mild mitral regurgitation can improve over time following revascularization, but moderate to severe mitral regurgitation is not well tolerated by the ischemic myocardium due to increased wall stress and volume load.

The optimal surgical correction for IMR depends on the underlying pathology as well as the clinical acuity and other co-morbidities. Intraoperative TEE is essential. Appropriate myocardial preservation using antegrade and retrograde blood cardioplegia is required. The acutely regurgitant mitral valve usually does not result in left atrial enlargement, and the exposure can be more difficult than with chronic mitral regurgitation. Often, a trans-septal approach through the right atrium provides improved exposure. A ruptured papillary muscle head causing anterior leaflet prolapse can often be repaired by attaching the ruptured head to an adjacent viable papillary muscle head with pledgeted sutures. Chordal transfer or replacement with synthetic PTFE sutures is also an option as long as the tissue is healthy enough to hold the sutures. Papillary muscle head rupture or papillary muscle elongation causing posterior leaflet prolapse can be repaired by quadrangular resection or sliding leaflet valvuloplasty. The Alfieri repair, using sutures to approximate a flail segment to the opposing normal leaflet and create a double orifice, has been used with mixed results, but can be an option when limiting the cross-clamp time is crucial.[83] When IMR is due to left ventricular dysfunction or dilatation with apical or lateral displacement of the papillary muscle, or if the papillary muscle infarction has been replaced by scar, the results of repair are less predictable and the valve should be replaced. IMR can be corrected by ring annuloplasty alone in the setting of annular dilatation with poor leaflet coaptation. IMR can occur associated with a left ventricular aneurysm involving a papillary muscle. The involved papillary muscle can be transferred to adjacent viable myocardium, or valve replacement can be performed along with aneurysmorrhaphy.

Despite favorable outcomes and expanding indications for mitral valve repair versus replacement for non-ischemic etiologies, the benefits of repair over replacement for IMR are not as clear.[84,86] Some surgeons favor valve replacement because it can be more expedient than a complex valve repair and because the elimination of regurgitation is more predictable. Retaining the subvalvular apparatus during valve replacement may account for improved outcomes due to preserved ventricular systolic function.[84] The literature has added to the controversy because of the diversity of reports on repair techniques and underlying mechanisms as well as imprecise definitions of IMR. Reported operative mortality rates for surgical correction of IMR range from 7% to 53%. Five-year survival for mitral valve repair and replacement ranges from 60% to 80%, whereas that for non-surgical treatment for moderate to severe IMR has been reported to be less than 20%. The incidence of re-operation for residual mitral regurgitation is low. Most patients show improvement in New York Heart Association (NYHA) functional class following surgical correction. Left ventricular dysfunction, preoperative cardiogenic shock and a non-structural mechanism of IMR are the most consistent indicators of poor outcomes.

KEY REFERENCES

Allen BS, Buckberg GD, Fontan FM, Kirsh MM, Popoff G, Beyersforf F, *et al.* Superiority of controlled reperfusion versus percutaneous transluminal coronary angioplasty in acute coronary occlusion. *J Thorac Cardiovasc Surg* 1993; **105**:864–84.

This multicenter study of patients with acute coronary occlusion (acute myocardial infarction) reports superior results in 156 patients using methods of controlled surgical reperfusion compared to prior reports using PTCA for reperfusion. With controlled surgical reperfusion, the authors observed a lower mortality (3.9%), fewer arrhythmias and improved functional recovery.

Allen BS, Okamoto F, Buckberg GD, Bagyi H, Young H, Leaf J, *et al.* Studies of controlled reperfusion after ischemia. XV. Immediate functional recovery after six hours of regional ischemia by careful control of conditions of reperfusion and composition of reperfusate. *J Thorac Cardiovasc Surg* 1986; **92**:621–35.

This landmark study fundamentally changes the approach to ischemia and reperfusion. No longer is the duration of ischemia (or time to reperfusion) the primary determinant of myocardial salvage after acute coronary occlusion. This study demonstrates that the method of reperfusion is of critical importance. Control of the conditions and composition of reperfusion enables immediate functional recovery, even after 6 hours of coronary occlusion. In contrast, reperfusion with normal blood produces infarction with severe dyskinesis after 2 hours of coronary occlusion.

Allen BS, Rosenkranz E, Buckberg GD, Davtyan H, Laks H, Tillisch J, *et al.* Studies on prolonged acute regional ischemia VI. Myocardial infarction with left ventricular power failure: a medical/surgical emergency requiring urgent revascularization with maximal protection of remote muscle. *J Thorac Cardiovasc Surg* 1989; **98**: 691–703.

This clinical report sounds the alarm, emphasizing that cardiogenic shock after acute myocardial infarction is a medical/surgical emergency requiring urgent revascularization. Attention to myocardial protective techniques and the remote myocardium is necessary for recovery from heart failure and patient survival.

Christenson Jan T, Simonet F, Badel P, Schmuziger M. Evaluation of preoperative intra-aortic balloon pump support in high risk coronary patients. *Eur J Cardiothorac Surg* 1997; **11**:1097–103.

This clinical study demonstrates the value of preoperative IABP support in patients with myocardial ischemia, acute infarction or left ventricular failure and the effectiveness of this modality in reducing mortality and improving outcomes in high-risk patients.

Rosenkranz ER, Okamoto F, Buckberg GD. Safety of prolonged aortic clamping with blood cardioplegia. III. Aspartate enrichment of glutamate-blood cardioplegia in energy-depleted hearts after ischemic and reperfusion injury. *J Thorac Cardiovasc Surg* 1986; **91**:428–35.

In this experimental study, the importance of substrate-enriched warm blood cardioplegia in hearts subjected to ischemia is demonstrated. The addition of glutamate and aspartate to blood cardioplegia enhanced functional recovery in energy-depleted hearts.

REFERENCES

1. Berry WH. Mechanisms of myocardial cell injury during ischemia and reperfusion. *J Card Surg* 1987; **2**:375–83.
2. Jennings RB, Schapner J, Hill ML. Effect of reperfusion late in the phase of reversible ischemic injury: changes in cell volume, electrolytes, metabolites, and ultrastructure. *Circ Res* 1985; **56**:262–78.
3. Buckberg GD. Protean causes of myocardial stunning in infants and adults. *J Card Surg* 1993; **8**(Suppl. 12):214–19.
4. Buckberg GD. Studies of controlled reperfusion after ischemia: when is cardiac muscle damaged irreversibly? *J Thorac Cardiovasc Surg* 1986; **92**:483–7.
5. Christenson JT, Simonet F, Badel P, Schmuziger M. Evaluation of preoperative intra-aortic balloon pump support in high risk coronary patients. *Eur J Cardiothorac Surg* 1997; **11**:1097–103.
6. Buckberg GD. Strategies and logic of cardioplegic delivery to prevent, avoid, and reverse ischemic and reperfusion damage. *J Thorac Cardiovasc Surg* 1987; **93**:127–39.
7. Sweeney MS, Frazier OH. Device-supported myocardial revascularization: safe help for sick hearts. *Ann Thorac Surg* 1992; **54**:1065–70.
8. Rosenkrantz ER, Vinten-Johansen J, Buckberg GD, Okamoto F, Edwards H, Bugyi H. Benefits of normothermic induction of blood cardioplegia in energy-depleted hearts with maintenance of arrest by multidose cold blood cardioplegic infusions. *J Thorac Cardiovasc Surg* 1982; **84**:667–77.
9. Beyersdorf F, Buckberg GD. Myocardial protection in patients with acute myocardial infarction and cardiogenic shock. *Semin Thorac Cardiovasc Surg* 1993; **5**:151–61.
10. Rosenkranz ER, Okamoto F, Buckberg GD, Robertson JM, Vinten-Johansen J, Bugyi H. Safety of prolonged aortic clamping with blood cardioplegia. III. Aspartate enrichment of glutamate-blood cardioplegia in energy-depleted hearts after ischemic and reperfusion injury. *J Thorac Cardiovasc Surg* 1986; **91**:428–35.
11. Allen BS, Okamoto F, Buckberg GD, Leaf J, Bugyi H. Studies of controlled reperfusion after ischemia. XII. Effects of 'duration' of reperfusate administrations versus reperfusate 'dose' on regional, functional, biochemical, and histochemical recovery. *J Thorac Cardiovasc Surg* 1986; **92**:594–604.
12. Follette DM, Fey K, Buckberg GD, Helly JJ, Steed DL, Foglig RP, *et al.* Reducing post-ischemic damage by temporary modifications of reperfusate calcium, potassium, pH, and osmolarity. *J Thorac Cardiovasc Surg* 1981; **82**:221–38.
13. Allen BS, Okamoto F, Buckberg GD, Acar C, Partington M, Bugyi H. Studies of controlled reperfusion after ischemia. IX. Reperfusate composition: benefits of marked hypocalcemia and diltiazem on regional recovery. *J Thorac Cardiovasc Surg* 1986; **92**:564–72.
14. Slogoff S, Keats A. Does perioperative myocardial ischemia lead to postoperative myocardial infarction? *Anesthesiology* 1985; **62**:107–14.
15. Braunwald E, Antman EM, Beasley JW, Califf RM, Cheitlin MD, Hochman JS, *et al.* ACC/AHA guidelines for the management of patients with unstable angina and non-ST-segment elevation myocardial infarction. *J Am Coll Cardiol* 2000; **36**:970–1062.
16. Influence of diabetes on 5-year mortality and morbidity in a randomized trial comparing CABG and PTCA in patients with multivessel disease: the Bypass Angioplasty Revascularization Investigation (BARI). *Circulation* 1997; **96**:1761–9.
17. Isom OH, Spencer FC, Firginbaum H, Cunningham J, Roe C. Prebypass myocardial damage in patients undergoing coronary revascularization: an unrecognized vulnerable period [Abstract]. *Circulation* 1975; **51**(2):119.
18. Bjessmo S, Ivert T. Troponin-T in patients with unstable and stable angina pectoris undergoing coronary bypass surgery. *Thorac Cardiovasc Surg* 2000; **48**(3):140–4.
19. Bjessmo S, Hammer N, Sandberg E, Ivert T. Reduced risk of coronary artery bypass surgery for unstable angina during a 6 year period. *Eur J Cardiothorac Surg* 2000; **18**:388–92.
20. Hanafy HM, Allen BS, Winkelmann JW, Ham J, Osimani D, Hart RS. Warm blood cardioplegia induction: an underused modality. *Ann Thorac Surg* 1994; **58**:1589–94.
21. Lazar HL, Philippides G, Fitzgerald C, Lancaster D, Sharmin RJ, Apstein C. Glucose–insulin–potassium solutions enhance recovery after urgent coronary artery bypass grafting. *J Thorac Cardiovasc Surg* 1997; **113**:354–60.
22. Cartier R. Systematic off-pump coronary artery revascularization: experience of 275 cases. *Ann Thorac Surg* 1999; **68**:1494–7.
23. Pasini E, Ferrari G, Cremora G, Ferrari M. Revascularization of severe hibernating myocardium in the beating heart: early hemodynamic and metabolic features. *Ann Thorac Surg* 2001; **71**:176–9.
24. Craver J, Murrah CP. Elective intraaortic balloon counterpulsation for high-risk off-pump coronary artery bypass operations. *Ann Thorac Surg* 2001; **71**:1220–3.
25. Lockowandt U, Owall A, Franco-Careceda A. Myocardial outflow of prostacycline in relation to metabolic stress during off-pump coronary artery bypass grafting. *Ann Thorac Surg* 2000; **70**:206–11.
26. DeWood MA, Spores J, Notske R. Medical and surgical management of myocardial infarction. *Am J Cardiol* 1979; **44**:1356–64.
27. Gunnar RM, Bourdillon PDV, Dixon DW, Fuster V, Karp R, Kennedy JW, *et al.* ACC/AHA guidelines for the early management of patients with acute myocardial infarction. *J Am Coll Cardiol* 1990; **16**:249–92.
28. Mehta, RH, Rathore SS, Radford MJ, Wang Y, Krumholz HM. Acute myocardial infarction in the elderly: difference by age. *J Am Coll Cardiol* 2001; **36**:736–41.
29. Tu JV, Pashos CL, Naylor CD, Chen E, Normand SL, Newhouse SL, *et al.* Use of cardiac procedures and outcomes in elderly patients with myocardial infarction in the United States and Canada. *N Engl J Med* 1997; **337**:139.
30. Lee DC, Oz MC, Weinberg AD, Lin SX, Ting W. Optimal timing of revascularization: transmural versus nontransmural acute myocardial infarction. *Ann Thorac Surg* 2001; **71**:1197–202.
31. Beyersdorf F, Maul F, Sarai K, Wendt T, Satter P, Buckberg GD, *et al.* Immediate functional benefits after controlled reperfusion during surgical revascularization for acute coronary occlusion. *J Thorac Cardiovasc Surg* 1991; **102**:856–66.
32. Von Segesser LK, Popp J, Amann FW, Turina MI. Surgical revascularization in acute myocardial infarction. *Eur J Cardiothorac Surg* 1994; **8**:363–9.
33. Allen BS, Buckberg GD, Fontan FM, Kirsh MM, Popoff G, Beyersdorf F, *et al.* Superiority of controlled surgical reperfusion

versus percutaneous transluminal coronary angioplasty in acute coronary occlusion. *J Thorac Cardiovasc Surg* 1993; 105:864–84.

34. Beyersdorf F, Mitrev Z, Sarai K, Eckel L, Klepzig H, Maul FD, *et al.* Changing patterns of patients undergoing emergency surgical revascularization for acute coronary occlusion: importance of myocardial protection techniques. *J Thorac Cardiovasc Surg* 1993; 106:137–48.

35. Vinten-Johansen J, Buckberg GD, Okamoto F, Rosenkranz ER, Bugyi H, Leaf J. Studies of controlled reperfusion after ischemia. V. Superiority of surgical versus medical reperfusion after regional ischemia. *J Thorac Cardiovasc Surg* 1986; 92:525–34.

36. Allen BS, Okamoto F, Buckberg GD, Bagyi H, Young H, Leaf J, *et al.* Studies of controlled reperfusion after ischemia. XV. Immediate functional recovery after six hours of regional ischemia by careful control of conditions of reperfusion and composition of reperfusate. *J Thorac Cardiovasc Surg* 1986; 92:621–35.

37. Allen BS, Buckberg GD, Schwariger M, Yeatman L, Tillisch J, Kawata N, *et al.* Studies of controlled reperfusion after ischemia. XVI. Consistent early recovery of regional wall motion following surgical revascularization after eight hours of acute coronary occlusion. *J Thorac Cardiovasc Surg* 1986; 92:636–48.

38. Buckberg GD, Beyersdorf F, Allen BS, Robertson JM. Integrated myocardial management: background and initial application. *J Card Surg* 1995; 10:68–89.

39. Lazar HL, Buckberg GD, Foglia RP, Manganaro AJ, Maloney JV Jr. Detrimental effects of premature use of inotropic drugs to discontinue cardiopulmonary bypass. *J Thorac Cardiovasc Surg* 1981; 82:18–25.

40. Bottner RK, Wallace RB, Visner WS, Stark KS, Recientes E, Katz NM, *et al.* Reduction of myocardial infarction after emergency coronary artery bypass grafting for failed coronary angioplasty with use of a normothermic reperfusion cardioplegia protocol. *J Thorac Cardiovasc Surg* 1991; 101:1069–75.

41. Shubrooks SJ, Nesto RW, Leeman D, Waxman S, Lewis SM, Fitzpatrick P, *et al.* Urgent coronary bypass surgery for failed percutaneous coronary intervention in the stent era: is backup still necessary? *Am Heart J* 2001; 142:190–6.

42. Reinecke H, Fetsch T, Roeder N, Schmidt C, Winter A, Ribbing M, *et al.* Emergency coronary bypass grafting after failed coronary angioplasty: what has changed in a decade? *Ann Thorac Surg* 2000; 70(6):1997–2003.

43. Lazar HL, Jacobs AK, Aldea GS, Shapira OM, Lancaster D, Sherwin RJ. Factors influencing mortality after emergency coronary artery bypass grafting for failed percutaneous transluminal coronary angioplasty. *Ann Thorac Surg* 1997; 64:1747–52.

44. Alvarez JM. Emergency coronary bypass grafting for failed percutaneous coronary stenting: increased costs and platelet transfusion requirements after the use of abciximab. *J Thorac Cardiovasc Surg* 1998; 115:462–3.

45. Berger PB, Stensrud PE, Daly RD, Grill D, Bell MR, Garratt KW, *et al.* Time to reperfusion and other procedural characteristics of emergency coronary artery bypass surgery after unsuccessful coronary angioplasty. *Am J Cardiol* 1995; 76:565–9.

46. Ladowski JS, Dillon TA, Deschner WP, DeRiso AJ 2nd, Peterson AC, Schatzlein MH. Durability of emergency coronary artery bypass for complications of failed angioplasty. *Cardiovasc Surg* 1996; 4:23–7.

47. Klatte K, Chaitman BR, Theroux P, Garard JA, Stocke K, Boyce S, *et al.* for the Guardian Investigators. Increased mortality after coronary artery bypass graft surgery is associated with increased levels of postoperative creatine kinase-myocardial band isoenzyme release. Results from the GUARDIAN Trial. *J Am Coll Cardiol* 2001; 38:1070–7.

48. Hekmet K, Clemens RM, Melhorn U, Geissler HJ, Kuhn-Regnier F, deVivie ER. Emergency coronary artery surgery after failed PTCA: myocardial protection with continuous coronary perfusion of beta-blocker-enriched blood. *Thorac Cardiovasc Surg* 1998; 46:333–8.

49. Beyersdorf F. Protection of evolving myocardial infarction and failed PTCA. *Ann Thorac Surg* 1995; 60:833–8.

50. Mooney MR, Arom KV, Joyce LD, Mooney JF, Goldenberg IF, Von Rueclen TJ, *et al.* Emergency cardiopulmonary bypass support in patients with cardiac arrest. *J Thorac Cardiovasc Surg* 1991; 101:450–4.

51. Beyersdorf F, Kirsh M, Buckberg GD, Allen BS. Warm glutamate/aspartate-enriched blood cardioplegic solution for perioperative sudden death. *J Thorac Cardiovasc Surg* 1992; 104:1141–7.

52. Lee KF, Mandell J, Rankin JS, Muhlbaier LH, Wechsler AS. Immediate versus delayed coronary grafting after streptokinase treatment: postoperative blood loss and clinical results. *J Thorac Cardiovasc Surg* 1988; 95:216–22.

53. Gersh BJ, Chesebro JH, Braunwald E, Lambrew C, Passamani E, Solomon RE, *et al.* Coronary artery bypass graft surgery after thrombolytic therapy in the Thrombolysis and Myocardial Infarction Trial, Phase II (TIMI II). *J Am Coll Cardiol* 1995; 25:395–402.

54. Boehrer JD, Kerieakes DJ, Navetta FI, Califf RM, Topol EJ, for the EPIC Investigators. Effects of profound platelet inhibition with c7E3 before coronary angioplasty on complications of coronary bypass surgery. *Am J Cardiol* 1994; 74:1166–70.

55. Lincoff AM, LeNarz LA, Despotis GJ, Smith PK, Booth JE, Raymond RE, *et al.* for the EPILOG and EPISTENT Investigators. Abciximab and bleeding during coronary surgery: results from the EPILOG and EPISTENT trials. *Ann Thorac Surg* 2000; 70:516–26.

56. Dyke CM, Bhatia D, Lorenz TJ, Marso SP, Tardiff BE, Hogeboom C, *et al.* Immediate coronary artery bypass surgery after platelet inhibition with eptifibatide: results from PURSUIT. *Ann Thorac Surg* 2000; 70:866–72.

57. Bracey A, Radovancevic R, Vaughn W, Ferguson J, Livesay JJ. Blood use in emergency coronary artery bypass after receipt of abciximab during angioplasty. *Transfusion* 1998; 38(Suppl.):68S.

58. Juergens CP, Yeung AC, Oesterle SN. Routine platelet transfusion in patients undergoing emergency coronary bypass surgery after receiving abciximab. *Am J Cardiol* 1997; 80:74–5.

59. Singh M, Nuttall GA, Ballman KV, Mullany CJ, Berger PB, Holmes DR Jr, *et al.* Effect of abciximab on the outcome of emergency coronary artery bypass grafting after failed percutaneous coronary intervention. *Mayo Clin Proc* 2001; 76:784–8.

60. Genoni M, Zeller D, Bertel O, Maloigne M, Turina M. Tirofiban therapy does not increase the risk of hemorrhage after emergency coronary surgery. *J Thorac Cardiovasc Surg* 2001; 122:630–2.

61. Mitka M. Results of CURE trial for acute coronary syndrome. *JAMA* 2001; 285:1828–9.

62. Goldberg RJ, Gore JM, Alpert JS, Osganian V, de Groot J, Bade J, *et al.* Cardiogenic shock after acute myocardial infarction: incidence and mortality from a community-wide perspective, 1975 to 1988. *N Engl J Med* 1991; 325:1117–22.

63. Hochman JS, Boland J, Sleeper LA, Porway M, Brinker J, Col J, *et al.*, and the SHOCK Registry Investigators. Current spectrum of cardiogenic shock and effect of early revascularization on mortality: results of an international registry. *Circulation* 1995; 91:873–81.

64. Prewitt RM, Gu S, Garber PJ, Ducas J, *et al.* Marked systemic hypotension depresses coronary thrombolysis induced by intracoronary administration of recombinant tissue-type plasminogen activator. *J Am Coll Cardiol* 1992; 20:1626–33.

65. Holmes DR, Berger PB, Bates E, Woodlief L, Topol EJ, Califf R, *et al.*, and the GUSTO Investigators. Predictors of mortality in cardiogenic shock: the GUSTO experience. *J Am Coll Cardiol* Special Issue February 1995. Program Abstracts 44th Annual Scientific Session, American College of Cardiology, 86A, Abstract No. 715-1.

66. Hochman JS. Cardiogenic shock: can we save the patient? *ACC Educational Highlights* 1996; **12**:1–5.

67. Anderson RD, Ohman EM, Holmes DR, Col I, Stebbins AL, Bates ER, *et al.*, and the GUSTO-I Investigators. Use of intraaortic balloon counterpulsation in patients presenting with cardiogenic shock: observations from the GUSTO-I study. *J Am Coll Cardiol* 1997; **30**(3):708–15.

68. Beyersdorf F, Acar C, Buckberg GD, Partington MT, Sjostrand F, Young HH, *et al.* Studies on prolonged acute regional ischemia, III. Early natural history of simulated single and multivessel disease with emphasis on remote myocardium. *J Thorac Cardiovasc Surg* 1989; **98**:368–80.

69. Beyersdorf F, Acar C, Buckberg GD, Partington MT, Okamoto F, Allen BS, *et al.* Studies on prolonged acute regional ischemic. V. Metabolic support of remote myocardium during left ventricular power failure. *J Thorac Cardiovasc Surg* 1989; **98**:567–79.

70. Allen BS, Rosenkranz E, Buckberg GD, Davtyan H, Laks H, Tillisch J, *et al.* Studies on prolonged acute regional ischemia. VI. Myocardial infarction with left ventricular power failure: a medical/surgical emergency requiring urgent revascularization with maximal protection of remote muscle. *J Thorac Cardiovasc Surg* 1989; **98**:691–703.

71. Sergeant P, Blackstone E, Meyms B. Early and late outcome after CABG in patients with evolving myocardial infarction. *Eur J Cardiothorac Surg* 1997; **11**:848–56.

72. Cooley DA. Postinfarction ventricular septal rupture. *Semin Thorac Cardiovasc Surg* 1998; **10**:100–4.

73. Honan MB, Harrell FE Jr, Reimer KA, Califf RM, Mark DB, Pryor DB, *et al.* Cardiac rupture, mortality and the timing of thrombolytic therapy: a meta analysis. *J Am Coll Cardiol* 1990; **16**:359–67.

74. Killen DA, Piehler JM, Borkon AM, Gorton ME, Reed WA. Early repair of postinfarction ventricular septal rupture. *Ann Thorac Surg* 1997; **63**:137–42.

75. Cooley DA, Belmonte BA, Zeis LB, Schnur S. Surgical repair of ruptured interventricular septum following acute myocardial infarction. *Surgery* 1957; **41**:930–7.

76. Madsen JC, Daggett WM Jr. Postinfarction ventricular septal defect and free wall rupture. In: *Cardiac Surgery in the Adult*, Edmunds LH Jr (ed.). New York: McGraw-Hill, 1997, 629–55.

77. DaSilva JP, Cascudo MM, Baungratz JF, Vila JHA, Macruz R. Postinfarction ventricular septal defect: an efficacious technique for early surgical repair. *J Thorac Cardiovasc Surg* 1989; **97**:86–9.

78. Skillington PD, Davies RH, Luff AJ. Surgical treatment for infarct-related ventricular septal defects: improved early results combined with analysis of late functional status. *J Thorac Cardiovasc Surg* 1990; **99**:798–808.

79. David TE, Dale L, Sun Z. Postinfarction ventricular septal rupture: repair by endocardial patch with infarct exclusion. *J Thorac Cardiovasc Surg* 1995; **110**:1315–22.

80. Seipelt RG, Schoendube FA, Vasquez-Jimenez JF, Doerge H, Voss M, Messmer BJ. Combined mitral valve and coronary artery surgery: ischemic versus non-ischemic mitral valve disease. *Eur J Cardiothorac Surg* 2001; **20**:270–5.

81. Gorman RC, McCaughan JS, Ratcliffe MB, Gupta KB, Stricher JT, Ferrari VA, *et al.* Pathogenesis of acute ischemic mitral regurgitation in three dimensions. *J Thorac Cardiovasc Surg* 1995; **109**:684–93.

82. Komeda M, Glasson JR, Bolger AF, Daughters GT II, MacIsaac A, Oesterle SN, *et al.* Geometric determinants of ischemic mitral regurgitation. *Circulation* 1997; **96**(9 Suppl.):II128–33.

83. Cohn LH, Rizzo RJ, Adams DH, Couper GS, Sullivan TE, Collins JJ Jr. The effect of pathophysiology on the surgical treatment of ischemic mitral regurgitation: operative and late risks of repair versus replacement. *Eur J Cardiothorac Surg* 1995; **9**:568–74.

84. David TE, Ho WC. The effect of preservation of chordae tendineae on mitral valve replacement for postinfarction mitral regurgitation. *Circulation* 1986; **74**(Suppl. I):116–20.

85. Fucci C, Sandrelli L, Pardini A, Torracca L, Ferrari M, Alfieri O. Improved results with mitral valve repair using new surgical techniques. *Eur J Cardiothorac Surg* 1995; **9**:621–7.

86. Rankin JS, Feneley MP, Hickey MS, Muhlbaier LH, Wechsler AS, Floyd RD, *et al.* A clinical comparison of mitral valve repair versus valve replacement in ischemic mitral regurgitation. *J Thorac Cardiovasc Surg* 1988; **95**:165–77.

87. Dion R, Benetis R, Elias B, Guennaoui T, Raphael D, Van Dyck M. Mitral valve procedures in ischemic regurgitation. *J Heart Valve Dis* 1995; **4**(Suppl. 2):124–31.

21

Surgery for the chronic complications of coronary disease

VINCENT M DOR

In the past 20 years there have been many advances in the understanding and treatment of myocardial infarction and chronic ischemia of the left ventricle. However, many studies have focused, perhaps unduly, on the patency of culprit arteries rather than the diseased left ventricular wall itself. Similarly, the concept of left ventricular remodeling was based largely on clinical, physiological and biological aspects, often with little attention to the anatomical disorder and its evaluation.

In the light of the recent advances in diagnosis and treatment (medical, endoluminal, surgical and mechanical) as well as understanding of the evolution of myocardial ischemia, ten important points may be identified relating to the role of surgery in the treatment of ischemic cardiomyopathy.

Clinically there is no standard typical case. A variety of presentations is encountered, from the dramatic acute transmural myocardial infarct, with necrosis and destruction of all the myocardium of the diseased area, followed by dyskinetic aneurysm, to the progressive loss of contractility of the left ventricular wall diseased by a long evolution of (sometimes silent) ischemia, and in between possibilities of combination of the two situations.

PATHOLOGICAL ANATOMY: THE LEFT VENTRICULAR WALL AFTER INFARCTION

Even though disease in the right coronary artery is the leading cause of infarction, the antero-apical septal region is the more common location for left ventricular scar, probably due to the detrimental effect of occlusion of left anterior descending (LAD) artery and its branches, compared with the consequences of occlusion of the right or circumflex arteries with their balanced anatomy.

After transmural infarction, the infarcted area is progressively necrotic, then fibrotic and, finally, often calcified. The remaining normal muscle is first normal, then hypertrophied and finally dilated. In such transmural lesions, there is a limit between sound area and scarred fibrous tissue, which is very often dyskinetic.

Since the standardization of the treatment of myocardial infarction in the acute phase by thrombolysis and angioplasty, these classical progressions are modified: the infarct is most of the time not transmural, as the sub-epicardial muscle is saved by recanalization, but the sub-endocardial muscle is necrosed.[1] Therefore, the left ventricular wall can show two different aspects in the same area: living myocardium (seen at surgery and during thallium scan) but an akinetic zone on echocardiogram or angiogram (and found inside the left ventricle after opening). Careful analysis of cardiac magnetic resonance images will be very helpful in the future in determining these two types of ventricular wall.

This partially scarred left ventricular wall can be dyskinetic or more often akinetic. It may be associated with mural thrombi or calcification. It is more important to determine the percentage of asynergic wall with abnormal myocardium, rather than the exact type of wall motion abnormality.[2,3]

PATHOPHYSIOLOGY: LEFT VENTRICULAR REMODELING

Gorlin demonstrated in 1967[4] that if more than 20% of left ventricular wall is diseased, the evolution of changes in the ventricle (due to the Starling and Laplace laws) will be progressive global akinesia. Gaudron[5] more recently showed that 20% of all myocardial infarcts follow this evolution to global cardiac insufficiency. Myocardial infarction is followed by complex and interrelated sequences of events termed *post-infarction left ventricular remodeling*.[6,7] Left ventricular remodeling describes the compensatory response of the cardiovascular system when faced with an acute loss of myocardial contractile function. Morphologically, the end result of these responses is that the infarcted ventricle is progressively spherically dilated. The Franck–Starling mechanism is beneficial in the early stage as ventricular dilatation maintains stroke volume, but progressively the dilatation of the ventricle has a detrimental effect on the surviving myocardium as it increases the wall tension (Laplace Law).

Cell necrosis initiates an inflammatory reaction with granulocyte infiltration and release of proteolytic enzymes.

Plasma concentration of several neurohormones is also increased after infarction. The *neurohormonal hypothesis*[8,9] postulates that neurohormones initially serve an adaptive role by maintaining cardiac output, but in the later stages the responses become pathological and contribute to adverse remodeling and progressive ventricular failure.

There is also an increase in sympathetic drive, which has both positive chronotropic and inotropic actions. While cardiac output is maintained, left ventricular loading increases, thereby aggravating infarct expansion. In addition, myocardial oxygen demand rises, precipitating further ischemia. Vasoconstriction and fluid retention are both features of activation of the renin–angiotensin axis, which serve to maintain blood pressure.

Left ventricular volume is a sensitive marker of post-infarction ventricular dysfunction, and left ventricular end-systolic volume is a very important predictor of prognosis after myocardial infarction.[10]

The problem for the moment is to know whether this deleterious secondary evolution of the ventricle due to this very complex biological reaction occurs only in the case of large diseased areas affecting more than 10% or 20% of the ventricular mass, or whether it can occur also with smaller scarred areas.

The present questions are:

- Will recanalization of the occluded arteries prevent this evolution?
- Can a surgical approach to diseased wall help to suppress this evolution?
- What is the optimal timing for recanalization and/or surgery to prevent this deleterious process?

CORONARY ARTERY RECANALIZATION

Immediately after coronary artery occlusion, irreversible cell necrosis can occur within minutes. Prompt reperfusion when myocytes are in a state of critical ischemia or are prenecrotic can reduce cell death and limit infarct size, and so increase survival. However, the potential benefit of recanalizing vessels supplying an infarcted and non-viable region remains controversial.[11] Nevertheless, coronary revascularization by endoluminal or surgical techniques has changed the treatment of myocardial ischemia, and re-opening of the artery during the acute phase of infarction has changed the prognosis of myocardial infarction. However, when there is fibrous myocardium resulting from chronic ischemia or when muscle has been totally destroyed by an infarct, revascularization itself has no effect. Consequently, it is clear that recanalization during the acute phase of infarction (by endoluminal revascularization, stenting or surgery) cannot be the sole therapy for left ventricular ischemic wall.

Recanalization is an essential treatment but not in itself sufficient to solve the whole problem, and weeks and months after infarction it can be a great disappointment to see patients with recanalized arteries but an asynergic left ventricular wall.

CONVENTIONAL, CLASSICAL, SURGICAL TECHNIQUES

Since Likoff in 1955,[12] Cooley in 1958[13] and others,[14] surgery of left ventricular aneurysm has been well described. Resection of exteriorized scarred tissues followed by a long linear suture is an easy and safe technique, accomplished on the beating or arrested heart. Changed left ventricular shape and hemodynamics give disappointing results, highlighted by the classical works of Froehlich[15] and Cohen,[16] and has led to a common view among cardiologists that surgery of left ventricular aneurysm has little effect on ventricular performance as only a small part of the dyskinesia is resected.

CIRCULAR REORGANIZATION OF THE LEFT VENTRICULAR WALL: LEFT VENTRICULAR RECONSTRUCTION

A more physiological reconstruction of the left ventricle was described in the 1980s. Jatene, in 1985,[17] presented a large experience using a technique of external circular reconstruction of the left ventricular wall associated with plication of the akinetic septum from inside the cavity. A patch was sometimes used (10%) to close the reorganized wall, and coronary revascularization was accomplished in 20% of cases.

In 1984, we used a patch inserted inside the ventricle on contractile muscle in order to exclude all akinetic, non-resectable areas and to rebuild the ventricular cavity as it was before the infarct, including revascularization of all diseased coronary arteries. A first series of 25 patients operated on with this technique was presented in 1985.[18] Following these two pioneering works, other similar techniques were described: endoaneurysmorrhaphy by Cooley in 1989[19] and tailored scar incision by Mickleborough in 1994.[20] All techniques aiming to improve the result of the classical linear suture are called left ventricular reconstruction or reshaping, or rebuilding . The word 'remodeling', normally applied to the spontaneous evolution of the infarcted ventricle, seems inappropriate for describing this surgery, which aims at *improving* the left ventricle.

Standard technique of endoventricular circular patch plasty (Figure 21.1)

Transesophageal echocardiography is used to assess the mitral valve. Surgery is conducted with a totally arrested heart. Coronary revascularization is accomplished first, then the left ventricular wall is opened at the center of the depressed area, the clots are removed, the endocardial scar is dissected and resected if the scar is calcified or if there is spontaneous or inducible ventricular tachycardia. In such circumstances, cryotherapy is applied in addition at the edge of the resection. In the case of mitral insufficiency, the valve is inspected by an atrial and, eventually, the ventricular approach, and, if required, a reconstructive procedure is performed (posterior annuloplasty, Goretex neochordae, Alfieri E-to-E suture, or mitral valve replacement if the posterior papillary muscle is totally diseased). The rebuilding of the left ventricular cavity is initiated by continuous suture of 2/0 monofilament passed at the

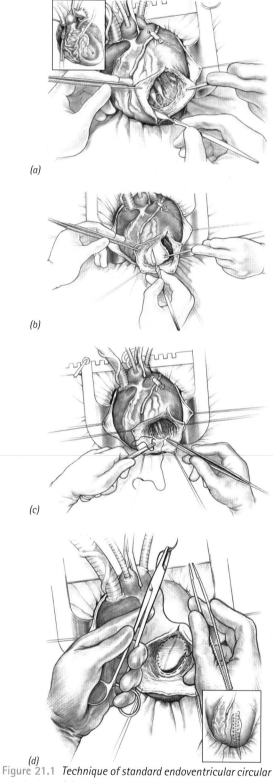

(a)

(b)

(c)

(d)

Figure 21.1 *Technique of standard endoventricular circular patch plasty. (a) Exposure of the lesions and opening of the anterior wall distally from left anterior descending sulcus. (b) Mobilization of scarred fibrous endocardium. (c) Endoventricular continuous circular suture ('Fontan trick'). (d) Endoventricular patch anchorage with the same suture and closure of excluded areas.*

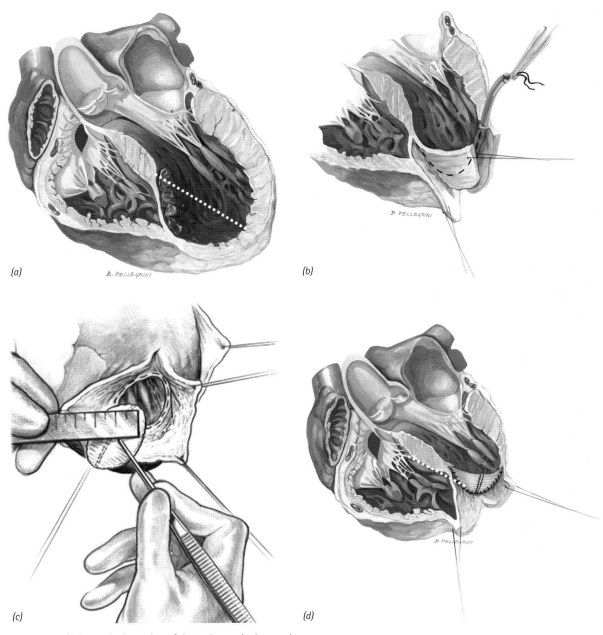

Figure 21.2 *Sizing and orientation of the endoventricular patch.*

limit between fibrous and normal muscle and tied over a balloon inflated inside the left ventricular cavity at the theoretical diastolic capacity of the patient (40–50 mL m^{-2} body surface area). The endoventricular circular suture, in addition to restoring the curvature of myocardium to what it was before the infarct, also helps in the selection of the shape, size and orientation of the patch. When the infarct scar is located in the antero-apical region, the septum and apex are more involved than the lateral wall. The suture is placed far back in the septum, excluding totally the apex and the posterior wall below the posterior papillary muscle base, and only a small portion of lateral wall above the antero-lateral papillary muscle base, so that the orientation of this new neck (and of the patch) is roughly aligned in the direction of the septum (Figure 21.2). A patch of Dacron is fashioned to the size of this neck and fixed to the 'clothesline' (the endoventricular circular suture) with the same suture. Excluded areas are either resected or, more often, sutured over the patch.

Alternatives

- Autologous tissue can be used instead of a synthetic patch: either a semicircle of the fibrous endocardial scar, mobilized with a septal hinge when this scar is

Posterior incision

Endocardectomy

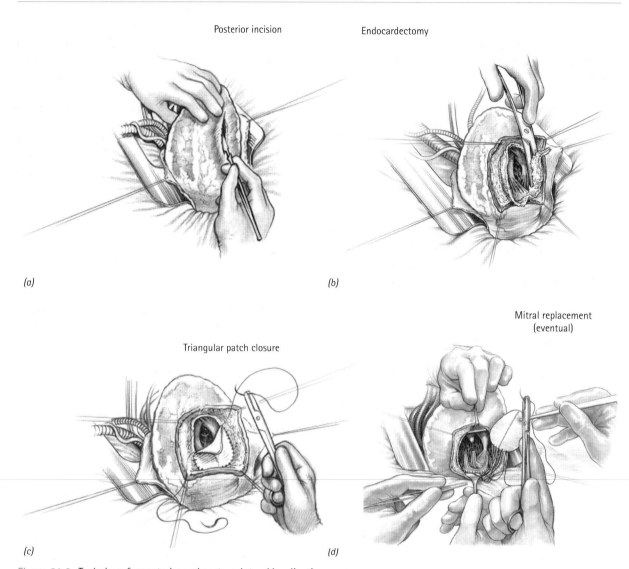

(a)

(b)

Triangular patch closure

Mitral replacement
(eventual)

(c)

(d)

Figure 21.3 *Technique for posterior and postero-lateral localization.*

tough, and without calcification or thrombi, or autologous pericardium (30% of the cases in our series).

- In the case of posterior or postero-lateral localization (Figure 21.3), a triangular patch, with its base fixed on the posterior or postero-lateral mitral annulus and on the posterior or antero-lateral papillary muscle base, enables a normal mitral geometry and normal left ventricular posterior wall to be reconstructed following extensive endocardectomy. If the posterior papillary muscle is totally involved in the resected scar, the mitral valve has to be replaced with a prosthesis, and this is easily achieved through the transventricular approach.

- When necrotic tissue is encountered during the repair of an acute mechanical complication of myocardial infarction (e.g. septal rupture or free wall perforation), the patch has to be inserted at

the boundary between sound and necrotic tissue using transmural U stitches reinforced with Teflon pledgets. The patch is anchored over the septal rupture, which is excluded from the left ventricular cavity.

Concomitant surgical problems

CORONARY REVASCULARIZATION

Revascularization of all significantly stenosed coronary arteries supplying the contractile area is mandatory. Revascularization of the infarcted area is almost always possible, even with a thrombosed LAD artery and even if the run-off is not opacified by homologous or heterologous collaterals on the preoperative coronary angiogram. Use of the internal thoracic artery is possible and at 1-year follow-up, more than 80% of these bypassed arteries are patent. Coronary revascularization was accomplished in our global series (reviewed in May 1998) in 97% of patients, with the internal thoracic artery being used in 90% of cases.

MITRAL INSUFFICIENCY

Mitral insufficiency is a common accompaniment of left ventricular scar, and the mitral valve must be assessed carefully before and during surgery (transesophageal echocardiography). When mitral regurgitation is quantified as grade II or more, or the mitral annulus is sized above 35 mm, a posterior annuloplasty is mandatory. We prefer the atrial approach with posterior annulus reduction using a Goretex strip. However, the transventricular approach is possible.[21] Some patients with associated degenerative mitral disease may need a more complete repair.

VENTRICULAR ARRHYTHMIAS

Spontaneous ventricular tachycardia (13% of patients in our series) and inducible ventricular tachycardia (25% in our series) are frequent and, in such circumstances, subtotal non-guided endocardectomy is conducted on all the endoventricular scar. Cryotherapy at the limit of this resection completes the surgical excision.

Applicability of this technique to extensive akinesia

This technique can also be used for extensive dyskinesia or akinesia. The extent of asynergy can be objectively measured by the centerline method and considered as large if it exceeds 50% of the left ventricular circumference.

Akinesia and dyskinesia should not be considered as different states for two reasons:

- In the same diseased left ventricle, 'there is a continuum between dyskinesia and asynergy', as Gorlin mentioned in 1967.[4]
- Dyskinesia progressively evolves towards progressive global dilatation and akinesia.

Patients with extensive left ventricular scar are clinically in congestive heart failure, with very often a mean pulmonary artery pressure above 25 mmHg, an ejection fraction (EF) below 30%, an end-diastolic volume index above 150 mL, and end-systolic volume index above 60 mL.

In such extensive lesions, surgery is accomplished with some modifications (Figure 21.4). Ventricular tachycardia is present in nearly 50% of cases. Mitral insufficiency has to be repaired in more than 30% of cases. The exclusion of all scarred areas leads to too small a left ventricular cavity, with a high risk of immediate or delayed diastolic non-compliance. The continuous suture is therefore placed above the limit of the sound muscle in the 'transitional'

fibrous area, and the use of a balloon inside the left ventricle, inflated at the estimated end-diastolic volume for the patient according to body surface area, is mandatory before tightening of the suture. The patch is often larger (3–4 cm in diameter) than in the usual technique.

The excluded septum often cannot be sutured to the lateral wall (because of the risk of damage to the revascularized anterior descending artery and the restraint of the right ventricle). In this event, the excess fibrous tissue is simply folded onto the patch. In such cases surgical glue is useful.

LEFT VENTRICULAR RECONSTRUCTION BY ENDOVENTRICULAR CIRCULAR PATCH PLASTY WORKS!

Based on a personal experience of more than 1000 cases, and confirmed by that of many other authors,[22–25] it can be said, in contradiction to the 'Froelich Law', that left ventricular reconstruction works and restores a more normal morphology and physiology to the ventricle.[26,27]

- Postoperative left ventricular cineangiograms show return to normal of the left ventricular shape, particularly in relation to the septal exclusion (Figure 21.5).
- Both systolic and diastolic function is improved: analysis of left ventricular EF shows that global EF (Table 21.1) and also theoretical contractile EF are improved (Figure 21.6, page 322). The mean increase of left ventricular EF is between 10 and 15 percentage points. This improvement in EF is noted for dyskinetic as well as for akinetic lesions (Table 21.2, page 322).
- Diastolic function is also improved, as is shown by analyzing the peak filling rate and the time of peak filling or the left portion of the pressure–volume loop (Figure 21.7, page 323).
- Ventricular arrhythmia, chiefly tachycardias (spontaneous or inducible), are controlled immediately and at later follow-up in 90% of cases.[28]

This technique is feasible with an acceptable risk. From 1984 to August 2001, 1011 patients with all indications were operated on, with 76 hospital deaths (7.5%). This risk was not the same for isolated left ventricular aneurysm as for global akinesia, nor for the patient with and the patient without congestive heart failure, nor for spontaneous or inducible ventricular tachycardia compared with normal rhythm. From 1987 to 2000 (Montecarlo experience), the hospital mortality for the cohort of 870 patients was 64 (7.4%). For those patients with very severely depressed pump function (EF <30%), mortality was 13% (44/341); for those with EF between 30% and 40%, mortality was 7% (16/227); and for those with EF >40%, mortality was

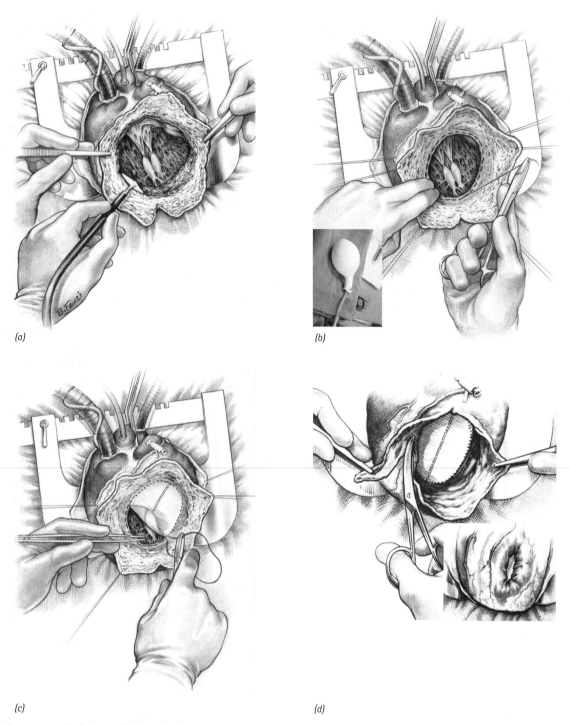

(a)

(b)

(c)

(d)

Figure 21.4 *Technique of left ventricular reconstruction for extensive asynergy. (a) Cryotherapy at the limit of endocardial resection. (b) The endoventricular suture and the balloon to check the diastolic volume. (c) Patch anchoring. (d) Resection and folding of excluded areas.*

1.3% (4/302). With increasing experience and improvement in the management of severely ill patients, and recognition of the importance of the remaining diastolic volume, operative risk for the recent series (1998–2000) was 4.8% (187 patients) and in the group with extensive akinesia it was 8%.

Actuarial survival at 10 years showed the influence of:

1 degree of congestive heart failure,
2 preoperative and postoperative systolic and diastolic volume,
3 preoperative left ventricular EF.

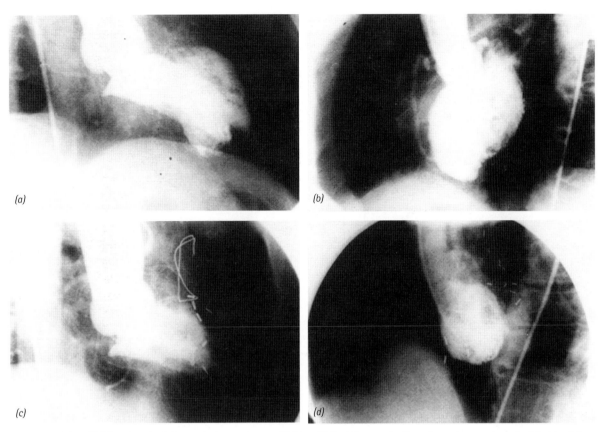

Figure 21.5 *(a) and (b) Preoperative left ventricular angiogram (right and left oblique projection of an antero-septo-apical dyskinesia). (c) and (d) The same patient postoperatively. Note the total disappearance of the septal akinesia.*

Table 21.1 *Patients with preoperative CI $<2.0\,L\,min^{-1}\,m^{-2}$ and EF$<30\%$ (n = 40)*

	Preoperative	Early postoperative	1 year postoperative
CI (L min^{-1} m^{-2}	1.71 ± 0.2	2.2 ± 0.5	2.5 ± 1/5
EF (%)	22 ± 6	40 ± 7	38 ± 7

CI, cardiac index; EF, ejection fraction.

More than 80% of patients were alive at 10 years when end-systolic volume index was below $90\,mL\,m^{-2}$ and New York Heart Association (NYHA) classification was II or III. Survival percentage fell towards 50% in patients with NYHA class IV, and end-systolic volume index $>120\,mL\,m^{-2}$.

THE 'WHYS AND WHEREFORES' OF ENDOVENTRICULAR CIRCULAR PATCH PLASTY

Left ventricular reconstruction enhances the beneficial, but partial, effects of coronary revascularization and of mitral valve repair (if necessary) by improving left ventricular function, for the following reasons.

- Septal scar is excluded.
- The left ventricular wall is reorganized. This suppresses the rise in wall tension in remote myocardial areas, and improves contraction of these areas. This is clearly shown by the analysis of pressure–volume curves.[29]
- The patch avoids excessive reduction of volume and maintains a reasonable physiological cavity in terms of diastolic capacity.

DISAPPOINTING RESULTS

Although operative and hospital mortalities are not prohibitive, in the case of extensive left ventricular akinesia and global dilatation, some disappointing late results were noted. In approximately 25% of such patients, there

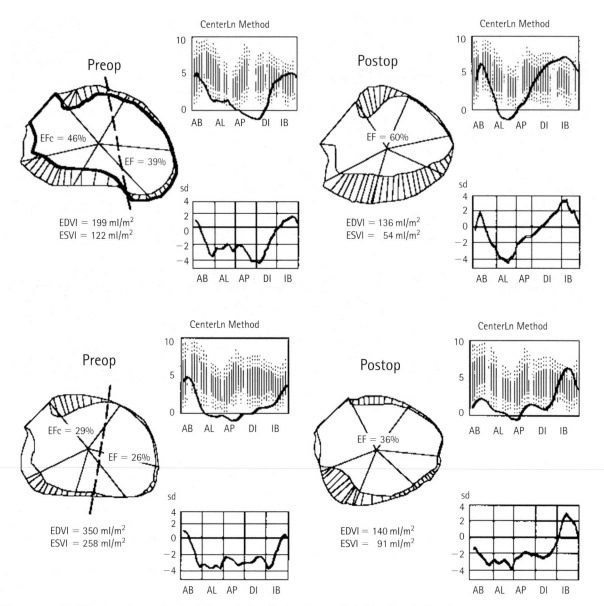

Figure 21.6 *Modification of postoperative left ventricular ejection fraction in dyskinetic and akinetic scars.*

Table 21.2 *Akinetic versus dyskinetic post-infarction scar*

	Small dyskinetic scar (n = 84)	Large dyskinetic scar (n = 41)	Small akinetic scar (n = 72)	Large akinetic scar (n = 48)
Preoperative EF	42 ± 11	26 ± 7	41 ± 10	25 ± 9
Postoperative EF	53 ± 11	45 ± 11	49 ± 13	41 ± 12
Hospital death (%)	4.8	12.2	0	12.5

EF, ejection fraction.

was a tendency after 1 year for an increase in pulmonary pressure, and secondary mitral insufficiency could occur.[30] The mechanism of the late failure is not clear. When the interval between infarction and left ventricular reconstruction is above 40 months, ventricular remodeling appears to continue in spite of surgery.[31] Moreover, diastolic volume or compliance and mitral competence must be assessed carefully. Since 1998, when the 'balloon sizing' of the remaining ventricle was applied and mitral annuloplasty was more widely used to maintain the annulus

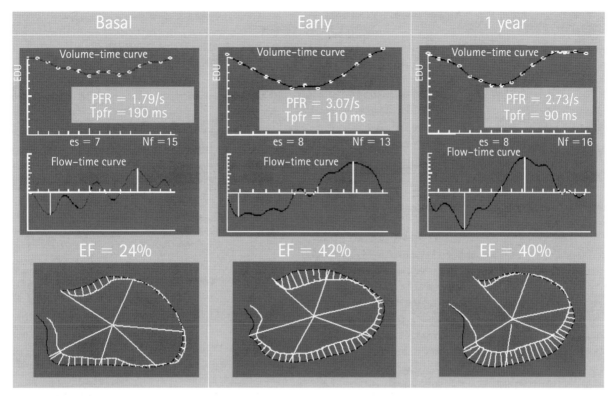

Figure 21.7 *Evolution of peak filling rate, 1 month and 1 year after left ventricular reconstruction.*

below 30 mm diameter, the tendency for late impairment fell from 25% to 10% in such patients among the last 200 cases of our series.

The continuation of left ventricular remodeling is influenced by mechanical, neurohormonal or autoimmune reactions. Following surgery, patients need to be protected with medical therapy including beta-blockers and ACE inhibitors to avoid this evolution.

WHAT SURGERY CAN DO FOR ISCHEMIC CARDIOMYOPATHY

Following coronary occlusion and myocardial infarction, restoration of arterial patency itself is not sufficient to improve the left ventricular performance. Thus, left ventricular morphology and left ventricular wall function must be assessed accurately by echocardiography, angiocardiography or computerized magnetic resonance imaging in the weeks and months following infarction and should be monitored regularly.

A permanent asynergic involvement of more than 50% of left ventricular circumference (totally or partially scarred, fibrotic, necrotic or ischemic), even after successful coronary revascularization, must be surgically reconstructed to avoid inevitable evolution to progressive global dilatation and irreversible akinesia.

Left ventricular reconstruction must be complemented almost always by complete coronary revascularization, in up to 30% of cases by the surgical treatment (endocardectomy plus cryotherapy) of spontaneous or inducible ventricular tachycardia, and in more than 25% by a curative (indeed preventive) surgical repair (annuloplasty) of mitral insufficiency.

Left ventricular reconstruction can avoid dilatation and end-stage left ventricular remodeling if it is applied in the early months (12 to perhaps 40 months) following an infarct.

Even in end-stage ischemic cardiomyopathy with congestive heart failure of grade 3 or 4, end systolic volume index above 60 mL, global EF below 30%, and often after failure of complete medical therapy, left ventricular reconstruction by endoventricular circular patch plasty is useful, with acceptable risk (less than 10% mortality), to slow down the remodeling and to avoid or delay heart transplantation or the need for mechanical assist device. Long-term outcome in such high-risk patients is encouraging (life expectancy above 50% at 10 years).[32]

FUTURE PROSPECTS

Better assessment of left ventricular morphology, and of the nature of the myocardial wall and its function, by careful analysis of computerized magnetic resonance imaging[33] is to be anticipated.

It may be possible to achieve recovery of dilated but non-scarred myocardium, by a combination of current surgical treatment (left ventricular reconstruction plus myocardial revascularization plus mitral repair) and new techniques presently under appraisal, such as left ventricular assist devices (which take over some cardiac function and suppress immune or autogenous hormonal reactions).

Results published by the German Heart Institute, Berlin,[34] and observations of Yacoub's group[35] show that in some cases of idiopathic cardiomyopathy following months of left ventricular assistance, sufficient improvement in left ventricular wall thickness and contraction can occur to allow the patient to be weaned from the assist device ('bridge to recovery'). Similar management may be possible in ischemic cardiomyopathy, where the left ventricular wall is not uniformly diseased – one part being a scar and one part being dilated with living, perfused myocardium. The synthesis of surgery (left ventricular reconstruction) for the scarred area and medical treatment with mechanical support for the dilated portion may well become a method for the treatment of severe endstage ischemic congestive heart failure in the future. The potential for adding cellular therapy to stimulate growth in the non-scarred, viable myocardium is a further possibility for complementing the surgical treatment strategy.

ventricular dimension and shape and geometric correlates of mitral regurgitation one year after surgery. *J Thorac Cardiovasc Surg* 2001; **121**:91–6.

Forty-four patients were studied to show the mechanisms of improvement in symptomatic patients following the Dor procedure, confirming the improvement in systolic pump function.

Dor V. The endoventricular circular patch plasty ('Dor procedure') in ischemic akinetic dilated ventricles. *Heart Fail Rev* 2001; **6**:187–93.

The author's unique experience involving 950 patients is reviewed, with results to 10 years.

Menicanti L, Di Donato M. The Dor procedure: what has changed after 15 years of clinical practice? *J Thorac Cardiovasc Surg* 2002; **124**:886–90.

Description of the Dor procedure as presently advocated in the light of experience of more than 2000 operations.

Menicanti L, Dor V, Buckberg GD, Athanasuleas CL, Di Donato M. RESTORE Group. Inferior wall restoration: anatomic and surgical considerations. *Semin Thorac Cardiovasc Surg* 2001; **13**:504–13.

Inferior wall infarction affects mitral valve function with a far greater frequency than does anterior wall infarction. The principles described for the Dor procedure in anterior scar are modified for inferior infarction, and management of the dysfunctional mitral valve is discussed.

CONCLUSION

Seventeen years after its inception, endoventricular circular patch plasty is confirmed as a good technique to reconstruct a scarred and dilated left ventricle following myocardial infarction. The technique is easily reproducible, efficient and safe, and must be considered as one of the major treatment strategies in the course of ischemic cardiomyopathy.

KEY REFERENCES

Di Donato M, Sabatier M, Dor V. RESTORE Group. Sugical ventricular restoration in patients with postinfarction coronary artery disease: effectiveness on spontaneous and inducible ventricular tachycardia. *Semin Thorac Cardiovasc Surg* 2001; **13**:480–5.

Ventricular tachyarrhythmias commonly accompany extensive scar. Their control is not solely attributed to cryoablation, but also to other favorable influences of the Dor procedure combined with revascularization.

Di Donato M, Sabatier M, Dor V, Gensini GF, Toso A, Maioli M, *et al.* Effects of the Dor procedure on left

REFERENCES

1. Bogaert J, Maes A, Van de Werf F, Bosmans H, Herregods MC, Nuyts J, *et al.* Functional recovery of subepicardial myocardial tissue in transmural myocardial infarction after successful reperfusion. *Circulation* 1999; **99**:36–43.
2. Zerhouni EA, Parish DM, Rogers WJ, Yang A, Shapiro EP. Human heart: tagging with MR imaging: a new method for noninvasive assessment of myocardial motion. *Radiology* 1988; **169**:59–63.
3. Kramer CM, Rogers WJ, Theobald TM, Power TP, Petruolo S, Reichek N. Remote noninfarcted region dysfunction soon after first anterior myocardial infarction: a magnetic resonance tagging study. *Circulation* 1996; **94**:660–6.
4. Klein MD, Herman MV, Gorlin R. A hemodynamic study of left ventricular aneurysm. *Circulation* 1967; **35**:614–30.
5. Gaudron P, Eilles C, Kugler I, Ertl G. Progressive left ventricular dysfunction after myocardial infarction. *Circulation* 1993; **87**:755–62.
6. Yousef ZR, Redwood SR, Marber MS. Postinfarction left ventricular remodeling: where are the theories and trials leading us? *Heart* 2000; **83**:76–80.
7. Braunwald E, Pfeffer MA. Ventricular enlargement and remodeling following acute myocardial infarction: mechanisms and management. *Am J Cardiol* 1991; **68** (Suppl. D):1–6D.
8. McAlpine HM, Morton JJ, Leckie B, Rumley A, Gillen G, Dargie HJ. Neuroendocrine activation after acute myocardial infarction. *Br Heart J* 1988; **60**:117–24.
9. Packer M. The neurohormonal hypothesis: a theory to explain the mechanism of disease progression in heart failure. *J Am Coll Cardiol* 1992; **20**:248–54.

10. White HD, Norris RM, Brown MA, Brandt PW, Whitlock RM, Wild CJ. Left ventricular end-systolic volume as the major determinant of survival after recovery from myocardial infarction. *Circulation* 1987; **76**:44–51.

11. Marber MS, Brown DL, Kloner RA. The open artery hypothesis: to open, or not to open, that is the question. *Eur Heart J* 1996; **17**:505–9.

12. Likoff W, Bailey CP. Ventriculoplasty: excision of myocardial aneurysm. *JAMA* 1955; **158**:915.

13. Cooley DA, Collins HA, Morris GC. Ventricular aneurysm after myocardial infarction: surgical excision with use of temporary cardiopulmonary bypass. *JAMA* 1958; **167**:557.

14. Mills NL, Everson CT, Hockmuth D. Technical advances in the treatment of left ventricular aneurysm. *Ann Thorac Surg* 1993; **55**:792–800.

15. Froehlich RT, Falsetti HL, Doty DB, Marcus ML. Prospective study of surgery for left ventricular aneurysm. *Am J Cardiol* 1980; **45**:923–31.

16. Cohen M, Packer M, Gorlin R. Indications for left ventricular aneurysmectomy. *Circulation* 1983; **67**:717–22.

17. Jatene AD. Left ventricular aneurysmectomy. Resection or reconstruction. *J Thorac Cardiovasc Surg* 1985; **89**:321–31.

18. Dor V, Kreitmann P, Jourdan J, Acar C, Saab M, Coste P. Interest of 'physiological' closure (circumferential plasty on contractile areas) of left ventricle after resection and endocardectomy for aneurysm of akinetic zone: comparison with classical technique about a series of 209 left ventricular resections (Abstract). *J Cardiovasc Surg* 1985; **26**:73.

19. Cooley D. Ventricular endoaneurysmorrhaphy: a simplified repair for extensive postinfarction aneurysm. *J Card Surg* 1989; **4**:200–5.

20. Mickleborough L, Maruyama H, Liu P, Mohamed S. Results of left ventricular aneurysmectomy with a tailored scar excision and primary closure technique. *J Thorac Cardiovasc Surg* 1994; **107**:690–8.

21. Menicanti L, Di Donato M, Frigiola A, Buckberg G, Santambrogio C, Ranucci M, *et al.* Ischemic mitral regurgitation: intraventricular papillary muscle imbrication without mitral ring during left ventricular restoration. *J Thorac Cardiovasc Surg* 2002; **123**:1041–50.

22. Jakob H, Zölch B, Schuster S, Iversen S, Hake U, Lippold R, *et al.* Endoventricular patch plasty improves results of LV aneurysmectomy. *Eur J Cardiothorac Surg* 1993; **7**:428–36.

23. Grossi E, Chimitz L, Galloway A. Endoventricular remodeling of left ventricular aneurysm: functional, clinical and electrophysiological results. *Circulation* 1995; **92**(Suppl. II):98–100.

24. Shapira O, Davidoff R, Hilkert RJ, Aldea GS, Fitzgerald CA, Shemin RJ. Repair of left ventricular aneurysm: long-term results of linear repair versus endoaneurysmorrhaphy. *Ann Thorac Surg* 1997; **63**:701–5.

25. Athanasuleas CL, Stanley AW, Buckberg GD, Dor V, Di Donato M, Siler W. RESTORE Group. Surgical anterior ventricular endocardial restoration (SAVER) for dilated ischemic cardiomyopathy. *Semin Thorac Cardiovasc Surg* 2001; **13**:448–58.

26. Dor V, Sabatier M, Di Donato M, Maioli M, Toso A, Montiglio F. Late hemodynamic results after left ventricular patch repair associated with coronary grafting in patients with postinfarction akinetic or dyskinetic aneurysm of the left ventricle. *J Thorac Cardiovasc Surg* 1995; **110**:1291–301.

27. Di Donato M, Barletta G, Maioli M, Fantini F, Coste P, Sabatier M, *et al.* Early hemodynamic results of left ventricular reconstructive surgery for anterior wall left ventricular aneurysm. *Am J Cardiol* 1992; **69**:886–90.

28. Dor V, Sabatier M, Montiglio F, Rossi P, Toso A, Di Donato M. Results of nonguided subtotal endocardectomy associated with left ventricular reconstruction in patients with ischemic ventricular arrhythmias. *J Thorac Cardiovasc Surg* 1994; **107**:1301–8.

29. Di Donato M, Sabatier M, Dor V, Gensini GF, Toso A, Maioli M, *et al.* Effects of the Dor procedure on left ventricular dimension and shape and geometric correlates of mitral regurgitation one year after surgery. *J Thorac Cardiovasc Surg* 2001; **121**:91–7.

30. Di Donato M, Sabatier M, Toso A, Barletta G, Baroni M, Dor V, *et al.* Regional myocardial performance of non-ischaemic zones remote from anterior wall left ventricular aneurysm. Effects of aneurysmectomy. *Eur Heart J* 1995; **16**:1285–92.

31. Louagie Y, Alouini T, Lesperence J, Pelletier LC. Left ventricular aneurysm complicated by congestive heart failure: analysis of long term results and risk factors of surgical treatment. *J Cardiovasc Surg* 1989; **30**:648–55.

32. Dor V. The endoventricular circular patch plasty ('Dor procedure') in ischemic akinetic dilated ventricles. *Heart Failure Rev* 2001; **6**:187–93.

33. Young A, Dougherty A, Bogen D. Validation of tagging with MR imaging to estimate material deformation. *Radiology* 1993; **188**:101–8.

34. Hetzer R, Müller J, Weng Y, Loebe M, Wallukat G. Midterm follow-up of patients who underwent removal of a left ventricular assist device after cardiac recovery from end-stage dilated cardiomyopathy. *J Thorac Cardiovasc Surg* 2000; **120**:843–55.

35. Yacoub M. Personal communication.

22

Combined procedures

THOMAS A ORSZULAK AND THOMAS C BOWER

CORONARY DISEASE COMBINED WITH VALVE DISEASE

Combined cardiac valve and coronary bypass operations are encountered in two circumstances:

1 with the primary diagnosis of valvular heart disease and a secondary diagnosis of coronary artery disease,
2 with the primary presentation of coronary artery disease and valvular heart disease as a secondary or unsuspected finding.

The former is the more common presentation of combined coronary and valvular procedures.

Both coronary and valve disease are increasing due to the aging population, and these co-diagnoses are therefore seen more frequently in senior age groups. In the US-based Society of Thoracic Surgeons (STS) database, for the 10-year period 1992–2001, there was a cumulative total of 1 852 497 open heart operations, a large majority (75.2%) of which were isolated coronary artery bypass grafting (CABG) procedures. Aortic and mitral valve surgery with or without CABG comprised a further 14.1% (Figure 22.1). As shown in Table 22.1, nearly half of these valve replacements were combined with CABG.

As can be seen from Figure 22.2, in US experience as recorded in the STS database, for those patients in whom CABG was undertaken in addition to valve replacement, the operative mortality was approximately doubled. The influence of coronary artery disease upon valve replacement was well described by Mullany et al.,[1] who demonstrated the negative influence of coronary artery disease upon mortality for aortic valve replacement (AVR). The

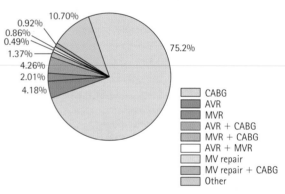

Figure 22.1 *Cardiac surgical procedures. Society of Thoracic Surgeons database January 1992–December 2001. For abbreviations, see text.*

Table 22.1 *Society of Thoracic Surgeons database, January 1992–December 2001: valve surgery ± CABG*

Procedure	Number	Percent
AVR alone	77 368	30.7
AVR ± CABG	78 980	31.4
MVR alone	37 249	14.8
MVR ± CABG	25 408	10.1
MV repair alone	15 974	6.3
MV repair + CABG	16 948	6.7
Total	251 927	100

Total patients = 1 852 497.
CABG, coronary artery bypass grafting; AVR, aortic valve replacement; MVR, mitral valve replacement; MV, mitral valve.

mortality was lowest when both diseases were treated operatively. If coronary artery disease was left ungrafted at the time of valve replacement, the mortality was highest, but even with complete revascularization, there was an increased operative mortality above that of isolated valve disease.

Table 22.2 demonstrates the operative figures from the Mayo Clinic between 1995 and 1999 for patients undergoing their first operation. The mitral figures include repair and replacement. All of these patient numbers are included in the National STS database and confirm the variability of mortality rates amongst institutions and reinforces the need for institutions to examine their own mortality rates. These results reflect a methodical approach to diagnosis and application to *appropriate* patient populations as well as a carefully conducted operation.

Investigations

A foolproof method of determining the threshold for valve replacement for mild to moderate disease at the time of CABG is elusive. There is little to discuss if there is critical, $<0.7\,\mathrm{cm}^2$, aortic stenosis, $<1.0\,\mathrm{cm}^2$ mitral stenosis or

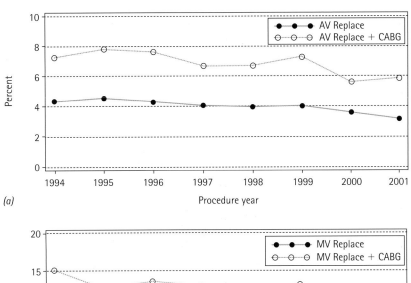

(a)

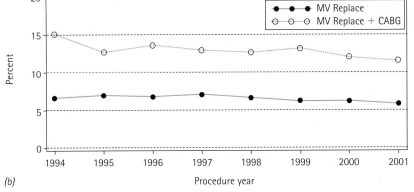

(b)

Figure 22.2 *Operative mortality for aortic and mitral valve replacement with or without CABG. US Society of Thoracic Surgeons database. (a) Risk-adjusted aortic valve operative mortality. (b) Risk-adjusted mitral valve operative mortality.*

Table 22.2 *Mayo Clinic mortality figures, 1995–1999: first-time procedures*

	Age <65		Age 65–75		Age >75		Total	
	Number	Operative mortality (%)	Number	Operative mortality (%)	Number	Operative mortality (%)	Number	Operative mortality (%)
Isolated CABG	1416	1.1	1607	1.7	752	4.9	3775	2.1
Isolated AVR	197	1.5	185	2.2	175	3.4	557	2.3
Isolated MVR or repair	331	0.0	177	2.8	61	3.3	569	1.2
AVR ± CABG	79	2.5	210	2.9	253	2.0	542	2.4
MVR/repair ± CABG	74	0.0	137	2.2	95	5.3	306	2.6

CABG, coronary artery bypass grafting; AVR, aortic valve replacement; MVR, mitral valve replacement.

severe grade 4 aortic or mitral regurgitation. It is obvious that the treatment of choice for severe disease is valve repair or replacement. There is some conflicting information regarding the safest approach to the mildly or moderately stenotic aortic valve when the original plan is CABG.[2–5] The major uncertainty relates to the operative risk to the patient when a repeat operation is needed for valve replacement following a previous CABG.[6,7] Obviously, if the risk of re-operation is high, it would have been prudent to replace the valve at the same time as the CABG was performed. If the re-operative risk is low, all decisions need to be balanced by the risk the valve prosthesis poses for the patient.

Let us first examine the diagnostic pathway of combined coronary and valve disease. History and physical examination remain the keystones in the evaluation of patients. Patients with combined coronary and valve disease are likely to present in a similar way to those with valve or coronary disease alone. However, they are likely to present earlier in their disease course. Owing to the myocardial demands caused by significant valve disease, symptoms occur when myocardial demand exceeds supply. It is easy to understand the impact of adding to the laboring, hypertrophied heart the restriction to delivery of blood supply and oxygen caused by obstructive coronary disease. The sub-endocardium is supplied by perforating vessels. As the myocardium hypertrophies, the supply line to the sub-endocardium lengthens. This intramyocardial supply line can lengthen to the point at which ischemia develops earlier during exertion. In addition, tachycardia shortens available time for coronary perfusion.

Basic technological methods for diagnosing valve disease beyond history and physical examination in patients with coronary artery disease include the echocardiogram, cardiac catheterization and chest x-ray. Echocardiography is the best method for providing evidence of valve disease, due to the amount of information that can be obtained from the echocardiogram, including the type and degree of valve disease, left ventricular pathology, shunts and aneurysms. It has become the practice in many areas of the USA for an echocardiogram to be performed before the patient is seen or examined by a physician. This aspect of the practice of medicine may cause some disquiet, but the return for the patient is significant. The current practice at our institution is to use echocardiography for defining valvular and ventricular pathology, and coronary arteriography for the elucidation of coronary disease. These complementary examinations provide the best information about the patient. When an equivocal finding is present, cardiac catheterization is required to define valvular dysfunction with greater precision.

The approach to combined valve and coronary disease varies with the degree and type of valve pathology involved. It is generally accepted that a patient with coronary stenoses of 50% or greater will receive a bypass graft to the affected vessel. There was an early reluctance to use the left internal thoracic artery (LITA) to the left anterior descending (LAD) coronary artery when left ventricular hypertrophy secondary to valve disease was present, due to concern about a mismatch of supply and demand. There is now general acceptance that the benefits of using the LITA far exceed the liabilities to the LAD circulation.[8] A word of caution is needed, however, with regard to patients coming to operation with acute ischemia. When unstable, the patient's internal thoracic artery *may* not be sufficient to relieve the oxygen depletion. In this circumstance, placing both the internal thoracic artery and a saphenous vein graft will cater for both the acute needs and late patency. The philosophy of complete revascularization applies equally to combined disease as it does to isolated coronary artery disease. The major concern during combined operations is the adequacy of myocardial protection.

Aortic valve

The majority of patients having AVR for aortic stenosis plus CABG at our institution are older than 65 years of age, which implies the senile form of aortic stenosis rather than the rheumatic or congenital (bicuspid) variety. In this age group, the decision to use an aggressive approach to the moderately stenotic valve is more easily made than for the younger age group.[9] The elderly are less tolerant of re-operations, and bioprostheses in this age group are very well tolerated and durable. On the other hand, young patients (under the age of 65 years) with mild to moderate aortic stenosis usually receive a mechanical valve, with its associated thromboembolic and anticoagulant limitations. The risk–benefit ratio of a mechanical prosthesis for mild or moderate disease versus the risk of an elective re-operation may favor the latter in the younger patient.

The presence of aortic regurgitation may be approached in a similar fashion in terms of the decision to repair or replace the valve. Repair is much less likely to be feasible for an aortic valve than for a regurgitant mitral valve. If the regurgitant valve can be repaired without increasing the risk of replacing it, repair should be performed. If there is mild aortic regurgitation, the valve should be left alone. This presumes that the aorta is of normal character and not aneurysmal or marfanoid. Moderate and severely regurgitant aortic valves for which there are no reparative options should be replaced at the time of revascularization.

Mitral valve

The mitral valve offers a different approach. The stenotic mitral valve is due to rheumatic fever in the majority of cases, given that we are dealing with an adult population. The occurrence of this is more frequent in women and is not usually associated with coronary artery disease. Some of the newer immigrant or challenged socioeconomic groups are young and have had recent rheumatic fever, and in this age group coronary artery disease is very unusual. In the non-smoking low-risk population, a coronary arteriogram is advised for men over the age of 50 and women over the age of 55 with mitral stenosis.

This is quite the opposite with mitral regurgitation. The uncertainty about mitral regurgitation combined with coronary artery disease is not related to those situations in which there is an anatomic abnormality of the valve such as ruptured chordae tendineae, prolapse, etc., but rather to the regurgitation of normal-appearing valves.[10,11] This phenomenon most commonly occurs with ischemic heart disease. Again, the cases of structural abnormality, such as ruptured papillary muscle, will require repair or replacement. Management of a structurally normal regurgitant valve may be less clear as a result of the variable degree of mitral valve impairment that occurs with myocardial ischemia.

When the valve is structurally normal and mild (grade 1–2) mitral regurgitation exists, usually nothing need be done for it. This situation rarely progresses and long-term consequences are uncommon. The more confusing clinical picture occurs with moderate to severe (grade 3–4) mitral regurgitation with coronary artery disease. This occurs due to a combination of events. Although the force of one event may dominate, there is often more than one factor involved.

There is obviously the impact of ischemic heart disease. This presents as either left ventricular dilatation, due to infarcted myocardium, ischemic hypokinetic myocardium, papillary muscle dysfunction or mitral annular dilatation, or a combination of all of these. A dilemma that presents when dealing with these situations is whether the mitral regurgitation will require repair or replacement, or whether revascularization alone will be enough to correct the regurgitation. Generally, when there is grade 1–2 mitral regurgitation without structural abnormalities, nothing is needed for the valve. Those situations in which there is a grade 3–4 regurgitation, on the other hand, will require intervention. The method of mitral correction in the majority of cases will be reparative. Any chordal rupture or mal-alignment may be corrected with chordal replacement or transposition. There will also be a significant number of situations in which an annuloplasty will correct severe mitral regurgitation. It is generally accepted that grade 3–4 will require some method of correction in addition to CABG (this alone will rarely, if ever, reduce severe mitral regurgitation).

The success or failure of repair can be determined in the operating room by transesophageal echocardiography, which has improved the decision-making process for this abnormality. In the event that the mitral regurgitation is still grade 2 or greater after a repair, it is necessary to re-institute cardiopulmonary bypass, re-inspect the valve and adjust the repair or replace the valve. The late results of combined CABG and mitral valve repair are unsatisfactory when there is significant residual mitral regurgitation. Late heart failure is the major cause of death. Significant mitral regurgitation combined with any residual ischemic myocardium will create a hopeless downward spiral.

Surgical strategy

The most pressing factors confronting a surgeon treating a patient with combined valvular and coronary heart disease are the sequence of the operation and, more importantly, the technique for myocardial protection. First, consider the conduct of CABG with mitral valve pathology. With the possibility of having to undertake valve replacement, it is best to complete the distal coronary anastomoses prior to approaching the valve. Elevation of the heart (necessary to expose the circumflex distribution) with a rigid prosthesis within the mitral annulus may lead to a rupture of the atrioventricular groove. The proximal anastomoses may then be constructed after closure of the atrial incision, relying on the native coronary circulation and any ITA graft for myocardial perfusion. Retrograde cardioplegia via the coronary sinus may also be utilized, especially if there is significant three-vessel disease. Each of the saphenous vein grafts can also be used as a delivery route for cardioplegia. It is not sufficient to rely on retrograde cardioplegia alone in these circumstances, due to the unpredictability of distribution, especially to the right ventricle.

When planning the approach to combined AVR and CABG, a similar sequence is followed. The majority of adult AVRs at our institution are in patients over the age of 65 years, and a bioprosthesis is preferred. By exposing the aortic valve, excising it and sizing the annulus first, the bioprosthesis can be rinsed while distal coronary anastomoses are performed. Following the final distal anastomosis, the valve is implanted and the aorta closed. The proximal graft anastomoses are performed either during cross-clamping or after removal of the cross-clamp, with a partial occluding clamp. It is important to assess the aortic root before cannulation and placement of the aortotomy to facilitate the placement of proximal anastomoses. In the event of a short aorta, it may be necessary to anastomose one of the grafts onto another graft to accomplish tension-free and kink-free grafts.

With AVR, retrograde coronary sinus perfusion has a final added advantage during closure of the aortotomy. The potassium can be removed from the cardioplegia during this last stage of the operation and flushed through the coronary sinus to back-bleed the coronaries of debris and air while the aortotomy is closed. The use of retrograde potassium-free blood cardioplegia will also clear metabolic

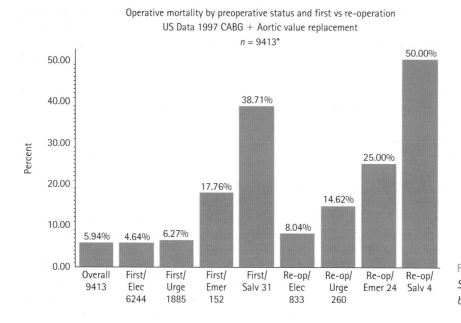

Operative mortality by preoperative status and first vs re-operation
US Data 1997 CABG + Aortic value replacement
$n = 9413^*$

Figure 22.3 *Society of Thoracic Surgeons database risk stratification by re-operation status.*

products and the heart will frequently begin to beat prior to removal of the cross-clamp. This is more evident when using normothermic or tepid (32–34°C) perfusion. **Nor**mothermic or tepid cardiopulmonary perfusion requires the use of blood, not crystalloid cardioplegia, and will require frequent (every 15 minutes) instillation.

In the placement of the proximal grafts onto the aorta with an aortotomy, it is prudent to avoid applying the partial occlusion clamp on the recently closed aortotomy itself. One reason for this is that the thickness of the aortotomy may prevent complete hemostasis of the field; another is that the clamp may fracture the Prolene suture, allowing later bleeding or suture-line disruption.

In general, the selection of valve type with combined CABG follows the same algorithm that is used for all patients. There is evidence, however, that for patients with moderate to severe diffuse coronary artery disease, very satisfactory valve durability may be achieved with a bioprosthesis. The most important aspect of this situation is to attempt complete revascularization with the valve procedure, and the type of prosthesis is secondary. In general for the selection of prosthesis type, it is important to take into account the patient's wishes, lifestyle and limitations. The patient's occupation, recreational activities, medications and reliability are also important considerations in this decision. The ultimate need for re-operation with a bioprosthesis can be mitigated by the relatively low re-operation risk when the surgery is done electively. There is still an increase of mortality from initial operation to reoperation, but when compared to the cumulative risk of anticoagulant-related bleeding and thromboemboli, any clear advantage of one over the other becomes clouded (Figure 22.3).

CORONARY DISEASE COMBINED WITH OTHER VASCULAR DISEASE

The need to combine cardiac and vascular operations is uncommon. In specific circumstances, carotid artery endarterectomy (CEA) or great vessel reconstructions are combined with CABG. Rarely, abdominal aortic aneurysm repairs (AAA) are combined with CABG.[12]

Coronary artery disease with carotid disease

The most common situation in which a combined procedure is considered involves patients with significant carotid and coronary artery disease. Options for surgical treatment include CEA followed by CABG; CABG followed by delayed CEA; or combined CEA and CABG.[13–20] However, management of these patients remains controversial. To date, no large, prospective, randomized clinical trial has been performed to determine which treatment approach is best.[21] Furthermore, most studies in the literature that address this topic are retrospective, have no uniform method for preoperative carotid artery screening, fail to define the severity of carotid stenosis, or have no routine independent postoperative neurological testing. All this makes data interpretation and comparison between treatment groups difficult. Therefore, combined versus staged operations are often dictated by surgeon preference and institutional experience.

Patients considered for combined operation are those in need of CABG who either have a symptomatic carotid stenosis, asymptomatic bilateral, pre-occlusive carotid lesions, or high-grade carotid artery stenosis with a contralateral carotid artery occlusion.[13–16,18–20] Only in specific circumstances are combined procedures offered to patients with a unilateral asymptomatic stenosis.[17]

Factors which affect the treatment decision include the age of the patient, past history of stroke, the severity and extent of carotid and coronary artery disease, the severity of symptoms in either territory, and left ventricular dysfunction.[13,15,18] Other critical issues include the risk and mechanism of stroke when CABG is performed alone; the incidence of carotid stenosis in patients undergoing CABG; the risk of myocardial infarction when CEA is performed alone; and the morbidity and mortality of combined versus staged procedures.[13,15]

The risk of stroke with CABG is low and ranges between 2% and 5%.[13,15,18,22] The Coronary Artery Surgery Study documented a postoperative stroke rate of 1.9%, with most strokes identified at least 24 hours after operation.[22] However, this stroke risk may have been underestimated, as only severe strokes were reported and patients were not routinely evaluated by a neurologist postoperatively.[22] Most strokes post-CABG occur in patients without significant carotid disease.[13] The cause of stroke during CABG is multifactorial. Emboli may occur from cross-clamping of the aorta, the bypass circuitry or the extracranial carotid or intracerebral circulation. Hypoperfusion during the pump run, or perioperative hemodynamic instability are other causes.[13,15,23,24] Two reviews found that 36–54% of post-CABG strokes were caused by emboli and were unifocal in location, whereas the remainder were related to hypoperfusion.[23,24]

The reported incidence of carotid stenosis greater than 70% in patients who required CABG ranges between 4% and 8.7%.[13,16,25–27] Female gender, diabetes mellitus, a history of stroke or transient ischemic attack and the presence of peripheral vascular or left main coronary artery disease increase the likelihood of underlying carotid disease.[16,20,26] The number of patients with symptomatic coronary artery disease and a 70% or greater carotid stenosis has increased, and is probably related to the advancing age of the coronary bypass population.[13,26] Importantly, one-half to two-thirds of strokes post-CABG in patients with significant carotid stenosis occur ipsilateral to the side of the lesion.[13] Nonetheless, prediction of which patients with carotid disease will sustain a perioperative stroke if treated by CABG alone is difficult. Ricotta *et al.* reported that 50% or greater carotid stenosis increased the perioperative stroke risk post-CABG sixfold.[28] The same group reported a 14.3% incidence of stroke in patients who did not have CEA first.[27] In contrast, other reports document stroke rates of only 0–3% in similar patient populations.[17,25]

Two clinical scenarios clearly increase stroke risk in patients with disease in both vascular beds. The first group is patients with carotid territory transient ischemic attacks or recent minor strokes related to a stenotic carotid artery.

These patients require CEA either prior to or together with CABG.[13,15] The other group is those with bilateral, asymptomatic, hemodynamically significant carotid stenoses or a high-grade stenosis together with a contralateral carotid artery occlusion.[13,15]

Most authors agree that patients who may require combined CEA and CABG are older and sicker than those who require operation for isolated disease, with an average age difference of 10 years.[18,29,30] The Cleveland Clinic and Massachusetts General Hospital groups note a higher association between patients with advanced carotid disease and those who have left main or three-vessel coronary artery disease or New York Heart Association Class III–IV angina pectoris.[18,29] Others report little correlation between the severity and extent of carotid and coronary artery disease.[15]

Brener and co-workers performed an extensive literature search to analyze the risk of myocardial infarction, stroke or death in patients who undergo isolated CEA or CABG, for those who have isolated CABG but have known carotid stenosis, and for those who have staged or combined procedures.[15] Patients without significant coronary artery disease who required CEA had a low incidence of myocardial infarction, stroke or death in three series reviewed by Brener's group.[15,20,29,31] The risk of myocardial infarction ranged between 0.8% and 2.0%, the risk of stroke ranged between 1.0% and 5.5%, and death occurred in less than 1% of patients.[20,30,31] In patients who had CABG without significant carotid disease, the incidence of myocardial infarction was 4.7%, the rate of stroke was 0.6–1.4%, and operative mortality ranged between 1.8% and 4.0%.[15,20,27,29] The risk of stroke or death in patients who had CABG with known carotid stenosis was more variable and ranged between 0.2% and 14.3% and 6.0% and 15.7%, respectively, in reported studies involving 20 or more patients.[13–15,25,28]

The same group also performed a meta-analysis of 35 studies in the literature which reported outcomes after staged versus combined operations.[15] Seventeen reports included more than 50 patients and seven had more than 100 patients. Patients who had CEA followed by CABG had an overall risk of myocardial infarction of 11.5%, risk of stroke of 5.3%, and risk of death of 9.4%. Patients with CABG followed by CEA had a myocardial infarction risk of 2.7%, a stroke rate of 10%, and a mortality rate of 3.6%. Finally, patients who had combined procedures had a risk of myocardial infarction of 4.7%, a stroke rate of 6.2%, and a mortality rate of 5.6%.[15] Comparison of outcomes between staged versus combined procedures showed the combined group and those who had CABG first had approximately the same risk of myocardial infarction and death. The combined group and CEA first group had the same probability of stroke. Patients who had CEA performed first had a higher risk of myocardial infarction and death, those who had

CABG performed before CEA had a higher risk of stroke.[15] However, the risk of stroke in the latter group may be lowered if the CEA is deferred for 1–2 months after the heart operation.[18]

There are flaws in such a meta-analysis, as noted by Brener et al.[15] For example, studies with poor outcomes may not have been published. Results may have been flawed by an intention-to-treat basis, so that patients who had staged procedures and sustained an adverse event or died may not have returned for the second operation. Many of the studies did not distinguish between unilateral versus bilateral carotid disease, nor did they define significant carotid stenosis. Finally, patient selection could have been biased by surgeon preference.[15]

At the Mayo Clinic, we reserve combined CABG/CEA for patients with symptoms in both territories or those who have high-grade, bilateral pre-occlusive carotid artery stenoses or a high-grade carotid stenosis together with a contralateral occlusion. It is our opinion that routine screening for carotid disease prior to CABG is not cost effective. However, patients over the age of 70, those with a cervical bruit or past history of stroke or carotid territory symptoms, and those with hypertension or diffuse vascular disease ought to be considered for duplex scan of the carotid arteries preoperatively.[13,15] This study is sensitive, specific and accurate for the detection of a ≥70% carotid stenosis in accredited vascular laboratories. Often, combination of a thorough physical examination and a duplex scan is all that is needed to plan CEA. If additional information is needed, magnetic resonance angiography using gadolinium with fluoroscopic-guided film sequencing provides imaging nearly equivalent to that of cerebral arteriography. The authors prefer to perform CEA prior to CABG in patients with symptomatic carotid disease or high-grade bilateral pre-occlusive stenoses in whom coronary symptoms are stable. Combined operations are offered to patients with symptoms in both vascular beds and to those with high-grade bilateral carotid stenoses in whom coronary symptoms are unstable. Such patients can expect a higher perioperative complication rate in contrast to those who require operation for disease confined to one territory.[13,15] The use of 'off-pump' CABG may help in the management of these patients, but current data for analysis are few.[17]

In summary, until prospective, randomized, clinical trials provide guidelines for management, the treatment of patients with both significant carotid and coronary artery disease should be based on the severity of preoperative symptoms and the experience and preference of the surgical teams. We generally prefer CEA prior to CABG in patients with symptomatic or high-grade asymptomatic carotid lesions in whom coronary symptoms are stable. Combined procedures are reserved for patients with symptoms in both territories and for those with pre-occlusive bilateral carotid artery stenoses.

Coronary disease combined with abdominal aortic aneurysm

We believe there is little role for combining CABG with AAA repair, except for the extraordinarily rare patient who has symptomatic CAD and AAA.[12] Less than 4% of patients who have required AAA at the Mayo Clinic have needed preoperative coronary artery intervention, with balloon angioplasty, stent placement or CABG.[32] This reflects improvement in anesthetic techniques and critical care and the use of perioperative beta-blockers prior to AAA repair. Patients in need of aneurysm repair who have a coronary stent placed usually have operation deferred for 3–4 weeks to reduce the risk of bleeding related to the use of glycoprotein IIb/IIIa platelet receptor inhibitors. Patients who require CABG prior to AAA repair often have the second operation deferred for 4–6 weeks. However, the authors are more aggressive in managing patients who require CABG and have a large (>6.0 cm) AAA. In these cases, we prefer to repair the AAA during the same hospitalization, if possible. This approach has evolved on the basis of anecdotal experience in a few patients who ruptured their large AAAs during the recuperative period after CABG and is not based on prospective data. The advent of endovascular stent graft repair of AAAs may allow earlier aneurysm repair after CABG regardless of aneurysm size. The choice for open versus endovascular AAA repair is dependent on the age of the patient, clinical status post-CABG and anatomical considerations. CABG and AAA repair have not been performed simultaneously at our institution. New techniques such as 'off-pump' CABG and endovascular stent graft repair of aneurysms offer surgeons other treatment approaches for these patients.

CORONARY DISEASE COMBINED WITH LUNG CANCER

A last consideration in combined procedures involves patients in whom cardiac disease is identified in conjunction with pulmonary disease, most notably carcinoma. Coronary disease needing intervention is not commonly seen in patients with concomitant lung cancer, and consequently there are no large series reported in the literature. The option of percutaneous coronary intervention prior to lung surgery should be kept in mind.[33]

Rao et al.[34] reported 15-year experience during which 30 patients had pulmonary resection combined with simultaneous cardiac surgery (CABG in 24), followed for 1–100 months (mean 22), with no increase in early or late morbidity and mortality. Danton et al.[35] reported simultaneous cardiac and pulmonary procedures in 13 patients (11 CABG), with acceptable operative morbidity and mortality. Most were operated on via standard median sternotomy, and lung resection was undertaken prior to heparinization and cardiopulmonary bypass in the majority. CABG was accomplished without cardiopulmonary bypass in two patients. The authors discuss the rationale for techniques and review previous literature.

In our institution, Piehler *et al.*[36] reported on an 18-year experience with 43 patients. The thrust of the report was that combined procedures are feasible but are associated with increased bleeding complications due to cardiopulmonary bypass. In such combined procedures, it is important to reverse anticoagulation before undertaking lung resection. This has been followed by a second report by Miller *et al.*[37] Over a 27-year period, 30 patients had combined coronary artery disease and lung carcinoma. It was found that although combined cancer and cardiac procedures can be accomplished, the completeness of the resection of the carcinoma via the sternotomy incision limited satisfactory node resection and significantly adversely affected late survival. It is felt that unless it is not possible, or the patient cannot tolerate a second procedure, the lesions should be approached separately. Unless the cardiac lesion is life threatening, the lung carcinoma should be approached first.

KEY REFERENCES

Akins CW, Hilgenberg AD, Vlahakes GJ, MacGillivray TE, Torchiana DF, Madsen JC. Results of bioprosthetic versus mechanical aortic valve replacement performed with concomitant coronary artery bypass grafting. *Ann Thorac Surg* 2002; **74**:1098–106.
This study of 750 patients having combined AVR and CABG with bioprosthetic and mechanical valves over 13 years confirmed the adverse influence of coronary disease on patients needing AVR. The study adds weight to the argument favoring the use of bioprostheses from an earlier age than generally recommended for AVR alone.

Borger MA, Fremes SE. Management of patients with concomitant coronary and carotid vascular disease. *Semin Thorac Cardiovasc Surg* 2001; **13**:192–8.
Up-to-date review of current thinking about combined carotid and coronary disease, taking account of the possibility of carotid stenting, which offers potential benefits in the near future.

Borger MA, Fremes SE, Weisel RD, Cohen G, Rao V, Lindsay TF, *et al.* Coronary bypass and carotid endarterectomy: does a combined approach increase risk? A meta-analysis. *Ann Thorac Surg* 1999; **68**:14–21.
A meta-analysis of 16 studies involving 844 combined and 920 staged patients with coronary and carotid disease. Results suggest that combined procedures may have higher stroke and death risk than staged procedures. The need for randomized trials is again emphasized.

Danton MHD, Anikin VA, McManus KG, McGuigan JA, Campalani G. Simultaneous cardiac surgery with pulmonary resection: presentation of series and review of literature. *Eur J Cardiothorac Surg* 1998; **13**:667–72.
Combined CABG and lung resection for neoplasm is rare. The authors report their own experience with 13 patients, discuss the therapeutic options and review previous literature.

REFERENCES

1. Mullany CJ, Elveback LR, Frye RL, Pluth JR, Edwards WD, Orszulak TA, *et al.* Coronary artery disease and its management: influence on survival in patients undergoing aortic valve replacement. *J Am Coll Cardiol* 1987; **10**:66–72.
2. Fiore AC, Swartz MT, Naunheim KS, Moroney DA, Canvasser DA, McBride LR, *et al.* Management of asymptomatic mild aortic stenosis during coronary artery operations. *Ann Thorac Surg* 1996; **61**:1693–7.
3. Hochrein J, Lucke JC, Harrison JK, Bashore TM, Wolfe WG, Jones RH, *et al.* Mortality and need for re-operation in patients with mild-to-moderate asymptomatic aortic valve disease undergoing coronary artery bypass graft alone. *Am Heart J* 1999; **138**:791–7.
4. Rahimtoola SH. Should patients with asymptomatic mild or moderate aortic stenosis undergoing coronary artery bypass surgery also have valve replacement for their aortic stenosis? *Heart* 2001; **85**:337–41.
5. Tam JW, Masters RG, Burwash IG, Mayhew AD, Chan KL. Management of patients with mild aortic stenosis undergoing coronary artery bypass grafting. *Ann Thorac Surg* 1998; **65**:1215–19.
6. Odell JA, Mullany CJ, Schaff HV, Orszulak TA, Daly RC, Morris JJ. Aortic valve replacement after previous coronary artery grafting. *Ann Thorac Surg* 1996; **62**:1424–30.
7. Sundt TM III, Murphy SF, Barzilai B, Schuessler RB, Mendeloff EN, Huddleston CB, *et al.* Previous coronary artery bypass grafting is not a risk factor for aortic valve replacement. *Ann Thorac Surg* 1997; **64**:651–7.
8. Gall S Jr, Lowe JE, Wolfe WG, Oldham HN Jr, Van TP III, Glower DD. Efficacy of the internal mammary artery in combined aortic valve replacement–coronary artery bypass grafting. *Ann Thorac Surg* 2000; **69**:524–30.
9. Cohen G, David TE, Ivanov J, Armstrong S, Feindel CM. The impact of age, coronary artery disease, and cardiac co-morbidity on late survival after bioprosthetic aortic valve replacement. *J Thorac Cardiovasc Surg* 1999; **117**:273–84.
10. Aklog L, Filsoufi F, Flores KQ, Chen RH, Cohn LH, Nathan NS, *et al.* Does coronary artery bypass grafting alone correct moderate ischemic mitral regurgitation? *Circulation* 2001; **104** (12 Suppl. I): I68–75.
11. Ryden T, Bech-Hanssen O, Brandrup-Wognsen G, Nilsson F, Svensson S, Jeppsson A. The importance of grade 2 ischemic mitral regurgitation in coronary artery bypass grafting. *Eur J Cardiothorac Surg* 2001; **20**:276–81.
12. Whittemore AD, Mannick JA. Simultaneous coronary bypass aortic surgery. In: *Aortic Surgery*, Bergan JJ, Yao JST (eds). Philadelphia: W.B. Saunders, 1989, 353–6.
13. Bilfinger T, Petersen M, Cicotta J. Coronary artery bypass grafting with carotid artery endarterectomy. In: *Practical Vascular Surgery*, Yao JST, Pearce WH (eds). Stamford, CT: Appleton and Lange, 1999, 147–60.
14. Brener BJ, Brief DK, Alpert J, Goldenkranz RJ, Parsonnet V. The risk of stroke in patients with asymptomatic carotid stenosis

undergoing cardiac surgery: a follow-up study. *J Vasc Surg* 1987; **5**:269–79.

15. Brener BJ, Hermans H, Eisenbud D. The management of patients requiring coronary artery bypass and carotid artery endarterectomy. In: *Surgery for Cerebrovascular Disease*, Moore WS (ed.). Philadelphia: W.B. Saunders, 1996, 278–87.

16. D'Agostino RS, Svensson LG, Neumann DJ, Balkhy HH, Williamson WA, Shahian DM. Screening carotid ultrasonography and risk factors for stroke in coronary artery surgery patients. *Ann Thorac Surg* 1996; **62**:1714–23.

17. Estes JM, Khabbaz KR, Barnatan M, Carpino P, Mackey WC. Outcome after combined carotid endarterectomy and coronary artery bypass is related to patient selection. *J Vasc Surg* 2001; **33**:1179–84.

18. Hertzer NR, Loop FD, Beven EG, O'Hara PJ, Krajewski LP. Surgical staging for simultaneous coronary and carotid disease: a study including prospective randomization. *J Vasc Surg* 1989; **9**:455–63.

19. Perler BA, Burdick JF, Minken SL, Williams GM. Should we perform carotid endarterectomy synchronously with cardiac surgical procedures? *J Vasc Surg* 1988; **8**:402–9.

20. Rizzo RJ, Whittemore AD, Couper GS, Donaldson MC, Aranki SF, Collins JJ Jr, *et al.* Combined carotid and coronary revascularization: the preferred approach to the severe vasculopath. *Ann Thorac Surg* 1992; **54**:1099–108.

21. Borger MA, Fremes SE, Weisel RD, Cohen G, Rao V, Lindsay TF, *et al.* Coronary bypass and carotid endarterectomy: does a combined approach increase risk? A meta-analysis. *Ann Thorac Surg* 1999; **68**:14–20.

22. Frye RL, Kronmal R, Schaff HV, Myers WO, Gersh BJ. Stroke in coronary artery bypass graft surgery: an analysis of the CASS experience. The participants in the Coronary Artery Surgery Study. *Int J Cardiol* 1992; **36**:213–21.

23. Blossom GB, Fietsam R Jr, Bassett JS, Glover JL, Bendick PJ. Characteristics of cerebrovascular accidents after coronary artery bypass grafting. *Am Surg* 1992; **58**:584–9.

24. Wijdicks EF, Jack CR. Coronary artery bypass grafting-associated ischemic stroke. A clinical and neuroradiological study. *J Neuroimaging* 1996; **6**:20–2.

25. Barnes RW, Nix ML, Sansonetti D, Turley DG, Goldman MR. Late outcome of untreated asymptomatic carotid disease following cardiovascular operations. *J Vasc Surg* 1985; **2**:843–9.

26. Berens ES, Kouchoukos NT, Murphy SF, Wareing TH. Preoperative carotid artery screening in elderly patients undergoing cardiac surgery. *J Vasc Surg* 1992; **15**:313–21.

27. Faggioli GL, Curl GR, Ricotta JJ. The role of carotid screening before coronary artery bypass. *J Vasc Surg* 1990; **12**:724–9.

28. Ricotta JJ, Faggioli GL, Castilone A, Hassett JM. Risk factors for stroke after cardiac surgery: Buffalo Cardiac–Cerebral Study Group. *J Vasc Surg* 1995; **21**:359–63.

29. Cambria RP, Ivarsson BL, Akins CW, Moncure AC, Brewster DC, Abbott WM. Simultaneous carotid and coronary disease: safety of the combined approach. *J Vasc Surg* 1989; **9**:56–64.

30. Vermeulen FE, Hamerlijnck RP, Defauw JJ, Ernst SM. Synchronous operation for ischemic cardiac and cerebrovascular disease: early results and long-term follow-up. *Ann Thorac Surg* 1992; **53**:381–9.

31. Beneficial effect of carotid endarterectomy in symptomatic patients with high-grade carotid stenosis. North American Symptomatic Carotid Endarterectomy Trial Collaborators. *N Engl J Med* 1991; **325**:445–53.

32. Elmore JR, Hallett JW Jr, Gibbons RJ, Naessens JM, Bower TC, Cherry KJ, *et al.* Myocardial revascularization before abdominal aortic aneurysmorrhaphy: effect of coronary angioplasty. *Mayo Clin Proc* 1993; **68**:637–41.

33. Ciriaco P, Carretta A, Calori G, Mazzone P, Zannini P. Lung resection for cancer in patients with coronary arterial disease: analysis of short-term results. *Eur J Cardiothorac Surg* 2002; **22**:35–40.

34. Rao V, Todd TR, Weisel RD, Komeda M, Cohen G, Ikonomidis JS, *et al.* Results of combined pulmonary resection and cardiac operation. *Ann Thorac Surg* 1996; **62**:342–6.

35. Danton MH, Anikin VA, McManus KG, McGuigan JA, Campalani G. Simultaneous cardiac surgery with pulmonary resection: presentation of series and review of literature. *Eur J Cardiothorac Surg* 1998; **13**:667–72.

36. Piehler JM, Trastek VF, Pairolero PC, Pluth JR, Danielson GK, Schaff HV, *et al.* Concomitant cardiac and pulmonary operations. *J Thorac Cardiovasc Surg* 1985; **90**:662–7.

37. Miller DL, Orszulak TA, Pairolero PC, Trastek VF, Schaff HV. Combined operation for lung cancer and cardiac disease. *Ann Thorac Surg* 1994; **58**:989–93.

23

The impact of coronary surgery on symptoms and prognosis

EUGENE H BLACKSTONE

From the unplanned reversed saphenous vein coronary artery bypass graft (CABG) to the left anterior descending coronary artery (LAD) by Garrett and colleagues in Houston,[1] to the unheralded internal thoracic artery (ITA) anastomosis to the LAD by Kolessov in Leningrad,[2,3] to the program of CABG by Favaloro and colleagues[4] in Cleveland made possible by the introduction of coronary angiography by Sones and Shirey[5] – all in the mid-1960s – CABG spread rapidly throughout the world. It has become far and away the most common heart operation. It accelerated the development of cardiac surgery expertise, stimulated research to increase the safety of managing the heart during cardiopulmonary bypass, fostered the expanding field of medical imaging, generated new business opportunities, propelled cardiac surgeons to prominent positions in hospitals, medical centers and universities, supported the finances of many institutions, and enriched a number of individuals. It was the target of the earliest attempts to measure, and announce publicly, institutional and surgeon-specific variance in medical outcomes.[6] It also gave birth to its competition, percutaneous coronary interventions, which have reduced the importance of CABG in the initial management of stenotic coronary artery disease.

Secure information about the early and long-term benefits, risks and limitations of CABG is now available. In part, this is because the prevalence of ischemic disease in developed countries made coronary revascularization a common procedure. Attention focused early, therefore, not just on its effectiveness in the relief of symptoms (favorable), but, because it did not claim to halt the progression of atherosclerotic coronary artery disease, also on its possible survival benefit (favorable),[7] cost–risk benefit (favorable),[8] total societal cost (prohibitive in some countries), and more acceptable, though not necessarily less costly, alternatives. Ubiquity of ischemic heart disease, cost of the operation, skepticism about its benefit, and alternatives made CABG one of the most studied medical procedures.

This chapter discusses time-related events occurring after CABG, interrelations among these events, and some of the risk factors modulating their occurrence.

Numerical and graphical presentation of these events is based largely on a series of 9600 consecutive patients undergoing first-time (primary) CABG at the Gasthuisberg University Hospital of the Katholieke Universiteit Leuven (KU Leuven) from the start of that institution's coronary surgery program in 1971 until 1 January 1992. The database was constructed and in-hospital data organized and entered systematically by Dr Sergeant and his collaborators.[9] An important aspect of Dr Sergeant's work was establishing a follow-up network, to ensure a regular stream of follow-up reports from referring specialists for updating outcomes in the database.[10] Reports are sent after each event, suspicion of event or regular visit. Supplementing this were two formal cross-sectional follow-up efforts, one of which had a common closing date of 1 January 1993 that achieved complete follow-up in 99.9%

of patients. These data are the subject of several published reports.[11–13] Many graphical depictions presented here are similar to those appearing in these reports; however, a number are novel to this chapter.

EVENTS AFTER CABG

Mortality

The most secure end-point following CABG is all-cause mortality.[14] It is not subject to interpretation and can be obtained by patient follow-up and verified using national death registries.

Overall, risk-unadjusted survival after CABG in the KU Leuven experience was 98%, 92%, 81%, 66% and 51% at 30 days, 5, 10, 15 and 20 years, respectively (Figure 23.1a).[13] The pattern of time-related survival consists of an initial small decrease immediately after operation, followed by a slow, gradual decline that becomes somewhat steeper after about 8–10 years.

This pattern of survival is best understood as being driven by a somewhat complex 'force of mortality' (hazard function; Figure 23.1b). The hazard function is the instantaneous risk of death.[15] It is analogous to the speed of an automobile; the survival function is somewhat analogous to the distance traveled.

Death after CABG is characterized by an initial period of high risk immediately after operation. This period of high risk is brief if the patient has few risk factors, but is increasingly prolonged as the number of risk factors increases.[16] (There is only a weak relation between duration of hospital stay after operation and duration of this period of high risk.) The consequence of this period of high risk is the initial drop in survival seen in Figure 23.1a.

Risk of death then falls to its lowest point about 1 year after operation (Figure 23.1b). Thereafter it rises steadily for as long as patients have been followed.

To put this pattern of risk into perspective, Figure 23.1 also displays survival and hazard functions for the general population. Numerical values for population survival and risk vary somewhat from country to country, of course. However, in developed countries, survival after CABG is about the same in pattern and magnitude as expected for similar age, sex and ethnicity in the general population, except for the initial period of high perioperative risk.

Return of angina

Sometimes forgotten in the emphasis that has been placed on the possible survival advantage of CABG is that the operation was devised to relieve angina and thereby improve the quality of life for patients with ischemic

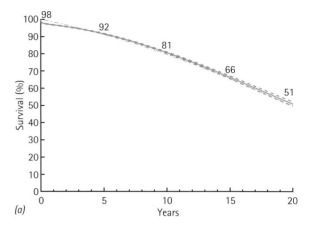

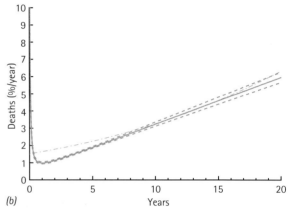

Figure 23.1 *Death after CABG (KU Leuven, 1971–1992, n = 9600). (a) Survival. The solid line is the survival estimate, and the dashed lines enclose confidence limits equivalent to 1 standard error. Numbers are percent survival at 30 days, 5, 10, 15 and 20 years after CABG. The dot-dash-dot line is survival in a population life table matched for age, sex and ethnicity. Note that this line is virtually superimposed on the patient cohort survival line. (b) Hazard. The solid line is the hazard estimate, and the dashed lines enclose confidence limits equivalent to 1 standard error.*

heart disease. When it is possible to revascularize the heart by CABG, it provides effective relief from the symptoms of angina.

Overall, non-risk-adjusted freedom from return of angina at 1, 5, 10, 15 and 20 years was 95%, 82%, 61%, 38% and 21%, respectively, in the KU Leuven experience (Figure 23.2a).[10] The trajectory of this time-related curve suggests that if patients survive long enough after CABG, return of angina is almost inevitable (Sergeant says 'immutable'[10]), but with a median interval to first occurrence of about 12 or more years.

Interestingly, there is a phase of early risk of return of angina after CABG that lasts for about 2 years (Figure 23.2b). After this relatively non-dramatic early phase (compared, e.g., to the early return of angina after classic balloon angioplasty), the hazard function for return of

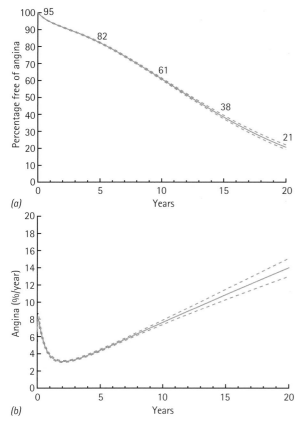

Figure 23.2 *First return of angina of any degree of intensity after CABG (KU Leuven, 1971–1992, n = 9600). The format of the figure is similar to that of Figure 23.1. (a) Freedom from angina. (b) Hazard.*

angina increases at a nearly linear rate across time (Sergeant says 'relentless'[10]).

Sergeant and colleagues defined 'return of angina' as the first recurrence of angina of any intensity and duration, unless it was associated on the same day with acute myocardial infarction or death.[10] In their study, intensity of first return of angina was classified as mild in 59% of patients. Thus first return of angina by their definition is a sensitive, though perhaps not specific, indicator of return of ischemic symptoms.

Conventional depictions of freedom from angina do not inform us of the longitudinal prevalence of angina of each degree of intensity in a cohort of patients. The author is only aware of the possible availability of yearly follow-up data within the Coronary Artery Surgery Study (CASS) registry that could be used to formulate such an estimate. However, at the time of the CASS study, appropriate methods for such a depiction – longitudinal data analysis techniques – had not yet been developed.[17,18]

COMPETING RISKS OF DEATH AND ANGINA

The depiction of return of angina (Figure 23.2a) should have more correctly (though, perhaps, obviously) been entitled 'freedom from return of angina among living patients'. That is, it is a true and valid estimate of the probability of return of angina if a patient survives to a given point along the horizontal axis. Although the depiction answers a useful question (and the author argues that it addresses the nature of the phenomenon of return of angina in a pure way), death simultaneously removes patients from being at risk of angina return. This is known as the problem of competing risks.[19] Therefore, another, and quite different, question may be asked: What net proportion of a group of patients undergoing CABG is anticipated to experience return of angina?

In such an analysis, at every moment in time, each patient can be in only one of three mutually exclusive categories:

1 alive without return of angina,
2 dead before return of angina,
3 having experienced return of angina.

The proportion of patients in all categories adds up to 100% at each moment in follow-up time. Hazard functions for death and return of angina operate simultaneously to move patients from the category 'alive without angina' into one of the other two categories (Figure 23.3a). The net result of these two simultaneously driving forces is the net proportion of patients in each category across time (Figure 23.3b).

Considering the palliative nature of the operation, Lytle, in discussing Sergeant and colleagues' experience, points out the remarkable fact that by 20 years, some 35% of the initial group of patients operated upon will not have experienced even a single recurrence of angina of even the mildest intensity.[10]

Myocardial infarction

Overall, non-risk-adjusted freedom from myocardial infarction at 30 days, 5, 10, 15 and 20 years after CABG was 97%, 94%, 86%, 73% and 56%, respectively (Figure 23.4a).[12] These figures include definite perioperative myocardial infarct confirmed by electrocardiogram and cardiac-specific enzyme elevation (CK-MB fraction >8% of total CK). Risk of infarction increases across time, nearly doubling every 5 years (1.1% per year at 5 years, 2.3% per year at 10 years, 4.2% per year at 15 years, and 6.7% per year at 20 years after surgery; Figure 23.4b).

Coronary re-intervention

Non-risk-adjusted freedom from either interventional cardiological or surgical coronary re-intervention 30 days, 5, 10, 15, and 20 years after CABG was 99.7%, 97%, 89%, 72% and 48%, respectively (Figure 23.5a).[11] Risk of re-intervention increases across time, nearly tripling from

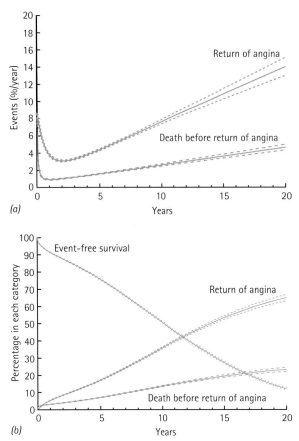

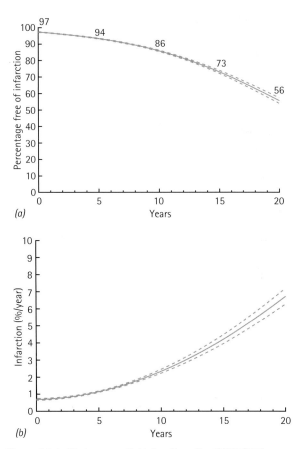

Figure 23.3 *Competing risks of return of angina and death before angina after CABG (KU Leuven, 1971–1992, n = 9600). (a) Hazard functions for return of angina and death before return of angina. The format of the figure is similar to that of Figure 23.1b. (b) Percentage of patients in each of three mutually exclusive categories, as determined by the driving forces of the hazard functions shown in (a). All patients begin in the category labeled 'event-free survival'. The two hazard functions act simultaneously on this category to transition patients from it into the category of 'return of angina' or 'death before return of angina'. The net result across time is known as the cumulative incidence function, which is labeled here 'Percentage in each category'.*

Figure 23.4 *First myocardial infarction after CABG (KU Leuven, 1971–1992, n = 9600). The format of the figure is similar to that of Figure 23.1. (a) Freedom from infarction. (b) Hazard.*

to the patient and to patent grafts, uncertainty as to the survival benefit of additional grafts (particularly if an ITA to the LAD coronary artery is widely patent), and other patient and physician decision-making factors. All introduce bias. This must be borne in mind when interpreting risk factors for re-intervention, because they may simply represent surrogate markers for systematic sources of bias.

Comment on events after CABG

Events other than mortality after CABG, such as return of angina, myocardial infarction and coronary re-intervention, are subject to underestimation. Their identification requires active patient follow-up, including the availability of information about patients who die before systematic follow-up commences. Passive information from health records is probably incomplete and not a good substitute. In addition, identification of myocardial infarction after CABG, particularly perioperative infarction, may differ among institutions according to the aggressiveness of monitoring and definition of the event. Sudden death could represent myocardial infarction rather than

5 to 10 to 15 years (Figure 23.5b). As with all events after CABG, there is a small elevation of hazard early after surgery, corresponding to the occasional patient who develops dramatic symptoms and signs of ischemia requiring re-intervention in the early postoperative period. These figures do not include re-interventions after the first.

Although re-intervention is a secure end-point, its interpretation is challenging. We do not know the *need* for re-intervention, only that it is performed. When ischemic events occur, decisions for or against re-intervention are tempered by life expectancy (perhaps lowering performance of re-interventions in the elderly), perceived ventricular mass at risk, increased risk of the procedure both

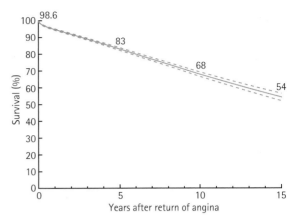

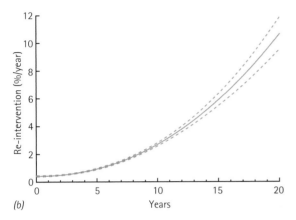

Figure 23.5 *First interventional cardiological or surgical coronary re-intervention after CABG (KU Leuven, 1971–1992, n = 9600). The format of the figure is similar to that of Figure 23.1. (a) Freedom from re-intervention. (b) Hazard.*

Figure 23.6 *Survival after return of angina (KU Leuven, 1971–1992,* n *= 9600). Depiction is as in Figure 23.1a.*

EVENTS AFTER RETURN OF ANGINA

Mortality

Survival after return of angina was 98.6%, 83%, 68% and 54% at 30 days, 5, 10 and 15 years, respectively (Figure 23.6).[10] Compared to overall survival after CABG (see Figure 23.1), these findings are considerably worse. However, patients are older – many considerably so – at the time of return of angina than at CABG. To adjust for this, we calculated a survival curve for each patient having return of angina using the multivariable equation for death after CABG,[13] conditional on survival to the day of return of angina. These curves were then averaged, and the resulting predicted survival curve had angina not returned was superimposed on the curve of observed deaths (Figure 23.7).[20] Compared to 83% observed survival at 5 years, expected survival was 87%; but 68% observed versus 70% expected at 10 years; and 57% observed versus 54% expected at 15 years. The inference is that angina appears to have a small adverse effect on survival early after its return, but thereafter the risk of mortality is as anticipated for similarly aged patients.

The inference that return of angina is rather benign must be tempered, however, by Sergeant and colleagues' finding that the more intense the grade of angina (particularly class 3 or 4) when it returns, the higher the *early* (only) mortality (about 12% in the first month for class 4).[10] This may be related to linkage between angina and infarction (see below), even though these depictions are of angina return without infarction the same day.

Myocardial infarction

Freedom from myocardial infarct after return of angina was 97% at 30 days and 92%, 82%, 71% and 62% at 1, 5, 10 and 15 years, respectively (Figure 23.8a).[10] Risk of

isolated arrhythmia. Return of angina is not just an event, but a graded intensity event and state of health, for which detection and methods of analysis are less well developed and employed than for discrete events (see above).

Interrelation of events after CABG

Return of angina, myocardial infarction and coronary re-intervention after CABG are only occasionally fatal (morbid events), may recur (repeating events), and occur in the context of inevitable mortality (competing risks). All negatively impact quality of life. They are generally analyzed and presented as isolated events, but they must in some ways be interrelated and interdependent. Thus, in this section we address such questions as:

- Is return of angina otherwise important?
- Does it increase risk of mortality?
- What is its relation to coronary re-intervention?
- Is myocardial infarction occurring after CABG serious?
- How is it related to re-intervention?
- Is return of angina often a precursor?

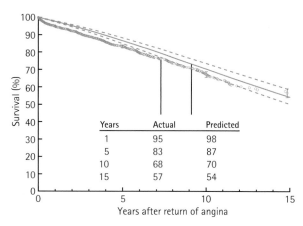

Years	Actual	Predicted
1	95	98
5	83	87
10	68	70
15	57	54

Figure 23.7 *Actual survival after return of angina compared to predicted survival had these same patients not experienced return of angina (KU Leuven, 1971–1992, n = 9600). Actual survival is depicted by circles, each representing a death; vertical bars represent asymmetric confidence limits equivalent to 1 standard error. Predicted survival is depicted by the solid line enclosed within 68% confidence limits (see text for method of construction).*

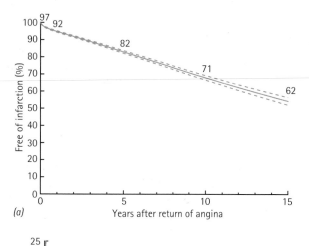

(a)

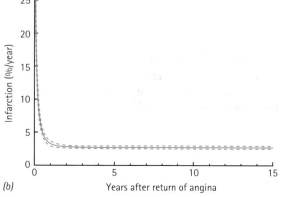

(b)

Figure 23.8 *Myocardial infarction after return of angina (KU Leuven, 1971–1992, n = 9600). The format of the figure is similar to that of Figure 23.1. (a) Freedom from infarction. (b) Hazard function for infarction after return of angina.*

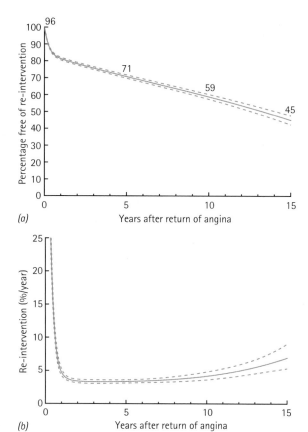

(a)

(b)

Figure 23.9 *Cardiological or surgical re-intervention after return of angina (KU Leuven, 1971–1992, n = 9600). The format of the figure is similar to that of Figure 23.1. (a) Freedom from re-intervention. (b) Hazard.*

infarction after return of angina (hazard) is particularly high during the first year after return of angina, falling subsequently to a constant risk of 2.7% per year (Figure 23.8b). This risk is considerably amplified when the intensity of angina at its return is anything other than mild (10–15% within 1 year compared to <5%).

Coronary re-intervention

One might anticipate a high prevalence of either cardiological or surgical re-intervention after return of angina, but 1-year freedom from re-intervention was 81% (Figure 23.9a). The incidence (hazard) was indeed highest in the first year after return of angina, but thereafter became more or less constant at about 4–5% per year (Figure 23.9b).

EVENTS AFTER MYOCARDIAL INFARCTION

Mortality

Early mortality is high when myocardial infarction occurs after CABG (Figure 23.10). Survival was 80%, 65%, 52%

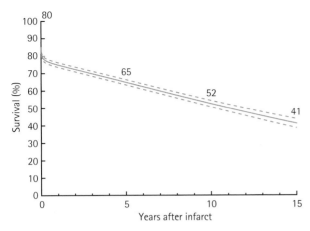

Figure 23.10 *Survival after myocardial infarction following CABG (KU Leuven, 1971–1992, n = 9600). The format of the figure is similar to that of Figure 23.1a.*

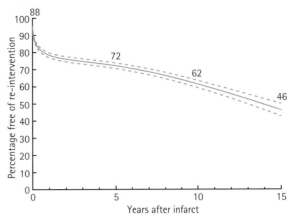

Figure 23.12 *Freedom from cardiological or surgical re-intervention after myocardial infarction following CABG (KU Leuven, 1971–1992, n = 9600). Presentation is as for Figure 23.1a.*

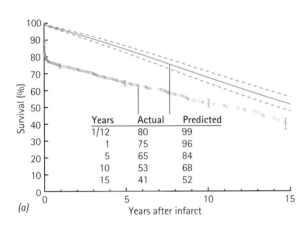

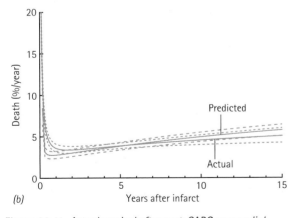

Figure 23.11 *Actual survival after post-CABG myocardial infarction compared to expected survival had these same patients not experienced an infarct (KU Leuven, 1971–1992, n = 9600). The format of the figure is similar to that of Figure 23.7. (a) Actual survival compared to expected survival. (b) Comparison of actual and expected hazard functions.*

and 41% at 30 days, 5, 10 and 15 years after post-CABG infarction.[12] However, compared to expected survival (calculated as described above; Figure 23.11a), patients surviving the early phase of high mortality after the infarct have a hazard function for death similar to that of patients who have not had an infarct (Figure 23.11b). Although this suggests an autoselection phenomenon, we did not have available for analysis either the size or myocardial location of the infarct, or mechanical and electrical sequelae of the infarct that might account for the pattern of risk.

Occurrence of angina

After a post-CABG myocardial infarction, freedom from occurrence of angina was 82%, 40%, 27% and 19% at 30 days, 5, 10 and 15 years, respectively.[12] This implies a considerably higher rate of occurrence, particularly early, than that for return of angina after CABG.

Coronary re-intervention

After a post-CABG myocardial infarction, freedom from cardiological or surgical coronary re-intervention was 88%, 72%, 62% and 46% at 30 days, 5, 10 and 15 years, respectively (Figure 23.12).[12]

EVENTS AFTER CORONARY RE-INTERVENTION

Mortality

Survival following first cardiological or surgical re-intervention after CABG was 95%, 87%, 73% and 58% at

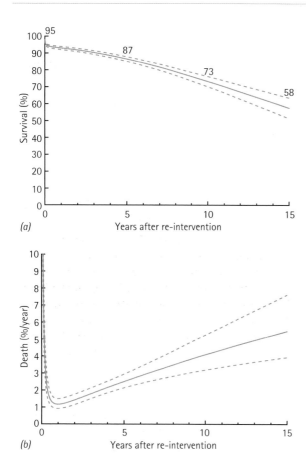

(a) Years after re-intervention

(b) Years after re-intervention

Figure 23.13 *Mortality after first cardiological or surgical coronary re-intervention following CABG (KU Leuven, 1971–1992, n = 9600). Presentation is as for Figure 23.1a. (a) Survival. (b) Hazard.*

30 days, 5, 10 and 15 years (Figure 23.13a).[11] Early risk is clearly higher than after primary CABG (Figure 23.13b), but thereafter is comparable to that observed after primary surgery.

Occurrence of angina

After surgical re-intervention, freedom from return of angina was about 10% lower at 5 and 10 years than after primary CABG.[11] However, as may be anticipated from the types of percutaneous interventions available at the time, return of angina after cardiological interventions occurred considerably sooner, with only 50% of patients free of angina at 1 year and 25% free at 5 years.

RISK FACTORS FOR EVENTS AFTER CABG

Specific risk factors for events after CABG have been established on the basis of numerous studies. Kirklin and

Barratt-Boyes[21] synthesized these into a set of general categories. The categories of risk factors include:

- severity of reduction of regional coronary flow reserve,
- number of myocardial regions with reduced coronary flow reserve,
- nature of the coronary atherosclerotic plaque,
- thrombotic and fibrinolytic milieu,
- aggressiveness of the atherosclerotic process,
- rate of progression of the coronary arterial stenosis,
- amount and distribution of myocardial scarring,
- secondary conditions,
- coexisting conditions (co-morbidity).

What is less well understood, despite many years of presenting and reporting results, is precisely how specific risk factors modulate the pattern of events across time, what a specific risk factor is and what it is not, and how specific risk factors become evident. Thus, this section first addresses these general issues before discussing some of the specific risk factors for events after CABG.

Risk factors: what they are, what they are not, and how they modulate risk

WHAT A RISK FACTOR IS AND WHAT IT IS NOT

A risk factor is a variable associated with outcome. It is not a mechanistic cause of the outcome. Some risk factors may indeed be causal mechanisms rather than general associations with outcome; establishing this causality is what randomized clinical trials attempt to do. Some risk factors may be surrogates or markers for a causal mechanism that has not been recorded or discovered. Some may be spurious. Thus, caution must be exercised in interpreting risk factors. The risk factors after CABG have been studied so intensely that most of the spurious ones have been weeded out.

In addition to randomized clinical trials, which have notoriously encompassed both a small part of the spectrum of ischemic heart disease and a relatively small number of patients, important techniques for analysis of clinical information have been developed that allow a semblance of testing for causal effects.[22,23] These are just beginning to make their way into the analysis of medical information and so have been applied to only a few analyses of CABG.[24]

Risk factors are identified by multivariable analysis, that is, by analyses that consider multiple variables simultaneously. Thus, risk factors might also be defined as that collection of factors identified by multivariable analysis.[25] The form of the multivariable model used may vary from logistic regression for hospital events to Cox proportional hazards methodology for follow-up events. Both methods are suboptimal for the analysis of events following CABG. Therefore, specifically for just such events, some 20 years ago my colleagues and I developed more appropriate methodology that has been employed for the data presented in this chapter.[26]

Methods for identifying risk factors from among a multitude of variables recorded are challenging and controversial. The issues may be resolved by emerging techniques that utilize computer-intensive data sampling.[27,28]

Multivariable analysis takes into account correlation among clinical variables. For example, women are smaller than men, and left main disease occurs more frequently in the presence of carotid disease. The magnitude of association of a given risk factor with outcome is the incremental risk remaining after taking into account all other variables in the model. (Some call this increment the 'independent' contribution of a risk factor. The author resists using this term because it has several statistical meanings, and physicians often confuse them.[29]) It is possible, therefore, that a variable may be associated with increased risk when analyzed by itself, but may not be identified as a risk factor *per se* because it does not contribute a sufficient increment of information about outcome over and above that already accounted for by other factors.

The ability to identify risk factors and estimate their multivariable contribution to risk with high reliability is dependent on the number of events available for analysis.[29] If the number of events is small or follow-up is short for even a large group of patients, risk factors may not be identified reliably. This is but one of the several factors that can lead to confusion when different groups report different risk factors.[30]

WHAT DOES A RISK FACTOR MODULATE?

For time-related events, the quantity that is modulated by risk factors is the hazard function (see, e.g., Figure 23.1b). Death after CABG may be characterized, for instance, by a period of rapidly diminishing high risk immediately after operation that eventually becomes an increasing hazard (see Figure 23.1b). However, this overall pattern of hazard and, consequently, overall survival pattern (or freedom from an event) for a group of patients is unlikely to be a good representation of expected risk for an individual patient. Some patients will have a number of co-morbidities; others will come to operation at an elderly age; others will have had prior myocardial damage from remote myocardial infarcts; some previously well patients will experience an acute infarction and come to the operating room in cardiogenic shock. All these factors will cause a patient's outcome to deviate from average. From a mathematical viewpoint, they all modulate the hazard function. The modulated hazard function generates a survivorship function that is different from the overall, non-risk-adjusted survivorship function.

Figure 23.14 depicts overall survival after CABG in the heterogeneous population taken from Figure 23.1. However, it then superimposes predicted survival of two

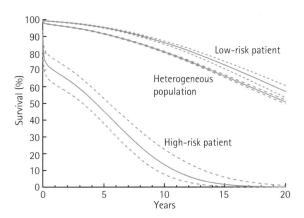

Figure 23.14 *Death after primary CABG according to different patient profiles (KU Leuven, 1971–1992,* n = 9600*). The center solid line is overall survival in the heterogeneous population, identical to that shown in Figure 23.1a. The highest set of curves is for a patient with a low-risk profile whose survival is predicted to be better than that of the heterogeneous group. The lower set of curves is for a patient with a high-risk profile: elderly, diabetic, with poor left ventricular function. (See text for details.)*

patients with different risk profiles, as described in the figure legend. The low-risk patient is expected to survive longer than the so-called 'average' patient; he is 65 years old, has chronic stable angina, three-system disease, well-preserved ventricular function, and no co-morbidities other than a history of smoking. The high-risk patient is 75 years old, also has three-system coronary artery disease, but, unlike the first patient, has unstable angina requiring preoperative stabilization, an ejection fraction of only 25%, and insulin-treated diabetes with important peripheral vascular disease.

These different patient profiles produce different prognostic patterns of time-related survival. The different patterns may impact recommendations for treatment, and they should play a prominent role in informed patient consent. The ability to generate such patient-specific predictions on the basis of analyses of clinical data has been available for a decade.[31] However, using risk factors to quantify the prognostic pattern for individual patients is rarely exploited, despite secure knowledge of both its potential and limitations.[32] Instead, prognostic models are locked in static publications, such as the ones reporting the risk factors from which figures for this chapter were generated. Publications are useful as a source for reporting prognostic factors, but unhelpful for generating predictions on a dynamic, clinically relevant, patient-specific basis.

Perhaps because of a misperception that refined knowledge of the nature of the relation of risk factors to outcome is unnecessary, little attention has been paid to the manner in which individual risk factors influence the pattern of hazard, and thereby the pattern of survival (prognosis) and freedom from other post-CABG events. Typical analyses of long-term events after CABG are based on the Cox proportional hazards multivariable model. This important statistical tool presumes that a single set of risk factors affects survival in a similar fashion across time. Some have argued that even if this is not a logical assumption, it is true enough for general purposes and for a general set of risk factors.[33]

A number of years ago, our group at the University of Alabama at Birmingham made the unsurprising observation that different risk factors affect different time frames of the pattern of survival. For example, factors representing the immediate preoperative condition of the patient have an impact on survival early after CABG. In contrast, co-morbid conditions, such as diabetes, influence late survival far more powerfully than early and intermediate-term survival. To discover these differences in risk factor influence, the period after surgery can be segmented and a Cox regression analysis performed separately for each segment.[34] However, the time segmentation is arbitrary.

Therefore, our group developed, programmed and distributed an effective and powerful alternative in the early 1980s.[26] The hazard function was decomposed in a fashion analogous to sending light through a prism to separate its individual color components. Figure 23.15 decomposes into three simple components the complex pattern of risk following CABG shown in Figure 23.1b. The first component predominates early after surgery; we called this the early hazard phase. The second component is a horizontal line, representing the constant hazard phase. The third component is a rising line (straight in this instance) that represents the late rising hazard phase. At every point along the time axis, the magnitude of the three components can be summed to produce overall hazard, as shown by the dashed line (identical to the solid line of Figure 23.1b).

The exact shape and magnitude of each hazard component is estimated from time-related follow-up data, not arbitrarily or from Kaplan–Meier estimates, as often supposed. That mathematical and statistical methods are able to discover these components should not be any more surprising than learning that similar, and even more complex, decomposition software is used daily to reconstruct magnetic resonance images.

For each phase of hazard, risk factors are identified and the magnitude of their incremental relation to outcome quantified.[26] In the early hazard phase, risk factors increase or decrease the area beneath the early hazard component. In the constant hazard phase, risk factors raise or lower the constant hazard value (horizontal line in Figure 23.15). In the late hazard phase, risk factors tilt the upward-sloping line (downward = less risk, upward = more risk). Consistently across all types of heart disease, from congenital to acquired, a different set of risk factors influences each

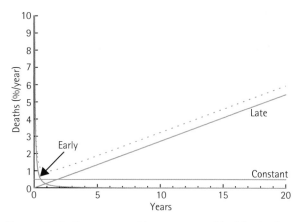

Figure 23.15 *Components of instantaneous risk of death after primary CABG (KU Leuven, 1971–1992, n = 9600). Three components (hazard phases) are depicted: (1) an early, rapidly falling hazard phase, (2) a constant hazard phase, and (3) a late, rising hazard phase. These components sum across time to the overall hazard function shown by the dotted line.*

hazard phase. Only occasionally does the same risk factor modify each hazard phase, and when it does, it rarely influences the phases equally. Patients with different risk factors, then, will have differently shaped hazard functions, because each hazard component will be different – more or less early risk, constant hazard risk, or late risk. This is what generates different prognostic patterns for each patient profile (see Figure 23.14), even though the identical risk factor equation is being used.

HOW DO RISK FACTORS BECOME EVIDENT?

There are three widespread misconceptions about risk factors and how they operate and, therefore, how they become evident.

The first misconception is that each risk factor for early risk (such as hospital mortality) adds incrementally to the absolute probability of survival. Thus, if five risk factors have been identified, and each increments risk by 5%, the overall risk will be 25%. A second, related misconception is that a risk (hazard) of a stated percentage per year translates into a reduction of survival or freedom from an event by that percentage each year. Thus, a 10% per year risk is assumed to result in 90% survival at the end of the first year, 80% at the end of the second, and 0% survival at 10 years. The third misconception is that reflectors of relative risk (such as odds ratios or hazard ratios) translate easily into absolute risk. Thus, a risk factor that doubles the risk of death is assumed to double the absolute risk of mortality.

Misconception 1: add risks

Starting with the Parsonnet score,[35] bolstered by deliberate and, in this author's opinion, misleading and misguided

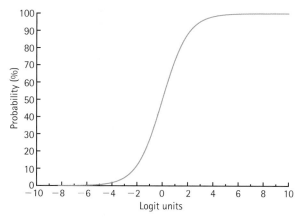

Figure 23.16 *Logit–probability relationship. The horizontal axis is a limitless scale of risk in so-called logit units, here shown only from −10 to +10. The vertical axis is probability of an event (here expressed as a percentage) on its naturally constrained axis from 0 to 100%. The solid sigmoid curve is the relation between logit units of risk and probability expressed by the logistic equation:* $P = 1/[1 + exp(−Z)]$ *where P is probability, Z is logit units, and exp is the natural exponential function. Logit units can also be thought of as units of the natural logarithm (Ln) of the odds ratio:* $Z = Ln[P/(1 − P)]$. *Similar sigmoid relations exist for hazard ratios and other expressions of risk.*

risk scoring systems proposed today, surgeons and even the public have been led to believe that risks 'add'. Despite rebuttal by respected statisticians such as Frank Harrell at The University of Virginia,[36] other statisticians must believe that medical personnel can only add. In their attempt to simplify, concepts of probability fundamental to both medicine and mathematics become confusing to physicians. Often the confusion is related to the difference between addition and multiplication.

The most useful diagram to keep in mind is the sigmoid-shaped relation between absolute risk and magnitude of a risk factor effect. Figure 23.16 illustrates one such sigmoid curve called the logit curve.[37] This curve demonstrates the relation between the absolute probability of an event and how it is modulated by change in the value of risk associated with a risk factor.

Suppose a risk factor's magnitude is 2 logit units. If a patient is 'positioned' at −8 on the logit unit axis, because of few risk factors, an increase of 2 logit units of risk by a surgical intervention imperceptibly elevates the absolute probability of experiencing an adverse event. This corresponds to the medical concept of 'robustness'. The number −8 represents mathematically the 'starting place' for this patient, but, more generally, a logistic regression analysis will generate an 'intercept' (a value pertaining when all factors in the analysis have a value of exactly zero) from which risk is incremented.

For example, imagine that a high-school football player is stabbed in the abdomen just outside your hospital emergency room. He is rushed to surgery with a lacerated inferior vena cava. Imagine that his injury increases his risk of dying by 2 logit units. However, his general condition leads us to be confident that he will survive this attack, because he has started 'far to the left' on the logit curve. Contrast this scenario with an elderly, insulin-dependent, atherosclerotic, cachetic, frail diabetic who is similarly attacked outside the emergency room. His co-morbidity has perhaps already placed him at −2 on the logit curve. He is a fragile patient. He, too, is rushed to the operating room. The same operation again imparts 2 logit units of risk. Yet we claim his prognosis is guarded because this increment of risk has increased his absolute probability of dying to a substantial 50%. In the third scenario we encounter a patient in advanced multisystem organ failure with oliguria and cardiogenic shock following a massive heart attack. The patient acutely ruptures his ventricular septum. We may elect not to operate because we believe this combination of pre-existing and acute factors, along with the added risk of operation, makes absolute risk very high and intervention futile. This patient is positioned too far to the right on the logit curve.

Thus, in a sense, risks add, but they do so on a special scale that is related to absolute risk in a sigmoid-shaped fashion representing the medical spectrum from robust, to frail, to futile.

For us, a particular disadvantage of Cox regression is that magnitude of risk factors are estimated, but not an intercept. This was one of the factors that drove us to mathematical models such as those described above, with intercepts providing reference points for interpreting the impact of risk factors on absolute risk.

Misconception 2: subtract survival risks

The relation between an expression of hazard, such as a linearized risk of 10% per year, and absolute survival probability is somewhat complex, but easily understood. Bear in mind that the only patients at risk of death are living patients.[38] Thus, if 90% of patients are alive at 1 year, and the risk of death is 10% (conversely, the probability of surviving is 90%), then approximately 90% of those alive will survive, and absolute survival at 2 years will be approximately 90% of 90%, or 81%, not 80% (obtained by multiplication, not subtraction). Even this is only approximate, because patients are not dying abruptly at exactly 2 years, but steadily along the way; the exact number is 81.9%. The same equation used to calculate compound interest on a mortgage is used, namely, the so-called negative exponential. According to this equation, survival is related to the exponential function (exp) of 10% multiplied by the time at risk, 2 years in this example. Thus, survival at 2 years with a 10% risk will be exp[−0.1 × 2 years], or 81.9%. Also, by 10 years, survival with a 10% per year loss will be 37%, not 0%.

Misconception 3: relative risk translates easily to absolute risk

A common way to express magnitude of long-term risk is as a hazard ratio. (As an aside, if the risk is not proportionate across time, which is usually the case, a hazard ratio is a meaningless statistic.) However, if the hazard ratio is a large number, such as 2, this does not mean that percent mortality will be doubled. If hazard is 10% per year without a risk factor and 20% per year with it, the hazard ratio is 2. Survival at 2 years with the risk factor would be 67% rather than 82%, an absolute survival difference of 15%. Let us say, however, that the underlying hazard is 0.05% per year. This means that at 10 years, survival will be 99.5%. If that rate is doubled to 0.1% per year, then survival will be 99.0% at 10 years. Doubling of the risk, as dramatic as that sounds, has decreased survival by only 0.5% in 10 years.

As we were admonished in childhood, twice nothing is still nothing. Twice near nothing is also still nearly nothing. Interestingly, this explains why relatively weak co-morbidities may greatly diminish survival when they exert their influence over a long period, and relatively strong early risks exerting influence for a brief time may have nearly imperceptible long-term impact.

Implications for identifying the effects of risk factors

These and other considerations lead to the following observations about the effects of risk factors.

- If a patient has no other risk factors, the effect of one risk factor is unlikely to be evident. For example, in a young low-risk patient, it may take many years before a benefit of bilateral ITA grafting becomes evident compared to single ITA grafting. These patients are positioned far to the left on the sigmoid curve relating magnitude of risk and absolute risk.
- A risk factor may not be evident in the presence of an overwhelming number of other risk factors. Thus, it is possible that the benefit of a procedure may not be evident in patients with cardiogenic shock or, if it is a long-term effect, in the elderly who are not expected to survive long enough to accrue benefit.
- Even a modest risk factor may become powerful in the face of a few other risk factors in the fragile, but not futile, patient. There is an important corollary in time-related survival. Imagine two risk factors of equal magnitude, one for early hazard phase risk and the other for late hazard phase risk. If the early hazard phase is small in magnitude and brief in duration, the early phase risk factors will have a minimal influence on prognosis. In contrast, the risk factor modifying an already large and prolonged late hazard phase will have a profound influence on ultimate prognosis.

Certain specific risk factors for events after CABG

Risk factors for events after CABG may be categorized as *patient* factors, *procedure* factors and *institutional* factors.[21]

Patient factors include:

- demography, severity and type of symptoms of ischemic heart disease,
- distribution of the coronary artery disease,
- size of coronary arteries and diffuseness of atherosclerotic disease,
- aggressiveness of the atherosclerotic process throughout the body,
- ventricular function,
- secondary acute conditions related to ischemic heart disease events,
- coexisting conditions.

Procedure factors relate to:

- decisions about conduits used for bypass,
- completeness of coronary revascularization,
- myocardial management during surgery,
- surgical support techniques (such as on-pump vs off-pump revascularization).

Institutional factors have received the greatest exposure in the lay press. They include many internal and external pressures and consequences of institutional decisions and organization, policies, financial support and practices (these have been called latent factors).[39] They include, of course, the surgeon and his or her team, cardiology, cardiac anesthesia, blood bank personnel, and multitudes of other persons. They also include the date of operation as a surrogate for possibly unrecognized temporal effects. Many of these variables are not recorded or considered in risk factor analyses.

As a generality (specifics given below), patient factors are the most powerful determinants of short-term and long-term prognosis. Severe symptoms such as uncontrollable unstable angina, secondary conditions such as cardiogenic shock, old age, severe left ventricular dysfunction and previous cardiac surgery contribute, for the most part, to early risk. Coexisting conditions and both younger and older age contribute powerfully to long-term prognosis and freedom from other events (late hazard phase). Procedural factors tend to contribute in only a small (even if statistically significant) way to early risks of various events; nevertheless, they become increasingly evident as determinants of outcome as time progresses because they act over a long period. Institutional factors tend to result in small differences in early outcome, important for quality assessment, but having little long-term effect as other factors come to dominate outcome.

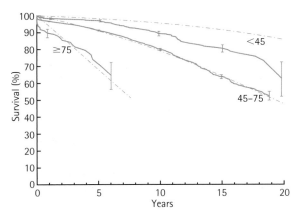

Figure 23.17 *Survival, stratified according to three age groups (KU Leuven, 1971–1992, n = 9600). The depiction is non-parametric Kaplan–Meier estimates connected by a solid line. Vertical bars represent asymmetric confidence limits equivalent to 1 standard error. Dot-dash-dot lines represent survival in the general US population matched for the age, ethnicity and sex of each patient (obtained by averaging individual survival curves for each patient in each group).*

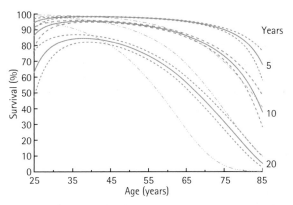

Figure 23.18 *Risk-adjusted survival at 5, 10 and 20 years according to the age of the patient at CABG. All risk factors other than age have been held constant. Dot-dash-dot lines indicate survival in the matched general population at 5 (single dot), 10 (double dot) and 20 (triple dot) years. Risk factor equation is based on data from KU Leuven, 1971–1992, n = 9600.*

The following are specific incremental risk factors with particularly interesting and important relationships to outcome.

AGE

The older the patient at CABG, the higher the early and late mortality (Figure 23.17). This is not surprising, because all-cause mortality in adults increases with increasing age. Thus, the question is whether the relation of age to survival after CABG is commensurate with that of the general population. As demonstrated in the figure in a simple, non-risk-adjusted fashion, CABG in young adults is associated simultaneously with both high long-term survival and worse age-specific survival in relation to their peers in the general population. Interestingly, in patients operated on between age 45 and 75, survival is similar to that of the general population from about 4 to 20 years after CABG. In the elderly, early mortality after surgery is high; however, in 6-month survivors, the risk of mortality is less than that in the general population, and this improved risk continues for at least the next 5 years (the maximum extent of follow-up data in these elderly patients was about 8 years). Similar favorable results in the elderly have been observed by others.[40]

Figure 23.17 relates to otherwise heterogeneous groups of patients within age groups. Thus, we have constructed Figure 23.18 to examine the risk-adjusted relation of survival and age in average-risk patients by holding values for all risk factors constant, so as to reveal the shape of the effect of age in isolation. The graph is based on the multivariable equation for mortality published by Sergeant and colleagues.[13] It has been solved for survival at 5, 10 and

20 years. Superimposed is expected survival at 5, 10 and 20 years in the general population of Caucasian men of the same age. Notice that survival after CABG is worse than expected in the general population for patients under about 45 years of age, mirroring the information observed in the risk-unadjusted Figure 23.17. However, for patients who have survived to develop coronary disease at an older age, but who have few risk factors, survival is substantially better after CABG than predicted for the general population.[41] At least one explanation of the higher than anticipated survival in the elderly is that these patients are highly selected, otherwise robust patients, with few co-morbid conditions.

Return of angina is more common in patients who were operated on at a young age, although the relation is somewhat weak. Counter-intuitively, freedom from re-intervention was higher in young patients in the KU Leuven experience (Figure 23.19), but lower in the Cleveland Clinic experience.[24] Freedom from re-intervention is also high for patients operated on at older ages, and this, too, is dissociated from the prevalence of return of anginal symptoms. This has led Sergeant and colleagues to be cautious in interpreting the otherwise hard end-point of coronary re-intervention, as described above.[11]

SEX

Whether women are at higher risk of adverse events following CABG has been debated for nearly 30 years. What seems reasonably clear is that women come to CABG with more risk factors than men, and may be expected, therefore, to have a higher mortality.[42,43] The once wide gap in hospital mortality between men and women has

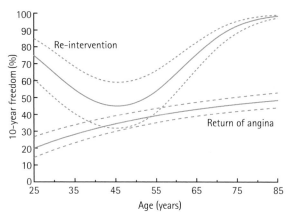

Figure 23.19 *Ten-year freedom from either return of angina or coronary re-intervention (cardiological or surgical) according to age at original CABG. All risk factors other than age have been held constant. Risk factor equations are based on data from KU Leuven, 1971–1992, n = 9600.*

narrowed[44] because of the general reduction in risk of CABG in high-risk patients. Adjustment for prevalence of risk factors and patient size,[45] at least in some settings,[46] is said to eliminate gender as a risk factor for early mortality.[47–49] Nevertheless, some have found that despite their increased number of risk factors, women receive less instruction than men in secondary disease prevention and are less likely to be referred for cardiac rehabilitation.[50] This may be due to either biases of healthcare workers or women's response to their ischemic heart disease and its treatment.[51]

In the long term, Sergeant and colleagues (as well as others[52]) found that women were more prone to have return of angina[10] and to receive re-intervention.[11] Compared to men, women have a lower perception of quality of life after CABG, less physical activity and more dyspnea.[53,54] Perhaps this issue has best been summarized by Robertson and colleagues, who analyzed the New Approaches to Coronary Intervention (NACI) registry:[55]

Additional studies are needed to evaluate the complex interplay of clinical, vessel and lesion characteristics on the success and complications of specific interventional techniques and to determine whether gender, per se, is a risk factor and whether gender-specific interventional strategies may be beneficial.

CORONARY DISEASE

One might suppose naively that complete revascularization by CABG neutralizes the influence of extent of native coronary artery disease. However, coronary artery disease is only palliated by CABG, so progression of native coronary artery disease is probably a time-related risk factor for late occurrence of myocardial infarction, late return of angina and late mortality. In addition, lesser coronary

disease at the time of CABG, and therefore fewer vessels bypassed, predisposes patients to later re-interventions.[11]

Left main disease is of particular interest. High-grade left main disease was a risk factor for early mortality in the KU Leuven experience.[13] Despite risk adjustment and propensity matching strategies, left main disease is a risk factor *per se* for hospital mortality in the Cleveland Clinic experience (Lytle and Blackstone, unpublished data). Scott and colleagues studied isolated left ITA to LAD grafting and found that survival in patients with any left main trunk disease was worse than if it were not present.[56] Perhaps this finding is related to underestimation of left main disease by angiography,[57,58] or perhaps it is simply a marker for more aggressive coronary disease. An interesting alternative speculation is that even after CABG, antegrade coronary blood flow may be of continuing importance for survival.

INCOMPLETE REVASCULARIZATION

Closely associated with the influence of extent of coronary artery disease is completeness of revascularization. There is no universally accepted definition of incomplete revascularization after coronary intervention. Faxon and colleagues defined it as restoration of perfusion to vessels judged bypassable that supply normal myocardium: 'functionally adequate revascularization'.[59] This definition is less stringent than that usually employed in presenting surgical revascularization. Sergeant's definition was quite stringent: non-revascularization of any epicardial vessel of any size, including vessels to portions of the myocardium that appeared akinetic or even dyskinetic.[13]

Scott and colleagues studied the reasons for incomplete revascularization, defined as failure to provide a graft to a coronary system containing an epicardial vessel with 50% or greater stenosis.[56] By this definition, some 25% of patients were incompletely revascularized at CABG. Forty-five percent of patients incompletely revascularized had small or severely diseased vessels that were believed unbypassable, and another 2.4% had lesions in a non-dominant right coronary artery system. For whatever reason, based on 25-year follow-up, patients with any degree of incomplete revascularization have a mortality that is considerably higher than that of patients with complete revascularization at initial CABG (Figure 23.20).

Incomplete revascularization may be a surrogate for small vessels with inadequate run-off, damaged myocardial segments, or extensive small-vessel disease, any of which could contribute to the difference in survival shown in Figure 23.20. Nevertheless, important lessons learned from Scott and colleagues' study of incomplete revascularization are:

1 an isolated left ITA to LAD graft cannot fully compensate for disease in other coronary artery systems,

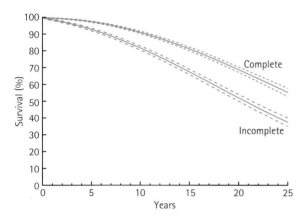

Figure 23.20 *Survival, stratified according to complete versus incomplete revascularization in patients receiving isolated left internal thoracic artery to left anterior descending coronary artery grafting (Cleveland Clinic, 1971–1997, n = 2067). The depiction is as in Figure 23.1a.*

2 unrevascularized high-grade circumflex lesions are more important than unrevascularized non-proximal right coronary artery disease,

3 small vessels may be of great importance,

4 the effect of incomplete revascularization on survival is not realized at all in the first year or so after CABG, and may not be identifiable statistically for even 5–10 years; therefore, statements about apparently benign effects of incomplete revascularization based on short follow-up should be received with skepticism.

LEFT VENTRICULAR DYSFUNCTION

Even the small power of the CASS randomized study in the 1970s identified patients with reduction in left ventricular function (generally because of previous myocardial infarction) and extensive coronary disease as benefiting most from CABG.[60] Risk-adjusted survival curves for a patient with a normal ejection fraction, one modestly depressed and one more severely depressed, are shown in Figure 23.21. Notice that ejection fraction must be depressed considerably before a substantial difference in survival is noted. Survival diminishes perceptibly (evident difference) below an ejection fraction of about 40% (Figure 23.22).

Sergeant and colleagues have found that patients with a previous infarct are prone to another one early after CABG,[12] as well as to early re-intervention.[11]

These matters, as well as those of managing ischemic mitral regurgitation and acute mechanical complications of myocardial infarction, are subjects of previous chapters.

CARDIAC CO-MORBIDITIES

The addition of uncorrected mild aortic valve regurgitation or of preoperative atrial or ventricular rhythm disturbances had a large and unexpected adverse survival impact in the

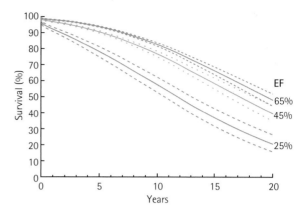

Figure 23.21 *Risk-adjusted survival after CABG in patients with identical risk factors except for ejection fraction (EF). Risk factor equation is based on data from KU Leuven, 1971–1992, n = 9600.*

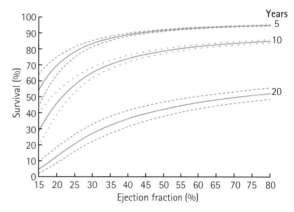

Figure 23.22 *Survival at 5, 10 and 20 years according to ejection fraction. These are risk-adjusted depictions in patients otherwise having the same risk factors. Risk factor equation is based on data from KU Leuven, 1971–1992, n = 9600.*

studies of Sergeant and colleagues.[61] Because of their rarity, these factors may not be considered in multivariable analyses, or the effective sample size (the number of events[29]) may be insufficient to provide either statistical power or computational tractability to quantify them. Thus, when faced with advising patients with rare risk factors about CABG, it is possible that available statistical models will underestimate both their early and late risk factors.

Re-operative coronary artery surgery has been studied less intensively than primary CABG (see Figure 23.13); however, the larger the number of re-operations, the higher the early risk, even after risk adjustment.[62,63] This has led to alternative surgical approaches to re-operations, the results of which are still being assessed.[64,65]

NON-CARDIAC CO-MORBIDITIES

These days, non-cardiac co-morbidities generally have little impact on early events after CABG, although they

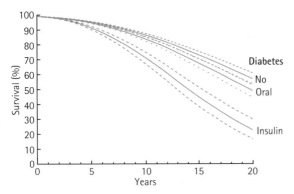

Figure 23.23 *Risk-adjusted survival after CABG according to diabetic status. Risk factor equation is based on data from KU Leuven, 1971–1992,* n = 9600.

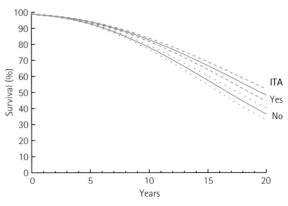

Figure 23.24 *Risk-adjusted survival after CABG according to use or not of an internal thoracic artery graft to the left anterior descending coronary artery. Risk factor equation is based on data from KU Leuven, 1971–1992,* n = 9600.

are likely to affect the prevalence of in-hospital complications, length of stay and cost.[66,67] They may dominate late events, however, quite possibly in a causal fashion.

High lipid levels are associated with higher late mortality,[13] late occurrence of myocardial infarction,[12] late return of angina[10] and late coronary re-interventions.[11] High lipid levels should, therefore, be a target for secondary prevention.[68] Chronic renal failure increases early mortality, but in the KU Leuven experience, high serum creatinine levels without dialysis are also associated with reduced late survival, return of angina and occurrence of myocardial infarction. Aggressiveness of the atherosclerotic process, as evidenced by peripheral vascular disease, increases the risk of late death, return of angina and incidence of coronary re-interventions.

The Bypass Angioplasty Revascularization Investigation (BARI) trial focused attention on diabetes as an important risk factor for events after coronary interventions.[69–71] Figure 23.23 shows the difference in survival for three patients with otherwise identical risk factors, except that one is a non-diabetic, another a diabetic treated with oral hypoglycemics, and the third is a diabetic treated with insulin. Survival is not greatly diminished in patients on oral hypoglycemics, unlike that reported for angioplasty,[72] but it is diminished substantially in insulin-treated diabetics. Sergeant and colleagues also found that diabetes increased the risk of late return of angina,[10] but did not identify a similar increased risk of re-intervention or infarction.

The CASS investigators, as well as virtually all other groups, have shown that mortality is increased in patients who are hypertensive, who are smokers at the time of CABG, who have reduced pulmonary function, or who are obese.[34]

INTERNAL THORACIC ARTERY GRAFTING

Although a number of surgeons had used the ITA as a conduit, the *New England Journal of Medicine* report from Loop and colleagues in 1986 captured the attention of surgeons, particularly in the USA, and made this the conduit

of choice for nearly all CABG operations.[73] Their study clearly demonstrated a survival advantage and greater freedom from subsequent myocardial infarction and re-operation in patients who had received an ITA graft versus only saphenous vein grafts. In the early days of CABG, some centers used the ITA more commonly in single-system disease, young patients and those with good ventricular function; such selection could give rise to exaggerated non-risk-adjusted survival benefits. Loop and colleagues attempted to risk adjust outcome to reveal the isolated benefit of ITA grafting. Today, more robust techniques would probably be employed, such as propensity matching.[22,23] Nevertheless, in patients followed sufficiently long to reveal it, the benefit of ITA grafting, particularly to the LAD, is universal. The presumed mechanism for superiority of the ITA as a conduit is its long-term patency.[73] Risk-adjusted benefit of ITA grafting on survival is shown in Figure 23.24.

Sergeant and colleagues found that ITA grafting is protective from early and late myocardial infarction and re-intervention,[11,12] as did Loop and colleagues.[73] However, they found that ITA grafting offered essentially no protection against return of angina.[10] Harder to interpret is the negative association between the proportion of grafts that are arterial conduits and the occurrence of re-intervention (Figure 23.25). It is possible that ITA grafts reduce the need for re-intervention. However, as stated earlier, this may reflect physician, surgeon and patient decision-making factors.

Lytle and colleagues at the Cleveland Clinic have demonstrated superior survival from the use of bilateral ITA grafting.[24,38] They were cognizant of the problem of patient selection when comparing outcomes after the use of one versus two ITA grafts. To meet this challenge, they studied only multisystem disease and used multivariable propensity score matching,[22,23] multivariable analysis and bootstrap resampling to mitigate against exaggerating the benefit.[74] Additionally, analysis of interactions revealed

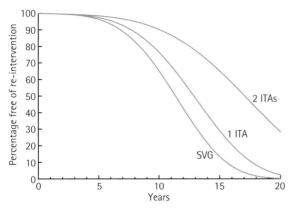

Figure 23.25 *Risk-adjusted freedom from re-intervention after CABG according to number of internal thoracic artery distals. (SVG, saphenous vein grafts only; 1 ITA, 1 internal thoracic artery graft; 2 ITAs, 2 internal thoracic artery grafts.) For clarity, no confidence limits are shown. However, confidence limits for freedom from re-intervention after two ITA grafts are widely separated from those for either one ITA or saphenous vein grafts. Risk factor equation is based on data from KU Leuven, 1971–1992, n = 9600.*

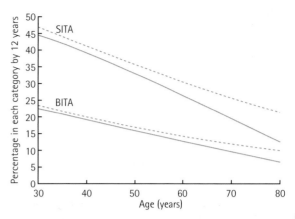

Figure 23.26 *Twelve-year competing (solid lines) and non-competing (dashed lines) analysis of re-intervention according to age at CABG and whether multisystem disease was managed by single internal thoracic grafting (SITA) or bilateral ITA grafting (BITA). The dashed lines are the complement of 12-year freedom from re-intervention as a function of age. They represent the probability of re-intervention were a patient to survive for 12 years. In contrast, the solid lines are the percentage of a cohort of patients initially undergoing CABG who are expected to be in the category 're-intervention' by 12 years, tempered by the competing risk of death that removes them from risk. Risk factor equation is based on data from the Cleveland Clinic, 1971–1991; bilateral ITA grafting n = 2001, single ITA grafting n = 8123.*

no patient subgroup that did not accrue a survival or freedom from re-intervention benefit from bilateral ITA grafting. Benefit was demonstrated even in high-risk patients for whom bilateral ITA grafting might be forgone by other groups. However, after quantifying benefit on a patient-by-patient basis, some patients were found whose survival benefit over the subsequent 12 years was small. Among these were young patients. This is understandable from the discussion above of the sigmoid-shaped relation between absolute, and expressions of relative risk (see Figure 23.16); further follow-up is predicted to demonstrate benefit among these patients over longer time frames.

Lytle and colleagues then addressed the matter of the benefit of bilateral ITA grafting in the elderly. This issue was answered negatively from the Belgium data,[13] perhaps because of lack of sufficient power and duration of follow-up. Lytle and colleagues found that the decreased incidence of re-intervention in the elderly was not simply a reflection of passive attrition of the elderly by death.[38] This was inferred from analysis of the simultaneous competing risk of death. Nevertheless, attrition by death progressively decreased the number of elderly patients who would be available for re-intervention (Figure 23.26).

DATE OF OPERATION

There is no doubt that early (in-hospital) risk of CABG for all subsets of patients has decreased during the last 35 years. It has been difficult to identify by multivariable analysis which changes have contributed to the improvement. Better forms of myocardial management have been assumed, but rarely proven, to contribute importantly; other changes include better CABG techniques,

better preoperative preparation, better postoperative care, and other factors that are rarely incorporated into databases (and that may be impossible to incorporate). Program monitoring in the state of New York[75] and collaborative quality improvement efforts of the Northern New England participants[76,77] have been credited with some of this improvement. It is unfortunate that causal inferences are elusive, because specific knowledge would be more valuable than the non-specific statement that mortality has generally improved across time.

A special assessment problem arises when one asks whether similar improvements have occurred late after CABG, or if a specific intervention, such as a form of myocardial management, has long-term benefit. Such questions are nearly impossible to answer because date of operation is confounded by duration of follow-up. The same confounding may be present if one attempts to assess the long-term benefits of any two methods that are instituted serially, as are most (presumed) improvements.

KEY REFERENCES

Blackstone EH, Naftel DC, Turner ME Jr. The decomposition of time-varying hazard into phases, each incorporating a separate stream of concomitant information. *J Am Stat Assoc* 1986; **81**:615–24.

This paper culminates a decade of work to find a suitable mathematical and statistical framework for analysis of surgical data. It was recognized that risk factors did not act uniformly across time, but that preoperative patient status dominated early outcome and co-morbidities dominated late outcome. This work capitalized on signal processing whereby white light is decomposed into separate colors. In this paper, three 'colors' are modeled as functions of a separate independent set of risk factors. Its mathematical nature allows time-related curves to be constructed based on each patient's individual characteristics.

D'Agostino RB Jr. Propensity score methods for bias reduction in the comparison of a treatment to a non-randomized control group. *Stat Med* 1998; **17**:2265–81.

A summary of work begun by Rosenbaum and Rubin on using balancing scores (the simplest being the propensity score) that brings scientific methodology and validity to the arena of non-randomized comparisons. It allows us to answer questions such as those concerning the influence of female gender on outcomes of CABG in the face of an impossibility to randomize gender. It also allows us to compare potentially randomizable alternatives to CABG operations, such as on-pump and off-pump surgery, with reduced selection bias.

Gordon T. Statistics in a prospective study: the Framingham study. In: *Proceedings of the American Statistical Association: Sesquicentennial Invited Paper Sessions*, Gail MH, Johnson NL (coordinators). Alexandria, VA: American Statistical Association, 1989, 719–26.

It was the Framingham investigators who coined the term 'risk factors'. This is a narrative of the thinking behind the concept. It is not just interesting history; it spells out the foundation of risk factor analyses and their use in improving patient care that is as germane today as it was in the 1960s.

Hannan EL, Siu AL, Kumar D, Kilburn H Jr, Chassin MR. The decline in coronary artery bypass graft surgery mortality in New York State. The role of surgeon volume. *JAMA* 1995; **18**:209–13.

Risk factors analysis, designed from the outset to understand heart disease and its treatment, improve patient care and suggest avenues of research, now becomes politicized and used to rank institutions and doctors in the lay press. It is claimed that this has improved early outcomes, and possibly it is true. It certainly has had a dramatic influence on healthcare systems and doctors. CABG was an easy target because surgeons have focused for years on outcomes, as they should have, but it came back to bite them.

Loop FD, Lytle BW, Cosgrove DM, Stewart RW, Goormastic M, Williams GW, *et al*. Influence of the internal-mammary-artery graft on 10-year survival and other cardiac events. *N Engl J Med* 1986; **314**:1–6.

This paper changed the operative strategy of coronary artery bypass grafting, at least in the USA. Since then, the finding that ITA grafting favorably affects long-term outcome has been repeatedly corroborated. It is one of the few surgical factors (incomplete revascularization being another) that clearly influences outcome.

Sergeant P, Blackstone E, Meyns B. Can the outcome of coronary bypass grafting be predicted reliably? *Eur J Cardiothorac* Surg 1997; **11**:2–9.

This paper asks the practical, though provocative, question as to whether the analyses of risk factors after CABG allow one accurately to predict outcome in future patients. The study shows that for most patients this is possible unless: (1) influential risk factors are not taken into account in the risk equations, (2) conditions are too rare to estimate their association with outcome, and (3) indications are extended to subgroups not considered by the equations. Survival in these types of patient is severely underestimated.

Sergeant P, Blackstone E, Meyns B. Is return of angina after coronary artery bypass grafting immutable, can it be delayed, and is it important? *J Thorac Cardiovasc Surg* 1998; **116**:440–53.

Dr Sergeant has built a remarkably rich database, entered most of the data himself, and established perhaps the best patient follow-up network in cardiac surgery anywhere, focused on identification and quantification of risk factors and their time-related influence on outcomes after CABG. This is but a sample of his group's many papers on risk factors for events after CABG.

REFERENCES

1. Garrett HE, Dennis EW, DeBakey ME. Aortocoronary bypass with saphenous vein graft: seven-year follow-up. *JAMA* 1973; 223:792–4.
2. Kolessov VI, Potashov LV. Operations on the coronary arteries. *Exp Chir Anaesth* 1965; 10:3.
3. Kolessov VI. Mammary artery–coronary artery anastomosis as method of treatment for angina pectoris. *J Thorac Cardiovasc Surg* 1967; 54:535–44.
4. Favaloro RG. Landmarks in the development of coronary artery bypass surgery. *Circulation* 1998; 98:466–78.
5. Sones FM Jr, Shirey EK. Cine coronary arteriography. *Mod Concepts Cardiovasc Dis* 1962; 31:735.
6. Hannan EL, Kilburn H Jr, O'Donnell JF, Lukacik G, Shields EP. Adult open heart surgery in New York State. An analysis of risk factors and hospital mortality rates. *JAMA* 1990; 264:2768–74.
7. National Heart, Lung, and Blood Institute Coronary Artery Surgery Study. A multicenter comparison of the effects of randomized medical and surgical treatment of mildly symptomatic patients with coronary artery disease, and a registry of consecutive patients undergoing coronary angiography. *Circulation* 1981; 63:II–81.
8. Weinstein MC, Stason WB. Cost-effectiveness of coronary artery bypass surgery. *Circulation* 1982; 66:III56–66.
9. Sergeant P, Flameng W, Suy R. The sequential internal mammary artery graft. Long term results of a consecutive series of 364 patients. *J Cardiovasc Surg (Torino)* 1988; 29:596–600.

10. Sergeant P, Blackstone E, Meyns B. Is return of angina after coronary artery bypass grafting immutable, can it be delayed, and is it important? *J Thorac Cardiovasc Surg* 1998; **116**:440–53.

11. Sergeant P, Blackstone E, Meyns B, Stockman B, Jashari R. First cardiological or cardiosurgical re-intervention for ischemic heart disease after primary coronary artery bypass grafting. *Eur J Cardiothorac Surg* 1998; **14**:480–7.

12. Sergeant PT, Blackstone EH, Meyns BP. Does arterial revascularization decrease the risk of infarction after coronary artery bypass grafting? *Ann Thorac Surg* 1998; **66**:1–11.

13. Sergeant P, Blackstone E, Meyns B. Validation and interdependence with patient-variables of the influence of procedural variables on early and late survival after CABG. K.U. Leuven Coronary Surgery Program. *Eur J Cardiothorac Surg* 1997; **12**:1–19.

14. Lauer MS, Blackstone EH, Young JB, Topol EJ. Cause of death in clinical research: time for a reassessment? *J Am Coll Cardiol* 1999; **34**:618–20.

15. Blackstone EH. Outcome analysis using hazard function methodology. *Ann Thorac Surg* 1996; **61**:S2–7.

16. Osswald BR, Blackstone EH, Tochtermann U, Thomas G, Vahl CF, Hagl S. The meaning of early mortality after CABG. *Eur J Cardiothorac Surg* 1999; **15**:401–7.

17. Diggle PJ, Heagerty PJ, Liang KY, Zeger SL. *Analysis of Longitudinal Data*. 2nd Ed. New York: Oxford University Press, 2002.

18. Blackstone EH. Breaking down barriers: helpful breakthrough statistical methods you need to understand better. *J Thorac Cardiovasc Surg* 2001; **122**:430–9.

19. David HA, Moeschberger ML. *The Theory of Competing Risks*. New York: Macmillan, 1978, 45–56.

20. Ferrazzi P, McGiffin DC, Kirklin JW, Blackstone EH, Bourge RC. Have the results of mitral valve replacement improved? *J Thorac Cardiovasc Surg* 1986; **92**:186–97.

21. Kirklin JW, Barratt-Boyes BG. *Cardiac Surgery*. New York: John Wiley & Sons, 1986, 293.

22. Rosenbaum PR, Rubin DB. The bias due to incomplete matching. *Biometrics* 1985; **41**:103–6.

23. D'Agostino RB Jr. Propensity score methods for bias reduction in the comparison of a treatment to a non-randomized control group. *Stat Med* 1998; **17**:2265–81.

24. Lytle BW, Blackstone EH, Loop FD, Houghtaling PL, Arnold JH, Akhrass R, et al. Two internal thoracic artery grafts are better than one. *J Thorac Cardiovasc Surg* 1999; **117**:855–72.

25. Gordon T. Statistics in a prospective study: the Framingham study. In: *Proceedings of the American Statistical Association: Sesquicentennial Invited Paper Sessions*, Gail MH, Johnson NL (coordinators). Alexandria, VA: American Statistical Association, 1989, 719–26.

26. Blackstone EH, Naftel DC, Turner ME Jr. The decomposition of time-varying hazard into phases, each incorporating a separate stream of concomitant information. *J Am Stat Assoc* 1986; **81**:615–24.

27. Breiman L. Bagging predictors. *Machine Learning* 1996; **26**:123–40.

28. Hastie T, Tibshirani R, Friedman J. *The Elements of Statistical Learning: Data Mining, Inference, and Prediction*. New York: Springer-Verlag, 2001.

29. Blackstone EH, Rice TW. Clinical–pathologic conference: use and choice of statistical methods for the clinical study, 'Superficial adenocarcinoma of the esophagus.' *J Thorac Cardiovasc Surg* 2001; **122**:1063–76.

30. Naftel DC. Do different investigators sometimes produce different multivariable equations from the same data? *J Thorac Cardiovasc Surg* 1994; **107**:1528–9.

31. ACC/AHA guidelines and indications for coronary artery bypass graft surgery. A report of the American College of Cardiology/American Heart Association Task Force on Assessment of Diagnostic and Therapeutic Cardiovascular Procedures (Subcommittee on Coronary Artery Bypass Graft Surgery). *J Am Coll Cardiol* 1991; **17**:543–89 and *Circulation* 1991; **83**:1125–73.

32. Harrell FE Jr, Lee KL, Matchar DB, Reichert TA. Regression models for prognostic prediction: advantages, problems, and suggested solutions. *Cancer Treat Rep* 1985; **69**:1071–7.

33. Smith LR, Harrell FE Jr, Rankin JS, Califf RM, Pryor DB, Muhlbaier LH, et al. Determinants of early versus late cardiac death in patients undergoing coronary artery bypass graft surgery. *Circulation* 1991; **84**:III245–53.

34. Myers WO, Blackstone EH, Davis K, Foster ED, Kaiser GC. CASS Registry: Long-term surgical survival. *J Am Coll Cardiol* 1999; **33**:488–98.

35. Parsonnet V, Dean D, Bernstein AD. A method of uniform stratification of risk for estimating the results of surgery in acquired heart disease. *Circulation* 1989; **79**:I3–12.

36. Harrell F. Regression coefficients and scoring rules. *J Clin Epidemiol* 1996; **49**:819.

37. Berkson J. Why I prefer logits to probits. *Biometrics* 1951; **7**:327–39.

38. Blackstone EH, Lytle BW. Competing risks after coronary bypass surgery: the influence of death on re-intervention. *J Thorac Cardiovasc Surg* 2000; **119**:1221–30.

39. Reason JT, Carthey J, de Leval MR. Diagnosing 'vulnerable system syndrome': an essential prerequisite to effective risk management. *Qual Health Care* 2001; **10**:II21–5.

40. Sollano JA, Rose EA, Williams DL, Thornton B, Quint E, Apfelbaum M, et al. Cost-effectiveness of coronary artery bypass surgery in octogenarians. *Ann Surg* 1998; **228**:297–306.

41. Cane ME, Chen C, Bailey BM, Fernandez J, Laub GW, Anderson WA, et al. CABG in octogenarians: early and late events and actuarial survival in comparison with a matched population. *Ann Thorac Surg* 1995; **60**:1033–7.

42. Salmon B. Differences between men and women in compliance with risk factor reduction: before and after coronary artery bypass surgery. *J Vasc Nurs* 2001; **19**:73–9.

43. Ott RA, Gutfinger DE, Alimadadian H, Selvan A, Miller M, Tanner T, et al. Conventional coronary artery bypass grafting: why women take longer to recover. *J Cardiovasc Surg (Torino)* 2001; **42**:311–15.

44. O'Rourke DJ, Malenka DJ, Olmstead EM, Quinton HB, Sanders JH Jr, Lahey SJ, et al. Improved in-hospital mortality in women undergoing coronary artery bypass grafting. Northern New England Cardiovascular Disease Group. *Ann Thorac Surg* 2001; **71**:507–11.

45. Fisher LD, Kennedy JW, Davis KB, Maynard C, Fritz JK, Kaiser G, et al. Association of sex, physical size, and operative mortality after coronary artery bypass in the Coronary Artery Surgery Study (CASS). *J Thorac Cardiovasc Surg* 1982; **84**:334–41.

46. Weintraub WS, Wenger NK, Jones EL, Carver JM, Guyton RA. Changing clinical characteristics of coronary surgery patients. Differences between men and women. *Circulation* 1993; **88**:II79–86.

47. Koch CG, Higgins TL, Capdeville M, Maryland P, Leventhal M, Starr NJ. The risk of coronary artery surgery in women: a matched comparison using preoperative severity of illness scoring. *J Cardiothorac Vasc Anesth* 1996; **10**:837–8.

48. Hammar N, Sandberg E, Larsen FF, Ivert T. Comparison of early and late mortality in men and women after isolated coronary artery bypass graft surgery in Stockholm, Sweden, 1980 to 1989. *J Am Coll Cardiol* 1997; **29**:659–64.

49. Jacobs AK, Kelsey SF, Brooks MM, Faxon DP, Chaitman BR, Bittner V, et al. Better outcome for women compared with men undergoing coronary revascularization: a report from the bypass angioplasty investigation (BARI). *Circulation* 1998; **98**:1279–85.

50. Caulin-Glaser T, Blum M, Schmeizl R, Prigerson HG, Zaret B, Mazure CM. Gender differences in referral to cardiac rehabilitation programs after revascularization. *J Cardiopulm Rehabil* 2001; 21:24–30.

51. Butterworth J, James R, Prielipp R, Cerese J, Livingston J, Burnett D. Female gender associates with increased duration of intubation and length of stay after coronary artery surgery. CABG Clinical Benchmarking Database Participants. *Anesthesiology* 2000; 92:414–24.

52. Jeffery DL, Vijayanagar RR, Bognolo DA, Eckstein PF. Results of coronary bypass surgery in elderly women. *Ann Thorac Surg* 1986; 42:550–3.

53. Herlitz J, Wiklund I, Sjoland H, Karlson BW, Karlsson T, Haglid M, *et al.* Relief of symptoms and improvement of health-related quality of life five years after coronary artery bypass graft in women and men. *Clin Cardiol* 2001; 24:385–92.

54. Westin L, Carlsson R, Erhardt L, Cantor-Graae E, McNeil T. Differences in quality of life in men and women with ischemic heart disease. A prospective controlled study. *Scand Cardiovasc J* 1999; 33:160–5.

55. Robertson T, Kennard ED, Mehta S, Popma JJ, Carrozza JP Jr, King SB III, *et al.* Influence of gender on in-hospital clinical and angiographic outcomes and on one-year follow-up in the New Approaches to Coronary Intervention (NACI) registry. *Am J Cardiol* 1997; 80:26–39K.

56. Scott R, Blackstone EH, McCarthy PM, Lytle BW, Loop FD, White J, *et al.* Isolated bypass grafting of the left internal thoracic artery to the left anterior descending coronary artery: late consequences of incomplete revascularization. *J Thorac Cardiovasc Surg* 2000; 120:173–84.

57. Bergelson BA, Tommaso CL. Left main coronary artery disease: assessment, diagnosis, and therapy. *Am Heart J* 1995; 129:350–9.

58. Isner JM, Kishel J, Kent KM, Ronan JA Jr, Ross AM, Roberts WC. Accuracy of angiographic determination of left main coronary arterial narrowing. *Circulation* 1981; 63:1056–64.

59. Faxon DP, Ghalilli K, Jacobs AK, Ruocco NA, Christellis EM, Kellett MA Jr, *et al.* The degree of revascularization and outcome after multivessel coronary angioplasty. *Am Heart J* 1992; 123:854–9.

60. Alderman EL, Bourassa MG, Cohen LS, Davis KB, Kaiser GG, Killip T, *et al.* Ten-year follow-up of survival and myocardial infarction in the randomized Coronary Artery Surgery Study. *Circulation* 1990; 82:1629–46.

61. Sergeant P, Blackstone E, Meyns B. Can the outcome of coronary bypass grafting be predicted reliably? *Eur J Cardiothorac Surg* 1997; 11:2–9.

62. Foster ED, Fisher LD, Kaiser GC, Myers WO. Comparison of operative mortality and morbidity for initial and repeat coronary artery bypass grafting: the Coronary Artery Surgery Study (CASS) registry experience. *Ann Thorac Surg* 1984; 38:563–70.

63. Noyez L, Touma IM, Skotnicki SH, Brouwer RM. Third-time coronary artery bypass grafting. *Ann Thorac Surg* 2000; 70:483–6.

64. Schutz A, Mair H, Wildhirt SM, Gillrath G, Lamm P, Kilger E, *et al.* Re-OPCAB vs. re-CABG for myocardial revascularization. *Thorac Cardiovasc Surg* 2001; 49:144–8.

65. Azoury FM, Gillinov AM, Lytle BW, Smedira NG, Sabik JF. Off-pump re-operative coronary artery bypass grafting by thoracotomy: patient selection and operative technique. *Ann Thorac Surg* 2001; 71:1959–63.

66. Silber JH, Williams SV, Krakauer H, Schwartz JS. Hospital and patient characteristics associated with death after surgery. *Med Care* 1992; 30:615–29.

67. Silber JH, Rosenbaum PR, Schwartz JS, Ross RN, Williams SV. Evaluation of the complication rate as a measure of quality of care in coronary artery bypass graft surgery. *JAMA* 1995; 274:317–23.

68. Loop FD. Coronary artery surgery: the end of the beginning. *Eur J Cardiothorac Surg* 1998; 14:554–71.

69. The BARI Investigators [Alderman EL, Brooks MM, Bourassa M, Califf RM, Chaitman BR, Detre K, *et al.*]. Seven-year outcome in the Bypass Angioplasty Revascularization Investigation (BARI) by treatment and diabetic status. *J Am Coll Cardiol* 2000; 35:1122–9.

70. Brooks RC, Detre KM. Clinical trials of revascularization therapy in diabetics. *Curr Opin Cardiol* 2000; 15:287–92.

71. Brooks MM, Jones RH, Bach RG, Chaitman BR, Kern MJ, Orszulak TA, *et al.* Predictors of mortality and mortality from cardiac causes in the Bypass Angioplasty Revascularization Investigation (BARI) randomized trial and registry. *Circulation* 2000; 101:2682–9.

72. O'Keefe JH, Blackstone EH, Sergeant P, McCallister BD. The optimal mode of coronary revascularization for diabetics. A risk-adjusted long-term study comparing coronary angioplasty and coronary bypass surgery. *Eur Heart J* 1998; 19:1696–703.

73. Loop FD, Lytle BW, Cosgrove DM, Stewart RW, Goormastic M, Williams GW, *et al.* Influence of the internal-mammary-artery graft on 10-year survival and other cardiac events. *N Engl J Med* 1986; 314:1–6.

74. Efron B, Tibshirani R. Bootstrap methods for standard errors, confidence intervals, and other measures of statistical accuracy. *Stat Sci* 1986; 1:54–77.

75. Hannan EL, Siu AL, Kumar D, Kilburn H Jr, Chassin MR. The decline in coronary artery bypass graft surgery mortality in New York State. The role of surgeon volume. *JAMA* 1995; 18:209–13.

76. O'Connor GT, Plume SK, Olmstead EM, Morton JR, Maloney CT, Nugent WC, *et al.* A regional intervention to improve the hospital mortality associated with coronary artery bypass graft surgery. The Northern New England Cardiovascular Disease Study Group. *JAMA* 1996; 275:841–6.

77. Malenka DJ, O'Connor GT. The Northern New England Cardiovascular Disease Study Group: a regional collaborative effort for continuous quality improvement in cardiovascular disease. *Jt Comm J Qual Improv* 1998; 24:594–600.

24

Predicting, evaluating and improving the results of coronary artery bypass surgery

STEPHEN K PLUME

The aims of this chapter are to describe methods that can help clinicians accurately estimate the risks of coronary surgery prospectively, evaluate results both retrospectively and in real time, and reduce the frequency of complications after surgery. It develops four recommendations:

1   select, understand and use objective prediction rules for preoperative risk assessment and for monitoring surgical results,
2   participate in a multi-institutional registry large enough to study infrequent outcomes,
3   adopt 'root cause analysis' to address individual adverse outcomes or near-misses,
4   maintain a time-ordered local registry of critical process and outcome measures, using statistical process control charts.

The underlying purpose is to help establish and nurture a climate of honest, relevant inquiry, in which curiosity about how things work is encouraged and determination to make things better is pervasive.

Use of personal, institutional and larger scale registries is emphasized as complementary to prospective randomized clinical trials (RCTs), the gold standard for scientific inquiry in clinical medicine. Sometimes RCTs are mandatory for isolating causal relationships and for making comparisons, but sometimes RCTs are unnecessary, inappropriate, impossible or inadequate.[1] Longitudinal observational studies can provide important insights about associations among existing practices and outcomes, about variation and about trends over time. They can help guide our efforts to improve the outcomes that we create and to reduce the human and economic costs of our care.

PREDICTING RESULTS: ESTIMATING THE RISKS OF CORONARY SURGERY

One example of the utility of observational studies is the development of quantitative clinical prediction rules. Many cardiac surgery databases have characterized large numbers of patients (often thousands, sometimes tens of thousands or even hundreds of thousands) and dozens of variables per patient. Regression and correlation analyses have made it possible to explore relationships among the variables, the variation inherent in differences among patients, practitioners and institutions, and changes that have occurred over time. Multivariate analyses and multiple regression techniques allow us to identify factors that contribute significantly to the frequency of important outcomes, to determine their absolute and relative weights, and to predict with reasonable accuracy the likelihood of various outcomes, given specific combinations of patient and process characteristics.

A good clinical prediction rule can do two important things for patients with coronary artery disease and for the clinicians who treat them.

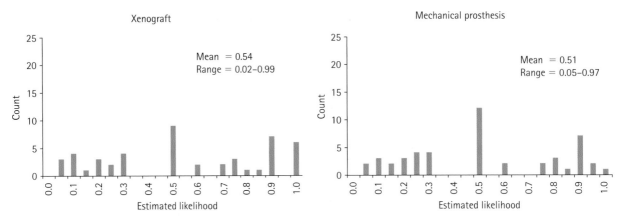

Figure 24.1 *Surgeons' estimates of the likelihood of sequelae from prosthetic heart valves used for aortic valve replacement.*

1 It can improve clinical decision-making by providing a realistic prospective assessment of the likelihood of complications that may attend myocardial revascularization.
2 It can calibrate personal or institutional clinical outcomes to a valid performance standard by comparing complication rates across risk-adjusted populations of patients, or by comparing observed results to what would be expected for a comparable group of patients.

Improving clinical decision-making

We owe patients our best assessment of the options they have and the risks they face.[2] It is well documented but not widely accepted that intuition alone, even among experts, is an unreliable guide for estimating probability.[3] It has been demonstrated that we all use cognitive heuristics: unconscious, personal, idiosyncratic mental shortcuts that simplify the task of integrating what we perceive and remember into judgment that we can act upon. The 'availability' heuristic, for example, includes the familiar tendency to extrapolate from a few characteristics to our most memorable experiences. Transposed to a coronary surgery decision-making setting, the availability heuristic might be at work if a surgeon's vivid memory of the spectacular ventricular rupture death of a morbidly obese patient with an open, infected sternotomy wound leads to over-estimating the risk of surgery in obese patients. Conversely, a proud memory of successfully revascularizing a markedly impaired heart in the setting of acute myocardial infarction may lead a surgeon to under-estimate the actual risk of such procedures. The 'representativeness' heuristic operates when we make inferences about a population, regardless of the size or representativeness of the sample. We intuitively generalize from the few to the many. The 'anchoring' heuristic biases our estimates towards our initial impression. The setting and sequence in which we learn prognostic information

influence our overall estimate of the likelihood of an outcome.

In complex decisions where multiple probability estimates must be combined, intuition can generate results inconsistent with our own beliefs. For example, when 50 experienced cardiac surgeons were asked to estimate the individual probabilities of 11 events associated with the use of mechanical or tissue valve prostheses, their responses were noteworthy both for wide variation of the estimates (Figure 24.1) and for the fact that half of the surgeons recommended a prosthesis different from that logically suggested by their own estimates.

Subjective cognitive factors can be seen at work in a comparison of UK and US physicians' judgments of probabilities of important outcomes. In a sample studied by Poses *et al.*, US physicians' estimates of the risk of complications after invasive cardiac procedures were higher than the estimates of UK physicians. Possible sources of their different perceptions of risk were hypothesized to be that the UK physicians were more risk-averse and were more uncomfortable with uncertainty.[4] In general, accuracy of subjective risk estimates is as poor in cardiac surgery as in other areas that have been studied.[5,6]

One cannot consciously decide not to be influenced by unconscious heuristics or not to make inaccurate intuitive calculations. The antidote to cognitive shortcuts is to anchor one's risk estimate on a value derived from objective data. Sometimes we feel impelled to adjust objective estimates in light of factors not included in the prediction rule. This is the clinician's prerogative, but a wise clinician is aware of the pitfalls of doing so. Calculating a statistically grounded patient-specific risk and sharing this information with the patient helps all parties make an adequately informed decision founded on objective assessment.

The language of probability

Independent of the issue of making reliable estimates of risk, a quantitative approach can improve communication

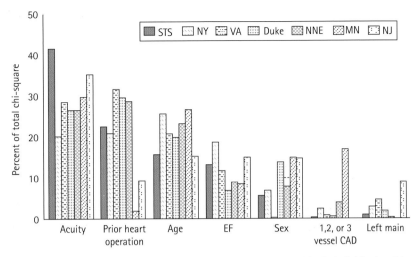

Figure 24.2 *Percentage of total chi-square contributed by each of the seven core variables in individual multivariable models from seven separate databases reflects the relative importance of these core variables in predicting mortality 30 days after CABG. CAD, coronary artery disease; EF, ejection fraction; Duke, Duke university; MN, Minnesota; NJ, New Jersey; NNE, Northern New England; NY, New York; STS, Society of Thoracic Surgeons; VA, Veterans Affairs. Reprinted with permission from the American College of Cardiology (Journal of the American College of Cardiology 1996; 28:1485).*

Table 24.1 *C-Index for each tested data set (core vs level 1 variables)*

	STS	NY	VA	Duke	NNE	MN	NJ
Core only	0.759	0.768	0.722	0.789	0.780	0.752	0.782
Core + level 1	0.795	0.839	0.748	0.818	0.796	NA	0.782
Difference	0.036	0.071	0.026	0.029	0.016	NA	0

STS, Society of Thoracic Surgeons; NY, New York; VA, Veterans Affairs; Duke, Duke University; NNE, Northern New England;
MN, Minnesota; NJ, New Jersey.
Reprinted with permission from the American College of Cardiology (*Journal of the American College of Cardiology* 1996; **28**:1486).

among participants in the clinical decision-making process. The everyday language of probability is imprecise and variable, among both physicians and lay persons. Asked to assign a numerical correlate to what they intended to convey in words, 10% of physicians intended 'infrequent' to imply less than 5% frequency of occurrence, but another 10% of physicians intended a number that was greater than 40%. 'Frequent', to some, meant a frequency that was less than 50%, and to others implied a frequency of greater than 85%. 'Majority' implied 50% or more to some, but 85% or more to others.[7] Quantifying our risk estimates clarifies the intent of our language, reducing misunderstanding among clinicians and between clinician and patient.[8]

Choosing a prediction rule

Which of the many available prediction rules for mortality and complications after coronary artery surgery should one use? Should we adopt, calibrate or customize an existing rule, or create a new rule?[9,10] The short answer is that the decision about which prediction rule to choose depends upon its intended use. Each prediction rule has characteristics that make it more or less appropriate for specific applications.

Jones *et al.* evaluated the performance of mortality risk estimates derived from seven large US datasets: Duke University, Minnesota, New Jersey, New York, Northern New England, Society for Thoracic Surgery, and Veterans' Affairs.[11] Seven 'core' variables (age, sex, left ventricular ejection fraction, urgency of operation, prior heart surgery, number of vessels with stenoses greater than 70%, presence of >50% stenosis of the left main coronary artery) predicted much of the risk, even though the contribution of each variable differed among models (Figure 24.2).

Despite these differences, the models performed quite similarly as estimators of risk, as judged by the area under the receiver operating characteristic (ROC) curve, which is a measure of a prediction rule's ability to discriminate between outcomes on the basis of the prognostic factors that it uses (Table 24.1).[12,13]

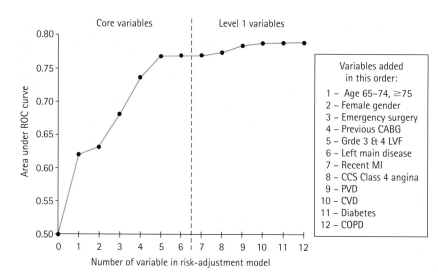

Figure 24.3 *Area under the ROC curve as more risk factors are included in a risk-adjustment model. Reprinted with permission from the American College of Cardiology (Journal of the American College of Cardiology 1997;* **30***:1321).*

A voluntary collaboration among 132 centers in ten European states documented that 128 of them could provide data judged to be 99+% accurate concerning 68 preoperative and 29 operative risk factors for 19 030 patients operated upon in the last few months of 1995. Multiple logistic regression analysis yielded a 17-element prediction rule for patients undergoing any procedure requiring cardiopulmonary bypass, not just for those receiving coronary artery bypass grafting (CABG) only. The Euroscore achieved areas under ROC curves ranging from 0.74 in Spain, where about half the patients received isolated CABG, to 0.87 in Finland, where nearly 80% of the patients received isolated CABG.[14] Additional information and a risk calculator can be accessed at http://www. euroscore. org/. While Jones *et al.*[11] demonstrate that several rules can be robust across test datasets, Roques *et al.*[14] show that a single rule from a large, diverse dataset is robust across a variety of applications.

Why isn't it better to include more variables?

Some factors that we know are clinically important contribute little additional predictive value to statistical risk models. In the datasets evaluated by Jones *et al.*, 13 'level 1' variables ('shown to have a likely relation to short-term CABG mortality') and 24 'level 2' variables ('not clearly shown to relate directly to short-term CABG mortality but with potential research or administrative interest') had a modest effect on the predictive capability of the statistical models.[11]

This phenomenon was studied by Tu *et al.*, who evaluated 12 variables available in an Ontario, Canada, regional database.[15] Six were 'core' and six were level 1 variables as defined by Jones *et al.* As is seen in Figure 24.3, the six core variables accounted for most of the risk. The six level 1 variables made little difference.

Inspecting the ROC curve, one might ask whether variable 6 ('left main disease') makes a significant contribution to the statistical model, and whether variable 9 ('peripheral vascular disease') should be substituted for it. Answering these questions would require re-evaluating the statistical model, because the correlation coefficient of each factor depends not only on what other factors are in the model, but also on the order in which factors are added to the model.

Reasons why a clinically significant factor may not be retained as a statistically significant variable in a database-derived clinical prediction rule include the following.

- Some issues that are obviously relevant for individual patients occur so infrequently that they do not emerge as predictive for the population as a whole. Consider the example of a patient who has coronary artery disease and a known malignancy. There are not enough such patients in a coronary surgery database to permit making any useful statistical inferences about such uncommon combinations of risk factors for the general population, however clear the clinical issue may seem for an individual patient. The Euroscore group decided that a variable must occur in at least 2% of patients in order to qualify for inclusion in the statistical analysis.[16]
- Some factors overlap in the realm in which they are predictive. If one factor is in a model, adding another may not improve its performance. Failure of the variable 'recent myocardial infarction' to appear in some stepwise logistic regression models is due partly to the infrequency of its occurrence (2.2% in the Ontario dataset) and partly to the inclusion of many such patients in a 'high acuity' category. Because there are other scenarios that contribute to 'high acuity', the 'recent myocardial infarction' variable may be subsumed within it and may become statistically, but not clinically, redundant. This does not mean that

recency of acute myocardial infarction cannot be studied separately and its relative risk, or odds ratio, for mortality determined.

Another example of this phenomenon is that including the variable 'body surface area' reduces the statistical impact of the variable 'sex' for predicting mortality after coronary artery surgery.[17] One possible explanation may be that there is a relationship between the size of the patient, the size of grafted vessels, blood flow, patency of grafts and mortality, and that women tend to be smaller than men. However, it may be advantageous to retain both variables until speculations about the role of hormones, or the role of biases that influence whether and when women are referred for coronary surgery,[18] have been resolved.

- Some variables are statistically significant in a model after adjusting for all of the other factors, especially when the dataset is large, but do not add materially to the predictive value of the equation. Whether to retain them (and therefore whether to continue to measure and collect the data) is a judgment about the trade-off between cost and utility of the information, and about the costs and risks of making changes in the data collection process, a challenge not to be underestimated.

Which statistical model should I use for estimating risk prospectively?

If our goal is to anchor our estimates in reasonable approximations as part of a preoperative decision-making process, it makes little difference which of the existing, validated rules one uses. Although risk estimates derived from different rules may vary by a large relative percentage, the absolute percentage estimates are similar enough to create a frame of reference that is appropriate for addressing the concerns of individual patients. Whether one rule estimates precisely 2.4% risk, another 3.6% and another 5.3% typically matters less, either to patient or clinician, than does an approximate but realistic sense of the magnitude of the risk. Even the best mortality prediction rules account for only about 70–90% of the variation in outcomes. No rule can prospectively identify individual non-survivors.[19]

Some practical issues for preoperative risk estimation are the availability, ease of use and perceived relevance of the prediction rule. One example of an easily used preoperative risk assessment tool derived from a logistic regression equation is shown in Table 24.2.[20] A simple scoring system assigns points to variables that are routinely available during the decision-making stage of clinical care. The points are the rounded-off odds ratios associated with each variable that occurs in the logistic regression model. The sums of the odds ratios are read off against

a table that relates them to predicted risks, on a scale that extends over the range in which nearly all of the patients lie. Table 24.2 is legible when reproduced onto a card that fits into a shirt pocket, and which can be used at the bedside or in conference or consultation. Such a form can be included in the medical record to document that a realistic preoperative risk assessment was carried out, and to inform other interested parties. Euroscore and Parsonnet estimates offer similar practical applicability for clinical decision-making. The issue to be resolved in any specific situation is whether the risk estimate and the elements upon which it is based are appropriate in context. There is an advantage in using one prediction rule consistently, so that interested parties become familiar with its definitions, logic and performance.

Numbers and decisions

Good clinical decision-making does not consist merely of arithmetic calculations. The risk estimate derived from an objective prediction rule is a useful fact to include in one's thinking about the decision at hand. Both clinicians and patients must use their own best judgment for deciding what to do with the information. Every risk prediction rule has important limitations:

1 There is an inherent imprecision in methodology that accounts for only 70–90% of observed risk. Rejoinder: prediction rules outperform intuitive estimates.
2 Any risk prediction rule embodies what happened in the past, necessarily ignoring what may have been learned in the interim. Rejoinder: if it can be demonstrated that outcomes are different now, the rule should be recomputed or at least calibrated.
3 A prediction rule assumes usual outcomes from usual care. It cannot discount risk in a way that recognizes conscious determination to modify care in order to achieve an 'unusual' (better than predicted) result. Rejoinder: all patients are treated with the intent to achieve the best possible result.
4 The prediction rule has almost never been developed in an identical clinical context. Rejoinder: empirically, existing rules work quite well.

EVALUATING THE RESULTS OF CORONARY SURGERY

Although many 'roughly right' objective risk estimates can be helpful for giving good clinical advice prospectively, retrospective evaluations of clinical performance are sensitive to details of risk adjustment methodology. In the emotionally and sometimes politically charged atmosphere in which report cards for performance of cardiac surgery are circulated, it can matter tremendously which

Table 24.2 *Northern New England Cardiovascular Disease Study Group: pre-operative estimation of risk of mortality, cerebrovascular accident (CVA) and mediastinitis (for use only in isolated CABG)*

Preoperative Estimation of Risk of Mortality, Cerebrovascular Accident, and Mediastinitis

For use only in isolated CABG surgery

Directions: Locate outcome of interest, e.g. mortality. Use the score in that column for each relevant preoperative variable, then sum these scores to get the total score. Take the total score and look up the approximate preoperative risk in the table below.

Patient or disease characteristic	Mortality score	CVA score	Mediastinitis score
Age 60–69	2	3.5	
Age 70–79	3	5	
Age ≥80	5	6	
Female sex	1.5		
EF <40%	1.5	1.5	2
Urgent surgery	2	1.5	1.5
Emergency surgery	5	2	3.5
Prior CABG	5	1.5	
PVD	2	2	
Diabetes			1.5
Dialysis or creatinine ≥2	4	2	2.5
COPD	1.5		3.5
Obesity (BMI 31–36)			2.5
Severe obesity (BMI ≥37)			3.5
Total Score			

Perioperative Risk

Total Score	Mortality %	CVA %	Mediastinitis %
0	0.4	0.3	0.4
1	0.5	0.4	0.5
2	0.7	0.7	0.6
3	0.9	0.9	0.7
4	1.3	1.1	1.1
5	1.7	1.5	1.5
6	2.2	1.9	1.9
7	3.3	2.8	3.0
8	3.9	3.5	3.5
9	6.1	4.5	5.8
10	7.7	≥6.5	≥6.5
11	10.6		
12	13.7		
13	17.7		
14	≥28.3		

Calculation of Mortality Risk: An 80-year-old female with an EF <40% who is having elective CABG surgery, has had no prior CABG surgery and has no other risk factors. Her total score = 5(age ≥80) + 1.5(Female) + 1.5(EF <40%) = 8. Because her total score = 8, her predicted risk of mortality = 3.9%.

Definitions:

EF <40% (Left ventricular ejection fraction): The patient's current EF is less than 40%.

Urgent: Medical factors require patient to stay in hospital to have operation before discharge. The risk of immediate morbidity and death is believed to be low.

Emergency: Patient's cardiac disease dictates that surgery should be performed within hours to avoid unnecessary morbidity or death.

PVD (Peripheral vascular disease): Cerebrovascular disease, including prior CVA, prior TIA, prior carotid surgery, carotid stenosis by history or radiographic studies, or carotid bruit. Lower-extremity disease including claudication, amputation, prior lower-extremity bypass, absent pedal pulses, or lower-extremity ulcers.

Diabetes: Currently treated with oral medications or insulin.

Dialysis or creatinine ≥2 : Peritoneal or hemodialysis dependent renal failure or creatinine ≥2 mg/dL.

COPD (Chronic obstructive pulmonary disease): Treated with bronchodilators or steriods.

Obesity: Find the approximate height and weight in the table below to classify the person as obese or severely obese. Obesity: BMI 31–36, Severe obesity: BMI ≥37.

Example: A patient 5'7" and weighing 200 lbs is classified as obese. If the patient weighed 236 lbs or more, he/she would be classified as severely obese.

Height (feet and inches)	Weight (lbs) Obesity BMI 31–36	Weight (lbs) Severe Obesity BMI ≥37	Height (feet and inches)	Weight (lbs) Obesity BMI 31–36	Weight (lbs) Severe Obesity BMI ≥37
5'0"	158–184	≥189	5'8"	203–236	≥244
5'1"	164–190	≥195	5'9"	209–243	≥250
5'2"	169–196	≥202	5'10"	215–250	≥258
5'3"	175–203	≥208	5'11"	222–258	≥265
5'4"	180–209	≥215	6'0"	228–265	≥272
5'5"	186–217	≥222	6'1"	235–273	≥280
5'6"	191–222	≥228	6'2"	241–280	≥287
5'7"	198–229	≥236	6'3"	248–288	≥296

Data set and definitions for dependent variables:
The regression models that generated the scores for these prediction rules were based on 7290 patients receiving isolated CABG surgery between 1996 and 1998. The dependent, variables and observed event rates are as follows: in-hospital mortality (2.93%); cerebrovascular accident, defined as a new focal neurological event persisting at least 24 hours (1.58%); and mediastinitis during the index admission, defined by positive deep culture and/or Gram stain and/or radiographic findings indicating infection and requiring re-operation (1.19%).

Northern New England Cardiovascular Disease Study Group 6/99.

Reprinted from *The Journal of the American College of Cardiology* 1999; **34**:1269, with permission from the American College of Cardiology.

prediction rule is used, and how it is applied, especially if the purpose is to compare surgeons or institutions.

Details matter in performance assessment

It is very important for evaluated individuals and institutions to understand how severity of patient illness affects mortality rates.[21] Those whose results are worse than average often believe that they are caring for a higher than average proportion of older and sicker patients, an explanation that is correct less often than it is invoked. Those doing the evaluation, and the public at large, often accept uncritically the conclusion that an observed difference in mortality rates reflects quality of care. Random variation within a sample and random variation that occurs over time are often poorly understood. Over-interpretation of random variation sometimes prompts misguided administrative or clinical measures.

Unwillingness to be judged by 'raw' or 'crude' rates has led to wide adoption of case-mix risk adjustment. Awareness that random variation can determine rank order has encouraged testing for statistically significant differences of outcomes among risk-adjusted populations. The criterion of statistical significance is usually based on the biomedical tradition of calculating that there is a less than 5% probability of erroneously accepting the null hypothesis that there is no difference. Whether this is a useful criterion is not discussed here, beyond noting that there are theoretical and practical dangers in choosing such a loose definition of statistical significance.

As a demonstration of how the choice of a prediction rule affects the interpretation of mortality rates, we return to the analysis of Tu et al.[15] Although core variables accounted for most of the risk of this population of patients, they did not have equal effects on risk-adjusted mortality rates of the institutions in the sample. As displayed in Figure 24.4, the factors that most influenced the risk-adjusted mortality rates of nine Ontario hospitals were emergency surgery, previous CABG, and poor left ventricular function. Age and sex were important determinants of outcome, but their lack of impact on risk-adjusted rates suggests that the populations were quite similar in these dimensions and that the factors operated similarly in each setting. This conclusion is supported by the demographic data. In contrast, adjusting for proportion of emergency or re-operative cases and for poor left ventricular function appears to differentiate results among the hospitals. Case-mix risk adjustment demonstrates that there are either differences in severity of illness or differences in the impact of severity factors on institutional mortality rates, and that the differences matter.

Designing or choosing the performance evaluation tool

When participation is optional, we should consider the 1996 recommendation of an expert panel that coronary artery surgery datasets should contain 'core' predictive variables ('unequivocally related to operative mortality') in order to permit comparisons of case mix and of outcomes across populations of patients.[11] This was reiterated in 1999 by the American College of Cardiology and American Heart Association Task Force on Practice Guidelines for Coronary Artery Bypass Graft Surgery.[20]

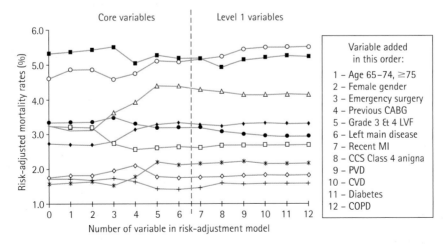

Figure 24.4 *Effect of adding more variables to risk-adjustment models on risk-adjusted mortality rates after CABG for the nine hospitals performing CABG in Ontario. Each* line *represents one hospital, whereas each* data point *represents that hospital's risk-adjusted mortality rate after a certain number of variables have been put into the model. Reprinted from* The Journal of the American College of Cardiology *1997; 30:1322, with permission from the American College of Cardiology.*

There are other important issues that should be resolved before deciding to participate in a database or choosing a prediction rule for performance assessment.

- Does one wish to use the definitions, format, data collection mechanisms, analytic methods and reporting capacity designed for a single institution, for a voluntary regional, national or international collaborative, or for a proprietary registry?
- Does one wish to be able to understand details of the risk-adjustment methodology, or is one content to use a proprietary, secret statistical modeling process?
- Is the patient population represented in the candidate database adequately comparable to one's own?
- Are the data and the prediction rules derived from them updated frequently enough to reflect current reality, given temporal changes in practice and in outcomes?
- Is the goal to sort and rank surgeons or programs, or is it to explore the consequences of practice variation and the causes of outcome variation?
- Do the primary users have commercial, administrative, fiscal and health policy interests, or are the primary users clinicians hoping to improve their own practice?
- Do the data handling methods and reporting format adequately protect patient and clinician confidentiality, if it is deemed important and legal to do so?

Institution-specific answers to questions like these carry practical implications. The challenge is to find sufficient common ground between one's own situation and the capacities, requirements and known shortcomings of the available options.

There is no alternative for most of us

In some countries, performance evaluation is both mandatory and outside the control of the clinicians and institutions that provide care. The hard fact is that clinical outcomes are demonstrably different within populations that appear to be comparable, even after adjusting for variations in prevalence of known risk factors. This reality, together with increasing public demand for and access to measures of treatment outcomes, explains the increasing focus on audits, registries, prediction rules, quality standards, safety standards and clinical process improvement that is being seen worldwide. Whatever misgivings clinicians may have, it seems clear that performance assessment is here to stay. Tu *et al.* describe a sound strategy for dealing with cardiac surgery report cards (Table 24.3).[22]

Surgeons could take comfort from the fact that neither the public nor the referring physicians pay much attention to report cards when they make specific care decisions.[23] While it cannot be doubted that public disclosure of performance data generates controversy, and that noteworthy

Table 24.3 *Tips for physicians in the report card era*

1	Don't shoot the messenger
2	Check that the results are risk-adjusted
3	Check the quality of the data prior to analysis
4	Ask if the authors have conflicts of interest
5	Know your outcomes before others do
6	Complete your charts carefully
7	Focus your practice
8	Learn from your colleagues
9	Ask for the full story of both process and outcomes
10	If you can't beat them, join them

Problems for clinical judgement: 4. Surviving in the report card era. Reprinted from *CMAJ*, 12 June 2001; **164**(12):1709–12, by permission of the publisher, © 2001 Canadian Medical Association.

improvement often ensues, it is interesting that the agents of improvement are the clinicians. It is our personal and professional pride and our commitment to our patients, not market or regulatory forces, that have driven widespread improvement of coronary surgery results.[24,25]

IMPROVING THE RESULTS OF CORONARY SURGERY

The aim of this section is to present three general and complementary strategies (root cause analysis, registry-based collaborative research, maintenance of a local registry) for identifying and changing the causal systems that create unwanted outcomes in coronary artery surgery. We seek an alternative to the view that complications are either due to human error or are inherent and inevitable, because our reality is that we work in complex systems for which such simple explanations do not suffice.

The problem of assuring clinical quality is often addressed through input standards (e.g. credentialing) and output reviews (e.g. audit). Improving quality has been thought to consist of holding clinicians and institutions accountable for their results. Poor performers are subjected to restriction or revocation of their right to practice, while good performers are labeled as 'preferred providers' or 'centers of excellence'. Students of human factors as determinants of performance generally de-emphasize this 'train and blame' strategy, on the grounds that system characteristics have an important causal role and are more tractable to improvement efforts.[26] Careful study of failures or complications in complex systems often reveals important inadequacies of system design, well beyond the capacity of individual practitioners to control.[27,28]

Perspective

'Every system is perfectly designed to get the results that it gets' – a phrase coined by a scholar of healthcare improvement leadership, Dr Paul Batalden. The key insight is that the waste and errors and near-misses that occur in a process are as intrinsic as are its intended results. Care always occurs in a context, within a constellation of personnel, equipment, methods, policies, measures and environment. From a systems perspective, complications of treatment are designed into the process of care, of which the human factor is only one element.[29] If we want fewer complications, we need to change our processes of care. Most of us are not accustomed to systematic assessments of our processes of care, or to continuous search for opportunities to improve. At present, most operating theater staff do not believe that their institutions handle errors well. Many senior staff deny the influence of well-established sources of error, and reject the importance of multiple sources of input from junior members.[30]

Typical, actual clinical vignettes

1   A seemingly uneventful multivessel revascularization for a patient with minimal risk factors and normal ventricular function was attended by initially moderate ('usual') and then increasingly intense inotropic support, culminating in fatal postoperative low cardiac output.
2   A difficult but apparently successful re-operation requiring a prolonged period of cardiopulmonary bypass ended in catastrophe when the patient collapsed while the chest was being closed, immediately after being given a unit of platelets.
3   A morbidly obese man died from acute pulmonary insufficiency on the second day after undergoing emergency revascularization. He had been extubated and subsequently transferred from the intensive care unit according to a surgeon-approved protocol, after evaluation by an experienced critical care pulmonary physician.
4   An anesthesiologist mistakenly administered phenylephrine instead of protamine, resulting in elevation of the blood pressure to over 300 mmHg. The patient experienced no apparent injury or requirement for extra care.

Whose fault?

These vignettes were chosen because they are typical of the ambiguity between person and process as the source of the problem. The following are a few of the many questions that they might raise.

1   Did the surgeon fail to protect the heart adequately during revascularization?
2   Was the platelet transfusion not indicated, or was compatibility testing inadequate?

3   Was the protocol for extubation inappropriate for a very obese patient, or was he mis-managed after transfer from the intensive care unit?
4   How did the medication error occur?

None of the direct participants in these vignettes was unqualified, inattentive, uncaring, over-tired or inexperienced. Each of the involved surgeons has a mortality rate below 3% for coronary revascularization. None of the cases resulted in an organized change in care, despite exhortations like 'Be more careful'. Exploration of the medication error revealed a typically complex sequence: the phenylephrine and the protamine were packaged in identical containers, easily recognizable as supplied by a particular manufacturer but not as being different compounds. The labels were printed in tiny script. A pharmacy technician had restocked the wrong bottle in the place reserved for protamine. This particular mistake had not occurred in thousands of similar cases performed over many years in that institution.

Every experienced coronary artery surgeon can recount a much larger inventory of similar catastrophes and near-misses. If we adopt our patients' desire for zero complications as our goal, assessment of our outcomes will need to expand beyond the traditional morbidity and mortality conference review of individual cases, and beyond calculations of whether we are performing outside two standard deviations from some standard. Instead, we need an effective assessment process that can help us understand what factors drive complication rates, how these factors operate, and how to reduce or eliminate their influence.

Safety and reliability are dynamic non-events

In medicine, as in many other areas, the usual question asked after a mishap is 'Whose fault is it?'. In high reliability industries such as military aviation and nuclear power, this question is rarely asked, and actual mishaps are not the only source of concern. For both mishaps and near-misses, the questions posed are 'What happened?', 'Why did it happen?', 'What are we going to do to prevent it from ever happening again?'. As Karl Weick and Kathleen Sutcliffe, students of organizational behavior, have written, 'Safety and reliability are *dynamic* non-events… Safety and reliability are complex outcomes that require continuous attention and effort' (emphasis in original).[31] There is considerable opportunity for improving clinical results by analyzing and changing our processes of care. Despite some controversy about the magnitude of the problem, a report from the United States Institute of Medicine has stimulated an intense interest in reducing the frequency of medical errors.[32]

Root cause analysis

Root cause analysis is an approach to improving safety in healthcare that has been adapted from the experience of the US National Aeronautics and Space Administration (responsible for the safety of astronauts) and of the US National Traffic Safety Board (which investigates air travel accidents). A recurrent finding is that airplane crashes, for example, routinely result from a confluence of causal chains that extend well upstream from crises that may or may not also have elements of 'pilot error'. Even when the latter can be identified, these often have their origins in poor communication, in certification or re-certification procedures, in over-scheduling, or in lack of training for crew resource management. The suggestion for cardiac surgeons, as for medicine in general, is that dependence on the good intentions, unflagging vigilance, excellent technical skills and all-encompassing knowledge of individual clinicians is a poor substitute for fail-safe mechanisms that we should embed in our processes of care.

According to the National Center for Patient Safety (NCPS) sponsored by the US Veterans' Affairs Administration, key elements of an effective healthcare safety program include the following.

- A mechanism for reporting errors and near-misses in a way that guarantees confidentiality to the person reporting a problem. Safety for the reporter is essential. For example, the previously successful voluntary reporting process of one national airline has had zero submissions for the many years since it permitted a single breach of confidentiality (Bagian J, personal communication). Trust that can be lost in an instant may not be regained in a decade, or more.
- A multidisciplinary project team that includes both the kinds of people involved in the problem (but not any of the individuals participating directly in the clinical episode being analyzed) and outside perspectives. Sometimes a person unfamiliar with the setting or the specific clinical problem can alert the team to issues that are invisible to those working in the environment.
- A clear chronological event sequence or flow chart, developed by the project team from available documents and from interviewing the directly involved parties.
- Systematic identification of probable causes and contributing factors. A checklist or cue card of possibly relevant questions is helpful. The NCPS version is available at http://www.va.gov/ncps/index.html. The only time it is appropriate to identify people as causes is when there is evidence of intentionally unsafe behavior.
- A focus on specific, measurable actions that can be taken to eliminate or reduce the frequency of the problem.

- Action and measurement. Doing an analysis and formulating a plan are the beginning, not the end, of effective change. To implement, evaluate and consolidate improvements require support from leadership, and real work.[33,34] The NCPS protocol includes explicit chartering of the root cause analysis team as well as formal acceptance or rejection of its report and recommendations. Acceptance implies time-bounded commitment by leadership to implement recommendations and follow up on results.

Coronary surgery is a particularly fruitful area for such an approach, because many of us already have considerable experience in thinking about how to organize reliable systems of cardiac care and because many coronary surgery programs have a tradition of teamwork and shared responsibility. Even so, widespread awareness of clinical anecdotes like those cited above, and empirical evidence of errors throughout healthcare, alert us to the need for intensifying our efforts to improve patient safety.[35]

Collaborative outcomes research

Every surgeon has idiosyncratic methods or techniques to accomplish revascularization, and every institution has distinctive patterns for the surgical management of coronary disease. While well aware that others have different ways of approaching the same task, individual surgeons believe strongly in their own rationales for their own processes. On the other hand, there is incontrovertible evidence that our results differ. It seems unlikely that each of the different methods, techniques and equipment that we use constitutes the best available care. Root cause analysis can often reveal why an intended result known to be achievable is not achieved, and can guide remedial action through system redesign. A different process, described below, is required when there is uncertainty or disagreement among professionals about how to achieve an intended result.

Desirable features of a clinical registry

A registry exploits variation in patient characteristics, in clinical practice and in outcomes to guide the search for better ways to achieve desired clinical results. The registry should be large enough to collect sufficient cases so that meaningful analyses of infrequent events can be conducted within reasonable time frames. A broad range of accepted approaches should be represented in the dataset. A good registry has well-documented, demonstrably effective operational definitions, i.e. definitions that provide consistent, reproducible counts and measures. Data elements to be collected should be those agreed upon by consensus to be worth the effort, because work perceived as useless will not be done well. Data collection should occur at the time, and by the persons to whom it matters, in the usual flow of work. This is especially important when there are inadequate resources to support a separate staff for gathering data. Expert statistical analysis, prompt feedback and collegial discussions of the findings and of their significance are important for discovering and disseminating useful findings. Representation of all types of participants (surgeons, cardiologists, anesthesiologists, nurses, perfusionists, administrators and others) helps assure that multiple perspectives contribute to a comprehensive understanding of the process of care, to sensible choice and definition of data elements, to shared interpretation and to broad acceptance of the findings. Participation must go beyond contributing data and receiving reports. Surprise, objection, disagreement and animated discussion in an atmosphere of openness and trust are the hallmarks of an effective collaborative effort to acquire new insights and achieve new levels of performance through the use of a clinical registry. Practitioners do not, and should not, readily modify or abandon clinical strategies that they believe in. They should, however, have the willingness and the means for challenging their own assumptions.

An example of a registry in action

In 1987, a national agency reported that risk-adjusted, institution-specific coronary artery surgery mortality rates for patients older than 65 years varied between 2.3% and 5.6% among the five hospitals offering cardiac surgery in Maine, New Hampshire and Vermont.[36] Skeptical about these findings, surgery and cardiology representatives of the institutions agreed to collect a core dataset for all patients operated upon in the region, representing 95% of all CABG surgery received by residents of these states. After 3 years, it became clear that differences in results were real, and could not be attributed to differences among patients.[37] Training in process observation and in process improvement concepts and tools was followed by a round of site visits and then by reports of process differences. Although no single cause could be identified, there was a subsequent sustained 24% drop in observed mortality rates despite progressive increase in predicted risk,[37] a rate of improvement twice that of the national trend.[38] A key finding from analysis of mode of death after CABG was that two-thirds of the deaths were attributable to postoperative heart failure, and that two-thirds of those who died from postoperative heart failure had normal ventricular function preoperatively. Further, most of the variation in surgeon-specific risk-adjusted mortality rates was accounted for by the incidence of postoperative heart failure.[39] Perioperative myocardial protection was an obvious leverage point for improving mortality

rates. More generally, if all sites could achieve the lowest rate of specific complications then current at some sites, the mortality rate for the region could drop to 1%, without new science or new technology.

Many findings have emerged from continuing analysis of this growing dataset. Confirming earlier reports, but not mirrored in the practice of the day, an acute survival benefit was documented from using the left internal thoracic artery for all classes of patients.[40] Over time, use of at least one internal thoracic artery has risen to above 90% in the region, compared to about 75% in the rest of the USA. Surgeons disagreed about the benefit of continuing aspirin therapy up to the time of surgery. Some insisted that patients discontinue aspirin at least 1 week before surgery, while others recommended continuation. Analysis of the database showed that there is an acute survival benefit associated with continuing aspirin, without any increase in re-exploration for bleeding, need for transfusion, or postoperative blood loss.[41] Most surgeons were surprised about the lack of impact of obesity on mortality rates following CABG.[42] The adverse effect of severe hemodilution on bypass was another surprise. There was a monotonic relationship between progressively more severe hemodilution below a packed cell volume of 25% and the incidence of death, stroke and need for intra-aortic balloon support. The problem appears to relate to the nadir hematocrit, not to the hematocrit at the end of bypass or at the end of the procedure.[43] Different prevention strategies (priming the pump with blood versus reducing the volume of the cardiopulmonary bypass circuit) are being evaluated. The presence of pre-existing peripheral vascular disease, even as a note concerning the past medical history or as a bruit noted during physical examination, conferred increased perioperative mortality risk.[44] It was learned that re-exploration for hemorrhage tripled operative mortality risk.[45] There is a definite, and reversible, adverse impact of tachycardia at the time of induction of anesthesia. Heart rates above 80 beats/min are associated with increased risk of adverse outcomes.[46]

Many other uncertainties and controversies in clinical practice are being studied. Over time, differences in institutional mortality rates have disappeared as the regional mortality rate has continued to drop. Changes in practice have not been mandated; they have occurred as understanding has diffused among the community of clinicians, which underscores the importance of active, broad participation and of prompt and clear feedback.

Recommendations

Participate actively in a clinical cardiac care registry whose avowed purpose is to improve patient care and whose relevance, size, structure, process and personnel make improvement a likely outcome. Track the 'core' variables recommended by Jones et al.[11] and other variables agreed upon by the participants, keeping in mind that trying to collect too many variables creates the risk of frustration and failure and adds expense beyond value. Foster inclusive participation: different kinds of clinicians, as well as other non-clinical personnel, are interdependent in creating outcomes, whether good or bad.

Local registries and statistical process control charts

Tracking and analyzing all the variables that are being contributed to a collaborative registry may exceed the interests or capacities that are available where a surgeon practices, and would be redundant to the larger effort. On the other hand, there are some outcomes and some process measures that are important enough to warrant monitoring at each site. There is a predictable benefit to be achieved from the ready availability of critical information. The selection may vary with the priorities of the program, and with the theories of causation that are current at a particular place and time. The easiest and most informative approach is to maintain a simple, time-ordered run chart of the chosen elements, partly because it provides a graphic sense of variation and of trends, and partly because it provides statistically valid early warning of important changes.

The central idea behind analyzing time-ordered data was developed by Bell Laboratories engineer Walter Shewhart in the 1920s[47] and has been elaborated in many areas outside medicine as the discipline of statistical process control.[48] Shewhart demonstrated that there are two classes of variation, classes that call for different types of intervention. Random variation that is observable in any process calls for deciding whether the average result is acceptable, and whether the amount of variation from that average is acceptable. Reducing the amount of random variation and centering a process at a different point require thinking about how the process is designed. Extreme variation of individual data points, on the other hand, calls for analysis of, and action on, the specific situation. Shewhart's recommendation is to use three standard deviations from the average as the criterion for extreme variation. He believed that this criterion is the empirically optimum trade-off between mistaking random variation for something special and failing to recognize instances that are special. A value that lies three standard deviations away from the average usually has an identifiable cause outside the usual interacting set of causes associated with the usual performance of a process. Less extreme variation, usually the result of random variation, is too often over-interpreted, and too often leads to managerial tampering that can be counterproductive.

Candidate outcome variables for local tracking include mortality, stroke, bleeding, infection, or any others that are of particular concern. Candidate process variables depend on local interests and theories. For example, one institution tracks return to cardiopulmonary bypass, having learned that return to bypass for any reason triples the mortality risk. Becoming aware of this changed the dynamic in the operating room, resulting in improved communication and coordination among surgeon, anesthesiologist and perfusionist. Learning that severe hemodilution on bypass increases the probability of death and stroke prompted the implementation of measures to prevent excessive hemodilution. As seen in Figure 24.5, a run chart is kept that tracks the percentage of patients with the lowest hematocrit while on cardiopulmonary bypass below 21%. There are many variations on the theme of local data collection. Shahian et al., describe an array of statistical process control charts adapted for use in cardiac surgery units.[49] The important common element is to measure, record and display what matters to the participants. Properly constructed control charts keep us aware and informed, and guide our interventions. The interested reader should consult Wheeler for details of the theory and mechanics of calculating natural process control limits from time-ordered data points, based on the principles laid out by Shewhart.[48]

Although this discussion, like much of our professional literature, has emphasized the traditional outcomes of mortality and morbidity, we should recognize that these statistics look at too narrow a spectrum. While our patients surely have intense interest in experiencing the lowest possible rates of death and complications, they have other concerns as well. Until cooperative registries begin to study outcomes in the other dimensions that matter to patients, local registries may be the best places to begin to collect a broader and more balanced set of measures, using the same methods as those discussed above. A 'value compass'[50,51] or 'balanced scorecard'[52] approach that tracks dimensions such as satisfaction with care, functional status and cost (broadly defined, not restricted to financial transfers) can provide important insights and can guide how we design care. As coronary surgery mortality rates begin to achieve a 'six sigma' standard (in statistical process control, this refers to a defect rate of 3 or fewer per thousand units produced, or 0.3%), safety will be assumed, not merely hoped for. We are appropriately called upon to remember that perioperative death and complications are only part of the spectrum of the burden of illness.

CONCLUSION

Mastery of clinical surgery is based on a structured educational process that depends heavily on apprenticeship

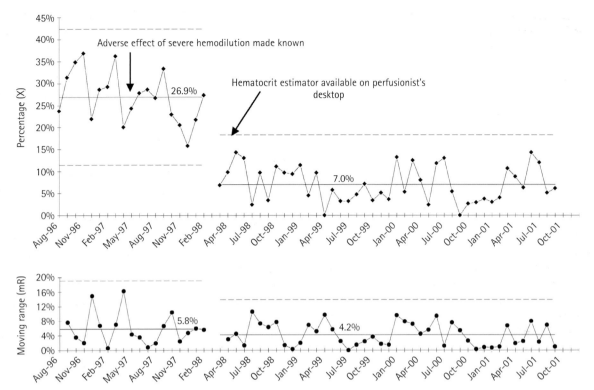

Figure 24.5 *Example of a control chart in a local registry; percentage of patients with lowest hematocrit <21% (XmR chart). 'XmR' control charts for sequential data values use the average moving range (the average absolute difference between successive values). Multiply the average moving range by 2.66 and add/subtract the result to/from the average of the individual data values to define the upper and lower natural process control limits of the process. Multiply the average moving range by 3.268 to define the upper control limit of the moving range. If all values lie within these limits, the process is said to be 'in control': there is a statistical basis for believing that future values will lie within these limits, if there is no change in the process. If there are values that lie outside the control limits, the process creating them is not 'in control', and there is no statistical basis for believing where future values will lie. Interpretation: a process change in April 1998 is indicated by two signals – the occurrence of a value below the previously established natural process control limits; and a series of eight values in a row below the previous process average, beginning at the same point. Note that presentation of data did not by itself have a discernable effect. Awareness of the data plus provision of an easy way to calculate and prevent hemodilution may account for the observed change.*

and on progressively independent responsibility, followed by a professional lifetime of reflection and learning. Methods like those outlined in this chapter, combined with appreciation of the interdependence of the elements of any system, can improve our ability to explore process – outcome relationships in coronary artery surgery. Thus armed, we can deliver the best care of which we are capable and, simultaneously, redesign the systems within which we work to become capable of delivering progressively better care.

KEY REFERENCES

Black N. Why we need observational studies to evaluate the effectiveness of health care. *BMJ* 1996; **312**: 1215–18.

A short, thoughtful, provocative editorial that challenges orthodox thinking about science and clinical medicine.

Kahneman D, Slovic P, Tversky A. *Judgment Under Uncertainty: Heuristics and Biases.* Cambridge: Press Syndicate of the University of Cambridge, 1982.

Twenty years after first publication, this collection remains a broad and persuasive documentation of the arenas in which intuitive judgments are not just fallible, but often systematically misleading.

O'Connor GT, Plume SK, Olmstead EM, Coffin LH, Morton JR, Maloney CT, *et al.* A regional prospective study of in-hospital mortality associated with coronary artery bypass grafting. The Northern New England Cardiovascular Disease Study Group. *JAMA* 1991; **266**(6):803–9.

Among the first articles emanating from the profession, rather than from presumably biased external sources, demonstrating that observed differences in clinical outcomes are not attributable solely to differences among patients. We the clinicians are part of the system of causes that are responsible for variable outcomes. See Donald Berwick's accompanying editorial.

Wheeler DJ. Advanced Topics in Statistical Quality Control. Knoxville, TN: SPC Press Inc., 1995.
Intimidating to readers who dread even simple mathematical notation; but also clear and authoritative in demonstrating why Shewhart's control charts are theoretically robust and practically useful.

REFERENCES

1. Black N. Why we need observational studies to evaluate the effectiveness of health care. *BMJ* 1996; **312**(7040):1215–18.
2. Bogardus ST Jr, Holmboe E, Jekel JF. Perils, pitfalls, and possibilities in talking about medical risk. *JAMA* 1999; **281**:1037–41.
3. Kahneman D, Slovic P, Tversky A. *Judgment Under Uncertainty: Heuristics and Biases.* Cambridge: Press Syndicate of the University of Cambridge, 1982.
4. Poses RM, De Saintonge DM, McClish DK, Smith WR, Huber EC, Clemo FL, *et al.* An international comparison of physicians' judgments of outcome rates of cardiac procedures and attitudes toward risk, uncertainty, justifiability, and regret. *Medical Decision Making* 1998; **18**:131–40.
5. Kong DF, Lee KL, Harrell FE Jr, Boswick JM, Mark DB, Hlatky MA, *et al.* Clinical experience and predicting survival in coronary disease. *Arch Intern Med* 1989; **149**:1177–81.
6. Pons JM, Borras JM, Espinas JA, Moreno V, Cardona M, Granados A. Subjective versus statistical model assessment of mortality risk in open heart surgical procedures. *Ann Thorac Surg* 1999; **67**:635–40.
7. Nakao MA, Axelrod S. Numbers are better than words. Verbal specifications of frequency have no place in medicine. *Am J Med* 1983; **74**:1061–5.
8. Kong A, Barnett GO, Mosteller F, Youtz C. How medical professionals evaluate expressions of probability. *N Engl J Med* 1986; **315**:740–4.
9. Ivanov J, Tu JV, Naylor CD. Ready-made, Recalibrated, or Remodeled? Issues in the use of risk indexes for assessing mortality after coronary artery bypass graft surgery. *Circulation* 1999; **99**:2098–104.
10. Iezzoni LI. Statistically derived predictive models. Caveat emptor. *J Gen Intern Med* 1999; **14**:388–9.
11. Jones RH, Hannan EL, Hammermeister KE, Delong ER, O'Connor GT, Luepker RV, *et al.* Identification of preoperative variables needed for risk adjustment of short-term mortality after coronary artery bypass graft surgery. The Working Group Panel on the Cooperative CABG Database Project. *J Am Coll Cardiol* 1996; **28**:1478–87.
12. Hanley JA, McNeil BJ. The meaning and use of the area under a receiver operating characteristic (ROC) curve. *Radiology* 1982; **143**:29–36.
13. Swets JA. Measuring the accuracy of diagnostic systems. *Science* 1988; **240**(4857):1285–93.
14. Roques F, Nashef SA, Michel P, Pinna Pintor P, David M, Baudet E, *et al.* Does EuroSCORE work in individual European countries? *Eur J Cardiothorac Surg* 2000; **18**:27–30.
15. Tu JV, Sykora K, Naylor CD. Assessing the outcomes of coronary artery bypass graft surgery: how many risk factors are enough? Steering Committee of the Cardiac Care Network of Ontario. *J Am Coll Cardiol* 1997; **30**:1317–23.
16. Roques F, Nashef SA, Michel P, Gauducheau E, de Vincentiis C, Baudet E, *et al.* Risk factors and outcome in European cardiac surgery: analysis of the EuroSCORE multinational database of 19030 patients. *Eur J Cardiothorac Surg* 1999; **15**:816–22; discussion 822–3.
17. O'Connor GT, Morton JR, Diehl MJ, Olmstead EM, Coffin LH, Levy DG, *et al.* Differences between men and women in hospital mortality associated with coronary artery bypass graft surgery. The Northern New England Cardiovascular Disease Study Group. *Circulation* 1993; **88**:2104–10.
18. Ayanian JZ, Epstein AM. Differences in the use of procedures between women and men hospitalized for coronary heart disease. *N Engl J Med* 1991; **325**:221–5.
19. Weightman WM, Gibbs NM, Sheminant MR, Thackray NM, Newman MA. Risk prediction in coronary artery surgery: a comparison of four risk scores. *Med J Aust* 1997; **166**:408–11.
20. Eagle KA, Guyton RA, Davidoff R, Ewy GA, Fonger J, Gardner TJ, *et al.* ACC/AHA guidelines for coronary artery bypass graft surgery: executive summary and recommendations: a report of the American College of Cardiology/American Heart Association Task Force on Practice Guidelines (Committee to Revise the 1991 Guidelines for Coronary Artery Bypass Graft Surgery). *J Am Coll Cardiol* 1999; **34**:1262–47.
21. Peterson ED, DeLong ER, Muhlbaier LH, Rosen AB, Buell HE, Kiefe CI, *et al.* Challenges in comparing risk-adjusted bypass surgery mortality results: results from the Cooperative Cardiovascular Project. *J Am Coll Cardiol* 2000; **36**:2174–84.
22. Tu JV, Schull MJ, Ferris LE, Hux JE, Redelmeier DA. Problems for clinical judgement: 4. Surviving in the report card era. *Can Med Assoc J* 2001; **164**:1709–12.
23. Schneider EC, Lieberman T. Publicly disclosed information about the quality of health care: response of the US public. *Qual Health Care* 2001; **10**:96–103.
24. Shahian DM, Yip W, Westcott G, Jacobson J. Selection of a cardiac surgery provider in the managed care era. *J Thorac Cardiovasc Surg* 2000; **120**:978–87.
25. Shahian DM, Normand SL, Torchiana DF, Lewis SM, Pastore JO, Kuntz RE, *et al.* Cardiac surgery report cards: comprehensive review and statistical critique. *Ann Thorac Surg* 2001; **72**:2155–68.
26. Lagasse RS, Steinberg ES, Katz RI, Saubermann AJ. Defining quality of perioperative care by statistical process control of adverse outcomes. *Anesthesiology* 1995; **82**:1181–8.
27. Reason J. *Human Error.* Cambridge: Cambridge University Press, 1990.
28. Vincent C, Taylor-Adams S, Stanhope N. Framework for analyzing risk and safety in clinical medicine. *BMJ* 1998; **316**(7138):1154–7.
29. Weinger MB, Pantiskas C, Wiklund ME, Carstensen P. Incorporating human factors into the design of medical devices. *JAMA* 1998; **280**:1484.
30. Sexton JB, Thomas EJ, Helmreich RL. Error, stress, and teamwork in medicine and aviation: cross sectional surveys. *BMJ* 2000; **320**(7237):745–9.
31. Weick K, Sutcliffe KM. *Managing the Unexpected: Assuring High Performance in an Age of Complexity.* San Francisco: Jossey-Bass, 2001.
32. Kohn LT, Corrigan JM, Donaldson MS (eds). *To Err is Human: Building a Safer Health System.* Washington, DC: National Academy Press, 1999.
33. Bagian JP, Gosbee JW. Developing a culture of patient safety at the VA. *Ambul Outreach* 2000; **Spring**:25–9.
34. Simmons JC. How root-cause analysis can improve patient safety. *The Quality Letter* 2001; **13**:2–12.
35. Casarett D, Helms C. Systems errors versus physicians' errors: finding the balance in medical education. *Acad Med* 1999; **74**:19–22.

36. O'Connor GT, Plume SK, Olmstead EM, Coffin LH, Morton JR, Maloney CT, *et al.* A regional prospective study of in-hospital mortality associated with coronary artery bypass grafting. The Northern New England Cardiovascular Disease Study Group. *JAMA* 1991; **266**:803–9.

37. O'Connor GT, Plume SK, Olmstead EM, Morton JR, Maloney CT, Nugent WC, *et al.* A regional intervention to improve the hospital mortality associated with coronary artery bypass graft surgery. The Northern New England Cardiovascular Disease Study Group. *JAMA* 1996; **275**:841–6.

38. Plume SK, O'Connor GT, Olmstead EM. As originally published in 1994: Changes in patients undergoing coronary artery bypass grafting: 1987–1990. Updated in 2000. Northern New England Cardiovascular Disease Study Group. *Ann Thorac Surg* 2001; **72**:314–15.

39. O'Connor GT, Birkmeyer JD, Dacey LJ, Quinton HB, Marrin CA, Birkmeyer NJ, *et al.* Results of a regional study of modes of death associated with coronary artery bypass grafting. Northern New England Cardiovascular Disease Study Group. *Ann Thorac Surg* 1998; **66**:1323–8.

40. Leavitt BJ, O'Connor GT, Olmstead EM, Morton JR, Maloney CT, Dacey LJ, *et al.* Use of the internal mammary artery graft and in-hospital mortality and other adverse outcomes associated with coronary artery bypass surgery. *Circulation* 2001; **103**:507–12.

41. Dacey LJ, Munoz JJ, Johnson ER, Leavitt BJ, Maloney CT, Morton JR, *et al.* Effect of preoperative aspirin use on mortality in coronary artery bypass grafting patients. *Ann Thorac Surg* 2000; **70**:1986–90.

42. Birkmeyer NJ, Charlesworth DC, Hernandez F, Leavitt BJ, Marrin CA, Morton JR, *et al.* Obesity and risk of adverse outcomes associated with coronary artery bypass surgery. Northern New England Cardiovascular Disease Study Group. *Circulation* 1998; **97**:1689–94.

43. DeFoe GR, Ross CS, Olmstead EM, Surgenor SD, Fillinger MP, Groom RC, *et al.* Lowest hematocrit on bypass and adverse outcomes associated with coronary artery bypass grafting. Northern New England Cardiovascular Disease Study Group. *Ann Thorac Surg* 2001; **71**:769–76.

44. Birkmeyer JD, Quinton HB, O'Connor NJ, McDaniel MD, Leavitt BJ, Charlesworth DC, *et al.* The effect of peripheral vascular disease on long-term mortality after coronary artery bypass surgery. Northern New England Cardiovascular Disease Study Group. *Arch Surg* 1996; **131**:316–21.

45. Munoz JJ, Birkmeyer NJ, Dacey LJ, Birkmeyer JD, Charlesworth DC, Johnson ER, *et al.* Trends in rates of reexploration for hemorrhage after coronary artery bypass surgery. Northern New England Cardiovascular Disease Study Group. *Ann Thorac Surg* 1999; **68**:1321–5.

46. Fillinger MP, Surgenor SD, Hartman GS, Clark C, Dodds TM, Rassias AJ, *et al.* The association between heart rate and in-hospital mortality after coronary artery bypass graft surgery. *Anesth Analg* 2002; **95**:1483–8.

47. Shewhart WA. *Economic Control of Quality of Manufactured Product.* New York: D. Van Nostrand Company Inc., 1931.

48. Wheeler DJ. *Advanced Topics in Statistical Process Control. The Power of Shewhart's Charts.* Knoxville, TN: SPC Press Inc., 1995.

49. Shahian DM, Williamson WA, Svensson LG, Restuccia JD, D'Agostino RS. Applications of statistical quality control to cardiac surgery. *Ann Thorac Surg* 1996; **62**:1351–8; discussion 1358–9.

50. Nelson EC, Splaine ME, Batalden PB, Plume SK. Building measurement and data collection into medical practice. *Ann Intern Med* 1998; **128**:460–6.

51. Nelson EC, Splaine ME, Godfrey MM, Kahn V, Hess A, Batalden P, *et al.* Using data to improve medical practice by measuring processes and outcomes of care. *Jt Comm J Qual Improv* 2000; **26**:667–85.

52. Kaplan RS, Norton, David P. *The Balanced Scorecard. Translating Strategy into Action.* Boston: Harvard Business School Press, 1996.

25

The role of risk factor modification

JOHN McMURRAY AND CHRIS J PACKARD

INTRODUCTION

Risk factor modification in the general population

Classic epidemiological surveys initiated in the 1960s and 1970s revealed three major, highly prevalent risk factors for coronary heart disease (CHD): cigarette smoking, raised blood pressure and elevated plasma cholesterol. Most notable among the surveys are the Framingham Study,[1] conducted over decades in a small town near Boston; the large-scale Multiple Risk Factor Intervention Trial (MRFIT) study, which involved more than 300 000 participants;[2] and in the UK, the British Regional Heart Study.[3] MRFIT demonstrated for both cholesterol and blood pressure the continuous, graded nature of the association between these factors and CHD risk (Figure 25.1). In each case the bulk of the population in most Western countries and in a growing number of developing societies is spread over the curve, with about three-quarters in the moderate to high risk range, with cholesterol >5.0 mmol L^{-1} and diastolic blood pressure >80 mmHg. Lowering cholesterol and blood pressure has been shown to reduce the risk of CHD, and so it follows that disease prevention programs (including drug therapy if they are to be effective) need to be directed to large numbers of individuals, with consequent strain on healthcare systems. Conceptually, CHD prevention strategies are divided into

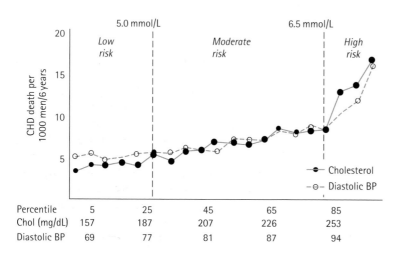

Figure 25.1 *Cholesterol, blood and coronary heart disease (CHD). Cholesterol and blood pressure have a continuous graded relationship to CHD mortality. Percentile refers to population cut-points. Arbitrary limits for low, moderate and high risks are denoted in mmol L^{-1} for cholesterol.[5,6] Figure adapted from reference 2. To convert mg dL^{-1} to mmol L^{-1} divide by 38.7.*

'primary', where subjects are asymptomatic members of the general population, and 'secondary', where patients exhibit signs or symptoms of CHD – myocardial infarction, angina – and thereby identify themselves as being in need of aggressive intervention.

The correct approach to primary prevention and risk factor modification in populations is a matter of current controversy and the subject of recent government guidelines in the UK.[4] The findings of the Framingham Study offer a way forward for physicians and public health bodies; equations have been produced[1] that calculate an individual's annual global CHD risk from a knowledge of demographic and lifestyle variables – age, gender, blood pressure, cholesterol levels, smoking habit and diabetes status (Table 25.1) – and this parameter can be used to prioritize people for treatment. The new National Cholesterol Education Program Adult Treatment Panel III (NCEP ATP III) guidelines[5] indicate that those with a risk of 2% or more per year are 'high risk' and require intensive intervention. This threshold is also promulgated in European guidelines,[6] but in the UK a figure of 3% per year is used.[4] The precise level chosen is secondary to the notion that a high-risk category of individuals who have not yet suffered a coronary event must be identified and those who fall within it given appropriate advice and treatment to prevent the first clinical manifestations of atherosclerotic disease.

Patients who present with established CHD need aggressive treatment not only to relieve any symptoms of ischemic coronary disease, but also to correct risk factors and so prevent future events. Intervention against major risk factors is as pertinent in secondary prevention as it is in primary prevention. Further investigation into the pathology of atherosclerosis and the accompanying thrombosis that leads to plaque growth and eventually an acute coronary event has led to the identification of a panoply of subsidiary risk factors (Table 25.1). Some, such as low density and high density lipoprotein and plasma triglyceride, add important details to known associations (i.e. that between total plasma cholesterol and risk), whereas others indicate that previously unrecognized mechanisms are at play in the etiology of CHD. Prime among these is inflammation; indeed, it has been suggested that atherosclerosis is fundamentally an inflammatory disease of the arterial wall.[7] Markers of chronic inflammation such as C-reactive protein (CRP) have been linked to the risk of first and recurrent myocardial infarction,[8,9] and of cerebrovascular disease.[10] There is still uncertainty as to whether high plasma CRP levels merely reflect the presence of widespread arterial disease or whether a heightened inflammatory state itself leads to the development of atherosclerotic lesions. In support of the latter scenario, evidence has been presented that a pro-inflammatory state can precede the clinical manifestation of arterial disease by 10 years.[8] Other elements of the infection–immunity pathways are becoming implicated as risk factors and potential causative agents in CAD. These include cell adhesion molecules that are expressed when endothelium binds circulating monocytes,[10,11] and macrophage-derived enzymes with potential pro-atherogenic properties.[12]

Table 25.1 *Major risk factors for coronary heart disease*

	High-risk categories
Classical	
Age	Men >45 years, women >55 years
Male gender	
Smoking	
Raised plasma (LDL) cholesterol	Cholesterol >5.0 mmol L^{-1}
Elevated blood pressure	>120/80 mmHg
Diabetes	
Family history of CHD	CHD in male <55, female <65
Low HDL cholesterol	HDLc <1.0 mmol L^{-1}
Obesity	BMI >30.0
New	
Pro-inflammatory factors	CRP >3 mg dL^{-1} (see references 8–10)
Fibrinogen	See reference 77
Lipoprotein(a)	Lp(a) >30 mg dL^{-1} (see reference 77)
Phospholipase A$_2$	See reference 12
Metabolic syndrome	See reference 5
Raised plasma triglyceride	Triglyceride >1.5 mmol L^{-1}
Small, dense LDL	See reference 78
Remnant lipoproteins	See reference 79
Homocysteine	Plasma level >14 μmol L^{-1} (see reference 80)

LDL, low density lipoprotein; CHD, coronary heart disease; HDLc, high density lipoprotein c; BMI, body mass index; CRP, C-reactive protein.

Risk factor modification after coronary artery surgery

Patients undergoing coronary artery bypass grafting (CABG) remain at high risk of cardiovascular events. For example, amongst the 1480 patients with a history of cardiac surgery randomized in the Clopidogrel versus Aspirin in Patients at Risk of Ischemic Events (CAPRIE) study, the *yearly* risk of vascular death, myocardial infarction, stroke or rehospitalization for ischemia was 22% in the aspirin group.[13] Clearly, in addition to graft failure, these individuals may develop new occlusions in ungrafted coronary vessels and in other arterial beds as the result of progression of the systemic atherosclerotic disease established by the time of surgery. Prior myocardial injury, present in many patients, increases the long-term incidence of heart failure. Concomitant hypertension, hypercholesterolemia and diabetes mellitus, also common in post-CABG patients, amplify the risk of adverse graft, arterial and myocardial events. Consequently, the medical management of the post-CABG patient includes not only interventions aimed at maintaining graft patency but also those targeted at reducing the progression of atherosclerosis elsewhere. Similarly, therapies to protect the damaged myocardium and treatments for concomitant 'aggravating' or 'accelerating' factors are often needed. Fortunately, many treatments have multiple actions, for example aspirin maintains graft patency and prevents arterial occlusion elsewhere; angiotensin-converting enzyme (ACE) inhibitors reduce the risk of both arterial occlusion and heart failure. Unfortunately, there is evidence that secondary prevention is neglected in these particularly high-risk patients.[14–16]

THERAPEUTIC APPROACHES IN REVASCULARIZED PATIENTS

Atherosclerosis has a multifactorial etiology and in patients with clinical manifestations of the disease it is essential to address all major risk factors with a combination of lifestyle changes and pharmacological agents. This therapeutic area is rich in clinical trials and it is possible in many instances to undertake true evidence-based medicine.

Hypertension

Hypertension is an important risk factor for future arterial occlusion, cerebral hemorrhage, heart failure and renal failure in any patient with CHD, including post-CABG patients. Indeed, hypertension has a particularly adverse prognostic impact in these post-surgery patients. In a Swedish observational study, the 5-year mortality rate in post-CABG patients with a history of hypertension was 16.9%, compared to 12.4% in patients with no such history ($P = 0.004$). Hypertensive survivors had more angina than non-hypertensives.[17]

There is a large body of clinical trial evidence to support the control of blood pressure as a means of preventing coronary and cerebrovascular disease. Classic studies using thiazide diuretics and beta-blockers showed that for a 5–6 mmHg reduction in diastolic blood pressure, there were reductions of about 16% in the risk of myocardial infarction and about 38% in the risk of stroke.[18] This was in line with the benefit predicted from epidemiology (see Figure 25.1).[19] Studies with calcium antagonists and ACE inhibitors have also shown significant risk reductions in a range of clinical end-points.[18] These were achieved in large part by the blood-pressure-lowering action of these

drugs, but possibly in the case of ACE inhibitors also through other ancillary effects (see below).

Cigarette smoking

The adverse impact of smoking on vascular outcome and non-vascular prognosis is well recognized in patients with and without CHD. Similarly, the vascular and other benefits obtained from smoking cessation are established.

Looking specifically at post-CABG patients, cigarette smoking is a powerful predictor of death, myocardial infarction, recurrence of angina and re-operation in most long-term series.[17,20–22] Similarly, as in other patients, smoking cessation is associated with a better prognosis than continued smoking after CABG. For example, in one recent study from Sweden, the 5-year mortality rate was 18.8% in smokers, 13.6% in ex-smokers and 12.5% in non-smokers ($P = 0.03$).[17] Consequently, there is good reason to actively promote smoking cessation in post-CABG patients, even using pharmacological aids (e.g. nicotine replacement therapy) as required.

Clotting: antiplatelet therapy

ASPIRIN

The use of aspirin in patients with CHD became widespread following publication of the Antiplatelet Trialists' Collaboration (ATC) in 1994.[23–25] This meta-analysis showed that antiplatelet therapy (mainly aspirin) reduced the risk of fatal and non-fatal vascular events in both 'low-risk' (primary prevention) and 'high-risk' (secondary prevention) populations. Clear-cut benefit was seen in 'high-risk' patients. For example, among 20 000 patients with a past history of myocardial infarction, 13% of patients receiving antiplatelet therapy suffered a vascular event, compared to 17% in the control group, i.e. a 2-year benefit of about 40 vascular events avoided per 1000 patients treated. Vascular events were defined as non-fatal myocardial infarctions, non-fatal strokes or vascular deaths. These events were, therefore, reduced by about one-quarter, and significantly so in all important subgroups of patients, for example middle-aged and older men and women, hypertensive and normotensive patients and diabetic and non-diabetic patients.

The ATC and others have also looked at the specific value of antiplatelet therapy in maintaining coronary graft patency.[24,26] When started 1 day preoperatively or on the day of surgery, aspirin is effective for up to 1 year in reducing the rate of saphenous vein occlusion. Approximately 90 occlusions are prevented per 1000 patients treated for an average of 7 months. The efficacy of aspirin beyond 1 year is uncertain. The addition of dipyridamole offers no further benefit over aspirin alone; neither are anticoagulants superior to aspirin. Aspirin does not improve internal mammary artery graft patency.[24,26]

CLOPIDOGREL

Clopidogrel is a thienopyridine derivative, related to ticlopidine, which inhibits platelet aggregation induced by adenosine diphosphate and as such is an effective alternative to aspirin. The evidence for this comes from two clinical trials.[27,28] The CAPRIE study[13,27] compared clopidogrel 75 mg to aspirin 325 mg (both taken once daily) in 19 185 patients with arterial disease (recent ischemic stroke, recent myocardial infarction or symptomatic peripheral arterial disease). The primary end-point was a composite of vascular death, myocardial infarction or ischemic stroke. After an average follow-up of 1.9 years, the annualized risk was 5.83% in the aspirin group and 5.32% in the clopidogrel group, a relative risk reduction of 8.7% ($P = 0.043$). Not surprisingly, given its mode of action and the dose used, aspirin caused more gastric side effects.[27]

The evidence that clopidogrel is an efficacious antiplatelet agent has recently been reinforced by the Clopidogrel in Unstable Angina to Prevent Recurrent Events (CURE) study.[28] In that study, clopidogrel *added* to aspirin significantly reduced major vascular events in patients with acute coronary syndromes (non-ST-segment elevation myocardial infarction and unstable angina). A loading dose of 300 mg followed by 75 mg daily of clopidogrel was given. The dose of aspirin was 75–325 mg daily alone or in combination and average follow-up was 9 months. A 20% relative risk reduction in cardiovascular death, myocardial infarction or stroke was found in the combination group. Treating 1000 patients for 9 months would thus prevent 28 major events in 23 patients at a cost of three life-threatening bleeds and three other transfusions. Clopidogrel is, therefore, a more expensive alternative to aspirin in aspirin-intolerant patients. The place of clopidogrel as an antiplatelet agent to use in addition to aspirin in the long term has yet to be determined.

There is no direct evidence concerning the effect of clopidogrel on coronary vein graft patency, though ticlopidine, sharing a similar mechanism of action to clopidogrel, is effective in maintaining patency. Furthermore, in the subset of 1480 patients with a prior history of cardiac surgery randomized into CAPRIE, the relative risk of vascular death was 43% lower in the clopidogrel group than in the aspirin group (reduced from 3.3% to 2%, $P = 0.03$).[13] The yearly rate of the combined end-point of vascular death, myocardial infarction, stroke or re-hospitalization was reduced from 52.9% in the aspirin group to 39.7% in the clopidogrel group (relative risk reduction 22.4%, $P = 0.001$). Though this is a retrospective subgroup analysis of CAPRIE, it does support the use of clopidogrel as an alternative to aspirin in intolerant patients.

Arrhythmia and cardioprotection

ANGIOTENSIN CONVERTING ENZYME INHIBITORS

Angiotensin converting enzyme inhibitors improve survival in patients with chronic heart failure and left ventricular systolic dysfunction.[29] These drugs also delay or prevent the onset of overt heart failure in patients with asymptomatic left ventricular systolic dysfunction (LVSD).[29] More recently, ACE inhibitors have been shown to be of value in patients with myocardial infarction and patients with arterial disease (or a high risk of arterial disease).[29–32]

Three large trials have shown that short-term, early use of ACE inhibitors (i.e. over the first few days and weeks after acute myocardial infarction) leads to a small but significant reduction in mortality (similar to that seen with intravenous beta-blockers), a conclusion supported by a recent meta-analysis.[30]

Clinical trials have also shown that ACE inhibitor therapy started in the first few days and weeks and continued long-term substantially reduced morbidity and mortality in *high-risk* myocardial infarction survivors.[31] The studies identified high-risk patients on the basis of having LVSD or evidence of acute heart failure complicating myocardial infarction, and showed that overall there was a 28% reduction in death, myocardial infarction and hospital admissions for heart failure in patients with left ventricular dysfunction after myocardial infarction treated with ACE inhibitors.[31] This equates to 70 patients having at least one event prevented for every 1000 patients treated. Consequently, all such high-risk myocardial infarction survivors should receive lifelong ACE inhibitor treatment.

We did not know, however, until recently whether other myocardial infarction survivors (i.e. those without LVSD or acute heart failure) should receive lifelong treatment with an ACE inhibitor. The Heart Outcomes Prevention Evaluation (HOPE) study has answered this question.[32] In HOPE, 9297 patients at high risk of vascular events (by virtue of having prior stroke/transient ischemic attack, CHD, peripheral arterial disease or diabetes plus another vascular risk factor) were randomized to placebo or ramipril (target dose 10 mg once daily). The primary end-point was a composite of cardiovascular death, myocardial infarction or stroke. After an average follow-up of 5 years, the cumulative event rate was 17.8% in the placebo group and 14% in the ramipril group ($P < 0.001$). All-cause mortality was also reduced (from 12.2% to 10.4%, $P = 0.005$), as was the need for 'revascularization procedures', e.g. percutaneous coronary angioplasty, coronary artery bypass surgery (from 18.3% to 16%, $P = 0.002$).[32] Collectively, therefore, these studies argue persuasively for treatment of all patients with coronary artery disease with an ACE inhibitor. Patients with significant myocardial damage and LVSD obtain particular benefit.

The role of ACE inhibitors in maintaining graft patency has not been specifically studied. However, in one relatively small trial (the Quinapril On Vascular Ace and Determinants of Ischemia – QUO VADIS – study), this type of treatment did reduce the risk of 'clinical ischemic events' in post-CABG patients.[33] Of 148 patents randomized to placebo or quinapril, started 1 month before surgery and continued for 1 year, 15% of the former and 4% of the latter (hazard ratio 0.23, $P = 0.02$) experienced such an event (myocardial infarction, stroke, recurrent angina pectoris or percutaneous revascularization).

It is also worth noting that 26% of the 9297 patients randomized in HOPE had a history of CABG.[32] Though a subgroup analysis has not been reported for these subjects, it is highly likely that the substantial benefit of ramipril, seen overall, was present in this subset of patients.

BETA-BLOCKERS

The long-standing evidence that beta-blockers reduce the risk of death and recurrent myocardial infarction in patients suffering a myocardial infarction has recently been reinforced by the Carvedilol Post Infarct Survival Control in Left Ventricular Dysfunction (CAPRICORN) study.[34] This trial focused on high-risk post-myocardial infarction patients with significant LVSD. These higher risk patients, many of whom also go on to develop acute heart failure, were probably excluded from the earlier beta-blocker trials. Recent trials had shown that ACE inhibitors substantially reduce morbidity and mortality in these patients. Consequently, CAPRICORN randomized patients with acute myocardial infarction complicated by LVSD to either placebo ($n = 984$) or carvedilol ($n = 975$), given in *addition* to full conventional therapy, including an ACE inhibitor. After an average follow-up of 1.3 years, 116 (12%) patients in the carvedilol group and 151 (15%) in the placebo group died, i.e. mortality was reduced by 23% ($P = 0.03$). Non-fatal re-infarction occurred in 34 (3%) in the carvedilol group and in 57 (6%) in the placebo group, i.e. 41% reduction ($P = 0.014$).[34] This important new trial reiterates the value of beta-blockers post-myocardial infarction, even in the modern era of myocardial infarction management.

The findings of the CAPRICORN are also consistent with those of new studies showing that beta-blockers result in a mortality relative risk reduction of about 35% in patients with heart failure and LVSD.[35] It is of particular note that beta-blockers reduce the risk of *sudden death* post-myocardial infarction and in congestive heart failure, something no other treatment does convincingly. Clearly, therefore, beta-blocker therapy should be continued after CABG in patients with prior myocardial infarction, LVSD or heart failure.

Two further comments are worth making about beta-blockers. These drugs appear to reduce the risk of death and acute coronary events in high-risk patients undergoing vascular surgery.[36] Recently, beta-blocker treatment has been shown to have a prophylactic benefit in preventing recurrent atrial fibrillation after cardioversion.[37] These additional properties may also be attractive in the treatment of CABG patients.

Lipid–lowering therapy

Cholesterol is insoluble in the aqueous medium of blood plasma and is transported with other lipids and key proteins in the form of lipoprotein complexes. These complexes fall into two families: those that contain apolipoprotein B (ApoB) as the major protein and those that contain apolipoprotein A (ApoA). ApoB-containing lipoproteins – chylomicrons, very low density lipoprotein (VLDL), low density lipoprotein (LDL) – carry triglyceride and cholesterol from sites of synthesis (liver) or absorption (gut) to tissues that utilize the lipids for energy production (skeletal muscle), storage (adipose tissue), cell membrane production or bile acid production (liver). ApoA-containing lipoproteins (high density lipoproteins, HDL) facilitate a 'reverse cholesterol transport' pathway, acquiring cholesterol from body tissues and carrying it back to the liver, the only organ capable of excreting the lipid in substantial quantities. Observations in the rural areas of developing countries, in young individuals and in primates, indicate that the body's needs for lipid can be met by a relatively low circulatory level of ApoB-containing lipoproteins, for example LDL cholesterol <2.0 mmol L^{-1}. In some people, concentrations above this are the result of inherited disorders, but in most (i.e. the bulk of the population in the USA and Europe – see Figure 25.1) are a consequence of surfeit. Diets high in saturated fat, and central adiposity, are major causes of raised LDL.

Lowering LDL and raising HDL in the bloodstream are the targets for lifestyle and pharmacological intervention. The evidence base for the benefits of LDL reduction is extensive; indeed, it is one of the most researched therapeutic approaches in medicine. A small number of clinical trials have been conducted to show that increasing HDL leads to reduced coronary morbidity and mortality, but the weight of evidence at present is not as strong as for LDL reduction. The relationship of plasma triglyceride and the particles that carry it – chylomicrons and VLDL – to risk has been a matter of controversy. Variation in plasma triglyceride is linked metabolically with change in HDL, and it is difficult in multivariate statistical models of trials to discern which perturbation – fall in triglyceride or rise in HDL – is responsible for the observed benefit. At present, reduction in plasma triglyceride *per se* is not a target in expert guidelines on lipid intervention.[5,6]

MECHANISM OF BENEFIT

The 'cholesterol hypothesis' – that lowering plasma (LDL) cholesterol would lead to a lower incidence of coronary disease – is now established as a fact. Over the last 7 years, publication of a series of trials has shown that treatment, especially with cholesterol synthesis inhibitors (statins), leads across a wide spectrum of subjects to reductions in angina, in the need for revascularization, in myocardial infarction, in sudden coronary death and in stroke.[38,39] Figure 25.2 depicts the major intervention studies, most of which are statin based but two used drugs of the fibrate class. Not shown is a large number of angiography-based studies, which explored the usefulness of lipid lowering in slowing the growth of atherosclerotic plaque and in some instances the potential for atherosclerosis regression. In general, in trials such as the Post Coronary Artery Bypass Trial (Post CABG study),[40] the Cholesterol Lowering Atherosclerosis Study (CLAS),[41] and the Familial Atherosclerosis Treatment Study (FATS),[42] treatment with lipid-lowering agents produced lesion stasis or slowed progression of disease as assessed by indices such as minimum lumen diameter. More impressive in these studies, however, was the reduction in the number of coronary events, which seemed out of all proportion to the decrease in atherosclerotic burden. These findings linked to new pathological studies have led to the important conclusion that the major determinant of risk of a coronary event is not plaque size but plaque fragility.

The effects of lipid regulation are now understood in terms of the net influence that treatment has on the stability of the cap of atherosclerotic plaques. It is postulated that plasma LDL reduction, especially by statins, leads to less 'damaged' (i.e. oxidized) LDL being present in lesions and hence less provocation of the inflammatory system.

A reduction in the number of inflammatory cells in a plaque allows smooth muscle cells to populate the cap, lay down collagen and hence stabilize the entire lesion. This may not be accompanied by a change in the size of the plaque, but will reduce dramatically the potential for rupture and the chance of precipitating an event. Statins have been suggested by some investigators to have serendipitously other anti-inflammatory and anti-thrombotic properties that may add to the benefits arising from simple reduction in LDL.[43]

STATINS IN PRIMARY AND SECONDARY PREVENTION

The results from clinical trials of lipid-lowering agents and the implications for coronary prevention in the general population have been the subject of several excellent reviews.[44,45] In summary, the West of Scotland Coronary Prevention Study (WOSCOPS)[46] and the Air Force/Texas Coronary Atherosclerosis Prevention Study (AF/Tex CAPS)[47] were primary prevention trials of pravastatin and lovastatin respectively. The former recruited hypercholesterolemic, high-risk men, and the latter men and women with low to normal cholesterol but a low HDL. Concordance between the results of these studies was remarkable. The end-points of cardiovascular mortality, non-fatal myocardial infarction and new hospitalizations for angina were reduced by about one-third by statin treatment. A similar fall was seen in the rate of revascularization (CABG, PTCA). This was achieved with no detectable adverse effect of drug therapy and, in the case of WOSCOPS, with a borderline significant reduction in total mortality.[46] The major secondary prevention trials recruited those with established disease who had high (Scandinavian Simvastatin Survival Study, 4S),[38] average (Long-term Intervention with Pravastatin in Ischemic Disease, LIPID),[48] or low (Cholesterol and Recurrent Events, CARE)[39] plasma cholesterol concentrations. The incidence of recurrent myocardial infarction was 20–40% less on statin treatment and, in the case of LIPID and 4S, cardiovascular and total mortality was substantially decreased. Other manifestations of coronary artery disease such as ischemic episodes and heart failure were also diminished by simvastatin in the 4S trial,[49] and subgroup analysis revealed that virtually all patients benefited from statin treatment.[50] Likewise, in the Pravastatin Pooling Project we found that men and women, those under and over the age of 65 years, diabetics and smokers all achieve the same relative risk reduction on treatment.[51] This observation has given rise to acceptance of the important principle that statin therapy should be directed towards those at highest absolute risk of an acute coronary event since such people will enjoy the greatest benefit and hence be the most cost effective to treat.[44] Virtually all patients attending for coronary surgery fall into this category.

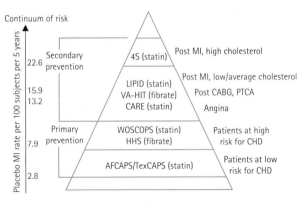

Figure 25.2 *Cholesterol-lowering trials in primary and secondary prevention. The trials are depicted in a pyramid to illustrate that at lower risk a greater proportion of the population is addressed as candidates for intervention. HHS, Helsinki Heart Study;*[76] *other abbreviations are explained in the text.*

Specific studies or elements of the major trials described above examined the effectiveness of lipid-lowering therapy in subjects with unstable angina, those with angiographically proven coronary artery disease and those who had coronary artery bypass surgery or cardiac transplantation. All again appear to benefit from LDL reduction with a statin. For example, 4S and LIPID included subjects who had angina but had not yet had a myocardial infarction and found that these individuals had a risk reduction equivalent to that seen for post-myocardial infarction patients. In the Atorvastatin versus Revascularization Treatment (AVERT) trial,[52] the question was posed as to whether medical therapy with a high-dose statin gave a comparable outcome to angioplasty in patients with angina. The study has been criticized for its design and lack of a control group, but the results showing less recurrent angina and fewer events in those randomized to statin suggest strongly that drug therapy should be instituted early once a diagnosis of angina is made. MIRACL (Myocardial Ischemia Reduction with Aggressive Cholesterol Lowering),[53] a trial of statin initiation immediately post-myocardial infarction, also provided evidence that lipid-lowering therapy should be begun as soon as a diagnosis of atherothrombotic arterial disease is made. However, statin treatment in post-angioplasty trials has so far failed to reduce the incidence of restenosis.[54] This may be due to a differing underlying cellular pathology in this induced arterial disease that is not responsive to lipid lowering or other statin effects.

CLINICAL TRIALS IN THE POST–CABG PATIENT

Trials that have specifically addressed the benefits of lipid-lowering therapy in patients who have undergone CABG include the Post CABG trial[40] and CLAS.[41] CLAS used a drug regimen of colestipol plus niacin and demonstrated after 2 years a reduction in atherosclerosis progression due to the 43% LDL reduction and 37% HDL increase. Further observations from this study were that new lesions were more prevalent in bypass grafts than native arteries, and that mild/moderate lesions (<50% stenosis) were more predictive of future coronary events than severe ones. The Post CABG trial randomized patients to moderate or aggressive lipid lowering; on-medication LDL levels in these groups were 2.4 mmol L^{-1} and 3.5 mmol L^{-1} respectively. Repeat angiography 4.3 years after baseline revealed the superiority of more aggressive treatment: 27% showed lesion progression versus 39% (P <0.001) in the moderate therapy group. Extended 7.5-year follow-up of trial participants revealed a 30% reduction in the rate of revascularization in the aggressively compared to moderately treated patients; further, there were 24% fewer clinical end-points in the former subjects.[55] Other recent studies confirm the substantial benefits of lipid correction in cardiac surgery preoperatively and postoperatively.[56,57]

STATINS AND CARDIAC TRANSPLANTATION

Raised cholesterol levels are common after transplantation and this increases the risks of vasculopathy and adverse coronary events. Thus, judicious use of statins to reduce the impact of hyperlipidemia is now accepted practice among transplant surgeons. Kobashigawa et al.[58] reported also that pravastatin had beneficial effects on the incidence of rejection causing hemodynamic compromise, on survival and on the incidence of vasculopathy. They suggested that the drug's effect was in part due to an influence on the natural T-cell killer activity (an observation that has not been reproduced consistently).[59] Reports have appeared documenting cases of rhabdomyolosis with statin when used in combination with other drugs (gemfibrozil, cylosporine) post-transplant.[60] Fortunately, these incidents are rare and their incidence may depend on the statin used. In this regard, pravastatin, with its general lack of drug–drug interaction and its independence of the cytochrome P450 mechanism for clearance, may be the statin of choice in transplanted patients.

Diabetes

Patients with type II diabetes suffer a particularly aggressive form of atherosclerosis. They appear to exist in a chronic inflammatory state, which predisposes them to lesion development. On presentation, diabetics often have unremarkable LDL levels but an elevation in plasma triglyceride and low HDL cholesterol. Intuitively, the best drug to correct the hyperlipidemia is a fibrate, which will produce clinical benefits as seen in the Veterans Affairs High-Density Lipoprotein Cholesterol Intervention (VA-HIT) trial.[61] However, statins have also been shown to be highly effective at reducing CHD risk in type II diabetics,[62,63] possibly due to their lipid-lowering and anti-inflammatory properties. Given the poor prognosis for the diabetic with established CHD (in 4S, 50% of diabetics who had had a myocardial infarction had a recurrent event within 5 years)[63] and post-coronary artery bypass,[64] the treatment of dyslipidemia and hypertension should be both immediate and aggressive. An argument can be made that all the type II diabetics should receive statin therapy unless contraindicated.

Hormone replacement therapy

Expectation was high that estrogen replacement in women would, in addition to relieving menopausal symptoms and the risk of osteoporosis, prevent CHD due to the LDL-lowering and HDL-raising properties of the hormone. However, trials such as the Heart and Estrogen/Progestin Replacement Study (HERS)[65] have shown that there is little CHD risk reduction with oral hormone replacement therapy (HRT). It appears that the potential benefits of the lipoprotein changes are offset by an increased thrombotic tendency. Therefore the current recommendation is that, while women on HRT should not stop their medication, those being considered for treatment should have their cardiovascular risk status taken into account; concomitant prescription of a statin may be indicated if there are pressing reasons to give HRT in women with CHD.

Atrial fibrillation

Atrial fibrillation, though usually transient, afflicts 20–30% of CABG patients in the first few days after surgery. If this persists in the longer term, oral anticoagulation may be indicated in order to reduce the risk of thromboembolism, particularly stroke. Guidelines on the indications for this form of treatment are widely available.[66] Broadly, warfarin is advocated in patients with any 'high-risk factor' (e.g. prior stroke/transient ischemic attack or thromboembolism, history of hypertension, LVSD, rheumatic mitral valve disease or age >75 years) or more than one 'moderate-risk factor' (e.g. age 65–75 years, diabetes mellitus, CHD). Clearly many, if not the majority, of patients undergoing CABG will have an indication for warfarin (with a target INR of 2.0–3.0) if atrial fibrillation persists. The drug of choice for ventricular rate control is a beta-blocker (because of the other potential benefits of such treatment in these patients) and *not* digoxin.[67] In the longer term, electrical cardioversion may be indicated.

Chronic heart failure

More patients with congestive heart failure due to LVSD are undergoing CABG. These patients have particularly high long-term rates of morbidity (hospitalization) and mortality. The beneficial effects of ACE inhibitors and beta-blockers in reducing these risks have been described earlier, as have the other favorable therapeutic actions of these agents. Patients with persistent signs and symptoms of congestive heart failure show a reduced risk of hospital admission and better survival if also given low-dose (25 mg) spironolactone once daily.[68] Digoxin may also be used, as a last resort, for symptom benefit and in order to reduce the risk of hospital admission.[69]

MANAGEMENT GUIDELINES

Learned societies and organizations around the world have generated guidelines that focus primarily on a single risk factor, for example raised blood pressure or elevated cholesterol, but few take a holistic, patient-centered approach. Thus the physician is often left to balance competing aims when attempting to practice evidence-based but practical intervention. There is a need to address systematically the optimum medical treatment of the post-revascularization or post-transplant patient. The following discussion sets out current guidelines on the correction of hypertension and hyperlipidemia and deals with acute and chronic problems that can follow coronary surgery.

Lifestyle

DIET

Adoption of a prudent diet is the cornerstone of coronary disease prevention. Nutritional guidelines are offered by both hypertension and hyperlipidemia expert groups.[5,6,18] It is unlikely in most cardiac surgery patients that diet alone will achieve therapeutic targets, and medical treatment as noted above should be started virtually immediately on referral. That said, an improved diet may have beneficial effects beyond cholesterol lowering and should not be neglected. Of particular interest in the coronary patient is the effect of fish and fish oils.[70]

ALCOHOL

Much has been written about the potential cardiac benefits of moderate alcohol consumption. It is an observation that alcohol intake has a U-shaped relationship to coronary risk, with a minimum around about 14 units per week.[71,72] Alcohol has HDL-raising properties, possibly through its action on circulating lipid transfer proteins,[73] but it also increases plasma triglyceride. It seems sensible to take a pragmatic approach, given the information available. Patients should be warned of the dangers of excessive alcohol consumption. Those who do not drink alcohol should not start. Moderate drinkers should be advised to limit their intake to one to two glasses of wine (or equivalent in units of alcohol) per day. Regular consumption at this level may indeed help reduce their risk of future coronary events.

EXERCISE

Most rehabilitation programs post-CABG include an exercise component.[74] Exercise increases the feeling of well-being and functional capacity, but there is no good evidence that it improves prognosis in terms of atherothrombosis risk. However, patients whose exercise training leads to a change in peak exercise capacity enjoy a better long-term outcome,[75] possibly due to more complete revascularization and better ventricular function.

Guide to hypertension treatment

International guidelines for the treatment of hypertension[18] lay out optimal lifestyle and drug-based approaches to blood pressure lowering. Weight reduction is important in those who are more than 10% overweight, and significant decreases in blood pressure can accompany weight losses of as little as 5 kg. Increased physical exercise, moderation of alcohol intake in overweight drinkers and reduced salt intake, especially in the elderly, have all been shown to be beneficial. These changes will also impact favorably on other risk factors such as raised cholesterol levels and insulin resistance. The principles of drug treatment are, where possible, to use agents tested in trials, start with low-dose regimens and use appropriate combinations to maximize hypotensive efficacy while minimizing side effects. In patients on a number of medications, once-a-day preparations will help improve compliance. Arterial pressure should be lowered to <140 mmHg systolic and <85 mmHg diastolic, in keeping with current guidelines (targets are <130/<80 mmHg in diabetics).

The choice of drug should be influenced by the aforementioned cardioprotective effects of ACE inhibitors and beta-blockers. Thereafter, thiazide diuretics are the drug of choice. Calcium-channel blockers should be used with caution in patients with LVSD, as they increase the risk of developing congestive heart failure and because there is still uncertainty about their prognostic effect in CHD. Alpha-adrenoreceptor antagonists (alpha-blockers) are probably a last resort in this patient population, as they may increase the risk of developing congestive heart failure compared with other antihypertensive agents.

GUIDE TO LIPID MANAGEMENT

Guidelines for lipid management in primary and secondary prevention have been published by many authorities worldwide, notably by National Cholesterol Education Program (NCEP) in the USA[5] and the European Atherosclerosis Society (EAS) in Europe.[6] All agree on the need for LDL lowering in subjects exhibiting signs or symptoms of coronary artery disease. Benefits are seen (as described above) in slowing atherosclerosis progression in native and grafted vessels, maintaining graft viability and preventing the first or recurrent coronary event. The weight of evidence indicates that treatment should be initiated as soon as the patient is diagnosed as suffering from atherosclerotic disease of any artery, ideally before surgery. Thus virtually all patients seen by cardiac surgeons for management of the clinical consequences of atherothrombotic arterial disease need lipid-correcting treatments, usually a drug. Most will have a plasma cholesterol above the treatment threshold of 5.0 mmol L^{-1} or a LDL cholesterol >3.0 mmol L^{-1} (130 mg dL^{-1}). A statin is the drug of choice for the vast majority of patients. Which one to use can depend on a number of factors, including evidence base and local policy. Some, such as atorvastatin, have less extensive trial evidence but are superior at LDL reduction; others, like pravastatin, have a wealth of clinical data relating to their safety and efficacy in a wide range of patients and conditions. The goal of treatment in current guidelines is to reduce LDL below 3.0 mmol L^{-1} (130 mg dL^{-1}). However, results from the Post CABG trial[40,55] have prompted many to adopt 100 mg dL^{-1} (about 2.5 mmol L^{-1}) as the goal in the CABG patient. This downward move in LDL target has often been reinforced by the results of the Heart Protection Study (HPS),[62] which examined benefits in specific subgroups, in particular patients whose starting LDL was <100 mg dL^{-1} as well as those in the 100–130 mg dL^{-1} range. In contrast to the findings of the CARE trial,[39] in which no decrease in risk was seen in those with an initial LDL <125 mg dL^{-1}, the risk reduction in HPS was uniform across all categories of LDL level.

Less clear at present is when to use fibrates, a separate class of lipid-lowering drugs with weaker LDL lowering than statins but greater effects on plasma triglyceride and HDL. The VA-HIT study[61] showed that fibrate treatment was effective in reducing coronary events in subjects with low HDL and low LDL. Thus drugs such as gemfibrozil and fenofibrate are options for patients with this lipid profile. They are also considered first-line agents for the treatment of hypertriglyceridemia. Fibrates can be used in combination with statins for patients with combined hyperlipidemia. However, as there have been reports of side effects with the lovastatin/gemfibrozil combination, it may be best to avoid giving these particular drugs together; results with other combinations indicate less of a potential problem.[60] More frequent monitoring of liver function tests and creatinine kinase (CK) is prudent when fibrates and statins are combined.

CONCLUDING REMARKS

Successful completion of a cardiac surgery procedure provides the patient with a new beginning. However, his or her propensity for atherothrombotic disease is unchanged unless steps are taken to alter lifestyle factors and to correct dyslipidemia and hypertension. The message of the preceding discussion is that there is a strong evidence base for aggressive medical intervention, and for some agents this should begin (if not already commenced) immediately following referral. A suggested approach is appropriate evaluation of the patient's risk factor status and adoption of the 'ABCD' of secondary prevention, i.e.:

- A – antiplatelet therapy, ACE inhibitor,
- B – beta-blocker, blood pressure control,
- C – cholesterol reduction, cigarette cessation,
- D – diet (exercise), diabetic control.

Compliance with medical therapy then becomes the key issue. The surgeon is in a unique position to reinforce this and to emphasize that, for a number of drugs, treatment is lifelong if the benefits of the operative procedure are not to be undone.

KEY REFERENCES

Furberg CD, Psaty B, Pahor M, Alderman M. Clinical implications of recent findings from the Antihypertensive and Lipid Lowering Treatment to prevent Heart Attack Trial (ALLHAT) and other studies of hypertension. *Ann Intern Med* 2001; **135**:1074–8.
An authoritative review including a meta-analysis of antihypertensive drugs showing that benefit may vary according to the class of drug used to lower blood pressure.

Gaw A, Packard CJ, Shepherd J (eds). *Statins: the HMG CoA Reductase Inhibitors in Perspective*. London: Martin Dunitz Ltd, 2000.
A useful book, reviewing the development of statins as lipid-lowering drugs. Chapters describe the major lipid trials and current guidelines for statin use.

Libby P. Atherosclerosis: the new view. *Sci Am* 2002; **286**: 46–55.
An excellent overview for the popular scientific press of the new paradigm for atherosclerosis. Inflammation is presented in the 'new view' as a fundamental mechanism involved in plaque initiation and plaque rupture.

McMurray JJ. Heart failure in 10 years time: focus on pharmacological treatment. *Heart* 2002; **88**(Suppl. 2):40–6.
The last decade has seen breakthroughs in the treatment of heart failure with ACE inhibitors, beta-blockers and spironolactone. This review describes future therapeutic strategies to blunt the projected rise in congestive heart failure over the coming years.

Straus SE, Majumdar SR, McAlister FA. New evidence for stroke prevention: a scientific review. *JAMA* 2002; **18**: 1388–95.
This review is a recent update of the 'state of the art' in stroke prevention. It includes a meta-analysis of trials on the primary and secondary prevention of stroke. Emphasis is placed on the benefits of blood pressure reduction, treatment of hyperlipidemia and use of anti-thrombotic therapy.

REFERENCES

1. Anderson KM, Wilson PWF, Odell PM, Kannel WB. An updated coronary risk profile. *Circulation* 1991; **83**:357–63.
2. Martin MJ, Hulley SB, Browner WS, Kuller LH, Wentworth D. Serum cholesterol, blood pressure and mortality: implications from a cohort of 361 662 men. *Lancet* 1986: **2**(8513):933–6.
3. Pocock SJ, Shaper AG, Phillips AN. Concentrations of high density lipoproteins, triglycerides and total cholesterol in ischaemic heart disease. *BMJ* 1989; **298**:998–1002.
4. Standing Medical Academy Committee. *The Use of Statins*. 11061 HCD Aug 97 (04). London: Department of Health, 1997.
5. Executive summary of the third report of the National Cholesterol Education Program (NCEP). Expert Panel on the detection, evaluation and treatment of high blood cholesterol in adults (Adult Treatment Panel III). *JAMA* 2001; **285**:2486–97.
6. Wood D, De Backer G, Faergeman O, Graham I, Marcia G, Pyorala K. Prevention of coronary heart disease in clinical practice: recommendations of the Second Joint Task Force of European and other Societies on Coronary Prevention. *Atherosclerosis* 1998; **140**:199–270.
7. Ross R. Atherosclerosis – an inflammatory disease. *N Engl J Med* 1999; **340**:115–26.
8. Ridker PM, Cushman M, Stampfer J, Tracy RP, Hennekens CH. Inflammation, aspirin and risks of cardiovascular disease in apparently healthy men. *N Engl J Med* 1997; **336**:973–9.
9. Ridker PM, Rifai N, Pfeffer MA, Sacks FM, Moye LA, Goldman S, *et al.* Inflammation, pravastatin and the risk of coronary events after myocardial infarction in patients with average cholesterol levels. Cholesterol and Recurrent Events (CARE) Investigators. *Circulation* 1998; **98**:839–44.
10. Ridker PM, Hennekens CH, Buring JE, Rifai N. C-reactive protein and other markers of inflammation in the prediction of cardio-vascular disease in women. *N Engl J Med* 2000; **342**:836–43.
11. de Caterina R. Endothelial dysfunctions: common denominators in vascular disease. *Curr Opin Lipidol* 2000; **11**:9–23.
12. Packard CJ, O'Reilly D, Caslake MJ, McMahon AD, Ford I, Cooney J, *et al.* Lipoprotein-associated phospholipase A_2, as an independent predictor of coronary heart disease. West of Scotland Coronary Prevention Study Group. *N Engl J Med* 2000; **343**:1148–55.
13. Bhatt DL, Chew DP, Hirsch AT, Ringleb PA, Hack W, Topol EJ. Superiority of clopidogrel versus aspirin in patients with prior cardiac surgery. *Circulation* 2001; **103**:363–8.
14. Allen JK, Blumenthal RS, Margolis S, Young DR. Status of secondary prevention in patients undergoing coronary revascularization. *Am J Cardiol* 2001; **87**:1203–6.
15. Irving RJ, Oram SH, Boyd J, Rutledge P, McRae F, Bloomfield P. Ten year audit of secondary prevention in coronary bypass patients. *BMJ* 2000; **321**:22–3.
16. EUROASPIRE II Study Group. Lifestyle and risk factor management and use of drug therapies in coronary patients from 15 countries; principal results from EUROASPIRE II Euro Heart Survey Programme. *Eur Heart J* 2001; **22**:554–72.
17. Herlitz J, Haglid M, Albertsson P, Westberg A, Karlson BW, Hartford M, *et al.* Short and long-term prognosis after coronary artery bypass grafting in relation to smoking habits. *Cardiology* 1997; **88**:492–7.
18. Guidelines Subcommittee. 1999 World Health Organization International Society of Hypertension Guidelines for the management of hypertension. *J Hypertens* 1999; **17**:151–83.
19. Collins R, Peto R, MacMahon S, Hebert P, Fiebach NH, Eberlein KA, *et al.* Blood pressure, stroke, and coronary heart disease. Part 2: Short-term reductions in blood pressure: overview of randomised drug trials in their epidemiological context. *Lancet* 1990; **335**:827–38.
20. Van Domburg RT, Meeter K, Van Berkel DF, Veldkamp RF, Van Herwerden LA, Bogers AJ. Smoking cessation reduces mortality after coronary artery bypass surgery: a 20 year follow-up study. *J Am Coll Cardiol* 2000; **36**:878–83.
21. Voors AA, Van Brussel BL, Plokker HW, Ernst SM, Koomer NM, Tijsse JG, *et al.* Smoking and cardiac events after venous coronary bypass surgery. A 15 year follow-up study. *Circulation* 1996; **93**:42–7.
22. Cavender JB, Rogers WJ, Fisher LD, Gersh BJ, Coggin CJ, Myers WO. Effects of smoking on survival and morbidity in patients randomized to medical or surgical therapy in the Coronary Artery Surgery Study (CASS): 10-year follow-up. *J Am Coll Cardiol* 1992; **20**:287–94.

23. Antiplatelet Trialists' Collaboration. Collaborative overview of randomised trials of antiplatelet therapy – I: Prevention of death, myocardial infarction, and stroke by prolonged antiplatelet therapy in various categories of patients. *BMJ* 1994; **308**:81–106.

24. Antiplatelet Trialists' Collaboration. Collaborative overview of randomised trials of antiplatelet therapy – II: Maintenance of vascular graft or arterial patency by antiplatelet therapy. *BMJ* 1994; **308**:159–68.

25. Antiplatelet Trialist's Collaboration. Collaborative overview of randomised trials of antiplatelet therapy – III: Reduction in venous thrombosis and pulmonary embolism by antiplatelet prophylaxis among surgical and medical patients. *BMJ* 1994; **308**:235–46.

26. Stein PD, Dalen JE, Goldman S, Theroux P. Anti-thrombotic therapy in patients with saphenous vein and internal mammary artery bypass grafts. *Chest* 2001; **119**(Suppl.);278–82S.

27. CAPRIE Steering Committee. A randomised, blinded trial of clopidogrel versus aspirin in patients at risk of ischemic events (CAPRIE). *Lancet* 1996; **348**:1329–39.

28. Yusuf S, Zhao F, Mehta SR, Chrolavicius S, Tognoni G, Fox KK. Effects of clopidogrel in addition to aspirin in patients with acute coronary syndromes without ST-segment elevation. *N Engl J Med* 2001; **345**:494–502.

29. Khalil ME, Basher AW, Brown EJ Jr, Alhaddad IA. A remarkable medical story: benefits of angiotensin-converting enzyme inhibitors in cardiac patients. *J Am Coll Cardiol* 2001; **37**: 1757–64.

30. ACE Inhibitor Myocardial Infarction Collaborative Group. Indications for ACE inhibitors in the early treatment of acute myocardial infarction: systematic overview of individual data from 100 000 patients in randomized trials. *Circulation* 1998; **97**:2202–12.

31. Flather MD, Yusuf S, Kober L, Pfeffer M, Hall A, Murray G, *et al.* Long-term ACE-inhibitor therapy in patients with heart failure or left-ventricular dysfunction: a systematic overview of data from individual patients. ACE-Inhibitor Myocardial Infarction Collaborative Group. *Lancet* 2000; **35**:1575–81.

32. Yusuf S, Sleight P, Pogue J, Bosch J, Davies R, Dagenais G. Effects of an angiotensin-converting-enzyme inhibitor, ramipril, on cardiovascular events in high-risk patients. Evaluation Study Investigators. The Heart Outcomes Prevention Evaluation Study. *N Engl J Med* 2000; **342**:145–53.

33. Oosterga M, Voors AA, Pinto YM, Buikema H, Grandjean JG, Kingma JH, *et al.* Effects of quinapril on clinical outcome after coronary artery bypass grafting (The QUO VADIS Study). *Am J Cardiol* 2001; **87**:542–6.

34. Dargie HJ. Effect of carvedilol on outcome after myocardial infarction in patients with left-ventricular dysfunction: the CAPRICORN randomised trial. *Lancet* 2001; **357**:1385–90.

35. Packer M. Current role of beta-adrenergic blockers in the management of chronic heart failure. *Am J Med* 2001; **110**(Suppl. 7A):81–94S.

36. Poldermans D, Boersma E, Bax JJ, Thomson IR, Paelinck B, van de Ven LL, *et al.* Bisoprolol reduces cardiac death and myocardial infarction in high-risk patients as long as 2 years after successful major vascular surgery. *Eur Heart J* 2001; **22**:1353–8.

37. Kuhlkamp V, Schirdewan A, Stangl K, Homberg M, Ploch M, Beck OA. Use of metoprolol CR/XL to maintain sinus rhythm after conversion from persistent atrial fibrillation: a randomized, double-blind, placebo-controlled study. *J Am Coll Cardiol* 2000; **36**:139–46.

38. Scandanavian Simvastatin Survival Study Group. Randomised trial of cholesterol lowering in 4444 patients with coronary heart disease: the Scandanavian Simvastatin Survival Study (4S). *Lancet* 1994; **344**:1383–9.

39. Sacks FM, Pfeffer MA, Moye LA, Rouleau JL, Rutherford JD, Cole TG, *et al.* The effect of pravastatin on coronary events after myocardial infarction in patients with average cholesterol levels. Cholesterol and Recurrent Events Trial investigators. *N Engl J Med* 1996; **335**:1001–9.

40. The Post Coronary Artery Bypass Graft Trial Investigators. The effect of aggressive lipid lowering of low-density lipoprotein cholesterol levels and low-dose anticoagulation on obstructive changes in saphenous-vein coronary-artery bypass grafts. *N Engl J Med* 1997; **336**:153–62.

41. Blankenhorn DH, Nessim SA, Johnson RL, Sanmarco ME, Azen SP, Cashin-Hemphill L. Beneficial effects of combined colestipol–niacin therapy on coronary atherosclerosis and coronary venous bypass grafts. *JAMA* 1987; **257**:3233–40.

42. Brown G, Albers JJ, Fisher ID, Schaefer FM, Lin JT, Kaplan C, *et al.* Regression of coronary artery disease as a result of intensive lipid-lowering in men with high levels of apolipoprotein B. *N Engl J Med* 1990; **323**:1289–98.

43. Rosenson RS, Tangney CC. Anti-atherothrombotic properties of statins: implications for cardiovascular event reduction. *JAMA* 1998; **279**:1643–50.

44. Shepherd J. Economics of lipid lowering in primary prevention: lessons from the West of Scotland Coronary Prevention Study. *Am J Cardiol* 2001; **87**(5A):19–22B.

45. La Rosa JC. Prevention and treatment of coronary heart disease: who benefit. *Circulation* 2001; **104**:1688–92.

46. Shepherd J, Cobbe SM, Ford I, Isles CG, Lorimer AR, MacFarlane PW, *et al.* Prevention of coronary heart disease with pravastatin in men with hypercholesterolemia. The West of Scotland Coronary Prevention Study Group. *N Engl J Med* 1995; **333**:1301–7.

47. Downs JR, Clearfield M, Weis S, Whitney E, Shapiro DR, Beere PA, *et al.* Primary prevention of acute coronary events with lovastatin in men and women with average cholesterol levels: results of AFCAPS/TexCAPS. Air Force/Texas Coronary Atherosclerosis Prevention Study. *JAMA* 1998; **279**:1615–22.

48. Long Term Intervention with Pravastatin in Ischaemic Disease (LIPID) Study Group. Prevention of cardiovascular events and death with pravastatin in patients with coronary heart disease and a broad range of initial cholesterol levels. *N Engl J Med* 1998; **339**:1349–57.

49. Pedersen TR, Kjekshus J, Pyorala K, Olsson AG, Cook TJ, Musliner TA, *et al.* Effect of simvastatin on ischemic signs and symptoms in the Scandanavian Simvastatin Survival Study (4S). *Am J Cardiol* 1998; **81**:333–5.

50. Miettinen TA, Pyorala K, Olsson AG, Musliner TA, Cook TJ, Faergeman O, *et al.* Cholesterol-lowering therapy in women and elderly patients with myocardial infarction or angina pectoris: findings from the Scandanavian Simvastatin Survival Study (4S.) *Circulation* 1997; **96**:4211–18.

51. Sacks FM, Tonkin AM, Shepherd J, Braunwald E, Cobbe S, Hawkins CM, *et al.* Effect of pravastatin on coronary disease events in subgroups defined by coronary risk factors: the Prospective Pravastatin Pooling Project. *Circulation* 2000; **102**:1893–900.

52. Pitt B, Waters D, Brown WV, van Boven AJ, Schwartz L, Title LM, Eisenberg D, *et al.* Aggressive lipid-lowering therapy compared with angioplasty in stable coronary artery disease. Atorvastatin versus Revascularization Treatment Investigators. *N Engl J Med* 1999; **341**:70–6.

53. Schwartz GG, Olsson AG, Ezekowitz MD, Ganz P, Oliver MF, Waters D, *et al.* Effects of atorvastatin on early recurrent ischemic events in acute coronary syndromes: the MIRACL study: a randomized controlled trial. *JAMA* 2001; **285**:1711–18.

54. Serruys PW, Foley DP, Jackson G, Bonnier H, Macaya C, Vrolix M, *et al.* A randomised placebo-controlled trial of fluvastatin for prevention of restenosis after successful coronary balloon angioplasty; final results of the Fluvastatin Angiographic Restenosis (FLARE) trial. *Eur Heart J* 1999; **20**:58–69.

55. Knatterud GL, Rosenberg Y, Campeau L, Geller NL, Hunninghake DB, Forman SA, et al. Long-term effects on clinical outcomes of aggressive lowering of low-density lipoprotein cholesterol levels and low-dose anticoagulation in the Post Coronary Artery Bypass Graft trial. Post CABG Investigators. Circulation 2000; 102:157–65.

56. Christenson JT. Preoperative lipid control with simvastatin reduces the risk for graft failure already 1 year after myocardial infarction. Cardiovasc Surg 2001; 9:33–43.

57. O'Rourke B, Babir M, Banner N, Yacoub M. Improved survival induced by long term statin therapy following cardiac transplantation correlates with lipid lowering effect. J Heart Lung Transplant 2002; 21:19–20.

58. Kobashigawa JA, Katznelson S, Laks H, Johnson JA, Yeatman L, Wang XM, et al. Effect of pravastatin on outcomes after cardiac transplantation. N Engl J Med 1995; 333:621–7.

59. Vaessen LM, van Miert PP, van Gelder T, Ijzermans JN, Weimar W. Reassuring effect of pravastatin on natural killer cell activity in stable renal transplant patients. Transplantation 2001; 1:1175–9.

60. Shek A, Ferrill MJ. Statin–fibrate combination therapy. Ann Pharmacother 2001; 35:908–17.

61. Rubins HB, Robins SJ, Collins D, Fye CL, Anderson JW, Elam MB, et al. Gemfibrozil for the secondary prevention of coronary heart disease in men with low levels of high-density lipoprotein cholesterol. Veterans Affairs High-Density Lipoprotein Cholesterol Intervention Trial Study Group. N Engl J Med 1999; 341:410–18.

62. Heart Protection Study Collaborative Group. MRC/BHF Heart Protection Study of cholesterol lowering with simvastatin in 20 536 high-risk individuals: a randomized placebo-controlled trial. Lancet 2002; 360:7–22.

63. Pyorala K, Pedersen TR, Kjekshus J, Faergeman O, Olsson AG, Thorgeirsson G. Cholesterol lowering with simvastatin improves prognosis of diabetic patients with coronary heart disease. A subgroup analysis of the Scandinavian Simvastatin Survival Study (4S). Diabetes Care 1997; 20:614–20.

64. Morris JJ, Smith LR, Jones RH, Glower DD, Morris PB, Muhlbaier LH, et al. Influence of diabetes and mammary artery grafting on survival after coronary bypass. Circulation 1991; 84(5 Suppl.): III275–84.

65. Hulley S, Grady D, Bush T, Furberg C, Herrington D, Riggs B, et al. Randomized trial of estrogen plus progestin for secondary prevention of coronary heart disease in postmenopausal women. Heart and Estrogen/progestin Replacement Study. (HERS) Research Group. JAMA 1998; 280:605–13.

66. Albers GW, Dalen JE, Laupacis A, Manning WJ, Petersen P, Singer DE. Anti-thrombotic therapy in atrial fibrillation. Chest 2001; 119(1 Suppl.):194–206S.

67. Fuster V, Ryden LE, Asinger RW, Cannom DS, Crijns HJ, Frye RL, et al. ACC/AHA/ESC guidelines for the management of patients with atrial fibrillation. Circulation 2001; 104:2118–50.

68. Pitt B, Zannad F, Remme WJ, Cody R, Castaigne A, Perez A, et al. The effect of spironolactone on morbidity and mortality in patients with severe heart failure. Randomized Aldactone Evaluation Study Investigators. N Engl J Med 1999; 341: 709–17.

69. The effect of digoxin on mortality and morbidity in patients with heart failure. The Digitalis Investigation Group . N Engl J Med 1997; 336:525–33.

70. Harris WS, Isley WL. Clinical trial evidence for the cardioprotective effects of omega-3 fatty acids. Curr Atheroscler Rep 2001; 3:174–9.

71. Rimm EB, Williams P, Fosher K, Criqui M, Stampfer MJ. Moderate alcohol intake and lower risk of coronary heart disease: meta-analysis of effects on lipids and hemostatic factors. BMJ 1999; 319:1523–8.

72. Hines LM, Rimm EB. Moderate alcohol consumption and coronary heart disease: a review. Postgrad Med J 2001; 77:747–52.

73. Liinamaa MJ, Hannuksela ML, Kesaniemi YA, Savolainen MJ. Altered transfer of cholesteryl esters and phospholipids in plasma alcohol abusers. Arterioscl Thromb Vasc Biol 1997; 17:2940–70.

74. Wenger NK, Froelicher ES, Ades PA, Berra K, Blumenthal JA, Certo CME, et al. Cardiac Rehabilitation: Clinical Practice Guideline No. 17. Rockville, MD: US Dept of Health and Human Services, Public Health Service, Agency for Health Care Policy and Research, National Heart, Lung, and Blood Institute; October 1995. AHCPR Publication No. 96-0672.

75. Vanhees L, Fagard R, Thijs L, Amery A. Prognostic value of training-induced change in peak exercise capacity in patients with myocardial infarcts and patients with coronary bypass surgery. Am J Cardiol 1995; 76:1014–19.

76. Frick MH, Elo O, Haapa K, Heinonen OP, Heinsalmi P, Helo P, et al. Helsinki Heart Study: primary-prevention trial with gemfibrozil in middle-aged men with dyslipidemia. Safety of treatment, changes in risk factors, and incidence of coronary heart disease. N Engl J Med 1987; 317:1237–45.

77. Cullen P, von Eckardstein A, Assman G. Diagnosis and management of new cardiovascular risk factors. Eur Heart J 1998; 19(Suppl. O): O13–19.

78. Griffin BA, Freeman DJ, Tait GW, Thomson J, Caslake MJ, Packard CJ, et al. Role of plasma triglyceride in the regulation of plasma low density lipoprotein (LDL) subfractions: relative contribution of small, dense LDL to coronary heart disease risk. Atherosclerosis 1994; 106:241–53.

79. Seman LJ, McNamara JR, Schaefar EJ. Lipoprotein(a) homocysteine and remnant like particles: emerging risk factors. Curr Opin Cardiol 1999; 14:186–91.

80. Verhoef P, Stampfer MJ, Rimm EB. Folate and coronary heart disease. Curr Opin Lipidol 1998; 9:17–22.

26

Management of refractory angina not amenable to conventional therapy

OH FRAZIER, EGEMEN TUZUN AND KAMURAN KADIPASAOGLU

INTRODUCTION

In recent years, improved medical and surgical therapy has permitted an increasing number of patients to survive cardiac events that would previously have been fatal. Some of these patients will develop advanced heart failure, characterized by severe coronary artery disease not amenable to standard surgical or interventional revascularization. Most patients (other than the relatively few, usually with diabetes mellitus, who have not undergone any previous attempts at cardiac revascularization) present with a history of one, two or (rarely) three coronary artery bypass graft (CABG) operations and/or multiple percutaneous transluminal coronary angioplasty (PTCA) procedures. With maximal anti-anginal therapy, the typical patient remains symptomatic owing to the presence of viable but underperfused (hibernating) myocardium. So far, heart transplantation has been considered the only definitive treatment for these patients. During the past decade, however, several other methods have emerged as therapeutic strategies for treating refractory angina. These include transmyocardial laser revascularization (TMLR), angiogenic therapy, urokinase therapy, and neurostimulation.

TRANSMYOCARDIAL LASER REVASCULARIZATION

The aim of TMLR is to establish channels between the left ventricular cavity and intramyocardial sinusoids, thereby restoring oxygenated blood flow to the ischemic myocardium (Figure 26.1).[1] The technique is based on the reptilian heart, in which the left ventricle is directly perfused from the left ventricular cavity.[1] In their seminal work on the myocardial microanatomy, Wearn and colleagues[2] demonstrated that the endocardium is a potential source of blood supply to the human myocardium via sinusoids. In the light of this finding, needle acupuncture,[3] intramyocardial implantation of T tubes,[4] and implantation of the internal mammary artery[5] were developed to perfuse ischemic segments of the heart. Enthusiasm for these approaches faded with the advent of CABG surgery[6] and PTCA.[7] Despite the success of these latter interventions, however, some patients with intractable angina pectoris are not optimal candidates for revascularization, owing to the distal, diffuse nature of their atherosclerotic involvement. In 1981, Mirhoseini and Cayton[1] proposed that a laser be used to create transmyocardial channels that could perfuse the ischemic myocardium from the

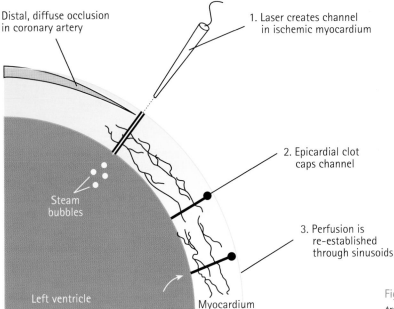

Distal, diffuse occlusion
in coronary artery

1. Laser creates channel
   in ischemic myocardium

2. Epicardial clot
   caps channel

Steam
bubbles

3. Perfusion is
   re-established
   through sinusoids

Left ventricle

Myocardium

Figure 26.1 *Schematic representation of transmyocardial laser revascularization.*

left ventricular cavity, and they did the initial animal experiments involving this technique. The first clinical operation was performed in 1986, by Okada and colleagues in Japan, using a low-power (80 W) CO_2 laser.[8] Since then, more than 6000 operations have been performed worldwide, using a variety of laser types and surgical approaches.

The late 1980s saw the introduction of the high-energy-beam laser. Because of the initial success of this technology in early clinical trials, other laser modalities were proposed for TMLR applications; these modalities included holmium: YAG (Ho:YAG) and excimer (Xe:Cl) lasers, argon lasers, and even radiofrequency devices. The CO_2 and Ho:YAG lasers are examples of infrared lasers, which interact with myocardial tissue by heating water molecules (producing a thermal effect). The Xe:Cl laser is an ultraviolet device that causes molecular dissociation.

In addition to using these new modalities, investigators applied TMLR by means of several different approaches, including a left thoracotomy, a sternotomy, and thoracoscopy as sole therapy or as an adjunct to CABG surgery, gene therapy or PTCA. In the standard sole therapy procedure, the heart is accessed by means of a limited anterolateral thoracotomy, and the laser probe is placed on the epicardial surface of the beating heart.[8] In adjunctive therapy, the laser can be used before, during, or after cardiopulmonary bypass. At our institution, it has also been used, on two occasions, on the day following the CABG procedure, after the patient's vital signs stabilized overnight.

The high-energy CO_2 laser yields an adjustable pulse of 20–60 J, with a pulse duration of 25–100 ms and a fixed peak power of 800 W. The recommended strategy is to drill approximately 1 laser channel per cm^2.[9] The high-energy pulse perforates the myocardium with a single shot, even at the low end (20 J) of the pulse spectrum. Although the relatively long pulse duration (50 ms) seems to cause thermal damage in myocardial tissue, reduction of the laser pulse energy to 20 J/pulse in areas of normal myocardium (without scarring or epicardial fat) prevents excessive collateral thermal injury and allows precision cutting. Ho:YAG and Xe:Cl lasers operate at low energy levels (1 J and 250 mJ/pulse) and require 10–20 pulses (Ho:YAG) or more than 40 pulses (Xe:Cl) to create a single transmyocardial channel.

Unfortunately, delivering repeated pulses to create a single channel has disadvantages. First, this approach makes it impossible to create a straight channel in the moving wall of the beating heart. Therefore, the long-term patency of the channel (which has a zigzag path) is compromised. Second, the heart is unavoidably hit during the T wave, when the myocardium is repolarizing, and is therefore most vulnerable electrically. The CO_2 laser's single pulse is synchronized with the R wave of the patient's electrocardiographic waveform. The maximum 100 ms long pulse stays safely away from the T wave, thus precluding arrhythmogenicity. The likelihood of premature ventricular contractions and ventricular tachycardias during the drilling of each channel is 68% with the Ho:YAG and Xe:Cl lasers but <1% with the CO_2 laser.[9] Clinical data support these findings, as the arrhythmogenic complications in Ho:YAG trials have far outweighed those obtained with the CO_2 laser.[10–12]

Because the pulse duration of the Ho:YAG and Xe:Cl lasers is many orders of magnitude shorter than that of the CO_2 laser, the peak power (energy delivered per unit time, i.e. pulse energy/pulse duration) is orders of magnitude different for each laser model. As opposed to the 1×10^3 W generated by the CO_2 laser, the peak powers of the Ho:YAG and Xe:Cl lasers can easily reach 10^3 and 10^6 W, respectively. Because the efficiency of ablation is not 100% for any of the lasers, some of this energy is converted to heat and dissipated in the adjacent tissue by means of conductive processes. The temperature of the tissue exposed to the excessive heat rises rapidly, vaporizing the water and forming a bubble that soon implodes and sends shock waves through the tissue. Traveling laterally, this acoustic wavefront imparts considerable structural damage to the myocardium and contributes to the traumaticity of the Ho:YAG and Xe:Cl lasers.[9] In contrast, ablation performed with the CO_2 laser is not explosive, so collateral structural damage is limited. Overall, the volumetric ablation associated with each channel is 6.5 times greater with the Ho:YAG than with the CO_2 laser.

In summary, because it offers a low-energy, high-power pulse, the CO_2 laser has advantages over its high-energy, low-power competitors in providing non-arrhythmogenic and non-traumatic drilling of straight, through-and-through channels in the cardiac muscle.

Sole TMLR with a CO_2 laser is performed via a left anterior thoracotomy.[13] One of the advantages of the Ho:YAG and Xe:Cl lasers is that their energy can be transmitted fiberoptically and is, therefore, suitable for percutaneous TMLR (PTMR).[9] Although PTMR seems to be cost effective and less traumatic to the patient, the created channels cannot be myocardial, so there is an ever-present risk of tamponade and arrhythmia.[14]

In 1998, the United States Food and Drug Administration (FDA) approved TMLR with the CO_2 laser as a sole treatment for patients with refractory angina secondary to diffuse end-stage coronary artery disease.[15] Patients amenable to TMLR usually present with Canadian Cardiovascular Society class III or IV stable angina that is refractory to maximum medical treatment, reversible ischemia of the left ventricular free wall, as documented by thallium-201 single-positron emission tomography (^{201}Tl:SPECT) or positron emission tomography (PET), and a coronary anatomy that is not conducive to CABG surgery or PTCA.[16,17]

For detecting hibernating muscle, the most common diagnostic techniques are nuclear medicine tests (T1: SPECT and/or PET) or low-dose dobutamine echocardiography (DE). For the identification of viable tissue, PET seems to have the highest sensitivity and specificity. Viability/perfusion mismatching in PET is strongly correlated with the recovery of left ventricular systolic function if complete revascularization is achieved.[18] Unfortunately, PET is an expensive modality that is not always available, and many centers rely on more readily available diagnostic techniques such as ^{201}Tl:SPECT or

DE. In a series of 27 consecutive patients who were being evaluated for TMLR at the Texas Heart Institute, an agreement between PET (taken as the standard) and DE was reached in 82% of the segments analyzed; this result was reduced to 68% when thallium was used. The accuracy and sensitivity of thallium can be increased by re-injection of the tracer at 4 or 12 hours, and valuable wall motion information can be obtained from DE.[19]

Clinically, patients whose primary complaint is stable angina seem to benefit more from TMLR than do those who have symptoms of unstable angina and/or congestive heart failure. According to a non-randomized, multi-center study by Horvath and colleagues,[16] patients with a left ventricular ejection fraction of <20% or a concurrent major illness (morbid arrhythmia, chronic obstructive pulmonary disease, congestive heart failure or unstable angina) are not good candidates for TMLR. Intraoperative transesophageal echocardiography is useful for confirming successful transmural laser penetration and for identifying the echocontrast presented by the bubbles of evaporated tissue in the left ventricle. Bleeding from some channels (which occurs in <1% of all cases) is easily controlled by temporary finger pressure or a 6-0 polypropylene epicardial suture.[16] The operation lasts for 2–2.5 hours, and the perioperative mortality is 3% for patients with chronic, disabling angina and 16% for those with unmanageable, unstable angina.[20] The latter percentage is reportedly decreasing significantly as investigators gain experience with the preoperative and postoperative management of these critically ill patients.[21]

Those who present with unstable angina are not suitable for this procedure because laser trauma to the myocardium (although minimized with the CO_2 laser) compromises the patient's clinical status because of edema, catecholamine discharge and fluid shifts, causing high perioperative and early postoperative morbidity.[20,21] Prophylactic intra-aortic balloon pumping[13] and maintenance of the electrolyte balance[21] have been proposed as effective preoperative and postoperative measures, respectively, for managing patients in unstable condition. Clinical trials suggest that TMLR significantly improves the angina class in 70–90% of patients who have no other treatment options. Almost 30% of these patients have remained completely free of symptoms 1 year postoperatively.[16,22] Relief of angina improved the quality of life, reduced the need for anti-anginal medications, and decreased the number of hospital admissions related to unstable angina at 1 year in patients treated with the CO_2 and Ho:YAG lasers.[16,20,22] However, at 3 years, the average angina class of patients treated with the Ho:YAG laser was significantly increased when compared to that of CO_2-laser-treated patients. In the Ho:YAG group, 30% of the patients improved by two angina classes, and 70% improved by one angina class compared to baseline values; in contrast, after treatment with the CO_2 laser, 65% of the patients

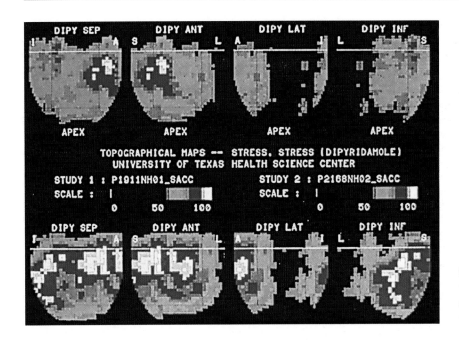

Figure 26.2 *Positron emission tomography scan showing improved sub-endocardial blood flow through the ischemic myocardial region.*

improved by two angina classes, and 23% improved by one angina class. Similarly, according to Lansing,[21] who used both CO_2 and Ho:YAG lasers as a single investigator, improvement was greater in the CO_2-laser-treated group than in the Ho:YAG group. Long-term follow-up of patients treated with the CO_2 laser shows that the average improvement in angina class often persists, or even grows, for up to 5 years.[17]

Two important questions are whether TMLR improves cardiac perfusion to the same degree as clinical status and whether a correlation exists between cardiac perfusion and anginal status. In patients treated with the CO_2 laser, Frazier and associates[23] demonstrated improved sub-endocardial blood flow through the ischemic myocardial region on PET scans (Figure 26.2). The accuracy of sub-regional PET was 89% when clinical symptomatology was taken as the gold standard.[23] A multicenter, randomized, controlled US trial with 192 patients at 12 sites resulted in significantly improved cardiac perfusion in TMLR recipients, compared to deteriorated cardiac perfusion in medically managed patients.[10] In a single-center, randomized, controlled trial of TMLR involving 188 patients in the UK, the authors reported improvement in angina at 12 months in the TMLR group compared with controls; however, although there was reduction in the number of left ventricular segments with reversible myocardial ischemia, this was seen in both treatment and control groups, with no significant difference between them.[24] Interpretation of the findings has been questioned.[25] In the other clinical trials that have used a CO_2 laser for TMLR (all of which were non-randomized, single-center studies), TMLR has had a positive effect on cardiac perfusion.[23,26]

This has not been the case with Ho:YAG trials, as none of them has documented any improvement in cardiac perfusion. Two randomized, multicenter, prospective trials, one involving 182 patients at 16 US centers, and the other involving 275 patients at 18 US centers, showed a lack of improvement in cardiac perfusion with the Ho:YAG laser in the surgical setting.[11,27] Furthermore, both trials documented significant arrhythmogenic complication rates (11% and 22%, respectively), which compare poorly with incidences of arrhythmia after use of the CO_2 laser (8%).[10] In addition, Burkoff and colleagues[11] reported a high rate of heart failure and myocardial infarction (28% and 15%, respectively, in the surgical Ho:YAG-treated group vs 11% and 9% in the medically managed group). Non-randomized, single-center trial of the Ho:YAG laser also failed to show improved cardiac perfusion.[27] There have been no reported trials of TMLR with the Xe:Cl laser.

The randomized clinical trials designed to assess the safety and efficacy of PTMR therapy include DIRECT,[28] which compares percutaneous laser myocardial revascularization and placebo therapy for refractory coronary ischemia in 298 patients at 14 participating US centers in a double-blinded fashion; PACIFIC (Potential Angina Class Improvement From Intramyocardial Channels),[12] which involves 221 patients at 12 US centers and one UK center; and BELIEF (Blinded Evaluation of Laser Intervention Electively for Angina Pectoris),[29] which involves 82 patients at one Norwegian center. The DIRECT study detected no differences in the outcomes in the PTMR and placebo groups and was stopped at 6 months. The PACIFIC and BELIEF studies showed an improvement of angina symptoms compared to the placebo groups at 12 and 6 months (34% in PTMR patients vs 13% in the medical group, respectively). However, this modest improvement in the collective anginal status failed to make up for a relatively excessive number of adverse clinical outcomes,

Table 26.1 *CO_2 and Ho:YAG trials (laser treatment versus medical management)*

Variable	Laser type			
	CO_2	CO_2	Ho:YAG	Ho:YAG
Study (reference)	Frazier *et al.* (10) 12 sites	Schofield (25) Single site	Burkhoff (11) 16 sites	Allen (27) 18 sites
Number of patients	192	188	182	275
Study design	Randomized, prospective	Randomized, prospective	Randomized, prospective	Randomized, prospective
Follow-up	12 months	12 months	12 months	12 months
Study end-points: primary	Angina, myocardial perfusion, freedom from MACE	Time on TMT	Time on TMT	Angina, treatment failure, perfusion
Study end-points: secondary	Mortality, morbidity	Perfusion, treatment failure	Angina, QOL, Perfusion, LVEF	Time on TMT, QOL
Improvement by ≥2 angina classes (% patients, laser vs MM)	72% vs 13%	25% vs 4%	61% vs 11%	76% vs 32%
Improvement in perfusion	20% improvement vs baseline	Reduction of ischemia and prevention of scar propagation	No change	No change
Perioperative mortality (laser vs MM)	3% vs 0%	5% vs 0%	1% vs 0%	5% vs 2%
1-year survival (laser vs MM)	85% vs 79%	89% vs 96%	95% vs 90%	84% vs 89%

CO_2, carbon dioxide laser; Ho:YAG, holmium:YAG laser; LVEF, left ventricular ejection fraction; MACE, major adverse cardiac events; MM, medical management; QOL, quality of life; TMT, treadmill test.

particularly in the PACIFIC trial.[12] These outcomes included death (PTMR group, 9%; medical group, 3%), heart failure or myocardial infarction (PTMR group, 29%; medical group, 18%), and total arrhythmias (PTMR group, 20%; medical group, 7%). Consequently, the FDA refused to approve the clinical use of PTMR in the USA but, rather, recommended further studies involving increased laser power and longer follow-up periods, thus terminating the hope of applying PTMR in the USA for some years to come. Tables 26.1 and 26.2 summarize the randomized single-center and multicenter trials using the CO_2 and Ho:YAG lasers.

Despite the overwhelming evidence of the beneficial clinical effects of TMLR, the technique's mechanisms of action have not been clearly documented. In earlier studies, the acute disappearance of angina was attributed to immediate direct perfusion of the ischemic myocardium from the ventricular cavity (as in the reptilian heart) through the laser channels.[30] However, the evidence of improved cardiac perfusion has consistently been criticized, mainly because of the small sample size and inaccurate diagnostic technique. Therefore, alternatively, the immediate benefit of TMLR (without concomitant improvement in myocardial perfusion) has been attributed to denervation of the epicardial sympathetic fibers by the laser and a resultant loss of afferent pain stimuli.[31] Several studies indicate that, particularly 3–6 months after the operation, myocardial perfusion improves in a way that is consistent with the gradual improvement seen in the patient's clinical condition.[23,26] This finding suggests that both laser and mechanical injuries create an inflammatory response that causes neovascularization by releasing angiogenic factors around the channels.[32]

To foster therapeutic angiogenesis, the concomitant use of vascular endothelial growth factor (VEGF) at the time of TMLR could provide better neovascularization than could be offered by TMLR alone.[33] Although a placebo effect is proposed as an alternative mechanism for the relief of angina, the persistence of pain relief with time[17] and the improvement of myocardial perfusion, as shown by PET,[26] suggest that these benefits are not purely psychosomatic.[16,17] The mechanism of TMLR is probably multifactorial, and further experimental work is needed to investigate the anti-ischemic effectiveness of this technique.

To investigate whether TMLR is a direct cause of increased cardiac perfusion, a multicenter US trial using high-resolution (1 mm) gated magnetic resonance imaging (MRI), with gadolinium as the contrast agent for perfusion and viability, is being designed. The end-points of the study will be cardiac function and perfusion both at rest and

Table 26.2 *Randomized percutaneous transmyocardial laser revascularization studies with the Ho:YAG laser*

Variable	Study (reference)		
	Leon *et al.* (28) DIRECT 14 sites	Oesterle *et al.* (12) PACIFIC 12 sites	Salem *et al.* (29) BELIEF 1 site
Number of patients	298	200	82
Study design	Double-blinded	Non-blinded	Double-blinded
Follow-up	6 months	12 months	6 months
Study endpoints: primary	30-day MACE 60-day TMT	Time on TMT	Angina, mortality, time on TMT
Study endpoints: secondary	–	Angina	–
Improvement in perfusion	NA	NA	NA
Improvement by ⩾2 angina classes (% patients, laser vs MM)	34% vs 42%	34% vs 14%	41% vs 12%
Perioperative mortality	0.7% in laser group	NA	1.2% in laser group; no data for MM group
1-year survival (% patients, laser vs MM)	98% vs 97%	93% vs 97%	97.6% in laser group; no data for MM group

CO$_2$, carbon dioxide laser; Ho:YAG, holmium:YAG laser; LVEF, left ventricular ejection fraction; MACE, major adverse cardiac events; MM, medical management; NA, non-applicable; QOL, quality of life; TMT, treadmill test.

under stress (with an adenosine challenge), along with scarring (denervation) of the laser-treated tissue. Simultaneously, European researchers are designing a multicenter trial, Laser-Supported Operations in CABG Patients (LASSO), to compare TMLR plus CABG to CABG surgery alone in stable and unstable patients.

In conclusion, TMLR with a CO$_2$ laser is an effective means of relieving angina that is not amenable to conventional revascularization.

ANGIOGENESIS AND GENE THERAPY FOR OTHERWISE UNTREATABLE ANGINA PECTORIS

De novo vascular development in the human embryo is associated with angioblasts and is termed *vasculogenesis*.[34] In contrast, the formation of new blood vessels from pre-existing microvascular networks, which can occur from the late fetal development period onwards, is termed *angiogenesis*.[34]

Physiologically, angiogenesis is a short-lived, strictly controlled process that in healthy females occurs during the menstrual cycle.[35] Angiogenesis also occurs in a variety of pathological conditions such as diabetic retinopathy and tumor development; in these cases, it persists long term.[35] Whether pathological or not, the angiogenic process is characterized by vasodilatation of the parent vessel, degradation of its basal membrane and extracellular matrix, endothelial migration towards the angiogenic stimulus, endothelial cell proliferation in the newly developing vessel, lumen formation, loop formation and new basal membrane formation. The final stage is incorporation of pericytes, and this step appears to regulate angiogenesis by inhibiting endothelial cell proliferation.[35]

The mediators that induce angiogenesis are known as 'angiogens' and are secreted from cells stimulated by hypoxia or ischemia.[34,35] Researchers have identified a large number of angiogens, any one of which appears capable of stimulating angiogenesis.[36] The most widely recognized and studied angiogens are fibroblast growth factors (FGFs) and VEGFs.[35] Acidic and basic fibroblast growth factors (aFGFs and bFGFs) are prototypes of the FGF family.[35] They induce proliferation of endothelial cells, smooth muscle cells, fibroblasts and myocytes, all of which carry high-affinity FGF receptors and play an important role in angiogenesis.[35] Because endothelial cells hold a large number of VEGF receptors, the mitogenic action of VEGF is selective for these cells.[35] VEGF is also known as 'vascular permeability factor', and it facilitates extravasation of the plasma proteins that favor endothelial and fibroblast cell migration.[35] Human VEGF is expressed as four isoforms (VEGF$_{121}$, VEGF$_{165}$, VEGF$_{189}$ and VEGF$_{206}$), which result from post-transcriptional splicing and are potential mediators of angiogenesis under ischemic conditions.[35,37] Other well-known angiogens include angiogenin, transforming growth factor α and β, and tumor necrosis factor-α.[36]

As regulating mechanisms, cells that secrete angiogenic factors to promote angiogenesis also produce inhibitors of angiogenic action such as angiostatin, thrombospondin-1 and platelet factor-4,[35] which are the so-called anti-angiogens.

In therapeutic angiogenesis, first proposed by Hockel and associates[38] in 1993, physicians administer angiogens to treat a large spectrum of ischemic conditions, including coronary and peripheral arterial diseases.[36] VEGF and FGF, the most common angiogens used therapeutically, are administered locally or systemically in the form of angiogenic protein or gene therapy.[36] In gene therapy, physicians deliver naked cDNA plasmids, cDNA coupled with lipophilic or hydrophilic agents, and adenoviral vectors encoding angiogenic proteins to the host cells to elicit angiogenesis.[36] For local therapy, the angiogen is delivered directly to the targeted tissue by means of intramuscular or intramyocardial injections, as in peripheral arterial disease or myocardial ischemia.[36] Alternatively, an angioplasty balloon catheter may be used to deliver angiogens into the arterial wall. For systemic therapy, angiogens are delivered directly via an intravenous or intra-arterial catheter.[36] Although more easily applicable than local therapy, the systemic approach is limited by the risk of hypotension, hyperproliferation of the retinal capillary plexus, and inappropriate angiogenesis in the synovium and in occult tumors.[35,36] Moreover, low perfusion of the ischemic regions may compromise the accessibility and efficacy of systemic therapy.[36]

The coronary collateral circulation has been shown to maintain myocardial viability and reduce infarct size after a myocardial infarction.[39] Once angiogenic factors were seen to enhance the development of collateral coronary vessels in animal models,[40] several clinical studies were initiated to stimulate coronary collateralization in regions of ischemic myocardium not amenable to PTCA or CABG surgery.[41,42] Naked protein or cDNA-encoding VEGF or FGF was delivered to the ischemic myocardium via a systemic intravenous injection,[43] a thoracotomy (for direct intramyocardial injection or intrapericardial delivery),[41] or a catheter-based technique (for intracoronary or transendocardial injection).[44]

In 1998, Schumacher and coauthors[45] announced the first successful clinical results of injecting aFGF into the myocardium as an adjunct to CABG surgery. Subsequent clinical studies in limited numbers of patients showed that FGF and VEGF injections increase coronary collateralization and improve anginal status, nitrate use and functional class.[41,46] Symes and colleagues[47] and Losordo and coworkers[48] showed that $VEGF_{165}$ injections can induce coronary collateral development, via a minithoracotomy or catheter-based technique, as sole therapy for refractory angina. These results were supported by angiography,[45] SPECT[48] and electromechanical mapping.[42] Conversely, in the FGF-2 Initiating Revascularization Support Trial (FIRST), a double-blind, placebo-controlled study that involved 337 patients, and in the VEGF in Ischemia for Vascular Angiogenesis (VIVA) study, which involved 178 patients, intracoronary injection of bFGF and high-dose VEGF failed to improve myocardial perfusion during objective tests.[43] Although the anginal class was lower in the high-dose VEGF group than in the placebo group, this finding

was not supported by objective testing. At this stage, the optimal dose regimen (single or repeated), delivery technique (local or systemic), delivery region (ischemic, non-ischemic, or both) and time necessary for developing new collaterals are not clear with these angiogenic agents.

Although a gold-standard technique for angiogenesis in humans is not yet available and progression to phase III clinical trials needs to be evaluated, therapeutic angiogenesis holds tremendous promise for the treatment of patients with refractory angina who do not respond to medical treatment and are not candidates for CABG surgery or PTCA.

LONG-TERM INTERMITTENT UROKINASE THERAPY IN PATIENTS WITH END-STAGE CORONARY ARTERY DISEASE AND REFRACTORY ANGINA PECTORIS

The therapeutic mechanisms of long-term intermittent urokinase therapy are based on improvements in rheological blood properties, thrombolysis and regression of coronary plaques.[49] Total peripheral vascular resistance is the product of a vascular component and a viscous component, which are combined in the following manner:

$$R \text{ (total peripheral resistance)} = \text{vascular resistance} \times \text{blood viscosity}$$

Thus, the flow properties of the blood are affected by the geometry of the vessels, perfusion pressure, endothelial functions, blood viscosity, hematocrit, plasma viscosity, red blood cell aggregation and red blood cell deformability.[50] Under normal conditions, blood viscosity does not strongly affect the flow properties in healthy coronary arteries.[51] In the post-stenotic microcirculation typical of severe coronary stenosis, however, blood viscosity (which is mainly determined by red cell aggregation and plasma viscosity) becomes the main determinant of flow-limiting resistance.[52] The fibrinogen concentration, which controls plasma viscosity, leads to an increase in blood viscosity and may limit oxygen delivery to the ischemic myocardium.[53] Therefore, it might be argued that, by using urokinase, a thrombolytic factor, to reduce fibrinogen concentrations, one might improve the rheological blood properties and increase microcirculatory flow.[54]

In a randomized dose–response trial, Leschke and colleagues[55] demonstrated that long-term, intermittent urokinase therapy ($3 \times 500\,000\,IU$ per week, intravenously, for 3 months) is clinically effective in patients with end-stage coronary artery disease and refractory angina. According to the treatment protocol, patients with a fibrinogen concentration $>300\,mg\,dL^{-1}$ at baseline were assigned to urokinase therapy. The therapy was discontinued when the target fibrinogen concentration of $200–250\,mg\,dL^{-1}$

was maintained. After 3 months of treatment, urokinase therapy decreased the fibrinogen levels by about 35%, plasma viscosity by 7% and red blood cell activation by 19%. [55]

Acute coronary syndrome appears to be related to thrombosis of an atherosclerotic lesion, as has been demonstrated angiographically[56] and pathologically[57] by several investigators. Although early thrombolytic therapy is very effective for reperfusing the occluded coronary artery, the incidence of residual thrombosis and the severity of the underlying coronary artery stenosis may cause re-occlusion.[58] Patients with multiple severe coronary stenoses are prone to recurrent episodes of thrombus formation because of impaired post-stenotic non-laminar flow and relative stasis of the blood.[50] Recurrent thrombus formation alternates with subsequent thrombus fragmentation to cause microinfarcts and/or lethal arrhythmias related to distal epicardial or collateral microembolization.[59] Recent studies of low-molecular-weight heparin in patients in clinically stable condition support the anti-ischemic efficacy of anti-thrombotic therapy for improving blood fluidity and inducing collateral angiogenesis to perfuse the ischemic myocardium.[60] As a potent anti-thrombotic and thrombolytic agent, low-dose urokinase has been found to be effective for improving myocardial perfusion in patients with refractory angina pectoris.[55]

The growth and extent of the atherosclerotic plaques in the coronary and carotid arteries are related to a high fibrinogen concentration,[61] which tends to accumulate into atherosclerotic plaques after repetitive plaque fissuring.[50] Even in a non-stenotic lesion, rupture of an atherosclerotic plaque may cause a coronary artery spasm and/or luminal thrombosis, producing a hemorrhage into the plaque and activating the thrombotic process.[59] Patients with critical coronary artery stenosis and impaired coronary blood flow are more prone to develop intracoronary thrombus after a plaque rupture.[50] It is likely that long-term urokinase therapy, which decreases fibrinogen levels by about 35% after treatment, may limit the thrombogenic stimulus and subsequent growth of the plaque.[55] This effect of long-term, intermittent thrombolytic therapy on plaque regression may explain the improvement in clinical symptoms that lasts for at least 3 months (average 12.7 ± 8.5 months) after the termination of urokinase therapy.[62]

Long-term, intermittent urokinase therapy involves a dosage of 3 × 500 000 IU per week for 3 months. Although major side effects such as gastrointestinal bleeding (0.8%) are uncommon, assessment of clinical symptoms and blood coagulation profiles every 2 weeks during treatment is recommended. Apart from the reduction in fibrinogen levels, studies have shown a 7% reduction in plasma viscosity, an 18% reduction in red blood cell aggregation, and an 18% reduction in plasminogen activity, which are consistent with the theory of increased blood fluidity.[55] The reduction in spontaneous angina and increase in exercise capacity correlate with objective signs of myocardial ischemia relief such as enhancement of myocardial perfusion on scintigraphy and electrocardiography.[55]

These data suggest that long-term urokinase therapy, in addition to conventional maximal medical treatment, is a safe, effective approach for treating refractory angina in patients with end-stage coronary artery disease.

NEUROSTIMULATION

According to the gate-control theory of pain transmission, pain impulses are carried by myelinated type-A and unmyelinated type-C fibers in peripheral nerves, and by the lateral spinothalamic tract in the spinal chord, to a pain center in the thalamus.[63] Type-C fibers inhibit the presynaptic neuron system and increase pain transmission to the first synaptic station in the spinal cord (the gate of which is opened), whereas activation of A fibers excites the system and reduces pain transmission to the next neuron chain (the gate of which is closed).[63] Neurostimulation therapy, in the form of transcutaneous electrical nerve stimulation (TENS) and spinal cord stimulation (SCS), was developed in response to this gate-control theory.[63] It is likely that both techniques excite the same group of afferent fibers, TENS doing so at the periphery and SCS at the level of the spinal cord.[64] After obtaining satisfactory results with TENS and SCS in peripheral vascular disease,[65,66] investigators showed that these techniques could also relieve otherwise intractable chronic angina pectoris.[67]

The mechanisms of action of neurostimulation are not completely known, but they probably involve a primary analgesic (indirect sympatholytic) and/or anti-ischemic (direct sympatholytic) effect.[49] A primary analgesic effect that may cause a secondary reduction in the adrenergic state is created with high-frequency stimulation of type-A fibers, which inhibits impulse transmission through type-C fibers and reduces the activation of central pain receptors.[49] According to the same mechanism, stimulation of the dorsal column suppresses cellular activity in the spinothalamic tract and inhibits the transmission of pain stimuli at the segmental level.[49,64] The reduction of anginal pain breaks the 'vicious circle', reduces psychological distress (a known trigger of angina), and reduces the myocardial oxygen demand by indirectly inhibiting sympathetic nervous activity.[68] This anti-anginal effect of neurostimulation is not masking an important warning signal, as maintained by some clinicians, but is raising the ischemic pain threshold and allowing the same symptoms to appear at a higher level.[68]

In an earlier report, the anti-ischemic effect of neurostimulation was related to an increased blood flow velocity at rest,[69] but subsequent studies have failed to confirm this finding.[70] The other possible mechanism of action is redistribution of the blood from non-ischemic areas to ischemic ones (the so-called Robin Hood effect).[68] With PET, Hautvast and colleagues[71] demonstrated that a redistribution of myocardial flow in favor of ischemic areas is a long-term effect of SCS, both at rest and in the presence of a high workload. This result is thought to be related to the adenosine-blocking effect of SCS.[71] Compared with patients having chronic stable angina, those with severe coronary artery disease have a high incidence of coronary collateralization. Adenosine plays an important role in a steal phenomenon in which blood is diverted by coronary collateral vessels to severely ischemic myocardial regions.[72]

After implanting a neurostimulator, many investigators have reported improved ST-segment analysis during exercise and stress echocardiography,[73] decreased anginal attacks and nitrate consumption, and an improved quality of life, which may persist for up to 10 years.[68] A placebo effect could not possibly account for these results.

Finally, it is possible that a direct sympatholytic effect is created by stimulation of the dorsal roots.[68,74] This effect would reduce the systemic epinephrine concentration, as well as the cardiac workload and myocardial oxygen demand.[68]

Some of these mechanisms of action were anticipated.[70,73] Recent clinical studies have confirmed that neurostimulation decreases the number and duration of anginal episodes, decreases sublingual nitrate use, increases the quality of life, and decreases angina-related hospital admission in patients with otherwise refractory angina.[49,68,75] Patients have also shown decreased ST-segment depression and improved lactate metabolism during exercise testing.[68]

For TENS treatment, two cutaneous electrodes are attached to the chest wall, one in the ipsilateral dermatome of the projected pain and the other in the contralateral dermatome. The intensity of stimulation changes according to each patient's pain threshold. Treatment is given for 1 hour at least three times a day and for an additional 10 minutes during angina episodes.[49]

The SCS device is implanted with the aid of local anesthesia, so that the patient and surgeon can cooperate during the perioperative test stimulation. Once a posterior midline thoracic incision has been made, the epidural space is punctured at the level of the sixth thoracic vertebra, and the tip of the electrode is placed at the level of the first or second thoracic vertebra. A pocket in the left upper abdomen is prepared for the stimulator, and the electrodes are connected by means of an extension lead. The stimulator is telemetrically programmed with two preset stimulation strengths, the stronger one being used for angina treatment and the weaker one being used for prophylaxis for at least 2 hours, four times daily. With the aid

of a magnet, the patient can switch between two preset stimulation strengths or can turn the stimulator on or off.[49,76] Neither TENS nor SCS worsens the mortality and morbidity or masks the symptoms of a new acute myocardial infarction.[76,77] Local skin irritation has been reported in some cases of TENS application.[77] The most common complications of SCS are electrode displacement, migration and fracture, and infection.[78] No tolerance or rebound is developed during SCS treatment.[78]

CONCLUSION

Over the past few decades, the advent of effective medical therapy, CABG surgery, and PTCA has improved the life expectancy of patients with severe coronary artery disease. However, this improvement is sometimes transient, and ischemic symptoms may recur. Complete revascularization may be impossible because of diffuse arteriosclerosis. In such cases, TMLR, angiogenesis, urokinase therapy or neurostimulation may be performed to improve myocardial perfusion. Although these techniques have proved safe and effective in a large number of cases, their usefulness needs to be confirmed in large, randomized clinical trials.

KEY REFERENCES

Horvath KA, Aranki SF, Cohn LH, March RJ, Frazier OH, Kadipasaoglu KA, *et al*. Sustained angina relief 5 years after transmyocardial laser revascularization with a CO_2 laser. *Circulation* 2001; **104**(12 Suppl. I):I81–4.

The clinical status and postoperative angina class of 78 patients with refractory angina pectoris who underwent CO_2 TMLR an average of 5 years ago (and up to 7 years) are reviewed in this study. There was a significant improvement in angina class in 77% of the patients at 1 year, and 68% of the patients had successful long-term (5 years) angina relief. Thus, TMLR with CO_2 laser as a sole therapy for refractory angina pectoris is an effective, long-term therapy for this group of patients. It is clear that this long-term efficacy is not related to the placebo effect.

Murray S, Collins PD, James MA. Neurostimulation treatment for angina pectoris. *Heart* 2000; **83**:217–20.

This article is a peer review of the neurostimulation techniques available for the treatment of refractory angina pectoris. The development, evidence of efficacy and current theories on mechanisms of action of the neurostimulation are clearly described.

Rosengart TK, Patel SR, Crystal RG. Therapeutic angiogenesis: protein and gene therapy delivery strategies. *J Cardiovasc Risk* 1999; **6**:29–40.

This article describes the advances in therapeutic angiogenesis based on recent reports. The authors review the complex mechanisms of action and delivery strategies of angiogenesis with a clear and systematic approach.

Schoebel FC, Frazier OH, Jessurun GAJ, De Jongste MJ, Kadipasaoglu KA, Jax TW, *et al*. Refractory angina pectoris in end-stage coronary artery disease: evolving therapeutic concepts. *Am Heart J* 1997; **134**:587–602.

The authors present in detail the three therapeutic approaches to refractory angina pectoris. The therapeutic effectiveness of long-term, intermittent urokinase therapy, TMLR and neurostimulation underlines the potential improvement of the coronary microcirculation for myocardial perfusion. Though the authors observe that further clinical and experimental data are needed, they conclude that these treatment modalities are promising for the treatment of end-stage coronary artery disease.

Schoebel FC, Jax TW, Fischer Y, Strauer BE, Leschke M. Anti-thrombotic effect in stable coronary syndromes: long-term intermittent urokinase therapy in end-stage coronary artery disease and refractory angina pectoris. *Heart* 1997; **77**:13–17.

This article is an overview of the role of long-term urokinase therapy in end-stage coronary artery disease and refractory angina pectoris. The clinical effectiveness of $3 \times 500\,000$ IU of urokinase per week in the improvement of angina symptoms and quality of life is described in the light of possible mechanisms of action such as improvement of rheological blood properties, thrombolytic potential and plaque regression.

REFERENCES

1. Mirhoseini M, Cayton MM. Revascularization of the heart by laser. *J Microvasc Surg* 1981; 2:253–60.
2. Wearn JT, Mettier SR, Klumpp TG, Zschiesche LJ. The nature of the vascular communications between the coronary arteries and the chambers of the heart. *Am Heart J* 1933; 9:143–64.
3. Sen PK, Udwadia TE, Kinare SG, Parulkar GB. Transmyocardial acupuncture. *J Thorac Cardiovasc Surg* 1950; 50:181–9.
4. Massimo C, Boffi L. Myocardial revascularization by a new method of carrying blood directly from the left ventricular cavity into the coronary circulation. *J Thorac Cardiovasc Surg* 1957; 34:257–64.
5. Vineberg AM. Development of an anastomosis between the coronary vessels and a transplanted internal mammary artery. *Can Med Assoc J* 1946; 55:117–19.
6. Kolessov VI. Mammary artery–coronary artery anastomosis as a method of treatment for angina pectoris. *J Thorac Cardiovasc Surg* 1967; 54:535–44.
7. Gruntzig A. Transluminal dilatation of coronary artery stenosis (Letter). *Lancet* 1978; 1:263.
8. Okada M, Ikuta H, Shimizu K, Horii H, Nakamura K. Alternative method of myocardial revascularization by laser: experimental and clinical study. *Kobe J Med Sci* 1986; 32:151–61.
9. Kadipasaoglu KA, Frazier OH. Transmyocardial laser revascularization: effect of laser parameters on tissue ablation

and cardiac perfusion. *Semin Thorac Cardiovasc Surg* 1999; 11:4–11.
10. Frazier OH, March RJ, Horvath KA. Transmyocardial revascularization with a carbon dioxide laser in patients with end-stage coronary artery disease. *N Engl J Med* 1999; 341:1021–8.
11. Burkhoff D, Schmidt S, Schulman SP, Myers J, Resar J, Becker LC, *et al*. Transmyocardial laser revascularisation compared with continued medical therapy for treatment of refractory angina pectoris: a prospective randomised trial. *Lancet* 1999; 354:885–90.
12. Oesterle SN, Sanborn TA, Ali N, Resar J, Ramee SR, Heuser R, *et al*. Percutaneous transmyocardial laser revascularization for severe angina: the PACIFIC randomized trial. *Lancet* 2000; 356:1705–10.
13. March RJ. Transmyocardial laser revascularization with the CO$_2$ laser: one year results of a randomized, controlled trial. *Semin Thorac Cardiovasc Surg* 1999; 11:12–18.
14. Kadipasaoglu KA, Sartori M, Masai T, Cihan HB, Clubb FJ Jr, Conger JL, *et al*. Intraoperative arrhythmias and tissue damage during transmyocardial laser revascularization. *Ann Thorac Surg* 1999; 67:423–31.
15. Ault A. FDA backs heart laser for angina. *Lancet* 1998; 351:1340.
16. Horvath KA, Cohn LH, Cooley DA, Crew JR, Frazier LH, Griffith BP, *et al*. Transmyocardial laser revascularization: results of a multicenter trial with transmyocardial laser revascularization used as sole therapy for end-stage coronary artery disease. *J Thorac Cardiovasc Surg* 1997; 113:645–54.
17. Horvath KA, Aranki SF, Cohn LH, March RJ, Frazier OH, Kadipasaoglu KA, *et al*. Sustained angina relief 5 years after transmyocardial laser revascularization with a CO$_2$ laser. *Circulation* 2001; 104(12 Suppl. I): I81–4.
18. Gould KL. Clinical cardiac positron emission tomography: state of the art. *Circulation* 1991; 84:I22–36.
19. Barasch E, Wilansky S. Dobutamine stress echocardiography in clinical practice with a review of the recent literature. *Tex Heart Inst J* 1994; 21:202–10.
20. Hattler BG, Griffith BP, Zenati MA, Crew JR, Mirhoeseini M, Cohn LH, *et al*. Transmyocardial laser revascularization in the patient with unmanageable unstable angina. *Ann Thorac Surg* 1999; 68:1203–9.
21. Lansing AM. Transmyocardial revascularization. Late results and mechanisms of action. *J Ky Med Assoc* 2000; 98:406–12.
22. Cooley DA, Frazier OH, Kadipasaoglu KA, Lindenmeir MH, Pehlivanoglu S, Kolff JW, *et al*. Transmyocardial laser revascularization: clinical experience with twelve-month follow up. *J Thorac Cardiovasc Surg* 1996; 111:791–9.
23. Frazier OH, Cooley DA, Kadipasaoglu KA, Pehlivanoglu S, Lindenmeir M, Barasch E, *et al*. Myocardial revascularization with laser. Preliminary findings. *Circulation* 1995; 92(9 Suppl. II): II58–65.
24. Schofield PM, Sharples LD, Caine N, Burns S, Tait S, Wistow T, *et al*. Transmyocardial laser revascularization in patients with refractory angina: a randomised controlled trial. *Lancet* 1999; 353:519–24.
25. Horvath KA, Kadipasaoglu KA. Transmyocardial laser revascularization (Letter). *Lancet* 1999; 353:1704.
26. Frazier OH, Cooley DA, Kadipasaoglu KA, Pehlivanoglu S, Barasch E, Conger JL, *et al*. Transmyocardial laser revascularization: initial clinical results (Abstract). *Circulation* 1994; 90(Suppl.):I640.
27. Allen KB, Dowling RD, Fudge TL, Schoettle GP, Selinger SL, Gangahar DM, *et al*. Comparison of transmyocardial revascularization with medical therapy in patients with refractory angina. *N Engl J Med* 1999; 341:1029–36.
28. Leon MB, Baim DS, Moses JW, Laham RJ, Knopf W, Reisman M, *et al*. A randomized blinded clinical trial comparing percutaneous laser myocardial revascularization (using Biosense LV mapping) vs

placebo in patients with refractory coronary ischemia (Abstract). *Circulation* 2000; **102**(Suppl. II):II565.

29. Salem M, Rotevatn S, Stavnes S, Brekke M, Pettersen R, Kulper K, *et al.* Blinded evaluation of laser intervention electively for angina pectoris (Abstract). *Circulation* 2001; **104**(Suppl. II):II565.

30. Cooley DA, Frazier OH, Kadipasaoglu KA, Pehlivanoglu S, Shannon RL, Angelini P. Transmyocardial laser revascularization. Anatomic evidence of long term channel patency. *Tex Heart Inst J* 1994; **21**:220–4.

31. Al-Sheikh T, Allen KB, Straka SP, Heimansohn DA, Fain RL, Hutchins GD, *et al.* Cardiac sympathetic denervation after transmyocardial laser revascularization. *Circulation* 1999; **100**:135–40.

32. Mueller XM, Tevaearai HT, Chaubert P, Genton CY, Von Segesser LK. Does laser injury induce a different neovascularization pattern from mechanical or ischemic injuries? *Heart* 2001; **85**:697–701.

33. Topol EJ, Serruys PW. Frontiers in interventional cardiology. *Circulation* 1998; **98**:1802–20.

34. Melillo G, Scoccianti M, Kovesdi I, Safi J, Riccioni T, Capogrossi MC. Gene therapy for collateral vessel development. *Cardiovasc Res* 1997; **35**:480–9.

35. Moulton KS, Folkman J. Angiogenesis in cardiovascular disease. In: *Molecular Basis of Cardiovascular Disease*, Chien KR, Breslow JL, Leiden JM, Rosenberg RD, Seidman CE (eds). Philadelphia: WB Saunders, 1999, 393–409.

36. Rosengart TK, Patel SR, Crystal RG. Therapeutic angiogenesis: protein and gene therapy delivery strategies. *J Cardiovasc Risk* 1999; **6**:29–40.

37. Thomas KA. Vascular endothelial growth factor, a potent and selective angiogenic agent. *J Biol Chem* 1996; **271**:603–6.

38. Hockel M, Schlenger K, Doctrow S, Kissel T, Vaupel P. Therapeutic angiogenesis. *Arch Surg* 1993; **128**:423–9.

39. Rentrop KP, Thornton JC, Feit F, Van Buskirk M. Determinants and protective potential of coronary arterial collaterals as assessed by an angioplasty model. *Am J Cardiol* 1988; **611**:677–84.

40. Harada K, Friedman M, Lopez JJ, Wang SY, Li J, Prasad PV, *et al.* Vascular endothelial growth factor administration in chronic myocardial ischemia. *Am J Physiol* 1996; **270**(5 Pt 2):H1791–802.

41. Rosengart TK, Lee LY, Patel SR, Sanborn TA, Parikh M, Bergman GW, *et al.* Angiogenesis gene therapy: phase I assessment of direct intramyocardial administration of an adenovirus vector expressing VEGF121 cDNA to individuals with clinically significant severe coronary artery disease. *Circulation* 1999; **100**:468–74.

42. Vale PR, Losordo DW, Milliken CE, Maysky M, Esakof DD, Symes JF, *et al.* Left ventricular electromechanical mapping to assess efficacy of phVEGF$_{165}$ gene transfer for therapeutic angiogenesis in chronic myocardial ischemia. *Circulation* 2000; **102**:965–74.

43. Kutryk MJB, Kassam SA, Stewart J. Angiogenesis: an emerging technology for the treatment of coronary artery disease. *Cardiol Rounds* 2001; **6**:1–8.

44. Vale PR, Losordo DW, Milliken CE, McDonald MC, Gravelin LM, Curry CM, *et al.* Randomized, single-blind, placebo-controlled pilot study of catheter-based myocardial gene transfer for therapeutic angiogenesis using left ventricular electromechanical mapping in patients with chronic myocardial ischemia. *Circulation* 2001; **103**:2138–43.

45. Schumacher B, Pecher P, von Spect BU, Stegmann T. Induction of neoangiogenesis in ischemic myocardium by human growth factors: first clinical results of a new treatment of coronary heart disease. *Circulation* 1998; **97**:645–50.

46. Pecher P, Schumacher BA. Angiogenesis in ischemic human myocardium: clinical results after 3 years. *Ann Thorac Surg* 2000; **69**:1414–19.

47. Symes JF, Losordo DW, Vale PR, Lathi KG, Esakof DD, Maysky M, *et al.* Gene therapy with vascular endothelial growth factor for

48. Losordo DW, Vale PR, Symes JF, Dunnington CH, Esakof DD, Maysky M, *et al.* Gene therapy for myocardial angiogenesis: initial clinical results with direct myocardial injection of phVEGF$_{165}$ as sole therapy for myocardial ischemia. *Circulation* 1998; **98**:2800–4.

49. Schoebel FC, Frazier OH, Jessurun GA, De Jongste MJ, Kadipasaoglu KA, Jax TW, *et al.* Refractory angina pectoris in end-stage coronary disease: evolving therapeutic concepts. *Am Heart J* 1997; **134**:587–602.

50. Koenig W, Ernst E. The possible role of hemorrheology in atherothrombogenesis. *Atherosclerosis* 1992; **94**:93–107.

51. Schmid-Schonbein H. Interaction of vasomotion and blood rheology in hemodynamics. In: *Clinical Aspects of Blood Viscosity and Cell Deformability*. Lowe GDO, Barbenel JC, Forbes CD (eds). Berlin: Springer-Verlag, 1981, 49–65.

52. Gordon RJ, Snyder GK, Tritel H, Taylor WJ. Potential significance of plasma viscosity and hematocrit variations in myocardial ischemia. *Am Heart J* 1974; **87**:175–82.

53. Wilhelmsen L, Svardsudd K, Korsan-Bengsten K, Larson B, Welin L, Tibblin G. Fibrinogen as a risk factor for stroke and myocardial infarction. *N Engl J Med* 1984; **311**:501–5.

54. Schoebel FC, Jax TW, Fischer Y, Strauer BE, Leschke M. Anti-thrombotic treatment in stable coronary syndromes: long-term intermittent urokinase therapy in end-stage coronary artery disease and refractory angina pectoris. *Heart* 1997; **77**:13–17.

55. Leschke M, Schoebel FC, Mecklenbeck W, Stein D, Jax TW, Muller-Gartner HW, *et al.* Long-term intermittent urokinase therapy in patients with end-stage coronary artery disease and refractory angina pectoris: a randomized dose-response trial. *J Am Coll Cardiol* 1996; **27**:575–84.

56. Holmes DR, Hartzler GO, Smith HC, Fuster V. Coronary artery thrombosis in patients with unstable angina. *Br Heart J* 1981; **45**:411–16.

57. Davies MJ, Thomas AJ. Thrombosis and acute coronary artery lesions in sudden cardiac ischemic death. *N Engl J Med* 1984; **54**:65–73.

58. Gash AK, Spann JF, Sherry S, Belber AD, Carabello BA, McDonough MT, *et al.* Factors influencing reocclusion after coronary thrombolysis for acute myocardial infarction. *Am J Cardiol* 1986; **57**:175–7.

59. Falk E. Unstable angina with fatal outcome: dynamic coronary thrombosis leading to infarction and/or sudden death: autopsy evidence of recurrent mural thrombosis with peripheral embolization culminating in vascular occlusion. *Circulation* 1985; **71**:699–708.

60. Quyyumi AA, Diodati JG, Lakatos EE, Bonow RO, Epstein SE. Angiogenic effects of low molecular weight heparin in patients with stable coronary artery disease: a pilot study. *J Am Coll Cardiol* 1993; **22**:635–41.

61. Broadhurst P, Kelleher C, Hughes L, Imeson JD, Raftery EB. Fibrinogen, factor VII clotting activity and coronary artery disease severity. *Atherosclerosis* 1990; **85**:169–73.

62. Schoebel FC, Leschke M, Stein D, Heins M, Pels K, Jax TW, *et al.* Chronic-intermittent urokinase therapy in refractory angina pectoris. *Fibrinolysis* 1995; **9**(Suppl. 1):121–5.

63. Melzack R, Wall PD. Pain mechanisms: a new theory. *Science* 1965; **150**:971–9.

64. Chandler MJ, Brennan TJ, Garrison DW, Kim KS, Schwartz PJ, Foreman RD. A mechanism of cardiac pain suppression by spinal cord stimulation: implications for patients with angina pectoris. *Eur Heart J* 1993; **14**:96–105.

65. Augustinsson LE, Carlsson CA, Holm J, Jivegard L. Epidural electrical stimulation in severe limb ischemia. Pain relief,

inoperable coronary artery disease. *Ann Thorac Surg* 1999, **68**:830–7.

increased blood flow, and a possible limb-saving effect. *Ann Surg* 1985; **202**:104–10.

66. Jacobs MJ, Jorning PJ, Joshi SR, Kitslaar PJ, Slaaf DW, Reneman RS. Epidural spinal cord electrical stimulation improves microvascular blood flow in severe limb ischemia. *Ann Surg* 1988; **207**:179–83.

67. Mannheimer C, Carlsson CA, Ericson K, Vedin A, Wilhelmsson C. Transcutaneous electrical nerve stimulation in severe angina pectoris. *Eur Heart J* 1982; **3**:297–302.

68. Murray S, Collins PD, James MA. Neurostimulation treatment for angina pectoris. *Heart* 2000; **83**:217–20.

69. Chauhan A, Mullins PA, Thuraisingham SI, Taylor G, Petch MC, Schofield PM. Effect of transcutaneous electrical nerve stimulation on coronary blood flow. *Circulation* 1994; **89**:694–702.

70. De Jongste MJ, Hautvast RW, Hillege HL, Lie KI. Efficacy of spinal cord stimulation as adjuvant therapy for intractable angina pectoris: a prospective, randomized clinical study. *J Am Coll Cardiol* 1994; **23**:1592–7.

71. Hautvast R, Blanksma P, DeJongste MJ, Pruim J, van der Wall EE, Vaalburg W, *et al*. Effect of spinal chord stimulation on myocardial blood flow assessed by positron emission tomography in patients with refractory angina pectoris. *Am J Cardiol* 1996; **77**:462–7.

72. Seiler C, Kaufmann U, Meier B. Intracoronary demonstration of adenosine induced coronary collateral steal. *Heart* 1997; **77**:78–81.

73. Ferguson RJ, Petitclerc R, Choquette G, Chaniotis L, Gauthier P, Huot R, *et al*. Effect of physical training on treadmill exercise capacity, collateral circulation and progression of coronary disease. *Am J Cardiol* 1974; **34**:764–9.

74. Murray S, Carson KGS, Ewings PD, Collins PD, James MA. Spinal cord stimulation significantly decreases the need for acute hospital admission for chest pain in patients with refractory angina pectoris. *Heart* 1999; **82**:89–92.

75. Andersen C. Does heart rate variability change in angina pectoris patients treated with spinal cord stimulation? *Cardiology* 1998; **89**:14–18.

76. Greco S, Auriti A, Fiume D, Gazzeri G, Gentilucci G, Antonini L, *et al*. Spinal cord stimulation for the treatment of refractory angina pectoris: a two year follow-up. *Pacing Clin Electrophysiol* 1999; **22**:26–32.

77. Mannheimer C, Carlsson CA, Emanuelsson H, Vedin A, Waagstein F, Wilhemsson C. The effects of transcutaneous electrical nerve stimulation in patients with severe angina pectoris. *Circulation* 1985; **71**:308–16.

78. de Jongste MJ, Nagelkerke D, Hooyschuur CM, Journee HL, Meyler PW, Staal MJ, *et al*. Stimulation characteristics, complications, and efficacy of spinal cord stimulation systems in patients with refractory angina: a prospective feasibility study. *Pacing Clin Electrophysiol* 1994; **17**(11 Pt 1):1751–60.

Index

Indexer: Dr Laurence Errington

Abbreviations: CABG, coronary artery bypass grafts; CAD, coronary artery disease; LV, left ventricle; MI, myocardial infarction; MR, magnetic resonance; MRI, magnetic resonance imaging; MRS, magnetic resonance spectroscopy; PTCA, percutaneous transluminal coronary angioplasty.